JL Berry

Potassium Channel Modulators

pharmacological, molecular
and clinical aspects

FRONTIERS IN PHARMACOLOGY & THERAPEUTICS

SERIES ADVISORS

FRONTIERS IN PHARMACOLOGY & THERAPEUTICS

Potassium Channel Modulators

pharmacological, molecular
and clinical aspects

edited by

Arthur H. Weston MSc, PhD

Leech Professor of Pharmacology
Smooth Muscle Research Group
Department of Physiological Sciences
University of Manchester, Manchester

Thomas C. Hamilton BSc, PhD, MRPharmS

Director, Cardiopulmonary Product Support
SmithKline Beecham Pharmaceuticals
Medicinal Research Centre, Harlow

OXFORD

BLACKWELL SCIENTIFIC PUBLICATIONS

LONDON EDINBURGH BOSTON

MELBOURNE PARIS BERLIN VIENNA

For G.A.

© 1992 by
Blackwell Scientific Publications
Editorial Offices:
Osney Mead, Oxford OX2 0EL
25 John Street, London WC1N 2BL
23 Ainslie Place, Edinburgh EH3 6AJ
238 Main Street, Cambridge
  Massachusetts 02142, USA
54 University Street, Carlton
  Victoria 3053, Australia

Other Editorial Offices:
Librairie Arnette SA
2, rue Casimir-Delavigne
75006 Paris
France

Blackwell Wissenschafts-Verlag
Meinekestrasse 4
D-1000 Berlin 15
Germany

Blackwell MZV
Feldgasse 13
A-1238 Wien
Austria

First published 1992

Set by Alden Multimedia, Northampton
Printed and bound in Great Britain
by Hartnolls Ltd, Bodmin, Cornwall

DISTRIBUTORS

Marston Book Services Ltd
P.O. Box 87
Oxford OX2 0DT
(*Orders*: Tel: 0865 791155
        Fax: 0865 791927
        Telex: 837515)

USA
Blackwell Scientific Publications, Inc.
238 Main Street
Cambridge, MA 02142
(*Orders*: Tel: 800 759-6102
        617 876-700)

Canada
Times Mirror Professional Publishing Ltd
5240 Finch Avenue East
Scarborough, Ontario M1S 5A2
(*Orders*: Tel: 800 268-4178
        416 298-1588)

Australia
Blackwell Scientific Publications
(Australia) Pty Ltd
54 University Street
Carlton, Victoria 3053
(*Orders*: Tel: 03 347-0300)

A catalogue record for this book is
available from the British Library

ISBN 0-632-03044-5

Contents

Contributors

L. A. Adams *Department of Medicine and Pharmacology, SJ-30, University of Washington School of Mediciine, Seattle, WA 98195, USA*

P-O. Andersson *Pfizer Central Research, Sandwich, Kent CT13 9NJ, UK*

J. M. B. Anumonwo *Department of Pharmacology, State University of New York Health Science Center at Syracuse, Syracuse, NY 13210, USA*

D. J. Beech *Department of Pharmacology and Clinical Pharmacology, St George's Hospital Medical School, Cranmer Terrace, London SW17 0RE, UK*

J. L. Berry *Department of Physiological Sciences, University of Manchester, Stopford Building, Oxford Road, Manchester M13 9PT, UK*

L. Birnbaumer *Department of Cell Biology and Physiology and Molecular Biophysics and the Division of Neurosciences, Baylor College of Medicine, Houston, TX 77030, USA*

T. B. Bolton *Department of Pharmacology and Clinical Pharmacology, St George's Hospital Medical School, Cranmer Terrace, London SW17 0RE, UK*

B. S. Brewster *Neuromuscular Unit, Department of Paediatrics and Neonatal Medicine, Royal Postgraduate Medical School, Hammersmith Hospital, Du Cane Road, London W12 0NN, UK*

T. J. Colatsky *Division of Cardiovascular and Metabolic Disorders, Wyeth-Ayerst Research, CN 8000, Princeton, NJ 08543, USA*

M. J. Dunne *Department of Biomedical Science, University of Sheffield, Western Bank, Sheffield S10 2TN, UK*

S. Duty *Department of Physiological Sciences, University of Manchester, Stopford Building, Oxford Road, Manchester M13 9PT, UK*

G. Edwards *Department of Physiological Sciences, University of Manchester, Stopford Building, Oxford Road, Manchester M13 9PT, UK*

J. M. Evans *SmithKline Beecham Pharmaceuticals, Medical Research Centre, Harlow, Essex CM19 5AD, UK*

L. C. Freeman *Department of Physiology, University of Rochester School of Medicine, Rochester, NY 14642-8642, USA*

R. W. Foster *Department of Physiological Sciences, University of Manchester, Stopford Building, Oxford Road, Manchester M13 9PT, UK*

M. Galvan *Marion Merrell Dow Research Institute, 16 rue d'Ankara, B.P. 447 R/9, 67009 Strasbourg Cedex, France*

M. L. Garcia *Department of Membrane Biochemistry and Biophysics, Merck Institute for Therapeutic Research, Rahway, NJ 08820, USA*

K. A. Green *Department of Physiological Sciences, University of Manchester, Stopford Bulding, Oxford Road, Manchester M13 9PT, UK*

M. S. Hadley *SmithKline Beecham Pharmaceuticals, Medical Research Centre, Harlow, Essex CM19 5AD, UK*

T. C. Hamilton *Director SmithKline Beecham Pharmaceuticals, Medical Research Centre, Harlow, Essex CM19 5AD, UK*

K. M. Houamed *Departments of Medicine and Pharmacology, SJ-30 University of Washington School of Medicine, Seattle, WA 98195, USA*

G. J. Kaczorowski *Department of Membrane Biochemistry and Biophysics, Merck Institute for Therapeutic Research, Rahway, NJ 08820, USA*

R. S. Kass *Department of Physiology, University of Rochester School of Medicine, Rochester, NY 14642-8642, USA*

W. M. Kwok *Department of Physiology, University of Rochester School of Medicine, Rochester, NY 14642-8642, USA*

M. A. Murray *Department of Physiological Sciences, University of Manchester, Stopford Building, Oxford Road, Manchester M13 9PT, UK*

Th. Noack *Department of Physiology, University of Marburg, Deutschhausstrasse 2, W-3550, Marburg, Germany*

O. Pongs *Zentrum für Molekulare Neurobiologie, Institute für Neurale Signalverarbeitung, Universität Hamburg, Martinistr. 52, Hans 42, W-2000 Hamburg 20, Germany*

R. C. Small *Department of Physiological Sciences, University of Manchester, Stopford Building, Oxford Road, Manchester M13 9PT, UK*

G. Stemp *SmithKline Beecham Pharmaceuticals, Medical Research Centre, Harlow, Essex CM19 5AD, UK*

P. N. Strong *Neuromuscular Unit, Department of Paediatrics and Neonatal Medicine, Royal Postgraduate Medical School, Hammersmith Hospital, Du Cane Road, London W12 0NN, UK*

B. L. Tempel *Geriatric Research, Education and Clinical Center, Seattle Veterans Affairs Medical Center, 1600 S Columbian Way, Seattle, WA 98108, USA; and Departments of Medicine and Pharmacology, SJ-30, University of Washington School of Medicine, Seattle, WA 98195, USA*

D. J. Trezise *Department of Physiological Sciences, University of Manchester, Stopford Building, Oxford Road, Manchester M13 9PT, UK*

A. C. Wareham *Department of Physiological Sciences, University of Manchester, Stopford Building, Oxford Road, Manchester M13 9PT, UK*

A. H. Weston *Department of Physiological Sciences, University of Manchester, Stopford Building, Oxford Road, Manchester M13 9PT, UK*

A. J. Williams *ICI Pharmaceuticals, Mereside, Alderley Park, Macclesfield, Cheshire SK10 4TG, UK*

M. G. Wyllie *Pfizer Central Research, Sandwich, Kent CT13 9NJ, UK*

Preface

The seeds of this book were sown, unknown to either of us, almost 10 years ago in 1982. At that time, Beecham Research Laboratories (now SmithKline Beecham) had recently synthesized a series of benzopyrans with *in vivo* hypotensive properties, but their mode of action was puzzling. Discussions between us led to the setting up of a collaborative project, partly funded by the Science and Engineering Research Council, with a young graduate student, Sheila Weir. An electrophysiological approach was adopted with the compound then known as BRL 34915 (cromakalim). Within a very short time, data from both our laboratories confirmed the involvement of K-channel opening in the vasorelaxant action of this agent.

Of course K-channel research did not begin with the discovery of the mode of action of cromakalim. For many years, electrophysiologists had appreciated the role and importance of K-channels in excitable cells. However, it is probably no exaggeration to say that the findings of the Beecham and Manchester groups with cromakalim were a major catalyst to the explosive growth of world-wide interest in the field of K-channels and their modulation by drugs.

Many other varied factors also combined to stimulate K-channel research during the 1980s. One of these was the realization that several existing, yet chemically diverse, molecules such as nicorandil, pinacidil, diazoxide and minoxidil also shared a mechanism of action similar to that of cromakalim. Thus chemists had a surfeit of information on which to base new structural developments. Furthermore, the pharmaceutical industry was also developing novel K-channel blockers for use as anti-dysrrhythmic agents and it was being realized that certain oral hypo-glycaemic drugs owed their effects to K-channel blockade in the pancreatic β-cell. Such pharmacological developments, together with advances in molecular biology and single-channel electrophysiology, all provided an unprecedented stimulus for K-channel research world-wide.

The purpose of this book is not to provide an encyclopaedia on all aspects of K-channel modulation. Instead, it is very much our personal view of some of the most important recent developments in K-channel research. As pharmacologists, we make no apology that many of the chapters are concerned with the mode of action of K-channel modulator drugs. However, we are sure that bioscientists of many disciplines will find this an invaluable source of reference and a stimulus to their own research.

One major problem in editing a work of this type has been K-channel nomenclature and the task of achieving standardization throughout the chapters has been difficult. As with many drug receptors, there is no agreed method of naming an ion channel in an abbreviated form and the scientific literature is currently awash with many different systems. We have thus adopted the basic guidelines laid down in the *Receptor Nomenclature Supplement of Trends in Pharmacological Sciences* (Watson & Abbott, 1992). In the absence of information from molecular biologists concerning the precise interrelationship between different K-channel types, the supplement provides a basis for a classification system and is updated annually. We have used the symbol K for a potassium *channel* and the symbol I for a *current*. Appropriate subscripts and prefixes define individual channels and currents. Thus BK_{Ca} and $I_{BK(Ca)}$ are used to describe the big conductance, calcium-dependent K-channel and its associated current, respectively. It is hard to believe that no such standardization already exists and that many investigators still use symbols such as I_K to signify both a current carried by K^+ and a K-channel. We hope that the rationalization in nomenclature suggested in this volume will become widely accepted.

The efforts of many have been involved in the production of this book. We thank all the contributors, not only for their submissions, but also for their patience. In an attempt to achieve some standardization, changes were necessary and all chapters were returned to authors for modifications. For various reasons, much of this editing was carried out in Manchester. Special thanks are due to Gill Edwards, Sarah Hughes, Christine Iron-monger and Kay Weston for their painstaking efforts.

Finally, one of us (AHW) would like to acknowledge the debt to his sources of funding for K-channel research. The Alexander von Humboldt Stiftung, the Japanese Society for the Promotion of Science, the Medical Research Council, the Science and Engineering Research Council, the Royal Society and the Wellcome Trust all provided funds variously for graduate studentships, apparatus and study visits to other laboratories. He also acknowledges the generous support which he has received from many companies within the pharmaceutical industry.

Arthur Weston, Tom Hamilton

Reference

Watson, S. & Abbott, A. (1982) Receptor nomenclature. *Trends in Pharmacological Sciences* **13**, S1–S36.

Chapter 1
Potassium channels in excitable cells: a synopsis
Th. Noack

Introduction

Using the sucrose-gap voltage-clamp technique or the classical two-electrode method, a good understanding of the membrane properties of many excitable cells had already been achieved by the late 1970s. However, neither technique could take into consideration the fact that most excitable tissues exhibit syncytial properties (Bolton *et al.*, 1981; Lammel 1981a,b) and thus the measured currents did not accurately reflect those flowing through the ionic channels of individual cell membranes. During the 1980s, investigation of the membrane properties and characteristics of excitable tissues has increased phenomenally. The main factor which enabled this tremendous development has been the introduction of the improved patch-clamp technique by Sakmann and Neher in 1981 (Hamill *et al.*, 1981).

The use of this methodology is much more demanding than earlier techniques and it is perhaps surprising that 'patch-clamping' has achieved such widespread popularity. Probably one reason for this is the fascination of observing ionic movements almost at a molecular level, which might also be the reason for the high impact of papers concerned with ionic channels. Such positive feedback could well explain the enormous number of papers dealing with the subject of ion channels published in the past 5 years.

The large number of additions to the observations dealing with the different types of ion channel described in the various tissues leaves the whole field more and more immense (Fig. 1.1). It thus makes sense to consolidate these observations from time to time and to reflect on the possible general principles which play a role in excitation processes and on

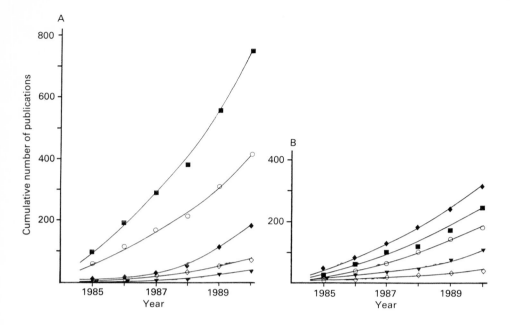

Fig. 1.1. Number of publications dealing with ionic channels/currents. A, Cumulative number of publications from the year 1985 to the year 1990 for the keywords *calcium current* or *calcium channel* in smooth muscle (■), cardiac muscle (○), skeletal muscle (◇), neurone (◆) and the pancreatic β-cell (▼). B, Cumulative number of publications for the same period for the keywords *potassium current* or *potassium channel*. The symbols in B refer to the meaning in A. (Source: Medline data base.)

those special mechanisms which seem to be organ-specific and which thus should not be generalized. The efforts of molecular biologists both to express and to transform ionic channels (*see* Chapters 2 and 3) have been a really positive development of recent years. Slight gene modification can completely change the activation, inactivation and pharmacological properties of ionic channels (Ruppersberg *et al.*, 1990) and close co-operation between physiologists, pharmacologists and molecular biologists is now an important factor in advancing knowledge in the field of membrane excitation. Such collaborative studies promise to yield important advances during the present decade.

Biophysical properties and nomenclature of K-channels in excitable tissues

If one compares the annual state of knowledge concerning excitation processes in cardiac muscle, skeletal muscle, smooth muscle, neurones and in the pancreatic β-cell, it can be shown that the most investigated tissues (from a numerical viewpoint) are smooth muscle, cardiac muscle and neurones (Fig. 1.1). A relatively small number of publications exists for skeletal muscle and the pancreatic β-cell. However, the relationship between those investigations on the subject of K- and Ca-channels/ currents is different in each tissue. In neurones and in the β-cell, twice the number of publications deals with K-currents compared with the number of investigations concerned with Ca-currents. For the three different muscle preparations the opposite is true with the number of publications concerning Ca-currents being two to three times larger than those involving K.

Although the number of publications dealing generally with ionic channels/currents in smooth muscle is large, the excitation and relaxation processes within the smooth muscle system are less well-understood than in other types of muscle. One reason for this is probably the relative diversity and specialization of smooth muscle-containing organs in the different species investigated (Golenhofen et al., 1970). This diversity is probably substantially linked to the presence of different types of ionic current component or to the extent to which individual currents are expressed in the various tissues. Furthermore, a mathematical description of the electrical activity of smooth muscle, similar to that available for nervous tissue (Hodgkin & Huxley, 1952) and also now available for cardiac muscle (Noble, 1975) is still lacking today for any of the types of smooth muscle.

Subdivisions of K-channels

Compared with the number of different types of Ca-channel so far identified (four types), a much larger number of K-channels (about 14) has been classified in excitable tissues during the last years. A recent overview was given by Watson and Abbott (1992) and the nomenclature used below has been adapted from this publication. The very large number of K-channels compared with Ca-channels may indicate that the characteristic and diverse electrical activity of different organs is closely associated with their complement of K-channels rather than with the presence of other ion conductances.

Potassium channels are usually broadly divided into four major groups:
1 voltage-dependent;
2 calcium-activated;
3 receptor-coupled;
4 metabolism steered.
Although such a subdivision is not without its limitations (because, e.g. Ca-activated channels are also voltage-dependent) it does indicate the experimental conditions under which the channel class can be investigated. The weakness of this classification is that some of the channels subdivided

in this way might be more or less identical (say from a structural or genetic viewpoint) within the different groups. Thus, an inappropriate or even a double classification could occur. At present, however, there is insufficient information available from molecular biologists to enable a true structural classification to be developed. In the future, such a system will probably supersede the rather arbitrary present subdivisions based on (usually) electrophysiological data.

Input and leakage conductances

If a membrane is investigated under ideal voltage-clamp conditions, the current measured reflects that which flows through the ionic channels of the membrane. The current values obtained for each clamped membrane potential are usually displayed graphically according to convention with the membrane potential (V) on the x-axis and the corresponding current (I) on the y-axis. Furthermore, potentials are defined as measured from intracellular to extracellular, the currents being positive when cations traverse the membrane in an outward direction.

To understand the basic electrical properties of a cell, its input conductance is of major importance. This conductance determines not only the zero current potential (ZCP) but also the range over which modulation of membrane potential can be induced by the activation or inactivation of the various current components. In some reports, the input conductance is termed 'leakage conductance' and the currents underlying this are sometimes crudely subtracted from other evoked currents. In this chapter the terms 'leakage current' and 'leakage conductance' are used in their proper form to describe the conductance which exists or the current which flows between pipette and membrane surface.

The input conductance consists usually of one or more outward components carried by K^+ together with inwardly directed components carried by Na^+ and/or Ca^{2+}. If attention is focused on the K-currents it seems useful to classify these components into those which seem to be activated negative to $-35\,mV$ and those which develop at potentials more positive than $-35\,mV$. Such a classification is useful, because a membrane which does not generate action potentials and spikes will not usually exhibit potentials positive to $-35\,mV$ under physiological conditions.

Analysis of the current–voltage relationships (I–V curves) of excitable cells measured using the whole-cell configuration shows that the slope of the I–V curves in the potential range between $-35\,mV$ and the actual K-equilibrium potential (E_K) is almost flat (Noble, 1975; Kwiecinski et al., 1984; Lammel et al., 1991). The net input conductance (dI/dV) is usually small and ranges between 0.15 and $0.5\,pS/\mu m^2$. Assuming a cell surface area of about $2000\,\mu m^2$ which is representative for cells from cardiac and smooth muscle and for neurones and the pancreatic β-cell, an overall input conductance of about 1 nS can be detected. For investigations in striated muscle, vesicles of 0.5–1 μm diameter are usually prepared. The input conductance of these artificial cells should be smaller than 1 nS.

A cellular input conductance of 1 nS means that a change in ionic current of only 10 pA would cause a membrane potential shift of about 10 mV. In the absence of voltage-clamping, the ZCP reflects the membrane potential at which the membrane current is zero. The term resting potential is difficult to define and sometimes misleading. In spontaneously active tissues there is no true resting level and in other tissues without spontaneous activity the measured membrane potential might be dependent on actual cell function and metabolism.

Potassium currents which are available in the voltage range of the physiological E_K (*see* Table 1.1)

Rectifying currents

In comparison with the low input conductance between E_K and -35 mV, this parameter increases 10-fold when the membrane is depolarized positive to 0 mV, a phenomenon termed outward rectification (Hodgkin & Huxley, 1952). The current(s) $I_{K(V)}$ producing outward rectification are discussed below. A similar dramatic increase of the input conductance is observed in those cells which express an inward rectifier K-channel (K_{IR}) at potentials more negative than E_K. The K_{IR} seems to be absent in some tissues, but in cardiac muscle, the inward rectifer current I_{K1}* shortens action potential duration and contributes to the input conductance (Kass *et al.*, 1990). In pancreatic β-cells an inwardly rectifying current inhibited by intracellular adenosine triphosphate (ATP) has been reported. The previously mentioned 'double classification' of ionic currents becomes obvious in this case (should such a current be designated $I_{K(ATP)}$ or $I_{K(IR-ATP)}$, for example?). The function of both inward and outward rectifiers is to keep the membrane potential within discrete limits.

Between these limits, defined by the potentials at which inward and outward rectification becomes effective, small current changes can produce quite large potential changes. This should be kept in mind when judging the results obtained with microelectrodes, especially in connection with putative K-channel openers (*see* (Chapter 13).

The necessity that living cells should fulfill their functions (information transport, tension development, exocrine secretion, etc.) with the maximum of energetic effectiveness makes shallow *I–V* curves desirable (Noble, 1975). On the other hand, the effective and precise control of cell

---

*By historical convention, the cardiac inward rectifier current is abbreviated to I_{K1} even though a more sensible designation would be $I_{K(IR)}$.

function could not be fulfilled by a large conductance channel in a given potential range in which neither inward nor outward rectification was exhibited by such a channel. Furthermore, the precise control of cell function should only be very little affected by those cytosolic messengers which exhibit a broad range of targets within the cell (non-specific messengers). Consideration of these aspects makes it doubtful for example that large conductance, Ca-activated K-channels (BK_{Ca}) really do take part in determining the input conductance of smooth muscle cells as recently proposed (Hu *et al.*, 1989).

M(uscarinic)-current ($I_{K(M)}$)

In some preparations the input K-conductance under non-stimulated conditions is reported to be carried by a channel population which shuts off under muscarinic stimulation. Such M(uscarinic)-currents ($I_{K(M)}$) are suppressed by acetylcholine or substance P. First described in sympathetic neurones (Brown & Adams, 1980), $I_{K(M)}$ was later shown to be present in the toad, *Bufo marinus* (Sims *et al.*, 1985), although in mammalian smooth muscle $I_{K(M)}$ has not yet been identified. The excitatory action of acetylcholine in these tissues is based on the opening of a non-selective cationic channel (Benham *et al.*, 1985). However, for a specific gastric region (guinea-pig fundus) it was recently reported that acetylcholine suppresses not only part of the K-input conductance but also a small component of a Na-conductance (Lammel *et al.*, 1991).

A-current ($I_{K(A)}$)

The very fast activating A-type current observed at step depolarizations positive to $-50\,mV$ with an inactivating time constant of about 50 ms was first described in neurones (Thompson, 1977) and was later shown to be present in other issues (crista terminalis of the heart: Giles & van Ginneken, 1985; portal vein: Beech & Bolton, 1989b). This current, which activates at potentials more positive than $-50\,mV$ seems to take part only in dynamic processes, e.g. during a fast repolarization and to counteract fast inward current movements. It also enables a faster recovery from inactivation for inward currents. The $I_{K(A)}$ seems to be present in the majority of fast repetitively-spiking cells but seems not to participate in the input conductance.

The composition of the input conductance

Taking into account the properties of those currents which are available near E_K, is it possible to identify those K-channels which are responsible for the shape of the $I-V$ curves in this potential range and thus for the input conductance of the cell? Unfortunately, an exact answer which is compatible with all tissue types remains elusive, one reason being that comprehensive data about the input conductance are rarely available for most tissues. However, in spite of these limitations, some relevant comments can be made.

As already mentioned, an inwardly rectifying K-channel (K_{IR}) is believed to comprise part of the input conductance in cardiac muscle (McAllister & Noble, 1966). Furthermore, in the pancreatic β-cell, two different types of K-channel are reported to be responsible for the input conductance. Both exhibit inward rectification and are sensitive to intracellular ATP (Findlay et al., 1985). In neurones, $I_{K(M)}$ which shuts off under muscarinic stimulation, forms a major part of the input conductance (Brown & Adams, 1980) and an $I_{K(IR)}$-current is also present in this tissue (Kandel & Tauc, 1966). Even in 1949, an inward rectifying current was identified in skeletal muscle (Katz, 1949) although whether this contributes specifically to the input conductance has not yet been determined. Whether this inward rectifier is ATP-sensitive is not clear since K_{ATP} in skeletal muscle exhibits usually large conductances (Woll et al., 1989; Weik & Neumcke, 1990).

In smooth muscle, an $I_{K(IR)}$-current has been reported in rabbit jejunum (Benham et al., 1987; Edwards & Hirst, 1988). However, such a current has only been reported in a relatively small number of smooth muscles. The non-inwardly rectifying current which underlies the input conductance in various smooth muscle tissues is neither completely blocked by 4-aminopyridine (5 mM) nor by tetraethylammonium (TEA; 10 mM; Noack et al., 1990; Lammel et al., 1991). Furthermore intracellular exchange of K^+ by Cs^+ does not completely inhibit the input conductance. Changing the concentration of intracellular Ca^{2+} ($[Ca^{2+}]_i$) over a wide range by varying the intracellular EGTA (ethylene glycol tetra-acetic acid) concentration or extrusion of $[Ca^{2+}]_i$ using extracellular EGTA has little effect on the input conductance in different smooth muscle preparations (Noack et al., 1990). From this it can be concluded that the channels which are responsible for the input conductance in these smooth muscles are relatively Ca-independent.

To date, the available evidence generally favours K_{IR} as the main factor which determines input conductance. However, inwardly-rectifying currents usually activate on hyperpolarizations negative to -50 mV and thus they cannot be the only component which underlies the input conductance in the voltage range between -90 and -30 mV. Furthermore, in smooth muscle, K_{IR}-channels are only rarely present. The difficulty in describing the channels responsible for the input conductance using the whole-cell clamp technique is probably related to the small size of the net currents involved. To describe these channels using single channel analysis could be extremely difficult because such channels probably only exhibit small unitary conductances and/or fast kinetics.

The action of K-currents available at depolarized membrane potentials
(*see* Table 1.1)

The K-channels available at potentials positive to $-35\,mV$ take part in the most complicated patterns of electrical activity in combination with those K-channels activated between -90 and $-35\,mV$ and those carrying the membrane current in an inward direction (e.g. Ca^{2+} or Na^{+}).

Inactivating K-currents

Under Ca^{2+}-free conditions, nearly every excitable tissue produces a delayed activating outward current on voltage-clamp depolarization (Noble & Tsien, 1969; Noma & Irisawa, 1976; Di Francesco *et al.*, 1979). This current usually inactivates in the following seconds and it is termed the delayed rectifier or $I_{K(V)}$. In some tissues $I_{K(V)}$ is increased by cyclic adenosine monophosphate (cAMP) or by activation of protein kinase C (PKC) (Tsien *et al.*, 1972; Tohse *et al.*, 1987; Walsh & Kass, 1988). However, the delayed outward current described in the early investigations can be subdivided into different currents which are carried by completely different K-channels (Noble & Tsien, 1969; Sanguinetti & Jurkiewicz, 1990). The single channel conductance for $I_{K(V)}$ as listed in Table 1.1 varies between 5 and 60 pS and such a large range is one indication that different K-channels are probably involved. Usually, inactivating and non-inactivating components can be identified using the appropriate holding potential. The former component may show some similarities to the neuronal A-current, but its inactivation is much slower and its threshold for activation is usually some 20 mV more positive than is characteristic for the A-current proper. The steep slope of $I–V$ relationships describing this component is due more to voltage-dependent activation than to simple outward rectification, which depends on both $[K^{+}]_i$ and $[K^{+}]_o$.

Non-inactivating Ca-independent K-currents

In a Ca^{2+}-free solution, the non-inactivating residual current component of $I_{K(V)}$ can itself be further subdivided using various K-channel blockers. In smooth muscle one such non-inactivating component consists of a high noise, delayed activating current while the other component shows no measurable delay of activation and exhibits a low noise current signal. Both components show outward rectification but only the high noise component can be suppressed by TEA (1–5 mM; Noack *et al.*, 1992).

Table 1.1. Summary of K-channels and currents. The channels and currents have been divided into groups according to their availability negative or positive to a membrane potential of $-35\,mV$. The given values for the single channel conductances are mostly referred to a symmetrical K-solution at $0\,mV$. If the solution has a quasi-physiological potassium gradient, the single channel conductance at $0\,mV$ will be lower than these values. Some K-channels and currents, the nature of which remains speculative, have not been included. Molecular biology should reveal whether non-specific cation channels should be regarded as variants of Na- or K-channels, respectively.

	Channel		
Type	Designation	Current	Conductance (pS)
Available negative to $-35\,mV$			
Inward rectifier	K_{IR}	$I_{K(IR)}$, (heart, I_{K1})	5–30
ATP-sensitive	K_{ATP}	$I_{K(ATP)}$	20–100
Big Ca^{2+}-activated*	BK_{Ca}	$I_{BK(Ca)}$	100–250
Intermediate Ca^{2+}-activated	IK_{Ca}	$I_{IK(Ca)}$	18–50
Small Ca^{2+}-activated	SK_{Ca}	$I_{SK(Ca)}$	6–14
Non-specific cation (Ca^{2+}-activated)	KNa_{Ca}	$I_{KNa(Ca)}$	25–30
M	K_M	$I_{K(M)}$	6
A	K_A	$I_{K(A)}$	20
Available positive to $-35\,mV$			
Delayed rectifier	K_V	$I_{K(V)}$	5–60
ATP-sensitive	K_{ATP}	$I_{K(ATP)}$	20–100
Sarcoplasmic reticulum	K_{SR}	$I_{K(SR)}$	150
Big Ca^{2+}-activated	BK_{Ca}	$I_{BK(Ca)}$	100–250
Intermediate Ca^{2+}-activated	IK_{Ca}	$I_{IK(Ca)}$	18–50
Small Ca^{2+}-activated	SK_{Ca}	$I_{SK(Ca)}$	6–14
Non-specific cation (Ca^{2+}-activated)	KNa_{Ca}	$I_{KNa(Ca)}$	25–30
M	K_M	$I_{K(M)}$	6
A	K_A	$I_{K(A)}$	20

*The availability of BK_{Ca} at potentials negative to $-35\,mV$ is a function of $[Ca^{2+}]_i$.

Unfortunately, because TEA (1–5 mM) also blocks large conductance Ca-activated K-currents, ($I_{BK(Ca)}$), the high noise component of $I_{K(V)}$ is sometimes inappropriately designated as Ca-dependent (Beech & Bolton, 1989a). It is now clear that blockade by TEA does not necessarily indicate the Ca-dependence of a particular current. Thus only the high noise component exhibits the proper specifications of a delayed rectifier ($I_{K(V)}$), i.e. a current which is Ca-independent, which shows delayed activation and which exhibits a I–V relationship described by the Goldmann–Hodgkin–Katz equation.

One of the most important components in determining the different patterns of electrical activity during depolarization seems to be the delayed rectifier $I_{K(V)}$. This slowly inactivating transient outward current is also sometimes termed I_{TO}. Its time-course of inactivation varies in the different tissues and it exhibits a voltage- and time-dependent recovery from inactivation (Noack *et al.*, 1990). The close relationship between $I_{K(V)}$ and $I_{K(A)}$ seems very obvious and improved terminology to describe and distinguish between these currents is long overdue.

Ca-dependent K-channels (K_{Ca})

Large conductance Ca-activated K-channels (BK_{Ca}; Table 1.1) have been reported for the pancreatic β-cell, skeletal muscle, neurones and smooth muscle but not for cardiac muscle. A large number of reports exists for this channel type which can be modulated by $[Ca^{2+}]_i$ and by the membrane potential. This channel is usually very sensitive to charybdotoxin and to TEA, although the former seems to be the more selective blocking agent. In smooth muscle, Ca^{2+} discharge from subplasmalemmal intracellular stores can induce large K-currents which may be carried by BK_{Ca}-channels (Benham & Bolton, 1986). In several tissues the possible function of the current associated with these channels ($I_{BK(Ca)}$) is probably closely associated with the repolarization phase of spikes (Adams *et al.*, 1982; Smith *et al.*, 1990) and regulation of Ca^{2+} entry (Rudy, 1988). This regulation might have functional relevance in the manner of a negative feedback mechanism which modulates voltage-activated Ca-currents.

K_{Ca} currents of a much smaller single channel conductance (6–14 pS) exist in skeletal muscle and in neurones (Marty, 1983; Cognard *et al.*, 1984; Romey & Lazdunski, 1984; Kawai & Watanabe, 1986). Such K-currents, which have not been reported in the pancreatic β-cell or in cardiac muscle, are usually selectively inhibited by apamin. From the excitatory action of apamin on some smooth muscle preparations the existence of similar small K_{Ca} channels has been claimed (Fedan *et al.*, 1984), although no voltage-clamp data exist to verify that these channels exist in smooth muscle. However, the ability of apamin to inhibit non-adrenergic non-cholinergic (NANC) relaxations and those mediated by noradrenaline in guinea-pig taenia caeci (Shuba & Vladimirova, 1980) provides further indirect evidence that such channels might exist in smooth muscle (*see* Chapter 7 for a further discussion of this topic). Small conductance K_{Ca}-channels in skeletal muscle and neurones are believed to prolong after-hyperpolarization (Romey & Lazdunski, 1984; Blatz & Magleby, 1986).

Conclusions

For the future it seems very important to carry out further investigations into the types of channel which underly the input conductance of the cell. As long as we know very little about the nature of this conductance, the extent of the complex interactions between its different components and how these determine observed patterns of electrical activity will remain speculative.

The conceptual subdivision of K-channels into those available for conduction in the potential ranges positive and negative to approximately $-35\,mV$ offers simple new insights into experimental problems. For example, there is much speculation at present about the type of K-channel which is opened by the agents known as the K-channel openers or activators. These drugs (see Chapter 13) produce sustained relaxation and membrane hyperpolarization of intact smooth muscle in both stimulated and quiescent circumstances. To be consistent with such observations it seems reasonable that the K-current activated by these agents should at least be (i) non-inactivating and (ii) available over a wide range of potentials and especially at those negative to $-35\,mV$. Single-cell experiments directed towards satisfying these criteria are to be recommended. The reader is referred to Chapters 7 and 14 for a further discussion of this interesting problem.

It can be anticipated that the ever-increasing amount of information about K-channels and currents will bring new insights into cell function and excitability. In parallel, however, it would be very worthwhile to update the system of describing such channels and currents in order to increase clarity and to prevent confusion. It is hoped that this book may provide the catalyst for such a process.

References

Adams, P. R., Constanti, A., Brown, D. A. & Clark R. B. (1982) Intracellular Ca^{2+} activates a fast voltage-sensitive current in vertebrate sympathetic neurones. *Nature* **246**, 746–749.

Beech, D. J. & Bolton T. B. (1989a) Two components of potassium current activated by depolarization of single smooth muscle cells from the rabbit portal vein. *Journal of Physiology* **418**, 293–309.

Beech, D. J. & Bolton T. B. (1989b) A voltage-dependent outward current with fast kinetics in single smooth muscle cells isolated from the rabbit portal vein. *Journal of Physiology* **412**, 397–414.

Benham, C. D. & Bolton, T. B. (1986) Spontaneous transient outward currents in single visceral and vascular smooth muscle cells of the rabbit. *Journal of Physiology* **381**, 385–406.

Benham, C. D., Bolton, T. B., Denbigh, J. S. & Lang, R. J. (1987) Inward rectification in freshly isolated single smooth muscle cells of the rabbit jejunum. *Journal of Physiology* **383**, 461–476.

Benham, C. D., Bolton, T. B. & Lang R. J. (1985) Acetylcholine activates an inward current in single mammalian smooth muscle cells. *Nature* **316**, 345–347.

Blatz, L. A. & Magleby, K. L. (1986) Single apamin-blocked Ca^{2+}-activated K^+ channels of small conductance in cultured rat skeletal muscle. *Nature* **323**, 718–720.

Bolton, T. B., Tomita, T. & Vassort, G. (1981) Voltage clamp and the measurement of ionic conductances in smooth muscle. In Bülbring, E., Brading, A. F., Jones, A. W. & Tomita, T. (eds), *Smooth Muscle: An Assessment of Current Knowledge*. Edward Arnold, London, pp. 47–63.

Brown, D. A. & Adams, P. R. (1980) Muscarinic suppression of a novel voltage-sensitive K$^+$ current in a vertebrate neurone. *Nature* **283**, 673–676.

Cognard, C., Traore, F., Potreau, D. & Raymond, G. (1984) Effects of apamin on the outward potassium current of isolated frog skeletal muscle fibers. *Pflügers Archiv* **402**, 222–224.

Di Francesco, D., Noma, A. & Trautwein, W. (1979) Kinetics and magnitude of the time-dependent potassium current in the rabbit sinoatrial node. *Pflügers Archiv* **381**, 271–279.

Edwards, F. R. & Hirst, G. D. S. (1988) Inward rectification in submucosal arterioles of guinea-pig ileum. *Journal of Physiology* **404**, 437–454.

Fedan, J. S., Hogaboom, G. K. & O'Donnel, J. P. (1984) Comparison of the effects of apamin, a Ca^{2+}-dependent K$^+$ channel blocker, and arylazido aminopropionyl ATP (ANAPP3), a P2-purinergic receptor antagonist, in the guinea-pig vas deferens. *European Journal of Pharmacology* **104**, 327–334.

Findlay, I., Dunne, M. J. & Petersen, O. H. (1985) ATP-sensitive inward rectifier and voltage and calcium-activated K$^+$ channels in cultured pancreatic islet cells. *Journal of Membrane Biology* **88**, 165–172.

Giles, W. R. & van Ginneken A. G. C. (1985) A transient outward current in isolated cells from the crista terminalis of rabbit heart. *Journal of Physiology* **368**, 243–264.

Golenhofen, K., von Loh, D. & Milenov, K. (1970) Elektrophysiologische Untersuchungen zur Spontanaktivität isolierter Muskelpräparate aus verschiedenen Abschnitten des Meerschweinchen-Magens. *Pflügers Archiv* **315**, 336–356.

Hamill, O. P., Marty, A., Neher, E., Sakmann, B. & Sigworth F. J. (1981) Improved patch-clamp techniques for high-resolution current recording from cells and cell-free membrane patches. *Pflügers Archiv* **391**, 85–100.

Hodgkin, A. L. & Huxley, A. F. (1952) A quantitative description of membrane current and its application to conductance and excitation in nerve. *Journal of Physiology* **117**, 500–544.

Hu, S. L., Yamamoto, Y. & Kao, C. Y. (1989) The Ca^{2+}-activated K$^+$ channel and its functional roles in smooth muscle cells of guinea-pig taenia coli. *Journal of General Physiology* **94**, 833–847.

Kandel, E. R. & Tauc, L. (1966) Anomalous rectification in the metacerebral giant cells and its consequences for synaptic transmission. *Journal of Physiology* **183**, 287–304.

Kass, R. S., Arena, J. P. & Walsh, K. B. (1990) Measurement and block of potassium channel currents in the heart: Importance of channel type. *Drug Development Research* **19**, 115–127.

Katz, B. (1949) Les constantes électriques de la membrane du muscle. *Archives de Science et Physiologie* **3**, 285–300.

Kawai, T. & Watanabe, M. (1986) Blockade of Ca^{2+}-activated conductance by apamin in rat sympathetic neurones. *British Journal of Pharmacology* **87**, 225–232.

Kwiecinski, H., Lehmann-Horn, F. & Rüdel, R. (1984) The resting membrane parameters of human intercostal muscle at low, normal and high extracellular potassium. *Muscle and Nerve* **7**, 60–65.

Lammel, E. (1981a) A theoretical study on the sucrose gap technique as applied to multicellular muscle preparations: I. Saline–sucrose interdiffusion. *Biophysical Journal* **36**, 533–553.

Lammel, E. (1981b) A theoretical study on the sucrose gap technique as applied to multicellular muscle preparations: II. Methodical errors in the determination of outward currents. *Biophysical Journal* **36**, 555–573.

Lammel, E., Deitmer, P. & Noack, Th. (1991) Suppression of steady membrane currents by acetylcholine in single smooth muscle cells of the guinea-pig gastric fundus. *Journal of Physiology* **432**, 259–282.

McAllister, R. E. & Noble, D. (1966) The time and voltage dependence of the slow outward current in cardiac Purkinje fibres. *Journal of Physiology* **186**, 632–662.

Marty, A. (1983) Ca^{2+}-dependent K channels with large unitary conductance. *Trends in Neuroscience* **6**, 262–265.

Noack, Th., Deitmer, P. & Golenhofen, K. (1990) Features of a calcium independent, caffeine sensitive outward current in single smooth muscle cells from the guinea-pig portal vein. *Pflügers Archiv* **416**, 467–469.

Noack, Th., Deitmer, P. & Lammel, E. (1992) Characterisation of membrane currents in single smooth muscle cells from the guinea pig gastric arteries. *Journal of Physiology* **451**, 387–417.

Noble, D. (1975) *The Initiation of the Heartbeat*. Oxford University Press, London, pp. 69–139.

Noble, D. & Tsien, R. W. (1969) Outward membrane currents activated in the plateau range of potentials in cardiac Purkinje fibres. *Journal of Physiology* **200**, 205–231.

Noma, A. & Irisawa, H. (1976) A time and voltage-dependent potassium current in rabbit sinoatrial node cell. *Pflügers Archiv* **366**, 251–258.

Romey, G. & Lazdunski, M. (1984) The coexistence in rat muscle cells of two distinct classes of Ca^{2+}-dependent K^+ channels with different physiological functions. *Biochemical and Biophysical Research Communications* **118**, 669–674.

Rudy, B. (1988) Diversity and ubiquity of K channels. *Neuroscience* **25**, 729–749.

Ruppersberg, J. P., Schröter, K. H., Sakmann, B., Stocker, M., Sewing, S. & Pongs, O. (1990) Heteromultimeric channels formed by rat brain potassium-channel proteins. *Nature* **345**, 535–537.

Sanguinetti, M. C. & Jurkiewicz, N. K. (1990) Two components of cardiac delayed rectifier K^+ current. *Journal of General Physiology* **96**, 195–215.

Shuba, M. F. & Vladimirova, I. A. (1980) Effect of apamin on the electrical responses of smooth muscle to adenosine 5'-triphosphate and to non-adrenergic, non-cholinergic nerve stimulation. *Neuroscience* **5**, 853–859.

Sims, S. M., Singer, J. J. & Walsh, J. V. (1985) Cholinergic agonists suppress a potassium current in freshly dissociated smooth muscle cells of the toad. *Journal of Physiology* **367**, 503–529.

Smith, P. A., Bokvist, K., Arkhammar, P., Berggren, P. O. & Rorsman, P. (1990) Delayed rectifier and calcium-activated K^+ channels and their significance for action potential repolarization in mouse pancreatic β-cells. *Journal of General Physiology* **95**, 1041–1059.

Thompson, S. H. (1977) Three pharmacologically distinct potassium channels in molluscan neurones. *Journal of Physiology* **265**, 465–488.

Tohse, N., Kameyama, M. & Irisawa, H. (1987) Intracellular Ca^{2+} and protein kinase C modulate K^+ current in guinea pig heart cells. *American Journal of Physiology* **253**, H1321–H1324.

Tsien, R. W., Giles, W. & Greengard, P. (1972) Cyclic AMP mediates the effects of adrenaline on cardiac Purkinje fibres. *Nature* **240**, 181–183.

Walsh, K. B. & Kass, R. S. (1988) Regulation of a heart potassium channel by PKA and C. *Science* **242**, 67–69.

Watson, S. & Abbott, A. (1992) Receptor nomenclature. *Trends in Pharmacological Sciences* **13**, S1–S36.

Weik, R. & Neumcke, B. (1990) Effects of potassium channel openers on single potassium channels in mouse skeletal muscle. *Naunyn-Schmiedeberg's Archives of Pharmacology* **342**, 258–263.

Woll, K. H. Lönnendonker, U. & Neumcke, B. (1989) ATP-sensitive potassium channels in adult mouse skeletal muscle: Different modes of blockage by internal cations, ATP and tolbutamide. *Pflügers Archiv* **414**, 622–628.

Chapter 2
Potassium channel genes: genomic complexity, molecular properties and differential expression

L. A. Adams, K. M. Houamed and B. L. Tempel

Introduction

Potassium channels constitute a family of integral membrane proteins which allow the conduction of K-currents in a variety of cell types, and which are important modulators of membrane excitability in neurones and other electrically polarized cells (Hille, 1984). A large number of these K-currents have been described electrophysiologically. They are known to vary significantly with respect to their kinetics and voltage dependence of activation and inactivation, gating properties, and pharmacological sensitivities to various agents (Rudy, 1988). This chapter explores the molecular mechanisms contributing to the functional diversity of K-channels. The first section includes a discussion of the genetic strategies used by two different species, flies (*Drosophila melanogaster*) and mice (*Mus musculus*) to generate multiple K-channel proteins with different electrophysiological properties. In the next section, the cell-specific expression of one of these channels in the central nervous system is described, and finally we discuss how various domains of the K-channel protein influence the physiological function of the channel itself.

The *Shaker* (*Sh*) mutants of *Drosophila* were originally described as fruit flies which shook their legs under ether anaesthesia, and demonstrated other behavioural abnormalities such as wing scissoring even when conscious. The discovery that *Sh* mutant larvae showed abnormally prolonged neurotransmitter release at the neuromuscular junction led to the proposal that defective K-channels in the nerve terminal membrane might be involved in the pathology of this mutant (Jan *et al.*, 1977). This was substantiated by subsequent intracellular recordings of the cervical giant axon in *Sh* mutants and normal *Drosophila*, which revealed that these mutants showed abnormally long delays in the repolarization of nerve action potentials; that this is due to an abnormal K-conductance was suggested by the ability of the K-channel blocker 4-aminopyridine (4-AP) to simulate the *Sh* phenotype in normal flies (Tanouye *et al.*, 1981). Using voltage-clamp analyses of flight muscles to identify more precisely which K-currents were involved, it was shown that the *Sh* mutation selectively affected the fast, transient K-current designated I_A (Salkoff, 1983).

The molecular characterization of K-channels has historically been hampered by the lack of a suitable ligand for biochemical purification purposes and by the fact that the protein is present at fairly low levels in most tissues. Thus, the identification of a chromosomal region from which a K-channel gene or genes might be isolated was particularly fortuitous. The *Sh* locus was identified by translocation mutation analysis as the polytene band 16F on the X chromosome (Tanouye *et al.*, 1981), and the technique of chromosomal walking was used to isolate 210 kb of genomic DNA from this locus. Clones spanning this region were used to screen translocation chromosomes from animals which had been characterized electrophysiologically in order to identify the chromosomal breakpoint which marked the transition between the presence or absence of I_A function and DNA spanning this breakpoint was used to probe genomic DNA from a number of different *Sh* mutants to determine where alterations in the mutant DNA might fall. The picture that emerged from these experiments was that *Sh* mutations were not clustered at a particular location, but were distributed over about 60 kb of DNA (Baumann *et al.*, 1987; Papazian *et al.*, 1987). When the coding regions within this large expanse of DNA were identified, it became clear that the *Sh* gene comprises a large and complex primary transcription unit which undergoes alternative exon splicing to generate multiple different secondary transcripts (Papazian *et al.*, 1987; Kamb *et al.*, 1987; Pongs *et al.*, 1988).

The likelihood that the DNA from the *Sh* locus indeed coded for a K-channel, or some portion thereof, was substantiated at this point by sequencing the cDNA clones designated ShA1 and ShA2 (Tempel *et al.*, 1987). Conceptual translation predicted a protein of 616 amino acids and a molecular mass of approximately 70 kDa. Hydropathy analysis suggested that the protein had a hydrophobic core comprised of seven membrane spanning domains and flanked at the amino (N) and carboxyl (C) ends by hydrophilic, presumably cytoplasmic ends. One of the putative membrane-spanning regions bore significant homology to the presumed voltage-sensing (S4) region of the Na-channel from the electric eel. Proof that these cDNA clones coded for K-channels was soon forthcoming, when it was shown that oocytes injected with ShA1 or ShB1 mRNA displayed transient outward currents carried by K^+. These currents, although differing somewhat from each other, each demonstrated pharmacological sensitivities, kinetic properties, and ion selectivities very similar to those described for the A-current in fly muscle (Timpe *et al.*, 1988b). These data were strongly supportive of the notion that the *Sh* locus of *Drosophila* codes for a transient, A-type K-channel (channel designation, K_A; current, I_A).

Potassium channel complexity

Fly *Sh* genes

As reviewed in Jan and Jan (1990), a number of genetic mechanisms can be used by a particular species to generate diversity of K-channel protein structure and electrophysiological function. These include: the existence of separate genes coding for different types of channel, the alternative splicing of one large gene to generate multiple, distinct protein products, and the combination of different subunits into homomultimeric or heteromultimeric structures with unique properties. Furthermore, different species may utilize these strategies in different ways. To illustrate this point, the following section will describe the mechanisms used to generate K-channel complexity in two species which provide a particularly interesting comparison: flies and mice.

The *Sh* data summarized above suggested a number of questions pertaining to the genomic complexity and potential multiplicity of K-channel genes and proteins. How many such genes exist in the fly genome, and how many different functional proteins can be generated from each gene? Do flies assemble subunits into both homomultimers and heteromultimers? Sequencing of additional *Sh*-related clones by the Jan group and others (Iverson *et al.*, 1988; Kamb *et al.*, 1988; Schwarz *et al.*, 1988) revealed that the predicted proteins had identical central core regions but different amino and carboxyl terminal ends. The central core region comprises eight common exons which are clustered within 10 kb of genomic DNA, while the exons coding for the variant ends are distributed over a much broader region of genomic DNA. Based on the uniqueness of their carboxyl and amino termini, four different predicted protein products coded for by the *Sh* locus have been identified.

Fly Shab, Shaw and Shal genes

The genomic complexity of fly K-channels does not stop with *Sh*, however. The observation that mutant flies in which the gene coding for the *Sh* K-channel is deleted still have A-type K-currents prompted the search for additional *Sh*-like genes. Three additional members of the *Sh* superfamily were soon isolated based on low-stringency hybridization of a *Sh* cDNA to an adult fly cDNA library (Butler *et al.*, 1989). These new members were named *Shab*, *Shaw* and *Shal*. They reside at different chromosomal loci and they have different patterns of expression during development. *Shab* and *Shal* genes can undergo splicing of primary mRNA transcripts to generate different protein products, but alternative splicing does not seem to be used as extensively in these genes as it is in *Sh*. The core region (S1–S6) is relatively highly conserved among all the fly K-channels, and structural variability is conferred by alterations in the N and C terminal flanking regions.

Fly *Sh* K-channels

Is this genomic complexity part of a strategy whereby channels with different electrophysiological properties are generated? It appears so. Evidence in support of this came first from the *Sh* family of genes, when mRNA from each of four classes of alternatively spliced *Sh* products (designated ShA, ShB, ShC and ShD), was injected into frog oocytes. Each transcript, when injected alone, directs the expression of a functional channel which conducts an A-type current (Timpe *et al.*, 1988a). The currents for ShA, ShB and ShD showed similar voltage dependence of activation, but different inactivation kinetics. Although the fast components of ShA, ShB and ShD inactivation are similar (10 ms), and most (95%) of ShB is inactivated during this initial period, ShA and ShD current remains and inactivates over a longer time course. Inactivation of ShC is yet slower than that of ShA. In addition, the four currents recover from activation at different rates: ShB and ShD fairly rapidly, ShA and ShC very slowly. Thus, the differences in the N and C terminal ends of proteins generated from the *Sh* locus generate kinetically distinct A-type K-currents.

The other *Drosophila* K-channel genes code for proteins with properties distinct from the *Sh* products. The *Shab* current has delayed rectifier properties (channel designation K_V; current $I_{K(V)}$) in that it is activated with a delay upon membrane depolarization to -40 mV, achieves maximal conductance slowly (300 ms at -40 mV), and shows sustained current over time. It is sensitive to tetraethylammonium (TEA) but not to (4-AP) (Pak *et al.*, 1991b). On the other hand, the *Shal* current is an A-type current which activates, inactivates, and decays within 200 ms, is not blocked by TEA, but is blocked by 4-AP (Pak *et al.*, 1991a).

In the experiments described above, a single species of mRNA was injected into an oocyte. Presumably, the channel formed was a homo-multimer of identical subunit types arranged according to some as yet unknown stoichiometry. The question of whether different subunit types can combine to form functional heteromultimeric channels can be addressed by injecting more than one species of mRNA into a single oocyte.

Experiments of this type suggest that, at least in the heterologous oocyte expression system, combinations of subunits can occur. For example, when two different *Sh* transcripts that express channels which differ markedly in their inactivation kinetics are co-injected into oocytes, the current expressed demonstrates an inactivation rate intermediate between the two homomultimeric channel currents (Aldrich, 1990; Isacoff *et al.*, 1990).

Thus it appears that the fly utilizes several different strategies to generate multiplicity and diversity of K-channels. Not only are there multiple K-channel genes in the fly genome, but each of these genes can be alternatively spliced to generate multiple protein products with kinetically distinct electrophysiological properties. There is evidence that subunits from different gene products may combine as homomultimeric or heteromultimeric structures, and that this affords an additional degree of functional variability. Next we will consider (taking the mouse as an example) whether mammals employ any or all of these strategies to generate K-channel diversity.

Mouse *Sh*-type K-channel genes

The isolation and cloning of the *Sh* gene provided the molecular tools to isolate and characterize K-channel genes from other species. Soon after *Sh* was cloned, the first mammalian K-channel gene was isolated from a mouse brain cDNA library based on sequence homology to the transmembrane region of the *Sh* clone ShA1 (Tempel *et al.*, 1988). The gene thus isolated, MBK1, shared 65% overall amino acid homology with the *Sh* proteins identified at that point, and even greater homology (95%) between some regions thought to be critical for channel function (i.e. S4). In contrast, the extent of nucleotide similarity was much lower, being less than 30% even in the S4 region. Tempel *et al.* hypothesized that evolutionary pressures had allowed the nucleotide sequence to diverge while selective pressures maintained the amino acid sequences critical for protein function.

MBK1 stands for mouse brain K^+-channel gene, number 1, a cDNA clone isolated from a mouse brain library. MK1 refers to the genomic clone which is intronless in the open reading frame and therefore identical to the coding sequence derived from the cDNA clone, MBK1. More recent nomenclature has renamed this gene mK_v 1.1. Northern blot analysis of MK1 expression revealed that, in contrast to the multiple transcripts generated from the *Sh* gene, MBK1 hybridized to a single band of about 8 Kb on a blot of mouse brain poly A^+ RNA. This raised the possibility that K-channel gene structure might differ between flies and mammals, and as more mouse K-channel genes were isolated and characterized, it became clear that this was the case. Two other members (MK2 and MK3)

Table 2.1. Tissue distribution of MK gene expression.

MK1	Brain, brainstem ≫ heart, skeletal muscle
MK2	Brain, brainstem
MK3	Thymus > brain
MK6	Brain (weak), brainstem (weak)

Tissues screened: brain, brainstem, heart, skeletal muscle, liver, kidney, spleen, thymus, testes.

of the *Sh*-related subfamily were isolated from a mouse genomic library using the full length MK1 cDNA as a probe (Chandy *et al.*, 1990), and an additional member, MK6, was isolated from a mouse brain cDNA library (Migeon *et al.*, 1992). On a Southern blot of mouse genomic DNA, MK1 hybridized strongly to three distinct bands, suggesting the possibility that each band represented a unique gene. When the genomic clones corresponding to each of these bands were sequenced, it became clear that the coding regions of MK1, MK2 and MK3 exist as single uninterrupted exons in the mouse genome. Although there are putative intronic sequences, identified by the presence of consensus sequences for splice donor and acceptor sites (Mount, 1982), these sequences are in the non-coding regions of the MK genes. The four genes show extensive amino acid homology in the transmembrane segments and in a portion of the amino terminus, but are more divergent in the C and extreme N termini, and in their non-coding regions. These three genes show different patterns of tissue expression by Northern blot analysis (Table 2.1), and they occupy distinct chromosomal loci. MK1, MK2 and MK3 are on mouse chromosomes 6, 3 and 3 respectively (Lock, submitted for publication); the chromosomal locus of MK6 is not yet established.

Mouse homologues of Shab, Shaw and Shal

Outside the *Sh* subfamily, mouse homologues of fly genes belonging to the *Shab*, *Shaw* and *Shal* subfamilies have now been identified. *mShab* and *mShal* have been sequenced and appear to be intronless (Pak *et al.*, 1991a,b). Four members of the *mShaw* subfamily have been described and named $K_V 3.1$, $K_V 3.2$, $K_V 3.3$ and $K_V 3.4$. In contrast to *mShab* and *mShal*, at least two of the *mShaw* genes contain introns: $K_V 3.3$ is encoded by at least two exons, one extending from S1 through the 3′ end and the other coding for the amino terminal sequence. The $K_V 3.4$ has a genomic structure similar to $K_V 3.3$ with its entire hydrophobic core contained in a single exon (Ghanshani *et al.*, 1990). The presence of transcripts of different sizes has not been established for $K_V 3.3$ or $K_V 3.4$, so it is still unclear whether the mouse utilizes alternative splicing of individual genes to generate multiple types of K_V-channel. It is evident, though, that the mouse generates multiple K-channels by expressing multiple genes.

Mouse K-channels have not been characterized as extensively as fly channels with respect to their electrophysiological properties. In oocyte expression studies, MK1, MK2 and MK3 direct the expression of currents of the delayed rectifier type, but they demonstrate some functional differences. MK2 is the slowest to activate, and although all are sustained outward currents, MK1 and MK2 persist for at least 2 s, whereas MK3 decays by about 50% within 600 ms. Mouse *Shab* also represents a delayed rectifier current, which activates and recovers from inactivation more slowly than its fly homologue, but otherwise is quite similar to *Shab* with respect to kinetic, voltage-sensitive and pharmacological properties (Pak *et al.*, 1991b). Similarly, the *mShaw* subfamily most likely codes for delayed rectifier currents. Although members of this mouse family have not been characterized electrophysiologically, the function of two of the genes, $K_V 3.1$ and $K_V 3.2$ can be inferred based on their homology to other channels. $K_V 3.1$ is identical to NGK2, isolated from a neuroblastoma-glioma cell line (Yokoyama *et al.*, 1989), and $K_V 3.2$ is similar to RkShIIIa (McCormack *et al.*, 1990), both of which express delayed rectifiers.

Recently, the mouse *Shal* (*mShal*) has been characterized electrophysiologically, and it appears to be the first of the mouse genes which does not code for a delayed rectifier. Mouse *mShal*, like the fly *Shal* (*fShal*), codes for a transient, A-type K-current, with activation occurring at about -60 mV, reaching peak current in 10 ms and having a fast component of decay of 23 ms. The current is insensitive to TEA but sensitive to 4-AP, which places it in the category of a classic I_A. Mouse *mShal* and *fShal* show a higher degree of interspecies structural and functional conservation than any of the other known K-channel proteins, sharing 82% amino acid similarity when the conserved core region (S1–S6) of the channel is considered. The conservation ends at a point toward the carboxyl end where alternative splicing occurs in *fShal* (Pak *et al.*, 1991a).

The examples provided by these two species suggest that common strategies may be used, albeit to different degrees, to generate K-channel diversity. Multiple genes certainly exist in both flies and mice. Alternative splicing of a gene to generate multiple transcripts is clearly used by flies and may be used by rodents as well. Finally, although direct evidence for this does not exist for mouse genes, subunit mixing may generate hetero-multimeric channel proteins in both flies and rodents (Ruppersberg *et al.*, 1990a; Christie *et al.*, 1990).

Cell-specific expression of MK1 in mouse brain

Regional distribution of MK1

The pattern of expression of MK1 in brain tissue offers additional insights about how diversity of function might be generated. *In situ* hybridization

Table 2.2. *In situ* hybridization analysis of MK1 expression in mouse brain.

Motor system
  Motor cortex
  Midbrain, pontine and medullary reticular formations
  Red nucleus
  Vestibular nucleus
  Ventral posterolateral nucleus of the thalamus
  Midbrain central grey
  Cerebellum (Purkinje cell layer)
  Olivary complex
  Pontine nuclei

Auditory system
  Cochlear nucleus
  Nucleus of the trapezoid body
  Olivary complex
  Lateral lemniscus
  Inferior colliculus
  Medial geniculate nucleus of the thalamus

Limbic system
  Septal nuclei
  Hippocampus
  Basolateral nucleus of the amygdala
  Diagonal band of Broca
  Stria medullaris

Olfactory system
  Piriform cortex
  Islands of Calleja

studies on sections of normal mouse brains using a probe directed against the 5′ untranslated region of the gene reveal that MK1 is not constitutively expressed in brain tissue; rather it is expressed in subpopulations of neurones which, in the cases we have examined, appear to be functionally related to one another (Adams *et al.*, submitted; *see also* Table 2.2). Thus, it appears in neurones from regions which comprise, variously, the auditory pathway, motor pathways, vestibular pathways, parts of the limbic system and olfactory system (Patton *et al.*, 1989). It is not expressed in the caudate and putamen and is only expressed at very low levels in the globus pallidus of the basal ganglia. It is not appreciably expressed in the hypothalamus, most of the amygdala is devoid of labelling, and labelling in the cortex is confined to two layers which probably correspond to layers III and V.

High density expression of MK1

In an attempt to understand why MK1 is expressed in this particular subpopulation of cells, we tried to identify what functional characteristics are common to cells expressing MK1, and compare these to cells in regions where MK1 is not expressed. One common feature is that cells in the regions where MK1 is expressed demonstrate very rapid firing rates. For example, large pyramidal motor neurones in the primary motor cortex and brainstem which are involved in generating voluntary movements may fire up to 500 spikes/s (Koike *et al.*, 1970; Takata *et al.*, 1982). Cells in the globus pallidus and substantia nigra of the basal ganglia which modulate motor activity, have higher resting rates of activity (> 50 spikes/s; DeLong, 1971) than cells in the caudate and putamen (2 spikes/s; Anderson, 1977). The Purkinje cells in the cerebellum, whose firing rates change with movement velocity and are able to code kinetic variables such as the rate of change of force or position, fire at rates between 100 and 200 spikes/s (Thach, 1968). As will be discussed in greater detail below, cells in the lower order neurones of the auditory pathway transmit information about incoming sound by phase-locking to the sinusoidal frequency of a sound wave as it is propagated into the inner ear. This requires that they are capable of firing at extremely high rates. Similarly, cells in the vestibular system often fire at very high rates and are capable of phase-locking to the sinusoidal pattern of head acceleration (Fernandez & Goldberg, 1971; Goldberg & Fernandez, 1971). Thus, MK1 is expressed in many of the CNS regions involved in processing frequency-coded information having a rapid kinetic component. In order to transmit frequency-coded information faithfully, it is important that the post-synaptic cell be able to follow the frequency of the presynaptic input. This in turn requires that the postsynaptic cell be able to terminate an action potential rapidly in order to be able to respond to the succeeding presynaptic spike.

Low density expression of MK1

In contrast, the regions where MK1 are not expressed to any significant extent, such as the amygdala and the hypothalamus, are involved in integrating sensory and environmental cues occurring over a long time period (Patton *et al.*, 1989). For example, among the functions of the hypothalamus are the governing of emotion, motivation, pituitary function, sexual behaviour and differentiation, and the regulation of temperature and cardiovascular responses. Neuroendocrine neurones in the hypothalamus involved in the phasic release of hormones occasionally increase their firing rate in response to some stimuli. Examples of these are paraventricular oxytocin neurones which respond to the suckling stimulus, and gonadotrophin releasing hormone neurones which increase their output to elicit the preovulatory surge of gonadotrophins from the pituitary. But even when maximally active, these do not generally fire at more than 30–40 spikes/s (Kesner *et al.*, 1986).

Clearly, these observations constitute only loose correlations between the functional properties of cells found in different regions of the brain and the expression of a particular channel type. The correlation makes some sense given the accepted notion that K_V-channels subserve the rapid repolarization of membrane potential following the generation of an action potential spike (Hille, 1984). It seems likely that the amount of delayed rectifier current present in a cell might be proportional to the rate of repolarization of the cell after an action potential, and might thereby determine not only the maximal firing rate of that cell, but perhaps more importantly, its ability to follow and reproduce the frequency component of the presynaptic stimulus.

Expression of MK1 in auditory pathways

To pursue this idea, we decided to assess the relative levels of MK1 expression in cells in different regions of the brain, reasoning that there might be higher levels of MK1 expression (on an individual cell basis) in cells which are called upon to fire more rapidly. The auditory pathway provides a unique system in which to examine this question, since there is known to be a shift in the response properties of neurones in progressively more rostral areas of the brain. As alluded to above, auditory processing by hair cells in the ear and by the lower order relay nuclei (including the cochlear nucleus, the nucleus of the trapezoid body, and the olivary complex) involves phase-locking of the electrical or synaptic output of the cell to the frequency of incoming sound. Cells which subserve this function must be able to maintain with great precision the pattern of incoming information, requiring rapid temporal resolution. In addition the cells often fire at extremely high rates and maintain this temporal resolution for short periods of time. In contrast, cells in the inferior colliculus and thalamus show less phase-locking ability (see E.W. Rubel chapter in Patton et al., 1989). We used semi-quantitative computerized image analysis to measure the density of autoradiographic grains (an index of mRNA levels) overlying individual cells in the cochlear nucleus, the olivary complex, the inferior colliculus, and the medial geniculate nucleus of the thalamus. We found that cells in the caudal region (cochlear nucleus and olivary complex) have twice the grain density of cells in the more rostral areas (inferior colliculus and thalamus; Adams et al., submitted). With the caveat that we have not rigorously identified that these cells are involved in auditory processing, it is nevertheless intriguing that cells which are known to entrain faithfully to very high frequency presynaptic input contain significantly higher levels of MK1 mRNA.

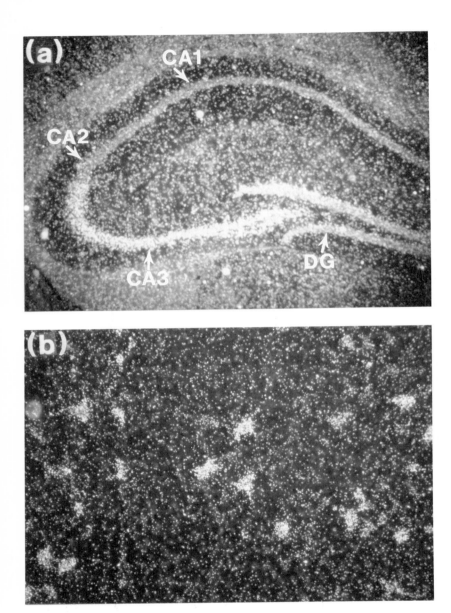

Fig. 2.1. *In situ* hybridization analysis of MK1 expression in cells in normal mouse brain. (a) MK1 expression in the hippocampus. Note the higher signal density over cells in the dentate gyrus (DG) and CA3 regions compared with CA1 and CA2. (b) Cells expressing MK1 in the pontine reticular formation. Computerized image analysis can be used to count the number of photographic grains overlying cells such as these (*see text*).

Structure–function studies

General features of K_A- and K_V-channels

The cloning of K-channels has enabled questions relating structure to function to be addressed on a molecular scale. Early models of K-channel topology assigned the N- and C-terminal domains to the cytoplasmic compartment of the cell. Hydropathy analysis of the predicted K-channel amino acid sequences revealed the presence of seven hydrophobic regions which, if they took the form of α-helices, would be of sufficient length to traverse the membrane (Tempel *et al.*, 1987). Since it appeared that this sequence was repeated fourfold (to yield a total of 28 membrane spanning segments) in Na- and Ca-channels, it was hypothesized that K-channels should consist of four subunits. Two of these putative transmembrane domains (termed S4 and H5) are of particular interest and will be discussed further here.

Since both K_A- and K_V-channels are activated by depolarization it was reasoned that an integral part of the channel molecule must constitute a dipole. Changes in the electrical potential across the membrane exert a moment on the dipole thereby causing a conformational change in the channel protein. Analysis of classical voltage-clamp experiments in squid and frog nerve fibres showed that the size of the dipole required for activation of K_V- channels was the equivalent of 4–6 elementary charges moving across the entire membrane electric field (reviewed in Hille, 1984). One of the transmembrane domains, termed S4, has the structure PxxPxxPxxPxxP, where x is a hydrophobic (neutral) amino acid, and P is an amino acid with a positively charged side chain (arginine or lysine). In many of the K-channel genes cloned to date the S4 region contains seven basic amino acids.

S4: the major voltage sensor for activation

The involvement of S4 in the voltage sensing mechanism underlying activation was first shown in Na-channels (Stühmer *et al.*, 1989). Point mutations in which basic residues were substituted with neutral or acidic residues affected the activation parameters of Na-channels in a predictable manner. Thus, as the net positive charge of S4 was decreased, the voltage sensitivity of activation decreased in an approximately linear fashion. Furthermore, the midpoint of the current–voltage (I–V) curve was shifted along the voltage axis in a positive direction when the basic residues postulated to be near the intracellular surface of the membrane were neutralized. Conversely, when those residues near the external surface of the membrane were neutralized the I–V curve shifted in a negative direction along the voltage axis. Such shifts are predicted by a model in which electrostatic interactions between charged structures modify the local electric field experienced by the voltage sensor.

Similar mutagenesis studies performed on K-channels (Logothetis *et al.*, 1991; Papazian *et al.*, 1991) also indicate that the S4 region contains a major part of the voltage-sensing apparatus. Although the data pertaining to mutations of the S4 region in K-channels suggest an important role for this locus in the voltage-sensing apparatus, they are not consistent with a simple electrostatic hypothesis. Mutations in the basic residues in the S4 region of *Sh* (Papazian *et al.*, 1991) and RCK1 (RC, rat cortex) (Logothetis *et al.*, 1991) resulted in altered voltage sensitivity as expected. However, some amino acid substitutions whereby charge was conserved (lysine to arginine and vice versa) also altered the voltage sensitivity. This unexpected result indicates that chemical interactions between side chains are also important in the potential sensing mechanism. Moreover, a mutation outside the S4 region (a conservative substitution in the S2 region of *Sh*) also affected the voltage sensitivity, indicating that S4 is not the sole voltage sensor for activation (Papazian *et al.*, 1991). The importance of chemical interaction of side chains and/or steric considerations in the voltage-sensing apparatus is also illustrated in Na-channels where a conservative substitution of a non-polar amino acid (leucine to phenylalanine) within S4 resulted in an approximately 25 mV depolarizing shift in the voltage dependence of activation (Auld *et al.*, 1990). Finally, mutations in S4 do not affect voltage sensitivity alone. A conservative substitution of arginine 368 to lysine in *Sh* channels slowed down the rate of recovery from inactivation approximately 2.5-fold (Papazian *et al.*, 1991). In conclusion, the S4 region represents a major part of the voltage sensor for activation of K-channels. Future work will show how this region senses membrane voltage changes, what other regions may be involved, and how the initial structural conformation brought about by the membrane voltage change effects opening of the K-channel.

The N- and C-termini: regulators of inactivation

Like Na-channels, some K-channels inactivate. Inactivation is an event whereby ion conduction ceases shortly after activation, despite a maintained stimulus. Inactivation can be fast (on a millisecond time scale) or slow (requiring seconds); these are probably mediated by distinct molecular processes. Classical work by Armstrong and colleagues showed that inactivation of Na-channels is probably due to a cytoplasmic portion of the channel, since intra-axonal administration of a proteolytic enzyme slowed or abolished inactivation without affecting other parameters (Armstrong *et al.*, 1973). This observation led to the development of the 'ball and chain' model of inactivation: a ball of positively charged amino acids, tethered to the channel but freely moving in the cytoplasm, moves into the inner channel mouth and blocks it, resulting in inactivation of the ionic current. Dialysis of squid axons with a quaternary ammonium derivative containing a long hydrophobic tail converted $I_{K(V)}$ into an I_A-like current (i.e. it introduced inactivation), suggesting that transient K-currents also inactivate by a ball and chain mechanism (Armstrong, 1969). This was substantiated by the observation that treatment of the intracellular side of the *Sh* channel with trypsin removed inactivation (Hoshi *et al.*, 1990). Molecular analysis has localized the linker region between repeats III and IV as being responsible for the rapid inactivation of Na-channels (Vassilev *et al.*, 1988; Stühmer *et al.*, 1989). Since K-channels are homologous to one of the four repeats of Na- and Ca-channels, the N- or C-terminus of a K-channel might correspond to the linker between two repeats in a Na-channel. Moreover, *Sh* channels which arise by alternative splicing display different rates of fast inactivation that could be correlated to the presence or absence of an N-terminal variant (Timpe *et al.*, 1988a). Aldrich and colleagues showed that mutations of a 19 amino acid stretch of the N-terminus of *Sh* profoundly influenced fast inactivation (Hoshi *et al.*, 1990). Additionally, in deletion mutants lacking inactivation, exposure of the intracellular side of the channel to a synthetic peptide of similar sequence to the deleted fragment restores inactivation (Zagotta *et al.*, 1990). Remarkably, exposing the inner mouth of a K_V-channel to this peptide introduces fast inactivation (Zagotta *et al.*, 1990). Therefore, rapid inactivation most likely is mediated by a structure in the (cytoplasmic) N-terminus that translocates and plugs the inner mouth of the channel. In contrast, slow inactivation appears to reside in the C-terminal end of K-channels. Slow inactivation, requiring several seconds, is seen in *Sh* channels after removal of fast inactivation and in some K_V channels. Mutations of one hydrophobic amino acid in the S6 region (Ala 463 in ShB) affected this slow inactivation. Thus, changing this amino acid to valine converted the slow inactivation of ShB to one like ShA, in which this position is normally occupied by a valine (Zagotta *et al.*, 1991). Similarly recovery from inactivation has been localized to the C terminus (Iversen & Rudy, 1990).

One of the remarkable features of K-channels is their ability to conduct large cation fluxes, yet rigorously to distinguish between closely related ion species. K-channels are among the most selective known, being at least 100 times less permeable to Na^+ than to K^+. The nature of the pore of K-channels has received a great deal of attention.

H5: the pore region

In Na-channels a mutation near the H5 region abolished the action of the pore blocking toxin tetrodotoxin (Noda *et al.*, 1989). In *Sh* channels the affinity of charybdotoxin, a pore-blocking K-channel inhibitor (*see*

Chapter 5), is diminished by replacing an acidic glutamate with a neutral glutamine or a basic lysine (MacKinnon & Miller, 1989). Additional evidence that H5 constitutes the entire or a major part of the pore is that charybdotoxin binding, external block by TEA, single channel conductance properties, selectivity among permeant cations, and block by internal TEA have all been localized to the H5 region (Mackinnon & Yellen, 1990; Hartman *et al.*, 1991; Yellen *et al.*, 1991; Yool & Schwarz, 1991). Recent data suggest that H5 spans the membrane twice, since mutations at either end of H5 appear to modify 'external' properties such as toxin and external TEA binding, while mutation near the middle affect 'internal' functions such as a block by internal TEA. Because H5 is not of sufficient length to cross the membrane twice if it is in the form of an α-helix, it has recently been proposed that H5 forms two antiparallel β-sheets that dip into the membrane. The pore therefore is envisaged as being formed by a β-barrel consisting of eight staves, two contributed by each subunit.

Importance of phosphorylation

An important physiological aspect of some ion channels is their ability to be modulated by cellular factors. The best understood mode of modulation is through phosphorylation–dephosphorylation reactions. For example, a hormone acting on its receptor may activate a kinase or a phosphatase and thereby increase or decrease, respectively, the level of cellular protein phosphorylation. Although most ion channels cloned to date contain consensus sequences for phosphorylation by protein kinases, a convincing demonstration of a function for these sequences has so far been lacking. Two recent studies indirectly indicate that cloned potassium channels may indeed be modulated by phosphorylation reactions. In one, a mammalian cell line transfected to express cloned K-channels exhibited rundown upon dialysis with patch-clamp micropipettes. Thus the density of K-currents diminished with time following dialysis, but this rundown was stopped or reversed if cyclic adenosine monophosphate was included in the patch pipette (Ruppersberg *et al.*, 1990b). One possible interpretation of this is that K-channels need to be phosphorylated in order to function. Another study has shown that when oocytes are co-injected with mRNA coding for a K-channel and a serotonin receptor (5HT$_{1c}$), activation of the serotonin receptor results in a long-term inhibition of the K-current, possibly by activating an endogenous phosphatase (Hoger *et al.*, 1991).

Summary

The above discussion is intended to give the reader an indication of recent progress in understanding structure–function relationships for K-channels. It may be concluded that the S4 region is the major voltage sensor for activation, the H5 region probably lines the pore, the N-terminus determines fast inactivation, and that the C end of the molecule influences the onset of slow inactivation and recovery from fast inactivation. Finally, the channel may need to be phosphorylated to function properly. This conclusion, although useful as a framework for further structure–function analysis, is almost certainly too simplistic. Channels, as oligomeric proteins are not 'modular'. Therefore assigning a function to a particular segment of a channel protein ignores the all too-important steric and long distance interactions with other parts of the channel. However, only by following this reductionist approach and making first approximations can we begin to understand how channels work and, subsequently make more sophisticated 'holistic' models to describe their behaviour.

Conclusions

We have reviewed the genetic approach used to clone the first K-channel gene from the *Sh* locus of *Drosophila* and have discussed the genomic strategies used in flies and mice to generate the diversity of K-channels observed in all species. In addition, we have provided original data on the regional distribution of the MK1 message in the mouse brain. All these data are of critical importance to the pharmacologist whose goal is to design drugs with high target specificity: first, channel diversity may provide specificity if drugs can be designed to distinguish between different gene products. Second, information of the distribution of specific isoforms may suggest their functional role and point to possible systems wherein side effects might be monitored.

At the molecular level, we have reviewed recent structure–function studies aimed at determining the physiological function of the various parts of the cloned K-channels. Sites in the predicted K-channel protein encoding voltage sensitivity, kinetic properties and sites of drug interaction have been suggested. While many of the functional properties of K-channels can be assigned to the cloned subunits discussed above, biochemical data recently reviewed elsewhere (Rehm & Tempel, 1991) suggest that other types of protein subunit may be involved in the function of K-channels expressed in brain. The convulsant snake neurotoxin, dendrotoxin, has been used to purify a brain protein (Rehm & Lazdunski, 1988; Parcej & Dolly, 1989) which conducts K^+ when reconstituted in lipid membranes (Rehm *et al.*, 1989b). That the 75 kDa glycoprotein subunit is encoded by a subset of the cloned K-channel genes has been shown immunologically using antibodies raised against synthetic peptides derived from the sequence of MK1 (Rehm *et al.*, 1989a) and biochemically by N-terminal amino acid sequence analysis of the 75 kDa band (Scott *et al.*, 1990; Newitt *et al.*, 1991). The functional role(s) of the other, co-purifying subunits of 35, 38 and 42 kDa is not known but may involve regulation or localization of the K-channel. A more complete understanding of how K-channels work will only be obtained when the identities of all the subunits of the mature channel are known.

The current interest and explosion of data on the molecular basis of K-channel function show no sign of abatement. In the coming years new K-channel types will be cloned and the functional role of the voltage-gated K-channels will be more closely defined.

Acknowledgements

This work was supported by grants from the National Multiple Sclerosis Society (L.A.A.), the Veterans Administration (B.L.T.), and NIH grant no. NS27206 (B.L.T.).

References

Aldrich, R. W. (1990) Mixing and matching. *Nature* **345**, 475–476.
Anderson, M. (1977) Discharge patterns of basal ganglia neurons during active maintenance of postural stability and adjustment to chair tilt. *Brain Research* **143**, 325–338.
Armstrong, C. M. (1969) Inactivation of potassium conductance and related phenomena caused by quaternary ammonium ions injected in squid axons. *Journal of General Physiology* **54**, 553–575.
Armstrong, C. M., Bezanilla, F. & Rojas, E. (1973) Destruction of sodium conductance inactivation in squid axons perfused with pronase. *Journal of General Physiology* **62**, 375–391.
Auld, V. J., Goldin, A. L., Krafte, D. S., Catteral, W. A., Lester, H. A., Davidson, N. & Dunn, R. J. (1990) A neutral amino acid change in segment II S4 dramatically alters the gating properties of the voltage-dependent sodium channel. *Proceedings of the National Academy of Sciences USA* **87**, 323–327.
Baumann, A., Krah-Jentgens, I., Muller, R., Muller-Holtkamp, F., Seidel, R., Kecskemethy, N., Casal, J., Ferrus, A. & Pongs, O. (1987) Molecular organization of the maternal effect region of the *Shaker* complex of *Drosophila*: Characterization of an I_A channel transcript with homology to vertebrate Na^+ channel. *European Molecular Biology Organization Journal* **6**, 3419–3429.
Butler, A., Wei, A., Baker, K. & Salkoff, L. (1989) A family of putative potassium channel genes in *Drosophila*. *Science* **243**, 943–947.
Chandy, G. K., Williams, C. B., Spencer, R. H., Aguilar, B. A., Ghanshani, S. & Tempel, B. L. (1990) A family of three mouse potassium channel genes with intron-less coding regions. *Science* **247**, 973–975.
Christie, M. J., North, R. A., Osborne, P. B., Douglass, J. & Adelman, J. P. (1990) Heteropolymeric potassium channels expressed in *Xenopus* oocytes from cloned subunits. *Neuron* **2**, 405–411.
DeLong, M. R. (1971) Activity of pallidal neurons during movement. *Journal of Neurophysiology* **34**, 414–427.
Fernandez, C. & Goldberg, J. M. (1971) Physiology of peripheral neurons innervating semicircular canals of the squirrel monkey. II. Response to sinusoidal stimulation

and dynamics of peripheral vestibular system. *Journal of Neurophysiology* **34**, 661–675.

Ghanshani, S., Pak, M., Strong, M., Dethlefs, B., Salkoff, L., Gutman, G. A. & Chandy, K. G. (1990) Shaw and *Shaker*-related potassium channel genes in mouse. *International Biophysics Congress*, Vancouver, BC.

Goldberg, J. M. & Fernandez, C. (1971) Physiology of peripheral neurons innervating semicircular canals of the squirrel monkey. I. Resting discharge and response to constant angular accelerations. *Journal of Neurophysiology* **34**, 635–660.

Hartman, H. A., Kirsch, G. E., Drewe, J. A., Taglialatela, M., Joho, R. H. & Brown, A. M. (1991) Exchange of conduction pathways between two related K^+ channels. *Science* **251**, 942–944.

Hille, B. (1984) *Ionic Channels of Excitable Membranes.* Sinauer, Sunderland, MA.

Hoger, J. H., Walter, A. E., Vance, D., Yu, L., Lester, H. A. & Davidson, N. (1991) Modulation of a cloned mouse brain potassium channel. *Neuron* **6**, 227–236.

Hoshi, T., Zagotta, W. N. & Aldrich, R. W. (1990) Biophysical and molecular mechanisms of *Shaker* potassium channel inactivation. *Science* **250**, 533–538.

Isacoff, E. Y., Jan, Y. N. & Jan, L. Y. (1990) Evidence for the formation of heteromultimeric potassium channels in *Xenopus* oocytes. *Nature* **345**, 530–534.

Iverson, L. E. & Rudy, B. (1990) The role of the divergent amino and carboxyl domains on the inactivation properties of potassium channels derived from the *Shaker* gene of *Drosophila*. *Journal of Neuroscience* **10**, 2903–2916.

Iverson, L. E., Tanouye, M. A., Lester, H. A., Davidson, N. & Rudy B. (1988) A-type potassium channels expressed from *Shaker* locus cDNA. *Proceedings of the National Academy of Sciences USA* **85**, 5723–5727.

Jan, L. Y. & Jan, Y. N. (1990) How might the diversity of potassium channels be generated? *Trends in Neurosciences* **13**, 415–419.

Jan, Y. N., Jan, L. Y. & Dennis M. J. (1977) Two mutations of synaptic transmission in *Drosophila*. *Proceedings of the Royal Society of London Series B* **198**, 87.

Kamb, A., Iverson, L. E. & Tanouye, M. A. (1987) Molecular characterization of *Shaker*, a *Drosophila* gene that encodes a potassium channel. *Cell* **50**, 405–413.

Kamb, A., Tseng-Crank, J. & Tanouye, M. A. (1988) Multiple products of the *Drosophila Shaker* gene may contribute to potassium channel diversity. *Neuron* **1**, 421–430.

Kesner, J. S., Kaufman, J. M., Wilson, R. C., Kuroda, G. & Knobil, E. (1986) The effect of morphine on the electrophysiological activity of the hypothalamic luteinizing hormone-releasing hormone pulse generator in the rhesus monkey. *Neuroendocrinology* **43**, 686–688.

Koike, H., Mano, N., Okada, Y. & Oshima, T. (1970) Repetitive impulses generated in fast and slow pyramidal tract cells by intracellularly applied current steps. *Experimental Brain Research* **11**, 263–281.

Logothetis, D. E., Liman, E. R., Weaver, F., Movahedi, S., Sattler, C., Koren, G., Nadal-Ginard, B. & Hess, P. (1991) Analysis of charge mutations in the S4 region of the delayed rectifier K channel RCK1. *Biophysical Journal* **59**, 196a.

McCormack, T., Vega-Saenz De Miera, E. C. & Rudy, B. (1990) Molecular cloning of a member of a third class of *Shaker*-family K^+ channel genes in mammals. *Proceedings of the National Academy of Sciences USA* **87**, 5227–5231.

MacKinnon, R. & Miller, C. (1989) Mutant potassium channels with altered binding of charybdotoxin, a pore-blocking peptide inhibitor. *Science* **245**, 1382–1385.

MacKinnon, R. & Yellen, G. (1990) Mutations affecting TEA blockade and ion permeation in voltage-activated K^+ channels. *Science* **250**, 276–279.

Migeon, M. B., Street, V. A., Demas, V. P. & Tempel, B. L. (1992) Cloning and characterization of MK6, a murine potassium channel gene. *Epilepsy Research* (in press).

Mount, S. M. (1982) A catalogue of splice junction sequences. *Nucleic Acids Research* **2**, 459–470.

Newitt, R. A., Houamed, K. M., Rehm, H. & Tempel, B. L. (1991) Potassium channels and epilepsy: Evidence that the epileptogenic toxin, dendrotoxin, binds to potassium channel proteins. *Epilepsy Research* **4**, 263–273.

Noda, M., Suzuki, H., Numa, S. & Stuhmer, W. (1989) A single point mutation confers tetrodotoxin and saxitoxin insensitivity on the sodium channel II. *FEBS Letters* **259**, 213–216.

Pak, M. D., Baker, K., Covarrubias, M., Butler, A., Ratcliffe, A. & Salkoff, L. (1991a) *mShal*, a subfamily of A-type K^+ channel cloned from mammalian brain. *Proceedings of the National Academy of Science USA* **88**, 4386–4390.

Pak, M. D., Covarrubias, M., Ratcliffe, A. & Salkoff, L. (1991b) A mouse brain homolog of the *Drosophila Shab* K^+ channel with conserved delayed-rectifier properties. *Journal of Neuroscience* **11**, 869–880.

Papazian D. M., Schwarz, T. L., Tempel, B. L., Jan, Y. N. & Jan, L. Y. (1987) Cloning of genomic and complementary DNA from *Shaker*, a putative potassium channel gene from *Drosophila*. *Science* **237**, 749–753.

Papazian, D. M., Timpe, L. C., Jan, Y. N. & Jan, L. Y. (1991) Alteration of voltage-dependence of *Shaker* potassium channel of mutations in the S4 sequence. *Nature* **349**, 305–310.

Parcej, D. N. & Dolly, J. O. (1989) Dendrotoxin acceptor from bovine synaptic plasma membranes. *Biochemical Journal* **257**, 899–903.

Patton, H. D., Fuchs, A. F., Hille, B., Scher, A. M. & Steiner, R. A. (eds) (1989) *Textbook of Physiology*, 21st edn. WB Saunders, Philadelphia.

Pongs, O., Kecskemethy, N., Muller, R., Krah-Jentgens, I., Baumann, A., Kiltz, H. H., Canal, I., Llamazares, S. & Ferrus, A. (1988) *Shaker* encodes a family of putative potassium channel proteins in the nervous system of *Drosophila*. *European Molecular Biology Organization Journal* **6**, 1087–1096.

Rehm, H. & Lazdunski, M. (1988) Purification and subunit structure of a putative K^+ channel protein identified by its binding properties of dendrotoxin I. *Proceedings of the National Academy of Sciences USA* **85**, 4919–4923.

Rehm, H. & Tempel, B. L. (1991) Voltage-gated K^+ channels of the mammalian brain. *Federation of American Societies for Experimental Biology* **5**, 164–170.

Rehm, H., Newitt, R. A. & Tempel, B. L. (1989a) Immunological evidence for a relationship between the dendrotoxin-binding protein and the mammalian homologue of the *Drosophila Shaker* K^+ channel. *FEBS Letters* **249**, 224–228.

Rehm, H., Pelzer, S., Cochet, C., Tempel, B. L., Chambaz, E., Trautwein, W., Pelzer, D. & Lazdunski, M. (1989b) Dendrotoxin-binding brain membrane protein displays a K^+ channel activity that is stimulated by both cAMP-dependent and endogenous phosphorylations. *Biochemistry* **28**, 6455–6460.

Rudy, B. (1988) Diversity and ubiquity of K channels. *Neuroscience* **25**, 729–749.

Ruppersberg, J. P., Schroter, K. H., Sakmann, B., Stocker, M., Sewing, S. & Pongs, O. (1990a) Heteromultimeric channels formed by rat brain potassium-channel proteins. *Nature* **345**, 535–537.

Ruppersberg, J. P., Schroter, K. H., Sakmann, B., Stocker, M., Sewing, S. & Pongs, O. (1990b) Regulation and interaction of rat brain potassium channel proteins. *Plfügers Archiv* **415** (Suppl. 1), R16.

Salkoff, L. (1983) Genetic and voltage-clamp analysis of a *Drosophila* potassium channel *Cold Spring Harbor Symposium on Molecular Biology* **48**, 221–231.

Schwarz, T. L., Tempel, B. L., Papazian, D. M., Jan, Y. N. & Jan, L. Y. (1988) Multiple potassium channel components are produced by alternative splicing at the *Shaker* locus in *Drosophila*. *Nature* **331**, 137–142.

Scott, V. E. S., Parcej, D. N., Keen, J. N., Findlay, J. B. C. & Dolly, J. O. (1990) Alpha-dendrotoxin acceptor from bovine brain is a K$^+$ channel protein. *Journal of Biological Chemistry* **265**, 20094–20097.

Stühmer, W., Conti, F., Suzuki, H., Wang, X., Noda, M., Yahagi, N., Kubo, H. & Numa, S. (1989) Structural parts involved in activation and inactivation of the sodium channel. *Nature* **339**, 597–603.

Takata, M., Fujita, S. & Kanamori, N. (1982) Repetitive firing in trigeminal mesencephalic tract neurons and trigeminal motoneurons. *Journal of Neurophysiology* **47**, 23–30.

Tanouye, M. A., Ferrus, A. & Fujita, S. (1981) Abnormal action potentials associated with the *Shaker* complex locus of *Drosophila*. *Proceedings of the National Academy of Sciences USA* **78**, 6548–6552.

Tempel, B. L., Jan, Y. N. & Jan, L. Y. (1988) Cloning of a probable potassium channel gene from mouse brain. *Nature* **332**, 837–839.

Tempel, B. L., Papazian, D. M., Schwarz, T. L., Jan, Y. N. & Jan, L. Y. (1987) Sequence of a probable potassium channel component encoded at *Shaker* locus of *Drosophila*. *Science* **237**, 770–775.

Thach, W. T. (1968) Discharge of Purkinje and cerebellar nuclear neurons during rapidly alternating arm movements in the monkey. *Journal of Neurophysiology* **31**, 785–797.

Timpe, L. C., Jan, Y. N. & Jan, L. Y. (1988a) Four cDNA clones from the *Shaker* locus of *Drosophila* induce kinetically distinct A-type potassium currents in *Xenopus* oocytes. *Neuron* **1**, 659–667.

Timpe, L. C., Schwarz, T. L., Tempel, B. L., Papazian, D. M., Jan, Y. N. & Jan, L. Y. (1988b) Expression of functional potassium channels from *Shaker* cDNA in *Xenopus* oocytes. *Nature* **331**, 143–145.

Vassilev, P. M., Scheuer, T. & Caterall, W. A. (1988) Identification of an intracellular peptide segment involved in sodium channel inactivation. *Science* **241**, 1658–1661.

Yellen, G., Jurman, M. E., Abramson, T. & MacKinnon, R. (1991) Mutation affecting internal TEA blockade identify a probable pore-forming region of a K$^+$ channel. *Science* **251**, 942–944.

Yokoyama, S., Imoto, K., Kawamura, T., Higashida, H., Iwabe, N., Miyata, T. & Numa, S. (1989) Potassium channels from NG 108-15 neuroblastoma–glioma hybrid cells. *FEBS Letters* **259**, 37–42.

Yool, A. J. & Schwartz, T. L. (1991) Alteration of ionic selectivity of a K$^+$ channel by mutation of the H5 region. *Nature* **349**, 700–704.

Zagotta, W. N., Hoshi, T. & Aldrich, R.W. (1990) Restoration of inactivation in mutants of *Shaker* potassium channels by a peptide derived from ShB. *Science* **250**, 568–571.

Zagotta, W. N., Hoshi, T. & Aldrich, R. W. (1991) Molecular separation of two inactivation processes in *Shaker* potassium channels. *Biophysical Journal* **59**, 2a.

Chapter 3
Cloning and pharmacology of voltage-gated potassium channels

O. Pongs

Introduction

Potassium channels play an important role in the transmission of electrical signals along the membrane of excitable cells (Hille, 1984; Adams & Galvan, 1986; Rudy, 1988). Probably they comprise the most diverse family of ion channels. Various cDNAs and genomic DNAs have been cloned which express expression system voltage-gated K-channels in the *Xenopus* oocyte (Iverson *et al.*, 1988; Stühmer *et al.*, 1988; Timpe *et al.*, 1988; Christie *et al.*, 1989; McKinnon, 1989, Frech *et al.*, 1989; Christie *et al.*, 1990; Stocker *et al.*, 1990; Swanson *et al.*, 1990; Wei *et al.*, 1990). The study of these K-channels has made it possible to correlate certain functional and structural aspects of voltage-gated K-channels. The response of K-channels to toxins and blockers varies widely. Some K-channels are insensitive to blockers like tetraethylammonium chloride (TEA), other K-channels are somewhat sensitive and still others are highly sensitive to blockade by this agent. The differing sensitivities have unleashed a search for amino acids in K-channel sequences which might confer insensitivity or sensitivity towards a certain K-channel blocker (MacKinnon & Miller, 1989; MacKinnon & Yellen, 1990). In the case of TEA, this search has been successful (MacKinnon & Miller, 1989; MacKinnon & Yellen, 1990). The information about the structure of binding sites of K-channel blockers can now be used to define the mouth of the K-channel pore and possibly the structure of the pore itself.

Several types of voltage-gated K-channel are essentially closed in hyperpolarized membranes*. The channels are activated upon depolarization and are converted into an open state (Hille, 1984). Open channels can relax back into closed channels or they become inactivated. The life-time of the open channel, the time-courses of activation and of inactivation are quite variable being an individual property of each particular K-channel. Obviously, changes in the rate of inactivation lead to the expression of a rapidly inactivating, a slowly inactivating or a virtually non-inactivating K-channel (Stocker et al., 1990). The availability of cloned K-channels and the possibilities of recombinant DNA techniques have allowed a detailed analysis of these K-channel properties. Furthermore, it has been possible to assign to particular K-channel domains particular functions concerning the opening and closing of K-channels.

Voltage-gated K-channel clones

General structure of K-channels

The derived protein sequences of K-channel clones exhibit a remarkable degree of similarity in primary structure which has been conserved during evolution (Yokoyama et al., 1989). The sequence similarities suggest that K-channels are members of a gene family.

The hydropathy profiles of the derived sequences always show six segments which have the potential to span the membrane. The segments are bordered by hydrophilic amino- and carboxy-terminal sequences varying greatly in length. The putative membrane spanning segments consist of five hydrophobic segments (S1, S2, S3, S5 and S6) and one positively charged segment (S4) (Pongs et al., 1988). A simple folding model of the K-channel protein predicts a membrane-inserted core domain (C) comprising segments S1 to S6, and amino- (N) and carboxy-terminal (T) domains facing the cytoplasmic side of the membrane (Fig. 3.1A). A more elaborate folding model has been proposed based on theoretical model building studies (Guy & Conti, 1990). The major difference between the simple and the complex model is that the sequence connecting segments S5 and S6 is inserted back into the membrane as illustrated schematically in Fig. 3.1B. Both folding models predict that only C domain sequences face the extracellular side of the membrane. This general picture of K-channel proteins makes several predictions concerning activation and inactivation gates as well as binding sites for K-channel blockers and toxins. The sensitivity or insensitivity of K-channels towards blockers binding from the outside of the channel should be determined by extracellularly-located sequences. In this case, the sequences would reside

---

*This statement does not apply to those K-channels which are voltage-independent or to those which are classed as inward rectifiers.

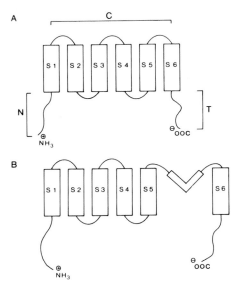

Fig. 3.1. Folding models proposed for membrane-inserted K-channel subunits. A, Based on hydropathy analyses (Pongs *et al.*, 1988) K-channel subunit proteins have possibly six membrane-spanning segments S1–S6 indicated as boxes. These segments are referred to as the C-domain. The N- and T-domains are located at the cytoplasmic side of the membrane. B, Based on theoretical calculations (Guy and Conti, 1990), the segments S5–S6 connecting sequence has been proposed to be inserted into the membrane such that the sequence has a bend in the middle allowing it to move in and out of the membrane as shown.

in the core domain, specifically in the loop regions connecting segments S1 and S2, S3 and S4, and S5 and S6.

Moreover, the physical gates of the K-channel are thought to be located intracellularly. Consequently, they should reside in intracellularly-located domains of the K-channel protein. Indeed, the available data suggest that the N-domain is a major determinant of the rate of inactivation and therefore should harbour the inactivation gate (Hoshi *et al.*, 1990).

Potassium channels are multimers

The general structure of voltage-gated K-channels is reminiscent of a single repeat unit of the voltage-gated Na- and Ca-channels (Pongs *et al.*, 1988; Jan & Jan, 1988, 1990). The latter channels have four internal repeats with similar topology, which are assumed to surround and to line the pore (Noda *et al.*, 1986). Potassium-channel proteins contain only one such repeat. Given the structural homologies between ion channels it is conceivable that K-channels have a quaternary structure consisting of four subunits (Isacoff *et al.*, 1990). Although the exact stoichiometry of

K-channel multimers is still a matter of conjecture, two separate lines of experiments strongly suggest that K-channels are in fact multimeric proteins. Gene dosage experiments have shown that the viable *Shaker* mutations belong to the antimorph type (Ferrus *et al.*, 1990). Genotypes in which several doses of the normal gene are combined with a single dose of the mutated *Shaker* K-channel gene, show the mutant phenotype. A simple interpretation of this type of mutation is that the abnormal gene product, interferes with the formation of functional multimeres. This hypothesis was tested by constructing transgenic flies expressing abnormal *Shaker* K-channel subunits in conjunction with wild type subunits (Gisselmann *et al.*, 1989). The altered subunits indeed interfere with normal *Shaker* K-channel function. Also, coexpression of mutant and wild type K-channel subunits in the *Xenopus* oocyte expression system leads to the formation of malfunctioning K-channels (Lichtinghagen *et al.*, 1991).

Furthermore, K-channel subunits are able to assemble into heteromultimers (Christie *et al.*, 1990; Isacoff *et al.*, 1990; Ruppersberg *et al.*, 1990). For example, RCK1,4 heteromultimeric K-channels are expressed after cotransfection of HeLa cells with the corresponding RCK1 and RCK4 cDNAs and after coinjection of the corresponding RCK1 and RCK4 cRNAs into *Xenopus* oocytes (Ruppersberg *et al.*, 1990). The heteromultimeric RCK1,4 channel mediates a transient K outward current, similar to the RCK4 channel but which inactivates more slowly, has a larger conductance and is more sensitive to block by dendrotoxin and TEA. The results which have been obtained with heteromultimers show that the homomultimeric and corresponding heteromultimeric K-channels have different kinetic and pharmacological properties. Thus it is conceivable that the coexpression of K-channel genes in a given cell and the possible assembly of heteromultimeres could be a further mechanism generating functional diversity of voltage-gated K-channels (Jan & Jan, 1990).

Domain-swapping between K-channels

The structure of voltage-gated K-channel subunits can be arbitrarily subdivided into N-, C- and T-domains. The corresponding domains of different K-channels apparently function interchangeably as independent functional units. This property allows domain-swapping between different K-channel subunits. Furthermore, the role of each K-channel domain in the assembled can be addressed. The N-, C- and T-domains of the *Drosophila Shaker* A2 protein were interchanged with the ones of the rat RCK1 protein (Stocker *et al.*, 1991). Both proteins form K-channels with markedly different kinetic and pharmacological properties; e.g. the *Shaker* channel activates rapidly, the RCK1 channel does not inactivate, the *Shaker* channel is dendrotoxin (DTX) resistant (Stocker *et al.*, 1990), the RCK1 channel is DTX sensitive (Stühmer *et al.*, 1989a). After introducing

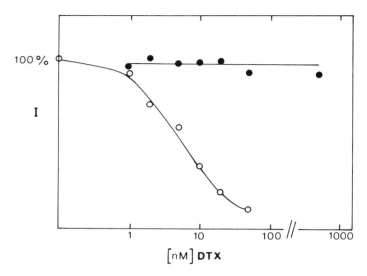

Fig. 3.2. Assignment of toxin-binding properties to the C-domain of K-channels. Chimeric *Shaker*/RCK1 K-channels were constructed which contain either the *Shaker* C-domain between RCK1 N- and T-domains (●) or the RCK1 C-domain between *Shaker* N- and T-domains (○). Chimeric K-channels were expressed in the *Xenopus* oocyte expression system. Dendrotoxin (DTX) was added to the bathing solutions at the concentrations indicated. The influence of DTX on peak outward currents I is shown. Outward currents in the absence of added DTX were normalized to 100%.

unique restriction enzyme cleavage sites at equivalent positions of both K-channel cDNAs, chimeric K-channels were constructed. The expressed chimeric K-channels were named SRR, SRS, RRS, RSR, SSR and RSS to indicate the domain composition of the chimeric K-channel forming protein, e.g. SRR is a combination of the N-domain of the *Shaker* A2 protein with the C and T domains of the RCK1 protein. All chimeric K-channel proteins mediated outward currents in the oocyte expression system (Stocker *et al.,* 1991). This indicated that the three domains can be swapped without loss of function. Thus, it was possible to correlate a particular function with the N-, C- or T-domain. Two major results have emerged from these studies. Firstly the rapid inactivation of K-channels is dictated by the nature of the N-domain. SRR channels inactivate rapidly like *Shaker* channels. Conversely, RSS channels do not inactivate rapidly. Secondly, the C-domain is responsible for the pharmacology of the K-channel. It defines the binding sites for TEA, 4-aminopyridine (4-AP), DTX, mast cell degranulating peptide (MCDP) and charybdotoxin (ChTX), e.g. RSR channels are resistant and SRS channels are sensitive to DTX (Fig. 3.2). The structures in the C-domain as well as in the N-domain which are responsible for the above properties have been delimited in subsequent studies to relatively small sequences and in some instances down to the level of single amino acids (MacKinnon & Yellen, 1990).

Definition of the inactivation gate of K-channels

The *Shaker* locus in *Drosophila* encodes a K-channel gene which gives rise to the expression of several different K-channel proteins (Kamb *et al.*, 1988; Pongs *et al.*, 1988; Schwarz *et al.*, 1988). Most markedly, the proteins differ in the sequences of their N-termini. For example, the 61 N-terminal amino acids of *Shaker* A2 protein are replaced by 16 different amino acids in *Shaker* D2 protein. The differing N-termini have profound effects on the electrophysiological properties of *Shaker* K-channels (Stocker *et al.*, 1990). *Shaker* A2 currents inactivate rapidly. In contrast, *Shaker* D2 currents do not inactivate rapidly at most test potentials studied. The differences in the gating behaviour of *Shaker* A2 and D2 K-channels might indicate a different interaction of the *Shaker* A- or D-N-terminus with the inactivation gate of the channel. This proposition has been tested in a series of elegant experiments which combined site-directed mutagenesis and single-channel patch-clamp recordings (Hoshi, *et al.*, 1990). These experiments have shown that a small region within the A-N-terminus has an important role in inactivation. A model was suggested where the A-N-terminus forms a ball that can swing into the open channel to cause inactivation. This model is known as the 'ball and chain' model for inactivation of ionic channels (Armstrong & Bezanilla, 1977). The K-channel inactivation ball has been proposed to consist of a hydrophobic core next to a positively charged region (Hoshi *et al.*, 1990). Both properties of the ball are apparently important for a hydrophobic and electrostatic interaction with the channel (Fig. 3.3).

Apparently, the N-terminal domain contributes to the threshold of activation of K-channels (Stocker *et al.*, 1991) although the critical region in the primary structure of the N-domain which might be involved has not yet been identified. Sequences of the C-domain also have a profound effect on the threshold of activation. Most notably, sequence alterations within a leucine zipper motif which connects segments S4 and S5 can shift the threshold of activation towards more depolarized membrane potentials (Lichtinghagen *et al.*, 1991).

Defining toxin-binding sites

The C-domain determines the pharmacological profile of a given chimeric K-channel. Given the general structural similarities among K-channels, possibly all K-channel blockers and toxins which bind from the outside interact with structures defined by C-domain sequences. The domain swapping experiments have been refined by interchanging between *Shaker*

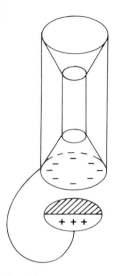

Fig. 3.3. Hypothetical model of the K-channel inactivation gate. The channel is depicted as a cylinder spanning the membrane (not shown). The extracellular side is on top, the intracellular one at the bottom. Negative charges at the inner mouth of the channel pore are indicated by $-$. The N-terminal inactivation gate is indicated as an ellipsoid. The shaded area symbolizes the hydrophobic side of the inactivation gate which supposedly plugs the core. Positive charges ($+$) are presumably facing towards the intracellular surface of the K-channel.

A2 and RCK1 proteins the putative extracellular loop sequences. The results showed that TEA, DTX and ChTX-binding sites are confined to the S5–S6 loop sequence (Stocker *et al.,* 1991).

The MCDP- and 4-AP-binding sites, on the other hand, could not be defined by these experiments. Site-directed mutagenesis studies also suggest that ChTX binding is targeted to the S5–S6 loop of K-channels (MacKinnon & Miller, 1989). More importantly, specific amino acid residues have been identified that affect the channel blockade by TEA (MacKinnon & Yellen, 1990). These studies proposed that variations of one of these identified amino acid residues among naturally occurring channels accounts for most of their differences in sensitivity to TEA (Table 3.1). This proposition has now been tested directly (Table 3.1). The results of these experiments indicate that TEA-resistant K-channels can indeed be converted into TEA-sensitive K-channels by single amino acid replacements at this particular site.

In this context, it is particularly interesting that some mutations change the single-channel conductance of the mutated versus the wild type channel (MacKinnon & Yellen, 1990). The results, however, argue against a simple electrostatic mechanism for the effect of the mutations on single-channel conductance. It cannot be rigorously excluded that these

Table 3.1. Tetraethylammonium sensitivities of K-channels.

K-channel	S5–S6 loop sequence	TEA (mM)
RCK1	M T T V G Y G D M Y P	0.6
RCK3	– – – – – – – – – H –	50
RCK4	– – – – – – – – – K –	>100
RCK4*	– – – – – – – – – Y –	0.6
Shaker wild type	– – – – – – – – – T –	27
Shaker*	– – – – – – – – – Y –	0.6
Shaker*	– – – – – – – – – K –	>200

Shown is a correlation between the presence and absence of a particular amino acid at position 449 (in one letter code) and the TEA-sensitivity of a given K-channel. *Shaker* data are from MacKinnon & Yellen (1990). M, methionine; T, threonine; V, valine; G, glycine; Y, tyrosine; D, aspartate; P, proline; H, histidine; K, lysine.
*Introduction of the indicated amino acid into the wild type sequence by site-directed mutagenesis.

mutations change the structure of the conduction pathway indirectly. However, combining all presently available data indicates that the toxin binding sites are located within the S5–S6 loop region. Thus, it is conceivable that the conduction pathway and the binding sites for K-channel blockers is determined by neighbouring amino acid side chains.

The voltage sensor

The positively charged segment S4 in the C-domain has been proposed as voltage sensor of voltage-gated ionic channels (Stühmer *et al.*, 1989b). Segment S4 contains a positively charged residue, arginine (Arg) or lysine (Lys), at every third position and usually hydrophobic residues (X) at the remaining positions. This Arg/Lys-X-X motif is repeated four to five times in S4 segments of voltage-gated ion channels. It has been suggested that segment S4 provides the charged gating particles that can move within the membrane and sense the membrane electric field. Movement of the gating particles produces a gating current which is a prerequisite for the transition of voltage-gated ionic channels from a closed to an open state (Hille, 1984). A combination of site-directed mutagenesis experiments and patch-clamp recordings has indicated that the positive charges in segment S4 are indeed involved in the voltage-sensing mechanism for activation of the voltage-gated sodium channel.

Acknowledgements

The work which is reported in this overview from my laboratory was carried out in close collaboration with W. Stühmer at the Max-Planck Institute of Biophysical Chemistry (Göttingen), with B. Sakmann and

J. P. Ruppersberg at the Max-Planck Institute of Experimental Medicine (Heidelberg) and with A. Ferrus at the Instituto Cajal (Madrid). Our work has been supported by grants from the Deutsche Forschungsgemeinschaft and from the EEC.

References

Adams, P. R. & Galvan, M. (1986) Voltage-dependent currents of vertebrate neurons and their role in membrane excitability. In Delgado-Escueta, A., Ward, A. A., Woodbury, D. M. and Porter, R., (eds) *Basic Mechanisms of the Epilepsies*. Raven Press New York.

Armstrong, C. M. & Benzanilla, F. (1977) Inactivation of the sodium channel. II. Gating current experiments. *Journal of General Physiology* **70**, 567–590.

Christie, M. J., Adelman, J. P., Douglass, J. & North, R. A. (1989) Expression of a cloned rat brain potassium channel in *Zenopus* oocytes. *Science* **244**, 221–224.

Christie, M. J., North, R. A., Osborne, P. B., Douglass, J. & Adelman, J. P. (1990) Heteropolymeric potassium channels expressed in *Xenopus* oocytes from cloned subunits. *Neuron* **4**, 405–411.

Ferrus, A., Llamazares, S., de la Pompa, J. L., Tanouye, M. A. & Pongs, O. (1990) Genetic analysis of *Shaker* gene complex of *Drosophila melanogaster*. *Genetics* **125**, 383–398.

Frech, G. C., VanDongen, A. M. J., Schuster, G., Brown, A. M. & Joho, R. H. (1989) A novel potassium channel with delayed rectifier properties isolated from rat brain by expression cloning. *Nature* **340**, 642–645.

Gisselmann, G., Sewing, S., Madsen, B. W., Mallart, A., Angaut-Petit, D., Müller-Holtkamp, F., Ferrus, A. & Pongs, O. (1989) The interference of truncated with normal potassium channel subunits leads to abnormal behaviour in transgenic *Drosophila melanogaster*. *EMBO Journal* **8**, 2359–2364.

Guy, H. R. & Conti, F. (1990) Pursuing the structure and function of voltage-gated channels. *Trends in Neurosciences* **13**, 201–206.

Hille, B. (1984) *Ionic Channels of Excitable Membranes*. Sinauer Associates, Sunderland, MA.

Hoshi, T., Zagotta, W. N. & Aldrich, R. W. (1990) Biophysical and molecular mechanisms of *Shaker* potassium channel inactivation. *Science* **250**, 533–538.

Isacoff, E. Y., Jan, Y. N. & Jan, L. Y. (1990) Evidence for the formation of heteromultimeric potassium channels in *Xenopus* oocytes. *Nature* **345**, 530–534.

Iverson, L. E., Tanouye, M., Lester, H. A., Davidson, N. & Rudy, B. (1988) Expression of A-type K channels from *Shaker* cDNAs. *Proceedings of the National Academy of Sciences USA* **85**, 5723–5727.

Jan, L. Y. & Jan, Y. N. (1988) Voltage-sensitive ion channels. *Cell* **56**, 13–25.

Jan, L. Y. & Jan, Y. N. (1990) How might the diversity of potassium channels be generated? *Trends in Neurosciences* **13**, 415–419.

Kamb, A., Tseng-Crank, J. & Tanouye, M. A. (1988) Multiple products of the *Drosophila Shaker* gene may contribute to potassium channel diversity. *Neuron* **1**, 421–430.

Lichtinghagen, R., Stocker, M., Wittka, R., Boheim, G., Stühmer, W. Ferrus, A. & Pongs, O. (1991) Molecular basis of altered excitability in *Shaker* mutants of *Drosophila melanogaster*. *EMBO Journal* **9**, 4399–4407.

MacKinnon, R. & Miller, Ch. (1989) Mutant potassium channels with altered binding of charybdotoxin, a pore-blocking peptide inhibitor. *Science* **245**, 1382–1385.

MacKinnon, R. & Yellen, G. (1990) Mutations affecting TEA blockade and ion permeation in voltage-activated K$^+$ channels. *Science* **250**, 276–279.

McKinnon, D. (1989) Isolation of a cDNA clone coding for a putative second potassium channel indicates the existence of a gene family. *Journal of Biological Chemistry* **264**, 8230–8236.

Noda, M., Ikeda, T., Suzuki, S., Takeshima, H., Takahaski, T., Kuno, M. & Numa S. (1986) Expression of functional sodium channels from cloned cDNA. *Nature* **322**, 826–828.

Pongs, O., Kecskemethy, N., Müller, R., Krah-Jentgens, I., Baumann, A., Kiltz, H. H., Canal, I., Llamazares, S. & Ferrus, A. (1988) Shaker encodes a family of putative potassium-channel proteins in the nervous system of *Drosophila. EMBO Journal* **7**, 1087–1096.

Rudy, B. (1988) Diversity and ubiquity of K channels. *Neuroscience* **25**, 729–750.

Ruppersberg, J. P., Schröter, K. H., Sakmann, B., Stocker, M., Sewing, S. & Pongs, O. (1990) Heteromultimeric channels formed by rat brain potassium-channel proteins. *Nature* **345**, 535–537.

Schwarz, T. L., Tempel, B. L., Papazian, D. M., Jan, Y. N. & Jan, L. Y. (1988) Multiple potassium-channel components are produced by alternative splicing at the *Shaker* locus in *Drosophila. Nature* **331**, 137–142.

Stocker, M., Pongs, O., Hoth, M., Heinemann, S., Stühmer, W., Schröter, K. H. & Ruppersberg, J. P. (1991) Swapping of functional domains in voltage-gated K$^+$ channels. *Proceedings of the Royal Society London, Series* B **245**, 101–107.

Stocker, M., Stühmer, W., Wittka, R., Wang, Y., Müller, R., Ferrus, A. & Pongs, O. (1990) Alternative *Shaker* transcripts express either rapidly inactivating or non-inactivating K$^+$ channels. *Proceedings of the National Academy of Sciences USA* **87**, 8903–8907.

Stühmer, W., Conti, F., Suzuki, H., Wang, X., Noda, N., Yahagi, N., Kubo, H. & Numa, S. (1989b) Structural parts involved in activation and inactivation of the sodium channel. *Nature* **339**, 597–603.

Stühmer, W., Ruppersberg, J. P., Schröter, K. H., Sakmann, B., Stocker, M., Giese, K. P., Perschke, A., Baumann, A. & Pongs, O. (1989a) Molecular basis of functional diversity of voltage-gated potassium channels in mammalian brain. *EMBO Journal* **8**, 3235–3244.

Stühmer, W., Stocker, M., Sakmann, B., Seeburg, P., Baumann, A., Grupe, A. & Pongs, O. (1988) Potassium channels expressed from rat brain cDNA have delayed rectifier properties. *FEBS Letters* **242**, 199–206.

Swanson, R., Marshall, J., Smith, J. S., Williams, B., Boyle, M. B., Folander, K., Luneau, Ch. J., Antanavage, J., Oliva, C., Buhrow, S. A., Bennett, C., Stein, R. B. & Kaczmarek, L. K. (1990) Cloning and expression of cDNA and genomic clones encoding three delayed rectifier potassium channels in rat brain. *Neuron* **4**, 929–939.

Timpe, L. C., Schwarz, T. L., Tempel, B. L., Papazian, D. M., Jan, Y. N. & Jan, L. Y. (1988) Expression of functional potassium channels from *Shaker* cDNA in *Xenopus* oocytes. *Nature* **331**, 143–145.

Wei, A., Covarrubias, M., Butler, A., Baker, K., Pak, M. & Salkoff, L. (1990) K$^+$ current diversity is produced by an extended gene family conserved in *Drosophila* and mouse. *Science* **248**, 599–603.

Yokoyama, S., Imoto, K., Kawamura, T., Higashida, H., Iwabe, N., Miyata, T. & Numa, S. (1989) Potassium channels from NG108-15 neuroblastoma–glioma hybrid cells. Primary structure and function expression from cDNAs. *FEBS Letters* **259**, 37–42.

Chapter 4
G proteins and the modulation of potassium channels

L. Birnbaumer

Introduction

The description of a receptor-sensitive signal-transducing adenylate cyclase system by Sutherland and coworkers in 1957 was expanded in the 1970s by the discovery that the system is regulated not only by hormones but also by guanosine triphosphate (GTP) (Rodbell *et al.*, 1971). Involvement of a GTP regulatory step in light perception was discovered in 1975 (Wheeler & Bitensky, 1977). The S49 cell mutant with a reduced capacity to synthesize cyclic adenosine monophosphate (cAMP) was described to the public in 1975 (Bourne *et al.*, 1975). This mutant, designated cyc^- was found to be affected in those aspects of cAMP formation which are dependent on GTP. By 1980, the GTP-binding component involved in light perception, originally called light-activated GTPase and now designated as transducin, and the GTP-binding regulatory component of adenylate cyclase, originally termed G/F or N and now designated as G_s, had both been purified (Kuehn, 1980; Northup *et al.*, 1980).

When compared, transducin and G_s were found to be quite similar. Both were activated by GTP under the influence of hormone and neurotransmitter receptors in the case of G_s and of light in the case of transducin. Furthermore, both were $\alpha\beta\gamma$ heterotrimers formed from homologous but distinct α subunits and apparently interchangeable β subunits (Manning & Gilman, 1983) associated with small γ subunits (Fung, 1983; Hildebrandt *et al.*, 1984). The α subunits of both types of G protein bound and hydrolysed GTP. The purified trimeric holoproteins dissociated on interaction with non-hydrolysable GTP analogues to give two products: a complex of the α subunit with the guanine nucleotide and a $\beta\gamma$ dimer. Of these two products it was established that the α subunits regulated the effector functions: adenylate cyclase for the α subunit of G_s (Northup et al., 1983) and the cAMP-specific phosphodiesterase for the α subunit of transducin (Fung et al., 1981). While it is now clear that $\beta\gamma$ dimers play a key regulatory role in what appears to be a receptor- and GTPase-dependent shuttling of the α subunit between effector and receptor, there is still considerable discussion as to whether $\beta\gamma$ dimers have an additional role as effector regulators analogous to that of α subunits.

Parallel to the in-depth studies on the biochemical and molecular basis of phototransduction and activation of adenylate cyclase, other studies led to the discovery that hormonal stimulation as well as hormonal inhibition of adenylate cyclase proceeded through intervening GTP-dependent steps (Hildebrandt et al., 1983). Furthermore, actions of hormones and neurotransmitters which modulated cell metabolism through means other than regulation of cAMP formation were also dependent on GTP binding. It is now recognized that a variety of processes occur with the obligatory participation of G proteins. These include the hormonal regulation of phosphoinositide hydrolysis by a C-type phospholipase which releases inositol triphosphate (IP_3) plus diacylglycerol (DAG) (Cockroft & Gomperts, 1985; Litosch et al., 1985), the activation of a phospholipase A_2 with consequential release of arachidonic acid (AA) (Murayama & Ui, 1985; Burch et al., 1986), the modulation of several types of K-channel (Yatani et al., 1987a; VanDongen et al., 1988), and at least two dihydropyridine-sensitive, voltage-gated Ca-channels (Yatani et al., 1987b, 1988). G proteins which regulate phospholipases are termed G_p (Cockroft & Gomperts, 1985) and those controlling K-channels are termed G_K (Breitwieser & Szabo, 1985). Smell receptors in cilia of the olfactory neuroepithelium activate adenylate cyclase through a unique 'olfactory' G protein, G_{olf}, the α subunit of which is highly homologous to that of G_s (Jones & Reed, 1989; see section on G proteins below).

Molecular diversity in signal transduction by G proteins

Receptors

About 80% of all known hormones and neurotransmitters, as well as many neuromodulators and other factors elicit cellular responses by combining with specific receptors coupled to effector functions by G proteins (Birnbaumer, 1990a,b; Fig. 4.1). Even though the primary messengers are many, the number of distinct receptors which mediate their actions is even larger, so that one can presently count about 100 distinct receptor types either as distinct gene products or as discrete pharmacological entities.

Receptors which are coupled to effector systems through G proteins all

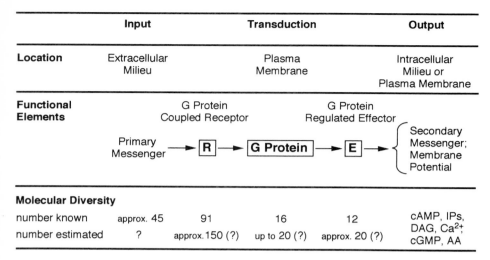

	Input	Transduction	Output
Location	Extracellular Milieu	Plasma Membrane	Intracellular Milieu or Plasma Membrane

Functional Elements

G Protein Coupled Receptor   G Protein Regulated Effector

Primary Messenger → R → G Protein → E → { Secondary Messenger; Membrane Potential

Molecular Diversity

number known	approx. 45	91	16	12	cAMP, IPs, DAG, Ca²⁺, cGMP, AA
number estimated	?	approx. 150 (?)	up to 20 (?)	approx. 20 (?)	

Key:
cAMP	- cyclic adenosine monophosphate
IPs	- inositol phosphates
DAG	- diacylglycerol
cGMP	- cyclic guanine monophosphate
AA	- arachidonic acid

Fig. 4.1. Flow of information through vertebrate G protein-dependent signal transduction systems.

belong to a common superfamily of 'opsin'-like proteins. These are characterized by a common structure which includes seven transmembrane domains with amino (N)- and carboxy (C)-termini located extracellularly and intracellularly respectively. As illustrated in Fig. 4.2, the relative lengths of the N- and C-termini and of the third intracellular loop vary considerably from receptor to receptor. Muscarinic acetylcholine receptors, especially the cardiac M_2-receptor, possess this basic structure. Typical effects of the M_2- receptor are the stimulation of an inwardly rectifying K^+ conductance, referred to in heart as the muscarinic K-channel or K_{ACh} (Breitwieser & Szabo, 1985; Pfaffinger et al., 1985) and inhibition of adenylate cyclase (Murad et al., 1962; Mattera et al., 1985).

Intervention of a G protein, or more precisely, of a GTP-regulatory step in the action of muscarinic receptors, was first discovered as a consequence of ligand binding studies. In these, agonist-induced displacement of antagonist binding to cardiac receptors was modified by GTP and GTP analogues (Berrie et al., 1979; Rosenberger et al., 1980). Dependence of muscarinic receptor-mediated inhibition of adenylate cyclase on a pertussis toxin (PTX)-sensitive G protein was shown by Kurose and Ui (1983). Involvement of GTP and of a PTX-sensitive step in the regulation of the atrial muscarinic K-channel was then shown in 1985 by Pfaffinger et al. (see below).

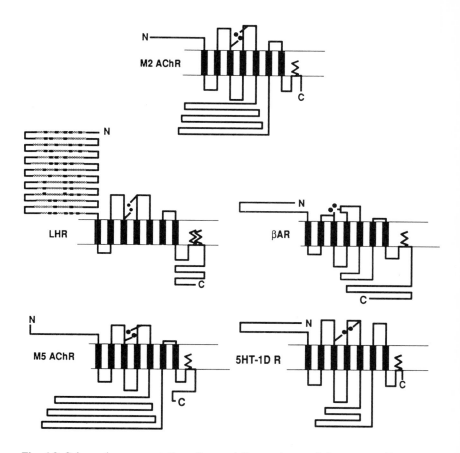

Fig. 4.2. Schematic representation of several G protein coupled receptors. Trans-membrane domains are presented as black boxes. The lengths of N-terminal chains, C-terminal chains, and of intracellular and extracellular loops are proportional to amino acid number as deduced from hydrophobicity plots. All receptors appear to have one conserved cysteine residue in each of the first and second extracellular loops, which are shown bonded by a disulphide bridge on the basis of studies with rhodopsin. In the C-terminal tail all have at least one cysteine which is depicted as a palmitoylated residue anchored in the membrane (on the basis of studies with the β-adrenoceptor: βAR). The longest extracellular domain is that of the N-terminus of the luteinizing receptor (LHR) which is depicted with its 14 imperfect homology repeats. The longest intracellular domain is that of the third intracellular loop of the M5 acetylcholine receptor (M5 AChR). Primary sequence information was from Peralta *et al.* (1987) for the human M2 acetylcholine receptor (M2 AChR), McFarland *et al.* (1989) for the rat LHR, Dixon *et al.* (1986), for the hamster β_2-adrenergic receptor (βAR), Liao *et al.* (1989) for the rat M5 AChR, and Levy *et al.* (1992) for the human serotonin 5HT-1D receptor (5HT-IDR).

G proteins

In comparison to receptors, the number of G proteins involved in receptor–effector coupling, based on the number of distinct α subunits, is small, probably not much more than 20. Of these only eight to 10 appear to have been purified to more than 95% purity. Based on the amino acid sequences of their α subunits, these G proteins can be separated into several groups:

1 G_s: represented by four isoforms (splice variants), all of which are substrates for cholera toxin (CTX), but not PTX, and derived from a single gene. G_s mediates stimulation of adenylate cyclase and L-type dihydropyridine sensitive Ca-channels in skeletal muscle and heart. Adenosine diphosphate (ADP)-ribosylation by CTX activates such G proteins due to partial blockade of the GTPase activity of their α subunit.

2 Three G_i proteins, all substrates for PTX (*see below*) and each encoded in a separate gene. These proteins modulate both K_{ACh} in heart and pituitary cells and the adenosine triphosphate (ATP)-sensitive K-channel (K_{ATP}) in pancreatic β-cells and cardiac ventricular muscle. G_i also appears responsible for inhibition of adenylate cyclase. Adenosine diphosphate-ribosylation by PTX blocks G_i interaction with receptors, i.e. causes receptor uncoupling, although the receptors can still be activated by non-hydrolysable analogues of GTP such as GTPγS or GMP-P(NH)P.

3 G_o, represented by two isoforms (splice variants), both of which are substrates for PTX, and derived like the G_s, from a single gene. G_o stimulates phospholipase C, both in *Xenopus* oocytes and in pituitary cell membranes, and hence has G_p-like activity.

4 One $G_{Z/X}$, insensitive to PTX, for which the gene is known but neither the protein nor its function is known.

5 Two highly homologous G_q-type proteins, G_q and G_{11}, insensitive to PTX and each derived from a separate gene. Like G_o, G_q has G_p-like activity.

6 Two classes of sensory G protein, one comprising two transducins, T-r, expressed in rod cells, and T-c, expressed in cone cells, and the other, G_{olf}, structurally related to the adenylate cyclase-stimulating G_s group.

Typical sets of G proteins are depicted in Fig. 4.3. In addition to distinct α subunits, there are at least four highly homologous β subunits and at least three γ subunits. It is the opinion of this author that $\beta\gamma$ dimers are fully interchangeable. In any given cell they constitute a heterogeneous pool of isoforms each of which interacts equally with any of the α subunits. In this case the number of functionally distinct G proteins would be equal to the number of distinct α subunits expressed in the cell of interest. If, however, there are $\beta\gamma$ combinations which prefer to interact with one type of α subunit, the number of functionally different G proteins would depend on whether or not individual $\beta\gamma$ combinations conferred distinct properties on the holo-G protein. For further information on molecular

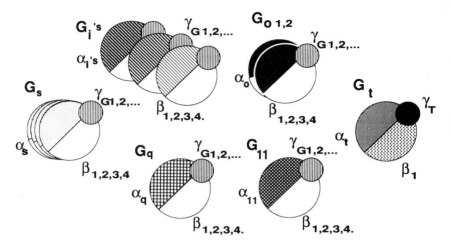

Fig. 4.3. Schematic representation of the subunit composition of typical vertebrate G proteins. G proteins have molecular weights (M_r) of 80 000–95 000. Except for transducin which is easily washed off membranes with low salt solutions, all other known G proteins are tightly bound to membranes and can only be extracted with detergents. All G proteins involved in receptor effector coupling, including transducin, comprise distinct $G\alpha$ subunits (M_r 39 000–50 000), one of four types of β subunit (β_{1-4}; $M_r = 35 000$–36 000) and one of four types of γ subunit (γ_T, and γ_{G1-3}; ($M_r = 7000$–10 000). One γ (type T) is water-soluble with a high proportion of charged amino acids. It is expressed only in retina and hence found in transducin γ_T. The other γ subunits are somewhat more hydrophobic and are found in all other G proteins. They are thought to play a role in anchoring G proteins to the plasma membrane. β and γ subunits have only been purified as dimers or complexed to α subunits as holo-G proteins. The relative abundance of β and γ subunits varies significantly from cell to cell. Extreme cases are retinal rod cells which have exclusively β_1 and γ_T and placenta which does not express β_1. Within any given tissue, the different α subunits interact with a common pool of $\beta\gamma$ dimers and $\beta\gamma$ heterogeneity is the same for each holo-G protein. G_s is depicted as a single $\beta\gamma$ dimer interacting with any one of four α_s splice variants; the two splice variants of G_o (Hsu *et al.*, 1990) are represented in similar form. The two families of highly homologous G_i proteins and highly homologous G_q/G_{11} proteins are presented as clusters of independent G proteins.

and signal transducing aspects of G proteins the reader is referred to articles by Lochrie and Simon (1988) and Birnbaumer (1990b).

Effectors

Unlike the G protein-coupled receptors or the G proteins proper, effectors for G proteins do not constitute a protein superfamily and are the least understood of the elements of the G protein-mediated signal transduction pathway. They include adenylate cyclase, the cAMP-specific phosphodiesterase of photoreceptor cells, phospholipases of the C, A_2 and possibly the D type. Various classes of ionic channel are effectors, including K_{ATP} and K_{ACh}

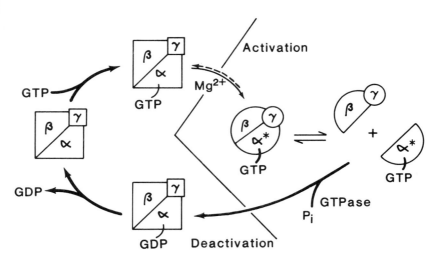

Fig. 4.4. Squares and semi-squares represent inactive conformations as they relate to modulation of effector functions. Circular and semi-circular shapes represent activated forms of the G protein. Activation is both GTP- and Mg^{2+}-dependent and stabilized by subunit dissociation to give an activated α^*GTP complex plus the $\beta\gamma$ dimer. α-subunit-mediated GTP hydrolysis leads to a α-subunit deactivation, increased affinity for $\beta\gamma$ and reassociation to give an inactive holo-G protein with GDP bound to it. Re-initiation of the activation cycle requires release of GDP and renewed binding of GTP. Specificity of action is encoded within the α subunit.

as well as voltage-gated Ca-channels and relatively non-selective monovalent cation channels such as the sinoatrial 'pacemaker' channel which carries the current designated I_f. (Yatani *et al.*, 1990). As a consequence of ion channel modulation, occupancy of G protein-coupled receptors by primary messengers leads not only to changes of intracellular second messengers — cyclic nucleotides, IP_3, DAG, AA and Ca^{2+} — but also of membrane potential, which itself is a potent regulator of cellular function (Fig. 4.1).

Mechanism of action of a G protein: molecular basis for receptor–effector coupling

GTPase-dependent regulatory cycle of a G protein catalysed by ligand occupied receptor

The mechanism by which binding of a ligand to a receptor is thought to increase or decrease the activity of an effector, with the intermediary participation of a G protein deserves some discussion. At the heart of receptor transduction lie two characteristic reactions of G proteins: (i) the binding of GTP followed by dissociation of the G protein to give a GTP α subunit complex (α^*GTP) plus $\beta\gamma$; and (ii) *in situ* hydrolysis of GTP, which leads to reassociation of G protein subunits (Fig. 4.4). In the

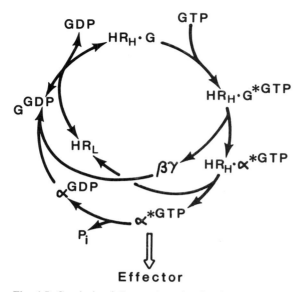

Fig. 4.5. Catalysis of G protein activation by hormone–receptor complex. The scheme incorporates three overlapping and mutually dependent regulatory cycles. (1) The G protein undergoes the cyclical dissociation–reassociation reaction, with the receptor interacting only with the trimeric form (G) of the G protein. (2) The G protein oscillates between GDP (G^{GDP}), nucleotide free and GTP (G^{GTP}) states, driven energetically forward by its capacity to hydrolyse GTP. (3) The hormone receptor (HR) intervenes as a catalyst by stabilizing an 'activated' GTP-liganded form of the G protein, ($HR_H \cdot G^{*GTP}$) which however, is no longer stable as a trimer and decomposes into free $\beta\gamma$ dimer plus $HR_H \cdot \alpha^{*GTP}$. This in turn, because of the absence of the $\beta\gamma$ portion of the G protein, loses its ability to stay associated with the receptor and decomposes further into activated α^{*GTP} plus the free form of the receptor (HR_L). The receptor is shown in two forms or states. One (HR_L) has a low affinity and the other (HR_H) has a high affinity for the agonist. These are the forms which the receptor adopts when it is free or associated with $\alpha\beta\gamma$, respectively. Although the assumption is made that regulation of the effector is possible only after $\beta\gamma$ and the receptor have dissociated, it is not yet known when the α subunit associates with the effector or acquires the capacity to hydrolyse GTP. In spite of these uncertainties, receptors could not act catalytically without subunit dissociation. Since the $\beta\gamma$ dimers are necessary for the interaction between G protein and receptor, their overall effect is to stimulate α activation. All G proteins involved in coupling receptors to effectors conform to this scheme.

test-tube, with isolated G proteins and GTP, this cycle proceeds only very slowly if at all. However, after substituting GTP analogues (GMP-P(NH)P or GTPγS) for GTP, the subunit dissociation reaction proceeds readily provided that the reaction is supplemented with Mg^{2+} (Fig. 4.4). This produces mixtures of $\beta\gamma$ dimers plus complexes of activated α subunit with G nucleotide and the activated α subunits can be isolated biochemically.

It is now accepted that the role of the receptor (Fig. 4.5) is to catalyse the activation reaction, i.e. binding of GTP followed by subunit dissociation and that effector stimulation (or inhibition) is due to its interaction with the α*GTP complex. In so doing, effectors act as monitors of the membrane levels of α*GTP complexes. On hydrolysis of GTP to GDP, the α subunit changes its conformation becoming α-GDP, which has low affinity for the effector from which it dissociates. The GTPase reaction is thus equivalent to an inactivation step. This is then followed by reassociation with $\beta\gamma$ to give a stable GDP-linked trimeric G protein ($\alpha\beta\gamma$-GDP) which interacts with the receptor to reinitiate the cycle. This occurs because in the presence of GTP the receptor promotes the formation of α*GTP $\cdot$ $\beta\gamma$ through a series of equilibrium reactions involving GDP dissociation, GTP binding and change in protein conformation. The cycle would come to a rest here if it were not that the 'starred' conformation of α has a low affinity for $\beta\gamma$, which therefore dissociates. This in turn leads to the release of the hormone–receptor complex. Thus, protein–protein interactions between receptor and G protein and between G protein and effector are based not only on the conformation of the individual subunits, but also on the protomer/oligomer state transitions of the G protein: the effector interacts with the monomeric α*GTP complex, while the receptor interacts with the trimeric forms of the G protein ($\alpha\beta\gamma$-GDP, $\alpha\beta\gamma$, $\alpha\beta\gamma$-GTP and α*GTP $\cdot$ $\beta\gamma$).

Consequences of the catalytic nature of receptor action

The receptor stimulated cycle (Fig. 4.5) allows the activated Gα*GTP to regulate the effector. At the same time the receptor which led to the formation of Gα*GTP is free to mediate the activation of another G protein by GTP. Two important consequences of this mechanism are: (i) that the receptor signal is amplified; and (ii) that receptor molecules of several types may be engaged simultaneously in activating the same G protein pool. Amplification has been convincingly demonstrated for phototransduction and for the β-adrenergic stimulation of adenylate cyclase. In the former, a single photon can lead to activation of up to 10 rhodopsin molecules (Fung *et al.*, 1981). In the case of β-adrenoceptors progressive chemical inactivation of the receptor results in a reduction in the rate, but not the extent, to which the membrane pool of G_s is activated (Tolkovsky & Levitzki, 1978). The second consequence leads to synergism between hormones at low concentrations but lack of additivity at high concentrations, such as may happen in tissues with multiple receptors of different ligand specificity but the same cellular action. Examples of this kind are found in fat and liver cells and in cardiac atria. In fat, adrenocorticotrophic hormone, β-adrenergic, secretin and glucagon receptors all summate with each other to induce cAMP-mediated lipolysis by catalysing the activation of G_s which stimulates adenylate cyclase (Birnbaumer &

Rodbell, 1969). In the liver, α_1-adrenergic, type-1a vasopressin and angiotensin II receptors co-operatively induce Ca^{2+}-mediated glycogenolysis by catalysing the activation of G_p. This leads to formation of the second messenger IP_3, which in turn causes release of Ca^{2+} from intracellular stores, and the subsequent activation of the phosphorylase system (Exton, 1988). In atria, muscarinic M_2, adenosine A_1 and in some species somato-statin and neuropeptide Y receptors have a bradycardic effect as a result of activation of K-channels stimulated by G_k (*see below*).

Direct regulation of ionic channels by G proteins

The inwardly rectifying muscarinic K-channel (K_{ACh})

Experiments leading to the discovery of G protein gating

The possibility of direct regulation of an ionic channel by a G protein, i.e. as shown in cell-free systems not involving soluble second messengers, emerged from studies on the mechanism by which muscarinic acetyl-choline receptors (mAChR) activate the atrial K-channels mediating vagal regulation of heart rate. Subsequently, ion channels which are directly gated either by G_i, G_o or G_s have been found.

G protein-gated K-channels are physiologically very relevant as mod-ulators of cellular function. Activation of these causes cells to hyper-polarize and they become less excitable. As a consequence, secretion or neurotransmitter release is attenuated in endocrine cells and in neurones from sympathetic and parasympathetic ganglia (Eccles & Libet, 1961; Hartzell *et al.*, 1977; Hill-Smith & Purves, 1978; Griffith *et al.*, 1981) and those of the central nervous system (Nakajima *et al.*, 1986). In the heart, such K-channels cause a decrease in heart rate (Trautwein & Dudel, 1958; Giles & Noble, 1976; reviewed by Hartzell, 1981, 1988).

Acetylcholine inhibits adenylate cyclase in heart membranes (Murad *et al.*, 1962; Kurose & Ui, 1983; Mattera *et al.*, 1985). In spite of this, the rapidity with which acetylcholine modifies K-channel activity suggested that a decrease in cAMP was not involved (Trautwein *et al.*, 1982; Nargeot *et al.*, 1983). This was first confirmed using the cell-attached patch con-figuration (Hamill *et al.*, 1981; Soejima & Noma, 1984) and subsequently by application of the whole-cell voltage clamp technique (Breitwieser & Szabo, 1985; Pfaffinger *et al.*, 1985). Direct regulation of the channel by a G_i-type G protein (G_k) was then proved in experiments with inside-out membrane patches (Codina *et al.*, 1987a,b; Yatani *et al.*, 1987a,c; Kirsch *et al.*, 1988; Mattera *et al.*, 1988).

Figure 4.6 summarizes the experimental approach used to demonstrate the direct (or membrane delimited) regulation of K_{ACh} by G_k. The cell-attached patch-clamp experiments showed that atrial muscarinic K-

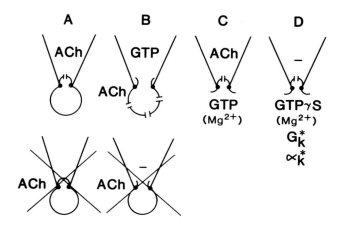

Fig. 4.6. Summary of experiments leading to the demonstration of direct (membrane delimited and independent of soluble second messengers and protein phosphorylation) G protein gating of a K-channel. A, Cell-attached patch: application of ACh to the pipette solution (*upper diagram*), but not to the bathing fluid (*lower diagram*) activates muscarinic K-channels within the patch. B, Whole-cell voltage-clamp: addition of GTP to the pipette solution (*upper diagram*) is required before addition of ACh to the bathing fluid can activate K-currents. C, Inside-out patch: ACh applied to the outer (pipette) surface requires GTP + Mg^{2+} to activate K-channels. D, Inside-out patch: K-channels can be directly activated in the absence of ACh by either GTPγS + Mg^{2+} or by activated G protein (G_k^*) or by resolved, activated α sub-units (α_i^*).

channels cannot be stimulated when acetylcholine is added to the bath, but they become activated when the agonist is applied onto the outer surface of the isolated membrane patch (i.e. in the pipette); Fig. 4.6A; Soejima & Noma, 1984. This indicates that the muscarinic receptors are in close proximity to the channel regulated by them and eliminates the possibility of a soluble, cytoplasmic second messenger as mediator of receptor activation. These experiments did not address the actual coupling mechanism involved. This could occur via direct receptor regulation of the channel (receptor–channel coupling) or receptor-induced G-protein activation (G protein–channel coupling). Alternatively, and possibly also through activation of a G protein, the receptor-mediated formation of a diffusible, yet membrane-delimited second messenger such as DAG could be involved.

The participation of a G protein in the coupling of cardiac muscarinic receptors to K-channels was established in the whole-cell voltage-clamp experiments in which atrial cells were 'perfused' with pipette solutions containing GTP or the GTP analogue GMP-P(NH)P (Fig. 4.6B; Breitwieser & Szabo, 1985; Pfaffinger *et al.*, 1985). Pfaffinger *et al.* (1985) established that acetylcholine was able to increase K-currents only when the pipette solution contained GTP and that PTX abolished this muscarinic response. This work indicated that a PTX-sensitive substrate was involved not only in the inhibition of adenylate cyclase but also in the opening of a K-channel linked to a cardiac muscarinic receptor.

In amphibian atrial cells Breitwieser and Szabo (1985) showed that acetylcholine induced a K-current (inwardly rectifying $I_{K(ACh)}$) and attenuated β-adrenergic receptor-induced increases in a specific Ca-current (the so-called slow inward I_{Ca}). The pipette/cytoplasm exchange (cell dialysis) was not extensive which allowed hormonal regulation of ionic currents without addition of GTP to the pipette solution. Addition of GMP-P(NH)P to the pipette had no effect unless hormones were added to the extracellular bathing fluid, presumably because of the inherent hysteresis (slowness) in the action of the nucleotide analogue in the absence of hormonal stimulation. Such slowness was accentuated by the prevailing low (submillimolar) intracellular Mg^{2+} concentrations. In the presence of hormones, the hysteresis in GMP-P(NH)P activation of G proteins was reduced as was the requirement for free Mg^{2+} so that agonist-induced, antagonist-resistant, persistent activation of ionic currents was obtained. Thus acetylcholine and isoprenaline induced persistent $I_{K(ACh)}$ and persistent I_{Ca} currents respectively.

These results indicate the involvement of a guanine nucleotide binding protein in the action of both types of receptor. Furthermore, the persistent nature of the acetylcholine response indicates that the G_i-type protein intervening between the muscarinic receptor and the K-channel, termed generically G_k (Breitwieser & Szabo, 1985), resembles the stimulatory G_s-type protein of adenylate cyclase. Specifically, the activation kinetics of G_k by GTP analogues are slow in the absence of hormonal stimulation and vice versa. In agreement with the postulate that muscarinic regulation of K-currents is independent of cAMP levels, stimulation of cells clamped using a GMP-P(NH)P-containing pipette in the presence of isoprenaline had no effect on the induction of K-currents by acetylcholine even though persistent effects of isoprenaline and therefore activation of G_s, were obtained (Breitwieser & Szabo, 1985).

Direct stimulation by human red blood cell G_i and its α subunit

A direct action of a G protein on the cardiac muscarinic receptor-sensitive K-channel was demonstrated in a cell-free system using inside-out membrane patches (Fig. 4.6C and D; Yatani et al., 1987a; Cerbai et al., 1988). In these experiments, addition of GTPγS or of an activated PTX-sensitive G protein purified from human erythrocyte membranes (hRBC) to the cytoplasmic face of the membrane resulted in K-channel activation. The effect of GTPγS required Mg^{2+} and proceeded with a lag, as expected from the activation kinetics of G proteins. The effect of the PTX-sensitive G protein pre-activated with GTPγS developed much faster. Since these studies were carried out in the absence of ATP (Yatani *et al.*, 1987a), they ruled out involvement of a phosphorylation reaction following stimulation of muscarinic receptors and functionally defined a G_k, i.e. a stimulatory regulatory G_i-type protein of a K-channel. Further studies with pituitary GH$_3$ cells showed the existence of a similar K-channel stimulated by a PTX-sensitive G protein modulated by somatostatin and muscarinic receptors (Yatani *et al.*, 1987c).

G protein-regulated K-channels in atrial and pituitary membranes are highly selective with respect to the G protein with which they interact. Highly purified G_s even at 100-fold higher concentrations than those needed to obtain half-maximal effects with G_i, had no effect on the K-channel (Yatani *et al.*, 1987a,c). Figure 4.7 summarizes many of the properties of receptor-mediated regulation of G_i-sensitive K-channels as seen in atrial and pituitary membrane patches. The experiments show that G protein regulation of K-channels by receptors is critically dependent on GTP and that activation of G_k by GTP requires the participation of an agonist-occupied receptor. Furthermore, the endogenous G_k is uncoupled from receptor regulation by PTX and such an uncoupled system is readily reconstituted by addition of exogenous, unactivated G_k, provided that GTP is present in the bath. Furthermore, resolved, GTPγS-activated α subunits of hRBC G_i (α_i^*) mimic the actions of GTPγS-activated G_i (G_i^*) with comparable potency, in contrast to resolved βγ dimers (Codina *et al.*, 1987a,b; Kirsch *et al.*, 1988). Thus, such experiments also indicate that the most plausible mechanism used by muscarinic receptors to stimulate G protein-gated K-channels is the catalysis of the activation of membrane G_k by GTP and the formation of activated free α_k^* which in turn acts as a mediator to stimulate the K-channel.

Properties of the G_i-stimulated K-channel

The microscopic kinetic properties of the G_i-sensitive K-channels have been measured and are typical of the muscarinic type of K-channel (Codina *et al.*, 1987a,b; Yatani *et al.*, 1987a,c; Cerbai *et al.*, 1988; Kirsch *et al.*, 1988). Once stimulated by G_i the channel open probability increases, with openings occurring in bursts and clusters of bursts as illustrated in Fig. 4.8. Frequency histograms of open times can be described by first order decay functions with time constants of about 1 ms and current amplitude frequency histograms show Gaussian distributions. Slope conductances obtained under symmetrical K$^+$ conditions (130–140 mM K$^+$) range from approximately 40 pS in guinea-pig atria to approximately 50 pS in pituitary GH$_3$ cells. It is not clear whether there are multiple genes for these channels or whether the above slightly different single channel conductances are due to cell-specific post-translational modifications of the same channel molecules. In each cell type the channels conduct very poorly in the outward direction (i.e. they inwardly rectify). In both systems the microscopic properties of the channels stimulated by receptor plus GTP are indistinguishable from those seen on stimulation by GTPγS or by exogenous addition of pre-activated G_i or its activated α subunit. Figure 4.8 also expresses channel activation data as cumulative NP values. When averaged over long periods of time, these allow a quantitative comparison of channel activity which is useful, for comparing the effects of increasing concentrations of holo-G or resolved α subunits.

Among the receptors which catalyse activation of G_k-type G proteins by GTP are the cardiac atrial muscarinic, adenosine and neuropeptide Y receptors (A. Yatani, L. Birnbaumer & A. M. Brown, unpublished), hippocampal $5HT_{1a}$ and $GABA_B$ receptors (Newberry & Nicoll, 1984; Andrade et al., 1986; Sasaki & Sato, 1987; Thalmann, 1988) and endocrine cell somatostatin and muscarinic receptors (Yatani et al., 1987c). The list is bound to grow and as shown below more than one type of K-channel may be involved. Moreover, while it is clear that atrial and pituitary cell receptors activate G_i-gated K-channels, studies in other cell types may reveal the involvement of G_o-gated conductances.

Identity of the G_k associated with $K_{(ACh)}$

Figure 4.9 illustrates that the GTPγS-activated forms of the α subunits of all three known G_i proteins are approximately equally effective in activating the atrial $K_{(ACh)}$ channel. These effects have also been obtained with recombinant α_i subunits, indicating that actions of these purified proteins are not due to contaminants (Yatani et al., 1988).

The following observations illustrate that the effects observed with each of the recombinant α_i subunits are intrinsic properties of the expressed molecules.

1 Boiling prior to addition to the bath obliterates the activity of each recombinant α_i.

2 *Threshold* concentrations of GTPγS for activation of atrial muscarinic K-channels in inside-out membrane patches (with 100 nM carbachol in the pipette) lie between 10 and 100 nM, which is at least 10 times the *maximum* GTPγS concentration added with saturating concentrations (1 nM) of any of the GTPγS-activated, partially purified and ultrafiltrated recombinant α_i preparations.

3 Prior addition of 100 μM GDPβS, which blocks the carbachol-mediated effects of 10 μM GTP, does not interfere with the effects of GTPγS-activated recombinant subtypes α_{i1}, α_{i2} or α_{i3}.

These data contrast with those obtained initially by Clapham, Neer and collaborators (Logothetis et al., 1987), who reported that bovine brain GTPγS-activated $\alpha_i(\alpha_{41}^*)$ and GTPγS-activated $\alpha_o(\alpha_{39}^*)$ subunits failed to stimulate atrial muscarinic K-channels, although, subsequently, stimula-

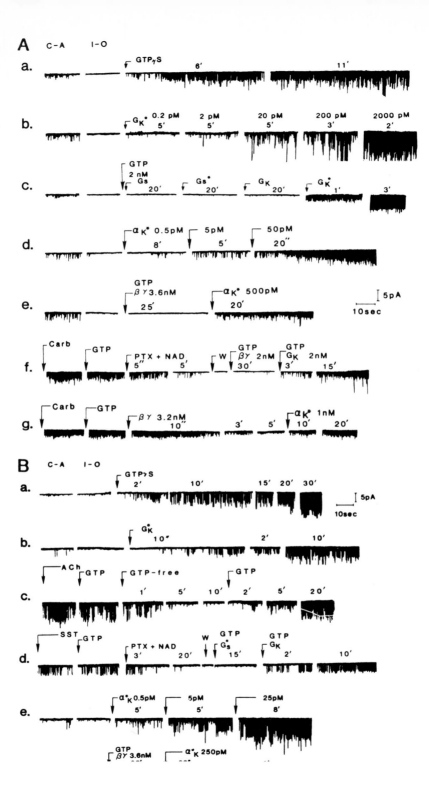

Fig. 4.7. (*Opposite*) Properties of G_k-mediated regulation of G protein sensitive K-channel as seen in inside-out membrane patches of guinea-pig atrial cells and GH$_3$ rat pituitary tumour cells. Each line represents a separate experiment in which single channel K-currents were recorded before (cell-attached; C-A) and after membrane patch excision to the inside-out configuration (I-O). Records were obtained at holding potentials between -80 and $-100\,mV$ and using symmetrical 130–140 mM KCl or K-methanesulphonate solutions. Numbers above the records denote time elapsed ('min, "sec) between the indicated additions and the beginning of the segment of record shown. Routinely, the first addition was made between 5 and 10 min after patch excision and subsequent additions were at 5–25 min intervals, depending on the purpose of the experiments. Five minute intervals were used when dose–response relationships were studied; 25-min intervals were used when substances added had no apparent effect. In some instances the bathing solutions were exchanged by perfusion at 1–2 ml/min.

A, Experiments with atrial membrane patches from adult guinea-pigs. Cells were freshly obtained by collagenase digestion. Experiment a: Stimulation of single channel K-currents by activation of the atrial G_k protein with GTPγS (100 µM in the bath). Experiment b: Stimulation of the atrial K-channels in a dose-dependent manner by exogenously added human erythrocyte pertussis toxin substrate (referred to as G_k), preactivated by incubation with GTPγS and Mg^{2+} (G_k^*) and dialysed, extensively to remove free GTPγS to ineffective levels. Threshold effects of G_k^*, were obtained with between 0.2 and 1 pM in separate membrane patches. Experiment c: the bathing solution contained 100 µM GTP throughout, each protein concentration was 2 nM. Lack of stimulatory effects of 2 nM of either non-activated or GTPγS-activated G_s or of non-activated G_k. Experiment d: Mimicry of the effect of GTPγS-activated holo-G_k (*see* experiment b) by equally low concentrations of the resolved GTPγS-activated α subunit of the protein (α_K^*). Experiment e: Lack of effect of resolved human erythrocyte βγ compared to an α_K^*-sensitive membrane patch. Experiment f: Stimulation of G_k-sensitive K-channels by the muscarinic receptor agonist carbachol (carb) present in the pipette throughout, maintenance of receptor-G protein effector coupling after patch excision into bathing solution with 100 µM GTP, and uncoupling of atrial G_k by treatment with PTX and nicotinamide adenine dinucleotide (NAD) added to the bathing solution. Lack of re-coupling effect of resolved human erythrocyte βγ and reconstitution of acetylcholine receptor-K-channel stimulation by addition of native unactivated human erythrocyte G_k in the presence of GTP. Note that this contrasts the result in experiment c and demonstrates that the exogenously added G_k requires receptor participation for activation by GTP. Experiment g: Inhibition of the carbachol- and GTP-driven muscarinic channel by exogenously added βγ dimers, and reactivation by persistently activated α_K^*.

B, Experiments with inside-out membrane patches from rat GH$_3$ pituitary tumour cells. Cells were grown as monolayers on cover slips and membrane patches excised from their upper membrane surface. Experiment a: effect of GTPγS added to the bathing medium. Experiment b: Representative time-course of activation of GH$_3$ cell K-channel by a saturating concentration (2 nM) of GTPγS-activated human erythrocyte G_k (G_k^*). Experiment c: Dependence on GTP and reversibility of receptor-mediated stimulation of G_k-sensitive K-channel. Acetylcholine (ACh) was present in the pipette solution throughout. 100 µM of GTP was present in the bathing medium, removed and re-added as shown. Experiment d: Stimulation of GH$_3$ cell G_k-sensitive K-channels by somatostatin (SST): demonstration of PTX sensitivity of the GH$_3$ G_k protein and reconstitution of the signal transduction pathway by addition of unactivated native human erythrocyte G_k in the presence of GTP. Experiments e and f: Mimicry of the effects of GTPγS-activated G_k by resolved GTPγS-activated α-subunit of human erythrocyte G_k and lack of effort of resolved, α-subunit-free βγ dimers. (Adapted from Yatani *et al.*, 1987a,c; Codina *et al.*, 1987a,b).

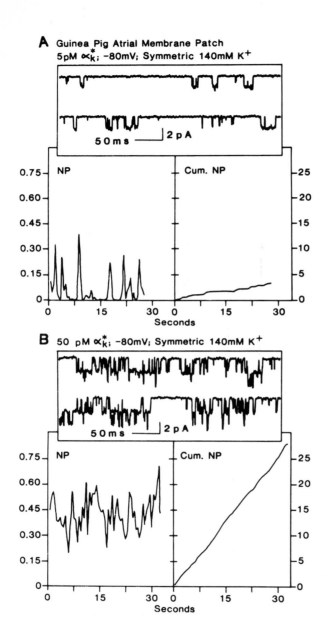

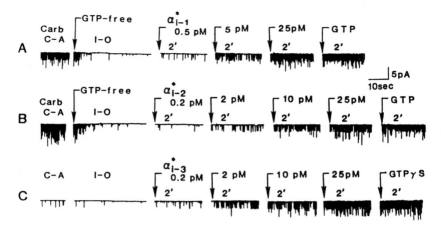

Fig. 4.9. Stimulation of single K-channel currents in guinea-pig atrial membrane patches by increasing concentrations of bovine brain α_i-1, A, and human erythrocyte α_i-2, B, and α_i-3, C. $G_i\alpha$-2 and $G_i\alpha$-3 were purified from human erythrocyte membranes as described by Birnbaumer *et al.* (1988). G_i-1 was purified by E. Padrell and R. Iyengar as described in Yatani *et al.* (1988c). Cell-attached (C-A) and inside-out (I-O) conditions are shown. Carbachol, GTP and GTPγS when present were 100 μM.

tion with the subunit was observed (Logothetis *et al.*, 1988). However, in a more recent publication by one of the co-authors it was reported that all α_i proteins stimulate the muscarinic K-channel (Kobayashi *et al.*, 1990). The reported stimulation by the α_o subunit (Logothetis *et al.*, 1987) may have been due to contamination by α_i proteins (Yatani *et al.*, 1987a).

Fig. 4.8. (*Opposite*) Single channel K$^+$ currents in guinea-pig atrial membranes after patch excision and addition of either 5 pM, A, or 500 pM, B, of GTPγS-activated resolved α subunit of G_k (α_k^*). Quantification of activity: NP and cumulative NP values. Records of single channel currents (top insets) are subdivided into consecutive 200 ms segments to quantify the proportion of time during which single channel currents are observed in each segment. The variation of these values per 200 ms, representing the product (NP) of the opening probability (P_o) of each of the channels present in the membrane patch and the number of channels in the patch (N), as a function of time are shown in the lower left panels. Lower right panels show cumulative NP values over the same time period (Cum NP) and are equivalent to a time course of channel activity. The slopes of the Cum NP curves (Cum NP/min) referred to maximum cumulative NP/min values, which can be elicited from the same membrane patch provide individual points which can serve to construct dose–response curves for the action of a G protein. Concentrations of G_k^* and α_k^* giving half-maximal stimulations of guinea-pig atrial K-channels vary between 5 and 60 pM with a mean of approximately 20 pM for either G_k^* or α_k^*.

The ATP-sensitive K-channel: a second G_i-gated K-channel

General properties of the ATP-sensitive K-channel/sulphonylurea receptor complex

It is now commonly accepted that an ATP-sensitive K-channel (K_{ATP}) is the 'glucose sensor' of pancreatic β cells and plays a key role in the regulation of membrane potential in this cell type. This results in modulation of the activity of voltage-gated Ca-channels, which upon activation promote first-phase secretory events. Insulin secretion is antagonized by hormones such as somatostatin of local origin and by adrenaline of adrenal origin, as well as by noradrenaline from local sympathetic innervation. The effects of somatostatin as well as those of the catecholamines, acting through α_2-adrenergic receptors, are blocked by PTX treatment. These agonists initiate a complex set of transmembrane events which includes reduction of adenylate cyclase activity (Katada & Ui, 1981), inhibition of L-type Ca-channels (Hsu *et al.*, 1990) and stimulation of K_{ATP} (Ribalet & Ciani, 1987; Ribalet *et al.*, 1989). It is not yet clear whether the different effects of these receptors are mediated by a single G protein.

K_{ATP} is blocked by sulphonylureas and it is likely, although not yet proven, that the sulphonylurea receptor may be the ATP-sensitive K-channel proper. As recently reviewed by Panten and his coworkers (Zunkler *et al.*, 1988, 1989; Panten *et al.*, 1989, 1990; U. Panten, personal communication), the regulation of this channel is complex, involving ATP, ADP, Mg^{2+}, channel phosphorylation and G proteins. Inhibition by ATP can be mimicked by the non-hydrolysable ATP analogue AMP-P(NH)P, and does not appear to involve a phosphorylation event. Inhibition by sulphonylureas requires ADP–Mg which appears to interact with the channel at a site allosteric to that of ATP. The binding affinity for sulphonylureas is decreased by Mg–ATP under phosphorylating conditions. Regulation by a G protein requires that the channel be first inhibited by ATP (or an analogue such as AMP-P(NH)P) and it may require prior phosphorylation, although this is uncertain. Figure 4.10 presents a diagram of factors relevant to the regulation of the sulphonylurea receptor/K_{ATP}.

Adenosine triphosphate-sensitive K-conductances are found not only in pancreatic β cells but also in a variety of other tissues, including skeletal, smooth and cardiac muscle. As reported by Noma (1983), a K_{ATP} with a unitary conductance of 65 pS can be readily identified in cell-attached as well as in inside-out membrane patches from guinea-pig and rabbit cardiac myocytes. This channel exhibits inward rectification, albeit less marked than that shown by K_{ACh}, from which it can also be readily distinguished by its larger conductance. The IC_{50} of ATP is approximately 0.1 mм.

In whole-cell voltage-clamp recordings from neonatal rat ventricular myocytes, the K-current increases with time, presumably due to gradual depletion

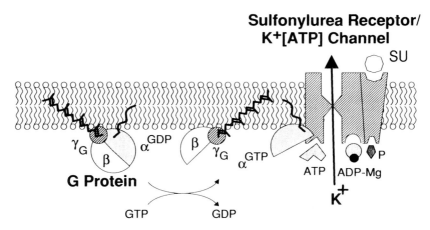

Fig. 4.10. Model of factors involved in the regulation of the K_{ATP}/sulphonylurea receptor complex and hypothetical mode of activation by a G_i protein. The K_{ATP}/sulphonylurea channel complex is depicted as a transmembrane protein with the G protein as a membrane-associated entity anchored to it by both a polyisoprenylated γ subunit and a myristoylated α_i-subunit. The affinity of the sulphonylurea (SU) is assumed to be decreased by phosphorylation (P); inhibition of K-channel activity may require occupancy of the intracellular SU regulatory site by ADP–Mg. Potassium-channel activity is assumed to be inhibited by occupancy of an additional regulatory site by ATP or AMP-P(NH)P, and activation by G_i (possibly by an α_i-GTP complex) is assumed to depend on prior occupancy of regulatory site by ATP or AMP-P(NH)P.

of ATP, and is inhibited by sulphonylureas like glibenclamide or tolbutamide. The rat myocyte K_{ATP} has a single channel conductance of 85 pS, mean open times of 1–2 ms and also exhibits inward rectification. These results are consistent with the existence in intact myocytes of an ATP- and sulphonyl-urea- sensitive K-channel, similar to that of pancreatic β cells. In cardiac myocytes, K_{ATP} can be activated by adenosine, which is known to act through receptors that are coupled to effectors by G proteins (Kirsch *et al.*, 1990).

Identity of G proteins which regulate K_{ATP}

Figure 4.11 illustrates the GTP-dependent activation by adenosine of K_{ATP} channels under inhibition by ATP or AMP-P(NH)P. In an outside-out membrane patch no effect of adenosine was obtained when GTP was omitted from the pipette (intracellular) solution. Both adenosine and the analogue cyclohexyladenosine (CHA) were effective when applied to the extracellular surface of inside-out membrane patches.

Addition of GTPγS to the cytoplasmic face of inside-out membrane patches activated K_{ATP} channels inhibited by ATP- or AMP-P(NH)P as expected if this channel were to be regulated by a G protein. Upon testing for the molecular identity of the G protein(s) which could have mediated

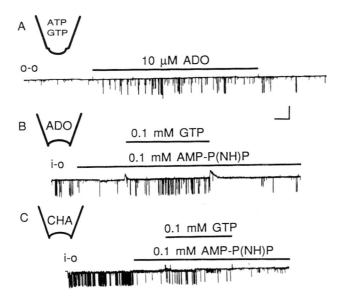

Fig. 4.11. Dependence on GTP of the effects of adenosine (ADO) and cyclohexyl-adenosine (CHA) on the K_{ATP}/sulphonylurea complex in excised membrane patches from neonatal rat ventricular myocytes. Recordings from (A) outside-out (o-o) patches were obtained with a pipette (intracellular) solution that included 140 mM KCl, 5 mM EGTA, 0.1 mM ATP, 0.1 mM GTP and 2 mM Mg^{2+} and a bath (extracellular) modified Tyrode solution (including 137 mM NaCl, 5.4 mM KCl, 2.0 mM $CaCl_2$, 1.0 mM $MgCl_2$, 10 mM glucose and 10 μM tetrodotoxin). Recordings from inside-out (i-o) membrane patches (B, C) were obtained with the pipette (extracellular) modified Tyrode and bath (intracellular) solutions described above. Membrane patches were perfused with bath solutions containing the indicated additives. Holding potential was − 80 mV, vertical and horizontal bars indicate 5 pA and 20 s, respectively. When present, CHA was 100 nM, ADO was 10 μM and ATP/GTP were 0.1 mM each. (Adapted from Kirsch *et al.*, 1990.)

the action of adenosine, it was established that any one of the G_i α subunits, but not those associated with G_s or G_o proteins could have been involved (Fig. 4.12).

It follows from all the studies so far described that G_i proteins are multifunctional. Not only do they inhibit adenylate cyclase, but they also activate both K_{ACh} and K_{ATP}. Moreover, with respect to these two K-channels, G_{i1}, G_{i2} and G_{i3} are isoforms, and all three act indistinguishably.

G protein gating as a tool to discover novel ionic channels: neuronal G_o-gated K-channels

One of the properties of the muscarinic K_{ACh} is that it is essentially silent in the absence of stimulation by an activated G_i protein (G_k). Thus, in the absence of activated G protein its open probability is close to zero. The

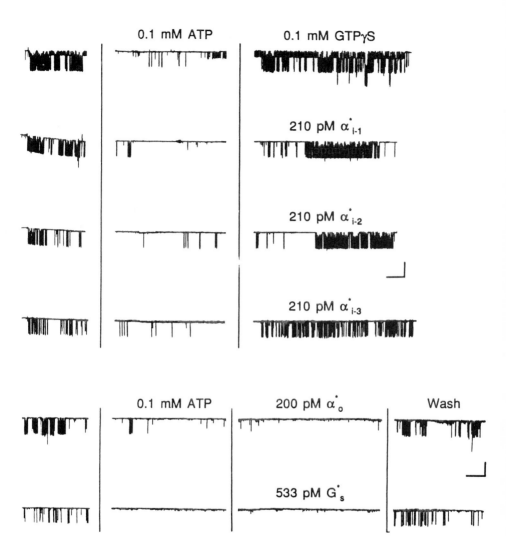

Fig. 4.12. Activation of the ATP-inhibited K_{ATP}/sulphonylurea complex by GTPγS and activated G_i with lack of effect of G_s or G_o, in inside-out membrane patches of neonatal rat ventricular myocytes. *Top four panels*: Sensitivity to GTPγS, α_{i1}, α_{i2} and α_{i3}. *Left*: K-channel currents after excision into ATP-free bath solution. *Middle*: K-channel activity after addition of 0.1 mM ATP. *Right*: K-channel activity after the indicated additives in the presence of ATP. All solutions contained 2.0 mM $MgCl_2$. *Bottom two panels*: Insensitivity to α_{o1} (α_o on the figure) and α_s. The design was the same as above, except that after failure to obtain a response with α_o^* and G_s^*, the viability of the channel in the patch was tested by removal of both the G protein α subunit and ATP (*Wash*). Solutions were as in Fig. 4.11; holding potential was −80 mV, vertical and horizontal bars indicate 5 pA and 20 s, respectively. (Adapted from Kirsch *et al.*, 1990.)

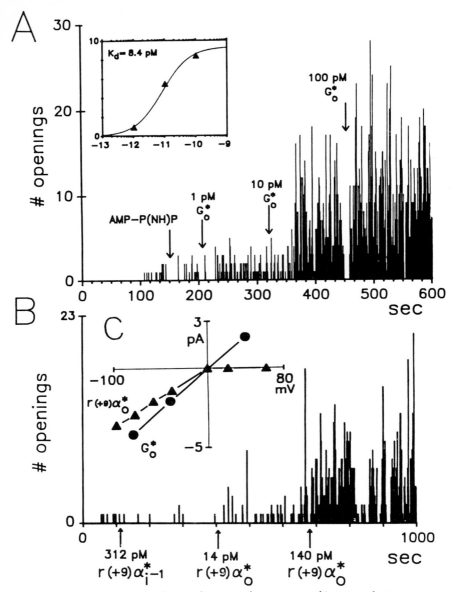

Fig. 4.13. Bovine brain G_o and *recombinant* α_o, but not *recombinant* $\alpha_i - 1$, gate single K-channel currents in hippocampal pyrimidal cells of neonatal rats. A, The effect of increasing concentrations of G_o^* on a 55 pS K-channel is shown by plotting the number of openings per 0.8 s as a function of time of continuous recording. *Inset*: Openings per 0.8 s averaged for 1 min as a function of G_o^* concentration. B, Lack of effects of 312 pM *recombinant* $\alpha_i^* - 1$, and stimulatory effect of increasing concentrations of *recombinant* α_o^* on a 40 pS K-channel, plotted as number of openings per 0.2 s as a function of the time of continuous recording shown. Single K-channel currents were recorded from excised inside-out membrane patches as in Fig. 4.7 in the presence of 0.2 mM AMP-P(NH)P. Holding potential was -80 mV and both pipette and bath solutions contained 140 mM K-methanesulphonate, 1 mM EGTA, 1 mM $MgCl_2$ and 10 mM Hepes adjusted to pH 7.4 with Tris-base. (Adapted from VanDongen *et al.*, 1988.)

possibility also exists that G_o proteins regulate K-channels. Hippocampal pyramidal cells, rich in G_o, have thus been studied for the potential presence of both G_i- and G_o-gated K-channels. Results with a highly purified preparation of one of the splice variants of bovine brain G_o, the GTPγS-activated G_{o1} (G_{o1}^*) has revealed the existence of several novel G_o-gated K-channels distinct from G_i-gated K-channels.

When purified bovine brain G_{o1}^* was applied to the cytoplasmic aspect of inside-out membrane patches of cultured hippocampal pyramidal cells, four new types of K-channel were identified. Three of these were non-rectifying with unitary conductances of 13, 40 and 55 pS respectively. The fourth was inwardly rectifying with a slope conductance of 40 pS. No such channel activities were observed with hRBC G_{i3}^* or hRBC α_{i3}^*. G_{o2}^* or α_{o2}^* have not yet been tested in this system. The effect of increasing concentrations of bovine brain G_o^* on the 55 pS-type K-channel is shown in Fig. 4.13A. In contrast to earlier observations with guinea-pig atrial membrane patches (Yatani *et al.*, 1987b) the hippocampal K-channel is highly sensitive to G_o^*. Significant activation was obtained at 1 pM and half-maximal effects were obtained at about 10 pM.

To confirm that the channels observed on addition of G_o^* were indeed gated by G_o and not by a contaminant, the G protein specificity of the channel was studied by addition of partially purified recombinant α^* molecules, including not only α_o (type 1) but also the three α_i subtypes. All four of the above-mentioned K-channel types were stimulated by recombinant α_o^*, under conditions in which prior addition of one of the recombinant α_i^* preparations, active on guinea-pig atrial muscarinic K-channels, had no effect. One such experiment, with a 40 pS inwardly rectifying K-channel is shown in Fig. 4.13B. The G_o-gated channels were stimulated in the absence of Ca^{2+} or ATP. The presence of AMP-P(NH)P, added routinely to inhibit the 70 pS K_{ATP}, and of EGTA did not interfere with the actions of G_o or *recombinant* α_o. Thus, in the hippocampal pyrimidal cells of the rat, G_o is a G_k, and the several K-channels gated by it differ from those present in atrial cells in various aspects including G protein specificity.

Effect of $\beta\gamma$ dimers: inhibition versus stimulation of K_{ACh} —a persisting controversy

Logothetis *et al.* (1987, 1988) and Kurachi *et al.*, (1989a) have reported that bovine brain as well as human placental $\beta\gamma$ dimers stimulate atrial K-channel activity. However, as shown in Fig. 4.7, $\beta\gamma$ dimers from hRBC have no stimulatory effects on either atrial or GH$_3$ G_k-gated K-channels in contrast to α_i. On the contrary, it was noted that when $\beta\gamma$ dimers were added at high (2–4 nM) concentrations to atrial membrane patches stimulated by carbachol in the pipette and with GTP in the bath, inhibition of

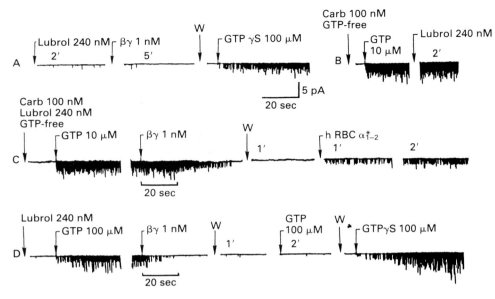

Fig. 4.14. Inhibition of G protein-gated K-channel activity by $\beta\gamma$ dimers. Inside-out membrane patches from adult guinea-pig atrial cells were exposed to the bathing solution (140 mM KCl, 2 mM MgCl$_2$, 5 mM EGTA, 10 mM Hepes-K, pH 7.4) containing the additives shown on the figure. The pipette solution was identical to the bathing solution and contained 100 nM carbachol (Carb) when indicated. The composition of bathing solution was changed by a concentration-clamp method. The Lubrol PX used to maintain $\beta\gamma$ dimers in suspension did not interfere with stimulation of activity by GTP (D) or GTP plus agonist (B, C). Furthermore, $\beta\gamma$ dimers had no effect on their own (A) but inhibited atrial K-channel stimulation by the membrane G_K (C, D). Inhibition was faster and was elicited with lower concentrations of $\beta\gamma$ dimers when the K-channels were operating under baseline conditions (GTP only, experiment D: cessation of activity after 16 s) than when they were stimulated by an agonist (carbachol plus GTP, experiment C: cessation of activity after 50 s). Numbers above records denote time elapsed in minutes between a solution change and the beginning of the record shown. (Adapted from Okabe *et al.*, 1990.)

signal transduction occurred. Although this result was obtained in only two of five initial experiments (Codina *et al.*, 1987a), it was later obtained consistently, especially when low concentrations of both GTP and carbachol were used (L. Birnbaumer, unpublished observations).

A typical set of results obtained with $\beta\gamma$ dimers is illustrated in Figs 4.14 and 4.15 (Okabe *et al.*, 1990). In these experiments, addition of $\beta\gamma$ dimers to inside-out membrane patches in which K-channels had been stimulated either by GTP alone (baseline activity) or by carbachol plus GTP (agonist-stimulated activity), resulted consistently in inhibition of K-channel activity. When added to silent patches in the absence of GTP, $\beta\gamma$ dimers had no effect under these conditions (Fig. 4.14; Codina *et al.*,

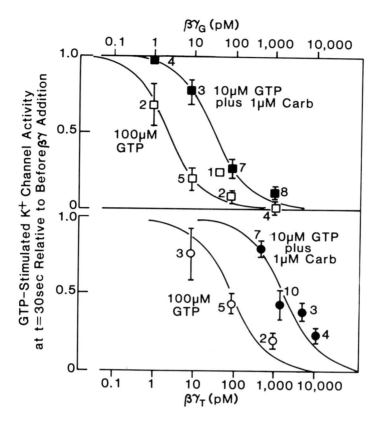

Fig. 4.15. Effect of agonist (carbachol) on the dose-dependent inhibition by $\beta\gamma$ dimers of GTP-dependent K-channel activities in inside-out guinea-pig atrial membrane patches by $\beta\gamma$ dimers. When 1 μM carbachol was present in the pipette, GTP was 10 μM; in the absence of carbachol, GTP was 100 μM. $\beta\gamma_G$: data obtained with $\beta\gamma$ dimers derived from either human erythrocytes, human placenta, or bovine brain were pooled. $\beta\gamma_T$: data obtained with $\beta\gamma$ derived from bovine rod outer segments. (Adapted from Okabe *et al.*, 1990.)

1987a; Kirsch *et al.*, 1988; Okabe *et al.*, 1990). Concentration–effect studies showed clearly that $\beta\gamma$ dimers were more potent at inhibiting agonist-independent than agonist-stimulated activity, and that this phenomenon applied not only to $\beta\gamma$ dimers suspended in Lubrol PX, such as those from human placenta, hRBC and bovine brain, but also to $\beta\gamma$ dimers presented to the patches in aqueous media, such as transducin $\beta\gamma$ (Fig. 4.15). Such findings had previously been observed in an homologous signal transduction system involving β-adrenoceptors (Cerione *et al.*, 1985; see also Birnbaumer, 1987). These results support the thesis that in intact membranes $\beta\gamma$ dimers act as suppressors of 'noise' generated by agonist-unoccupied receptors.

The inhibitory effects of $\beta\gamma$ dimers just described contrast with the stimulation obtained by Clapham, Neer, and their collaborators (Logothetis *et al.*, 1987, 1988; Kim *et al.*, 1989). The reasons for the discrepancy are not understood but they are not due to the detergent used, since inhibition was also obtained in the absence of Lubrol PX using water-soluble $\beta\gamma$ dimers from transducin (Fig. 4.15). The claim that $\beta\gamma$ dimers may be acting by stimulation of AA formation (Kim *et al.*, 1989), conflicts with the data of Kurachi *et al.* (1989b). These workers showed that the effects of AA and its metabolites required bath addition of GTP and were abolished on addition of GDPβS. Nevertheless, the stimulatory effects of $\beta\gamma$ dimers occurred in the absence of GTP (Logothetis *et al.*, 1987, 1988; Kim *et al.*, 1989), which dissociates the stimulatory effects of $\beta\gamma$ dimers (Kim *et al.*, 1989; Logothetis *et al.*, 1987, 1988) from the effects of AA (or its metabolites) (Kurachi *et al.*, 1989b).

Conclusions

The present chapter summarizes most of the evidence which relates to G protein-mediated modulation of two types of G_i-gated K-channel and of a class of G_o-gated K-channels. In all cases the effects appear to be independent of phosphorylation or of the formation of classical second messengers such as cAMP or IP$_3$. Thus, G proteins seem to direct protein–protein interaction, as opposed to the formation of intermediary and diffusible membrane-delimited second messengers. However, involvement of such second messengers cannot be totally excluded. Even if diffusible second messengers are not involved in the action of the G proteins, this does not preclude the possibility that K-channels could be additionally regulated by second messengers and/or phosphorylation, as seems to be the case for K_{ATP}. Full resolution of the biochemical mechanisms by which K-channels are modulated awaits full purification of the channel protein(s), and its incorporation into lipid bilayers together with the purified G protein(s). While this is currently not possible, molecular cloning and subsequent overexpression of the channel proteins, should aid in this aim.

Acknowledgements

Supported in part by NIH research grants to LB (DK-19318, HD-09581, HL-45198, and HL-37044) and to Arthur M. Brown (HL-39262) and by the Baylor Diabetes and Endocrinology Research Center grant DK-27685.

References

Andrade, R., Malenka, R. C. & Nicoll, R. A. (1986) A G protein couples serotonin and GABA$_B$ receptors to the same channels in hippocampus. *Science* **234**, 1261–1265.
Berrie, C. P., Birdsall, N. J. M., Burgen, A. S. V. & Hulme, E. C. (1979) Guanine

nucleotides modulate muscarinic receptor binding in the heart. *Biochemical and Biophysical Research Communications* **87**, 1000–1005.

Birnbaumer, L. (1987) Which G protein subunits are the active mediators in signal transduction. *Trends in Pharmacological Sciences* **8**, 209–211.

Birnbaumer, L., Codina, J., Mattera, R., Yatani, A., Graf, R., Olate, J., Sandford, J. & Brown, A. M. (1988) Receptor-effector coupling by G proteins: purification of human erythrocyte Gi-2 and Gi-3 and analysis of effector regulation using recombinant alpha sub-units synthesized in *Escherichia coli*. *Cold Spring Harbor Symposia on Quantitative Biology* **53**, 229–239.

Birnbaumer, L. (1990a) Transduction of receptor signal into modulation of effector activity by G proteins: the first 20 years or so . . . *FASEB Journal* **4**, 3178–3188.

Birnbaumer, L. (1990b) G proteins in signal transduction. *Annual Review of Pharmacology and Toxicology* **30**, 675–705.

Birnbaumer, L. & Rodbell, M. (1969) Adenylyl cyclase in fat cells. II. Hormone receptors. *Journal of Biological Chemistry* **244**, 3477–3482.

Bourne, H. R., Coffino, P. & Tomkins, G. M. (1975) Selection of a variant lymphoma cell deficient in adenylate cyclase. *Science* **187**, 750–752.

Boyd, A. E., Aguilar-Bryan, L., Bryan, J. *et al.* (1991) Sulfonylurea signal transduction. *Recent Progress in Hormone Research* **47**, 299–317.

Breitwieser, G. E. & Szabo, G. (1985) Uncoupling of cardiac muscarinic and beta-adrenergic receptors from ion channels by a guanine nucleotide analogue. *Nature* **317**, 538–540.

Burch, R. M., Luini, A. & Axelrod, J. (1986) Phospholipase A_2 and phospholipase C are activated by distinct GTP-binding proteins in response to alpha$_1$-adrenergic stimulation in FRTL5 cells. *Proceedings of the National Academy of Sciences USA* **83**, 7201–7205.

Cerbai, E., Kloeckner, U. & Isenberg, G. (1988) The α subunit of the GTP binding protein activates muscarinic potassium channels of the atrium. *Science* **240**, 1782–1784.

Cerione, R. A., Staniszewski, C., Caron, M. H., Lefkowitz, R. J., Codina, J. & Birnbaumer, L. (1985) A role for N$_i$ in the hormonal stimulation of adenylate cyclase. *Nature* **318**, 293–295.

Cockroft, S. & Gomperts, B. D. (1985) Role of guanine nucleotide binding protein in the activation of polyphosphoinositide phosphodiesterase. *Nature* **314**, 534–536.

Codina, J., Grenet, D., Yatani, A., Birnbaumer, L. & Brown, A. M. (1987a) Hormonal regulation of pituitary GH$_3$ cell K$^+$ is mediated by its *alpha* subunit. *FEBS Letters* **216**, 104–106.

Codina, J., Yatani, A., Grenet, D., Brown, A. M. & Birnbaumer, L. (1987b) The α subunit of the GTP-binding protein G$_k$ opens atrial potassium channels. *Science* **236**, 442–445.

Eccles, R. M. & Libet, B. (1961) Origin and blockade of the synaptic responses of curarized sympathetic ganglia. *Journal of Physiology* **157**, 484–503.

Exton, J. H. (1988) Role of phosphoinositides in regulation of liver function. *Hepatology* **8**, 152–166.

Fung, B. K-K. (1983) Characterization of transducin from bovine retinal rod outer segments. I. Separation and reconstitution of the subunits. *Journal of Biological Chemistry* **256**, 10 495–10 502.

Fung, B. K-K., Hurley, J. B. & Stryer, L. (1981) Flow of information in the light-triggered cyclic nucleotide cascade of vision. *Proceedings of the National Academy of Sciences USA* **78**, 152–156.

Giles, W. & Noble, S. J. (1976) Changes in membrane currents in bullfrog atrium produced by acetylcholine. *Journal of Physiology* **261**, 103–123.

Griffith, W. H., III, Gallagher, J. P. & Shinnick-Gallagher, P. (1981) Sucrose-gap recordings of nerve-evoked potentials in mammalian parasympathetic ganglia. *Brain Research* **208,** 446–451.

Hamill, O. P., Marty, A., Neher, E., Sakmann, B. & Sigworth, F. J. (1981) Improved patch-clamp techniques for high resolution current recording from cells and cell-free membrane patches. *Pflügers Archiv* **391,** 85–100.

Hartzell, H. C. (1981) Mechanisms of slow postsynaptic potentials. *Nature* **291,** 539–544.

Hartzell, H. C. (1988) Regulation of cardiac ion channels by catecholamines, acetylcholine and second messenger systems. *Progress in Biophysics and Molecular Biology* **52,** 165–247.

Hartzell, H. C., Kuffler, S. W., Stickgold, R. & Yoshikami, D. (1977) Synaptic excitation and inhibition resulting from direct action of acetylcholine on two types of chemoreceptors on individual amphibian parasympathetic neurones. *Journal of Physiology* **271,** 817–846.

Hildebrandt, J. D., Codina, J., Risinger, R. & Birnbaumer, L. (1984) Identification of a *gamma* subunit associated with the adenylyl cyclase regulatory proteins N_s and N_i. *Journal of Biological Chemistry* **259,** 2039–2042.

Hildebrandt, J. D., Sekura, R. D., Codina, J., Iyengar, R., Manclark, C. R. & Birnbaumer, L. (1983) Stimulation and inhibition of adenylyl cyclases is mediated by distinct proteins. *Nature* **302,** 706–709.

Hill-Smith, I. & Purves, R. D. (1978) Synaptic delay in the heart: An ionophoretic study. *Journal of Physiology* **270,** 31–54.

Hsu, W. H., Rudolph, N., Sanford, J. *et al.* (1990) Molecular cloning of a noval splice variant of the alpha sub-unit of the mammalian G_o protein. *Journal of Biological Chemistry* **265,** 11220–11226.

Hsu, W. H., Xiang, H., Rajan, A. S., Kunze, D. L. & Boyd, A. E. (1991) Somatostatin inhibits insulin secretion by a G-protein-mediated decrease in Ca^{2+} entry through voltage-dependent Ca^{2+} channels in the beta cell. *Journal of Biological Chemistry* **266,** 837–843.

Jones, D. T. & Reed, R. R. (1989) G_{olf}: An olfactory neuron specific-G protein involved in odorant signal transduction. *Science* **244,** 790–795,

Katada, T. & Ui, M. (1981) Islet-activating protein; a modifier of receptor-mediated regulation of rat islet adenylate cyclase. *Journal of Biological Chemistry* **256,** 8310–8317.

Kim, D., Lewis, D. L., Graziadei, L., Neer, E. J; Bar-Sagi, D. & Clapham, D. E. (1989) G protein $\beta\gamma$-subunits activate the cardiac muscarinic K-channel via phospholipase A_2. *Nature* **337,** 557–560.

Kirsch, G., Codina, J., Birnbaumer, L. & Brown, A. M. (1990) Coupling of ATP-sensitive K^+ channels to purinergic receptors by G-proteins in rat ventricular myocytes. *American Journal of Physiology* **259,** H820–H826.

Kirsch, G., Yatani, A., Codina, J., Birnbaumer, L. & Brown, A. M. (1988) The *alpha* subunit of G_k activates atrial K^+ channels of chick, rat and guinea pig. *American Journal of Physiology* **254** (*Heart Circulation Physiology* 23), H1200–H1205.

Kobayashi, I., Shibasaki, H., Tohyama, K., Kurachi, Y., Itoh, H., Ui, M. & Katada, T. (1990) Purification and characterization of five different α subunits of guanine nucleotide binding proteins in bovine brain membranes. Their physiological properties concerning the activities of adenylate cyclase and atrial muscarinic K^+ channels. *European Journal of Biochemistry* **191,** 499–506.

Kuehn, H. (1980) Light-induced, reversible binding of proteins to bovine photoreceptor membranes. Influence of nucleotides. *Neurochemistry* **1,** 269–285.

Kurachi, Y., Ito, H., Sugimoto, T., Katada,T. & Ui, M. (1989a) Activation of atrial muscarinic K^+ channels by low concentrations of $\beta\gamma$ subunits of G rat brain protein. *Pflügers Archiv* **413,** 325–327.

Kurachi, Y., Ito, H., Sugimoto, T., Shimizu, T., Miki, I. & Ui, M. (1989b) Arachidonic acid metabolites as intracellular modulators of the G protein-gated cardiac K⁺ channel. *Nature* **337**, 555–557.

Kurose, H. & Ui, M. (1983) Functional uncoupling of muscarinic receptors from adenylate cyclase in rat cardiac membranes by the active component of islet-activating protein, pertussis toxin. *Journal of Cyclic Nucleotide and Protein Phosphorylation Research* **9**, 305–318.

Levy, F. O., Gudermann, T., Perez-Reyes, E. Birnbaumer, M. & Birnbaumer, L. (1992) Molecular cloning of a human serotonin receptor (S12) with a pharmacological profile resembling that of SHT_{ID} subtype. *Journal of Biological Chemistry* **267**, 7553–7562.

Liao, C-F., Themmen, A. P. N., Joho, R., Barberis, C., Birnbaumer, M. & Birnbaumer, L. (1989) Molecular cloning and expression of a fifth muscarinic acetylcholine receptor (M5-mAChR). *Journal of Biological Chemistry* **264**, 7328–7337.

Litosch, I., Wallis, C. & Fain, J. N. (1985) 5-Hydroxytryptamine stimulates inositol phosphate production in a cell-free system from blowfly salivary glands. Evidence for a role of GTP in coupling receptor activation to phosphoinositide breakdown. *Journal of Biological Chemistry* **260**, 5464–5471.

Lochrie, M. A. & Simon, M. I. (1988) G protein multiplicity in eukaryotic signal transduction systems. *Biochemistry* **27**, 4957–4965.

Logothetis, D. E., Kim, D., Northup, J. K., Neer, E. J. & Clapham, D. E. (1988) Specificity of action of guanine nucleotide-binding regulatory protein subunits of the cardiac muscarinic K⁺ channel. *Proceedings of the National Academy of Sciences USA* **85**, 5814–5818.

Logothetis, D. E., Kurachi, Y., Galper, J., Neer, E. J. & Clapham, D. E. (1987) The $\beta\gamma$ subunits of GTP-binding proteins activate the muscarinic K⁺ channel in heart. *Nature* **325**, 321–236.

McFarland, K. C., Sprengel, R., Phillips, H. S., Köhler, M., Rosemblit, N., Nikolics, K., Segaloff, D. L. & Seeburg, P. H. (1989) Lutropin–choriogonadotropin receptor: An unusual member of the G protein-coupled receptor family. *Science* **245**, 494–528.

Manning, D. R. & Gilman, A. G. (1983) The regulatory components of adenylate cyclase and transducin. A family of structurally homologous guanine nucleotide-binding proteins. *Journal of Biological Chemistry* **258**, 7059–7063.

Mattera, R., Pitts, B. J. R., Entman, M. S. & Birnbaumer, L. (1985) Guanine nucleotide regulation of a mammalian myocardial receptor system. Evidence for homo- and heterotrophic cooperativity in ligand binding analyzed by computer assisted curve fitting. *Journal of Biological Chemistry* **260**, 7410–7421.

Mattera, R., Yatani, A., Kirsch, G. E., Graf, R., Olate, J., Codina, J., Brown, A. M. & Birnbaumer, L. (1988) Recombinant α_i-3 subunit of G protein activates G_k-gated K⁺ channels. *Journal of Biological Chemistry* **264**, 465–471.

Murad, F., Chi, Y.-M., Rall, T. W. & Sutherland, E. W. (1962) Adenyl cyclase. III. The effect of catecholamine and choline esters on the formation of adenosine 3′,5′-phosphate by preparations from cardiac muscle and liver. *Journal of Biological Chemistry* **237**, 1233–1238.

Murayama, T. & Ui, M. (1985) Receptor-mediated inhibition of adenylate cyclase and stimulation of arachidonic acid release in 3T3 fibroblasts. Selective susceptibility to islet-activating protein, pertussis toxin. *Journal of Biological Chemistry* **260**, 7226–7233.

Nakajima, Y., Nakajima, S., Leonard, R. J. & Yamagucchi, K. (1986) Acetylcholine raises excitability by inhibiting the fast transient potassium current in cultured hippocampal neurons. *Proceedings of the National Academy of Sciences USA* **83**, 3022–3026.

Nargeot, J., Nerbonne, J. M., Engels, J. & Lester, H. A. (1983) Time course of the increase in the myocardial slow inward current after a photochemically generated concentration jump of intracellular cAMP. *Proceedings of the National Academy of Sciences USA* **80,** 2395–2399.

Newberry, N. R. & Nicoll, R. A. (1984) Direct hyperpolarizing action of baclofen on hippocampal pyramidal cells. *Nature* **308,** 450–452.

Noma, A. (1983) ATP-regulated K⁺ channels in cardiac muscle. *Nature* **305,** 147–148.

Northup, J. K., Sternweis, P. C., Smigel, M. D., Schleifer, L. S., Ross, E. M. & Gilman, A. G. (1980) Purification of the regulatory component of adenylate cyclase. *Proceedings of the National Academy of Sciences USA* **77,** 6516–6520.

Northup, J. K., Smigel, M. D., Sternweis, P. C. & Gilman, A. G. (1983) The subunits of the stimulatory regulatory component of adenylate cyclase. Resolution of the activated 45 000-dalton (alpha) subunit. *Journal of Biological Chemistry* **258,** 11 369–11 376.

Okabe, K., Yatani, A., Evans, T., Ho, Y-K., Codina, J., Birnbaumer, L. & Brown, A. M. (1990) βγ dimers of G proteins inhibit muscarinic K⁺ channels in heart. *Journal of Biological Chemistry* **265,** 12 854–12 858.

Panten, U., Burgfeld, J., Goerke, F., Rennicke, M., Schwanstecher, M., Wallasch, A., Zunkler, B. J. & Zemen, S. (1989) Control of insulin secretion by sulfonylureas, meglitinide and diazoxide in relation to their binding to the sulfonylurea receptor in pancreatic cells. *Biochemical Pharmacology* **38,** 1217–1229.

Panten, U., Heipel, C., Rosenberger, F., Scheffer, K., Zunkler, B. J. & Schwarstecher, C. (1990) Tolbutamide-sensitivity of the adenosine 5′-triphosphate-dependent K⁺ channel in mouse pancreatic B-cells. *Naunyn-Schmiedeberg's Archives of Pharmacology* **342,** 566–574.

Peralta, E. G., Winslow, J. W., Peterson, G. L., Smith, D. H., Ashkenazi, A., Ramachandran, J., Schimerlik, M. I. & Capon, D. J. (1987) Primary structure and biochemical properties of an M₂ muscarinic receptor. *Science* **236,** 600–605.

Pfaffinger, P. J. , Martin, J.M., Hunter, D. D., Nathanson, N. M. & Hille, B. (1985) GTP-binding proteins couple cardiac muscarinic receptors to a K channel. *Nature* **317,** 536–538.

Ribalet, B. & Ciani, S. (1987) Regulation by cell metabolism and adenine nucleotides of a K channel in insulin-secreting B cells (RIN m5F). *Proceedings of the National Academy of Sciences USA* **84,** 1721–1725.

Ribalet, B. Ciani, S. & Eddlestone, G. T. (1989) Modulation of ATP-sensitive K channels in RINm5F cells by phosphorylation and G proteins. *Biophysical Journal* **55,** 587A.

Rodbell, M., Birnbaumer, L., Pohl, S. L. & Krans, H. M. J. (1971) The glucagon-sensitive adenyl cyclase system in plasma membranes of rat liver. V. An obligatory role of guanyl nucleotides in glucagon action. *Journal of Biological Chemistry* **246,** 1877–1882.

Rosenberger, L. B., Yamamura, H. L. & Roeske, W. R. (1980) Cardiac muscarinic cholinergic receptor binding is regulated by Na⁺ and guanyl nucleotides. *Journal of Biological Chemistry* **255,** 820–823.

Sasaki, K. & Sato, M. (1987) A single GTP-binding protein regulates K⁺-channels coupled with dopamine, histamine and acetylcholine receptors. *Nature* **325,** 259–262.

Schlegel, W., Wuarin, F., Zbaren, C. & Zahnd, G. R. (1985) Lowering of cytosolic free Ca²⁺ by carbachol, a muscarinic cholinergic agonist, in clonal pituitary cells (GH3 cells). *Endocrinology* **117,** 976–981.

Soejima, M. & Noma, A. (1984) Mode of regulation of the ACh-sensitive K-channel by the muscarinic receptor in rabbit atrial cells. *Pflügers Archiv* **400,** 424–431.

Thalmann, R. H. (1988) Evidence that guanosine triphosphate (GTP)-binding proteins control a synaptic response in brain: Effect of pertussis toxin and GTPγS on the late inhibitory postsynaptic potential of hippocampal CA_3 neurons. *Journal of Neuroscience* **8**, 4589–4602.

Tolkovsky, A. M. & Levitzki, A. (1978) Mode of coupling between the β-adrenergic receptor and adenylate cyclase in turkey erythrocytes. *Biochemistry* **17**, 3795–3810.

Trautwein, W. & Dudel, J. (1958) Zum Mechanismus der Membranwirkung des Acetylcholin an der Herzmuskelfaser. *Pflügers Archiv* **266**, 324–334.

Trautwein, W., Taniguchi, J. & Noma, A. (1982) The effect of intracellular cyclic nucleotides and calcium on the action potential and acetylcholine response of isolated cardiac cells. *Pflügers Archiv* **392**, 307–314.

VanDongen A., Codina, J., Olate, J., Mattera, R., Joho, R., Birnbaumer, L. & Brown, A. M. (1988) Newly identified brain potassium channels gated by the guanine nucleotide binding (G) protein G_o. *Science* **242**, 1433–1437.

Wheeler, G. L. & Bitensky, M. W. (1977) A light-activated GTPase in vertebrate photoreceptors: Regulation of light-activated cyclic GMP phosphodiesterase. *Proceedings of the National Academy of Sciences USA* **74**, 4238–4242.

Yatani, A., Codina, J., Brown, A. M. & Birnbaumer, L. (1987a) Direct activation of mammalian atrial muscarinic K channels by a human erythrocyte pertussis toxin-sensitive G protein, G_k. *Science* **235**, 207–211.

Yatani, A., Codina, J., Imoto, Y., Reeves, J. P., Birnbaumer, L. & Brown, A. M. (1987b) A G protein directly regulates mammalian cardiac calcium channels. *Science* **238**, 1288–1292.

Yatani, A., Codina, J., Sekura, R. D., Birnbaumer, L. & Brown, A. M. (1987c) Reconstitution of somatostatin and muscarinic receptor mediated stimulation of K^+ channels by isolated G_k protein in clonal rat anterior pituitary cell membranes. *Molecular Endocrinology* **1**, 283–289.

Yatani, A., Mattera, R., Codina, J., Graf, R., Okabe, K., Padrell, E., Iyengar, R., Brown, A. M. & Birnbaumer, L. (1988) The G protein-gated atrial K^+ channel is stimulated by three distinct G_i α-subunits. *Nature* **336**, 680–682.

Yatani, A., Okabe, K., Codina, J., Birnbaumer, L. & Brown, A. M. (1990) Heart rate regulation by G proteins acting on the cardiac pacemaker channel. *Science* **249**, 1163–1166.

Zunkler, B. J., Lins, S., Ohno-Shosaku, T., Trube, G. & Panten, U. (1988) Cytosolic ADP enhances the sensitivity to tolbutamide of ATP-dependent K^+ channels from pancreatic B-cells. *FEBS Letters* **239**, 241–244.

Zunkler, J. B., Trube, G. & Panten, U. (1989) How do sulfonylureas approach their receptor in the B-cell plasma membrane? *Naunyn-Schmiedeberg's Archives of Pharmacology* **340**, 328–332.

Chapter 5
High conductance calcium-activated potassium channels: molecular pharmacology, purification and regulation

M. L. Garcia and G. J. Kaczorowski

Introduction

General features of Ca^{2+} homeostasis

Many different cellular processes have evolved to regulate those signal transduction pathways in which Ca^{2+} is used as an intracellular mediator. In addition, these processes are necessary for efficiently controlling Ca^{2+} homeostasis. In electrically excitable tissues such as skeletal, cardiac and smooth muscles, as well as in neuroendocrine cells, a variety of well-defined ion transporting systems exists (Fig. 5.1). These include Ca^{2+} influx pathways (e.g. voltage and receptor-operated Ca-channels), Ca^{2+} efflux pathways (e.g. plasmalemmal Ca–ATPase and Na–Ca exchange), and Ca^{2+} sequestration mechanisms (e.g. organelles like the sarcoplasmic reticulum and mitochondria) which directly influence the concentration of free intracellular Ca^{2+}. Among those ion flux pathways which indirectly modulate Ca^{2+} homeostasis are K-channels. These channels provide a repolarization pathway for depolarized cells, and help maintain resting potential. If cells become hyperpolarized due to the opening of K-channels, Ca^{2+} influx through voltage-dependent channels is blunted and

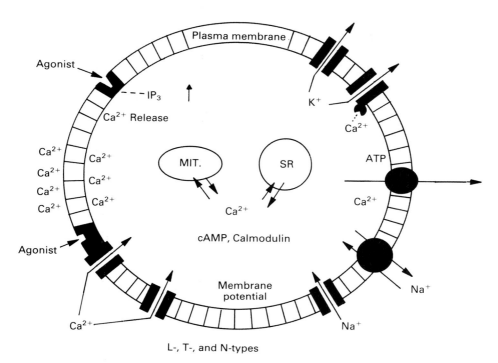

Fig. 5.1. Schematic view of pathways controlling cellular ion flux. In both electrically excitable and non-excitable cells, ion channels and transporters are signal transduction mechanisms; they modulate electrical patterns of activity and trigger the generation of second messengers (e.g. Ca^{2+}). In addition, these pathways control ionic homeostasis by keeping resting levels of Ca^{2+} low, and by maintaining Na^+ and K^+ gradients. MIT: mitochondria; SR: sarcoplasmic reticulum.

Ca^{2+} efflux through electrogenic Na–Ca exchange is stimulated leading to net overall lowering of cytoplasmic Ca^{2+} levels.

Ionic calcium-activated K-channels (channel designation, K_{Ca}; current $I_{K(Ca)}$) are distributed in a wide variety of both electrically excitable and non-excitable cells (Schwartz & Passow, 1983; Petersen & Maruyama, 1984; Blatz & Magleby, 1987). There are several distinct subtypes comprising this class of K-channel, and these differ in their single channel conductance, Ca^{2+}-sensitivity, voltage-dependency, and pharmacological properties. The most common distinguishing feature among this group is the unitary conductance of the channel which ranges from a few to several hundred picosiemens (pS).

The BK_{Ca}-channel

The so-called large conductance K_{Ca} also known as the maxi-K or BK channel (channel designation BK_{Ca}; current $I_{BK(Ca)}$) has a very large conductance (150–300 pS), and is maximally activated by both voltage and micromolar levels of Ca^{2+} (Latorre et al., 1989). Binding of this cation on the inner surface of the channel shifts the voltage dependency of gating and allows the channel to open at more negative membrane potentials. In the absence of other divalent cations, binding of 2–4 Ca^{2+} are required for channel opening. In the presence of millimolar levels of intracellular ionic magnesium (Mg^{2+}), the Hill coefficient for Ca^{2+} increases to 6, with a concomitant increase in Ca^{2+} affinity. BK_{Ca} channels are found in neurones, striated and smooth muscle, kidney tubules, the choroid plexus, blood cells such as platelets and B-lymphocytes, and in endocrine and exocrine glands. These channels are particularly abundant in many types of smooth muscle; e.g. vascular, airways, uterine, bladder and gastro-intestinal smooth muscle (Benham et al., 1985; Inoue et al., 1985; McCann & Welsh, 1986; Singer & Walsh, 1986; Williams et al., 1988; Kume et al., 1989; Kitamura et al., 1989; Hu et al., 1989; Klöckner et al., 1989; Vazquez et al., 1989; Toro et al., 1990). They are not present in cardiac tissue. Since BK_{Ca} channels function to repolarize cells following membrane depolariz-ation and elevation of intracellular Ca^{2+}, they have been implicated in regulation of neuroendocrine secretion, in control of muscle contractility, in movement of ions across epithelial tissues and in a variety of diverse cellular processes. One interesting feature of these channels is the com-bination of high conductance and extreme cation selectivity. Perhaps this large conductance is due to both the presence of fixed negative charges in the mouth of the channel which collect K^+, and the existence of a multi-ion pore (Latorre et al., 1989). The molecular pharmacology of BK_{Ca} is relatively undeveloped because of the paucity of selective high affinity probes for this protein. However, with the finding that crude venom of the Old-World scorpion Leiurus quinquestriatus would block this channel (Miller et al., 1985), it has become possible to discover and purify a number of unique high affinity peptidyl inhibitors and use these agents to characterize the biochemical, pharmacological and physiological proper-ties of BK_{Ca}. One such agent is charybdotoxin (ChTX), and the study of this toxin is largely responsible for our knowledge of the pharmacology of this large conductance K-channel.

IK_{Ca}- and SK_{Ca}-channels

A number of different intermediate to small conductance Ca^{2+}-activated K-channels exist and these can be broadly divided into two categories. voltage-dependent K-channels such as those found in neurones from Aplysia and Helix (channel designation IK_{Ca}; current $I_{IK(Ca)}$), voltage-independent K-channels present in muscle, erythrocytes and some sensory neurones (channel designation SK_{Ca}; current $I_{SK(Ca)}$). In general, these channels are very sensitive to levels of intracellular Ca^{2+}. The SK_{Ca}-channel present in rat skeletal muscle exhibits a conductance of 12 pS and accounts for the after-hyperpolarization in myotubes (Blatz & Magleby, 1986). It is very sensitive to inhibition by apamin, a peptidyl toxin isolated from bee venom (Habermann, 1972). Noteworthy is the fact that while apamin does not block high conductance BK_{Ca}-channels, ChTX will inhibit some smaller conductance K-channels. The latter toxin will block a 35 pS IK_{Ca} channel found in *Aplysia* neurones (Hermann & Erxleben, 1987) and a 40 pS IK_{Ca} present in red blood cells (Wolff *et al.*, 1988), although neither of these channels is sensitive to inhibition by apamin.

Voltage-dependent channels: K_A and K_V

Much information has recently been obtained regarding the structure and function of voltage-dependent K-channels (for example K_A and K_V; *see* Chapters 2 & 3). This has come largely through molecular biology efforts (Jan & Jan, 1990). With the cloning of the K-channel responsible for the '*Shaker*' phenotype in *Drosophila*, it has become possible to identify genes for other K-channels that share homology with *Shaker* through low stringency hybridization techniques (Temple *et al.*, 1988; Christie *et al.*, 1989; McKinnon, 1989; Stühmer *et al.*, 1989). Expression cloning has also been used to identify novel voltage-dependent K-channels (Takumi *et al.*, 1988; Frech *et al.*, 1989; Folander *et al.*, 1990; Pragnell *et al.*, 1990). However, limited structural information is available for K_{Ca}-channels since these have not been successfully identified by low stringency hybridization protocols, and they have been difficult to expression clone (Ashcroft *et al.*, 1988; Lu *et al.*, 1990). Although some similarities may exist in the pharmacological properties of individual members from these classes of channel, significant differences in primary structure must undoubtedly be present. If this issue cannot be resolved using molecular biology techniques, then biochemical approaches must be employed to purify the target protein of interest to homogeneity and define its molecular characteristics. With the advent of toxin probes for K_{Ca}-channels such a strategy has become possible. This review will focus on studies directed at developing the molecular pharmacology of the high conductance BK_{Ca} of smooth muscle, purification of the protein and assessment of its role in the physiology of selected smooth muscle tissues. Similar studies have been attempted with the apamin-sensitive SK_{Ca}-channel (for a review see Garcia *et al.*, 1991), but they will not be the subject of this report.

Molecular pharmacology of BK_{Ca}

Use of ChTX as a probe for BK_{Ca} and other channels

Venom derived from the scorpion *Leiurus quinquestriatus* var. *hebraeus* contains many distinct peptidyl modulators of voltage-dependent Na- and K-channels. The active component of *Leiurus* venom which inhibits K_{Ca} is ChTX (Miller *et al.*, 1985), and this venom was originally shown to block the high conductance BK_{Ca} present in mammalian skeletal muscle when added at the external surface of the channel. Charybdotoxin inhibition of BK_{Ca} is characterized by records in which bursts of channel activity are interdispersed between periods when the channel is quiescent. During these bursts of activity, gating kinetics and unitary conductance appear normal. Therefore, the silent periods have been interpreted as times when toxin is bound to the channel and blocks the ion conduction pathway. Since ChTX binding is a completely reversible reaction, dissociation of toxin allows normal channel activity to resume because channel gating kinetics are faster than toxin association. Charybdotoxin binding to BK_{Ca} can be described as a bimolecular reaction because the average blocked time of the channel is independent of toxin concentration, while the average time the channel spends in the active state is inversely proportional to the concentration of ChTX (Smith *et al.*, 1986).

Purification and synthesis of ChTX

Charybdotoxin has been purified to homogeneity from crude scorpion venom by a number of different laboratories all using combinations of ion exchange and reversed-phase chromatographic techniques (Gimenez-Gallego *et al.*, 1988; Valdivia *et al.*, 1988; Luchesi *et al.*, 1989; Strong *et al.*, 1989; Schweitz *et al.*, 1989a). The complete 37 amino acid primary structure of this toxin has been deduced by amino acid sequence analysis (Gimenez-Gallego *et al.*, 1988), and later confirmed by three independent laboratories (Luchesi *et al.*, 1989; Strong *et al.*, 1989; Schweitz *et al.*, 1989a). This consensus structure differs from that of a previously-reported partial sequence of the carboxyl (C)-terminus of the toxin (Valdivia *et al.*, 1988). Charybdotoxin is a 4.3 kDa, highly basic peptide (i.e. overall net charge of $+5$ at physiological pH) which has a blocked amino (N)-terminus in the form of pyroglutamic acid and six cysteine residues (Fig. 5.2). The N-terminal residue can be removed by treatment with pyroglutamate aminopeptidase, and this allows sequence determination by automated Edman degradation. The highly basic nature of ChTX is due to the presence of four lysine, three arginine and one histidine residue, with only a single glutamic acid moiety. These basic residues play an important role in the mechanism by which ChTX inhibits BK_{Ca} activity (see below).

Recently, two laboratories have reported the chemical synthesis of ChTX (Sugg *et al.*, 1990b; Lambert *et al.*, 1990). In the study by Sugg *et al.*, this synthesis was accomplished using a solid phase Fluorenyl methyloxy carbonyl (FMOC) pentafluorophenyl ester methodology. Oxidation of the synthetic peptide yields biologically active material which is indistin-

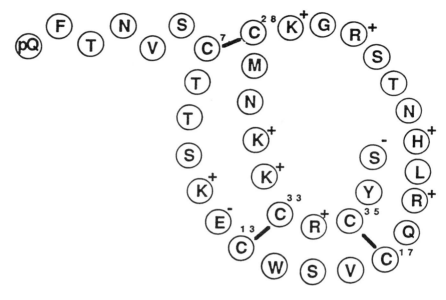

Fig. 5.2. Structure of ChTX. Proposed secondary structure of ChTX indicating the assignment of the three disulphide bonds in the toxin as determined after enzymatic digestion of oxidized peptide. (Reprinted with permission from Sugg *et al.* (1990) *Journal of Biological Chemistry* **265**, 18 745–18 748.)

guishable from native toxin. Further proof that the synthetic material has folded properly is provided by proteolytic digestion experiments with oxidized material which produce identical patterns for synthetic and native ChTX. These peptide fragments were isolated and used to assign the three disulphide bridges in ChTX (i.e. Cys_7–Cys_{28}, Cys_{13}–Cys_{33} and Cys_{17}–Cys_{35}) by analysis of their respective amino acid contents (Fig. 5.2). Since data obtained from both species are indistinguishable, the synthetic toxin must have folded properly. The experimentally-derived disulphide bonding pattern differs from one previously postulated by Gimenez-Gallego *et al.* (1988), which was based on sequence homologies between ChTX and α-bungarotoxin, a peptide blocker of the acetylcholine receptor whose 3-dimensional X-ray structure is known. The current prediction is that ChTX is a highly compact structure with clusters of positively charged residues and a C-terminus which is buried within the peptide. Such a model is consistent with the poor reactivity of the C-terminal carboxyl group, and also with the difficulties encountered in iodinating Tyr^{36} (Vazquez *et al.*, 1989), the penultimate residue from the C-terminal end of the peptide. This notion is also consistent with the solution structure of ChTX predicted from nuclear magnetic resonance (NMR) experiments, although there are some differences in the model structure proposed in two independent studies (Lambert *et al.*, 1990; Massefski *et al.*, 1990).

Types of ion channel susceptible to ChTX

Charybdotoxin has been investigated for its ability to inhibit a number of different types of ion channels. It has no affect on Na- or Ca-channels (Miller *et al.*, 1985; Hermann & Erxleben, 1987; Gimenez-Gallego *et al.*, 1988; Sands *et al.*, 1989), but does inhibit BK_{Ca} with nM-range potency in a wide variety of tissues, including skeletal muscle (Anderson *et al.*, 1988; Valdivia *et al.*, 1988), cultured kidney epithelia (Guggino *et al.*, 1987), aortic smooth muscle (Vazquez *et al.*, 1989), GH_3 anterior pituitary cells (Gimenez-Gallego *et al.*, 1988) and brain (Reinhart *et al.*, 1989). The K_i for block of channel activity is typically approximately 2 nM under conditions of normal physiological salt concentrations (Gimenez-Gallego *et al.*, 1988). In the study with brain where four types of K_{Ca} were detected after incorporating synaptic plasma membrane vesicles into planar lipid bilayers (Reinhart *et al.*, 1989), three channels were blocked (i.e. 242, 135 and 76 pS K_{Ca} channels monitored in symmetrical 150 mM K^+), whilst the fourth (236 pS) was insensitive to ChTX. This is the only BK_{Ca}-channel reported to be insensitive to ChTX. The selectivity of ChTX as an inhibitor of BK_{Ca} has been challenged (Schweitz *et al.*, 1989b). However, to date this toxin has been shown to block only one other class of K-channel; namely, an inactivating, voltage-dependent K-channel of the K_V type present in neurones (Christie *et al.*, 1989; Schneider *et al.*, 1989; Schweitz *et al.*, 1989b) and T-lymphocytes (Sands *et al.*, 1989; Price *et al.*, 1989). It has no effect on other types of K-channel (e.g. cardiac delayed or inwardly rectifying K-channels, adenosine triphosphate (ATP)-sensitive K-channels, neuronal A-type K-channels), especially the channel responsible for the *Shaker* phenotype in *Drosophila* (Oliva *et al.*, 1991) or the apamin-sensitive SK_{Ca} (Pennefather *et al.*, 1989).* This last point has caused some confusion since reports are present in the literature that ChTX will inhibit the *Shaker* and SK_{Ca} channels (MacKinnon *et al.*, 1988, 1990; Goh & Pennefather, 1987). However, the effects observed by these workers are due to contaminants in the ChTX preparations used since synthetic ChTX does not possess these properties.

Inhibition of BK_{Ca} by ChTX: mechanistic studies

The mechanism by which ChTX inhibits BK_{Ca} has been the subject of intense study. Most experiments have been carried out with channels from skeletal muscle reconstituted into artificial lipid bilayers (Anderson *et al.*,

*The view that blockade of voltage-dependent K-channels by ChTX is restricted to K_V-type channels may be controversial (*see* Chapter 11).

1988; MacKinnon & Miller, 1988). Measurements of toxin association and dissociation kinetics indicate that ChTX binding is voltage-dependent and influenced by the conformational state of the channel. Charybdotoxin binds to both open and closed states of BK_{Ca} but its affinity is higher for the open state, and this is reflected by an increase of sevenfold in the association rate of the peptide. Depolarization of the membrane enhances toxin dissociation rates by e-fold per 28 mV, but association kinetics are not affected by voltage if the channel's open probability is maintained constant as variations are made in the voltage parameter. Toxin association kinetics are highly dependent on the ionic strength of the medium, and decrease by 2 orders of magnitude when salt concentrations are increased from 20 to 300 mM. These results suggest that negatively charged residues are located within the ChTX receptor on BK_{Ca}. The effects of voltage on ChTX dissociation kinetics are not direct, but rather are related to its effects on K^+ entering the channel from the internal medium. Binding of K^+ at a site located along the ion conduction pathway destabilizes ChTX at its receptor. As the internal K^+ concentration is increased, dissociation of ChTX increases, and as the membrane is depolarized, internal K^+ more effectively promotes toxin dissociation. Other channel substrates such as Rb^+ behave in a similar fashion, while impermeant ions like Na^+, Li^+, and Cs^+ do not. These data have been used to propose a model for toxin inhibition of BK_{Ca} in which ChTX binds to acidic amino acid residues at the external pore of the channel to block the ion conduction pathway by direct physical occlusion.

Such a model is supported by two different lines of evidence. First, when the effects of externally applied tetraethylammonium ion (TEA) were monitored on ChTX blocking kinetics, it was found that TEA and ChTX behave as competitive blockers of BK_{Ca} (Miller, 1988). In these experiments, TEA affected the association kinetics of ChTX in exact proportion to its blocking of single channel currents, but had no effect on toxin dissociation kinetics. Because the TEA binding site is located at the external pore of the ion conduction pathway (Villarroel et al., 1988), it follows that the ChTX receptor is similarly placed. Second, in an effort to demonstrate that negatively charged residues comprise the ChTX binding site, chemical modification of amino acid side chains on BK_{Ca} was attempted with the carboxyl group selective reagent trimethyloxonium (TMO) ion, which esterifies free carboxyl functionalities with a methyl group (MacKinnon & Miller, 1989; MacKinnon et al., 1989). Alkylation of BK_{Ca} by TMO results in decreased single channel conductance, a shift in the voltage activation curve to more depolarized potentials and a pronounced reduction in the affinity of ChTX. As an indication of specificity, the effects of TMO are prevented if BK_{Ca} is treated with a methylating reagent in the presence of toxin. Moreover, modification by TMO not only causes a reduction of the k_1 of ChTX, but also significantly reduces the ionic

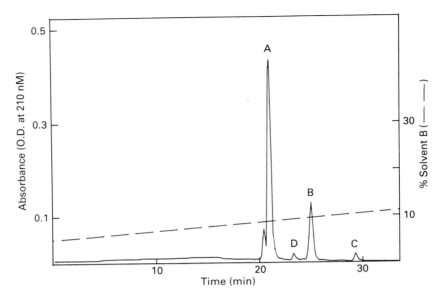

Fig. 5.3. High performance liquid chromatography profile of ChTX after iodination. The ChTX was subjected to iodination by employing the Iodo-Gen method. The iodination mixture was injected onto a C_{18} reversed-phase column and eluted in the presence of a linear gradient of organic solvent. The migration of various iodinated derivatives of ChTX is indicated: A, ChTX; B, monoiodotyrosine ChTX; C, mono-iodohistidine ChTX; D, diiodotyrosine ChTX. (Reprinted with permission from Vazquez *et al.* (1989) *Journal of Biological Chemistry* **264**, 20 902–20 909.)

strength dependency for toxin inhibition of channel activity. These findings imply that surface charges in the mouth of BK_{Ca} attract ChTX through an electrostatic interaction.

ChTX contains a single Tyr penultimate from its C-terminus, and this residue is a potential site for iodination. Using protocols employing either Iodo-Gen or lactoperoxidase/glucose oxidase methods, it has been possible to radiolabel ChTX with $Na^{125}I$ to high specific activity (Vazquez *et al.*, 1989; Luchesi *et al.*, 1989). In one study (Vazquez *et al.*, 1989), monoiodinated toxin was separated from the other products of the reaction mixture by reversed phase high-performance liquid chromato-graphy (HPLC) techniques (Fig. 5.3). Sequence analysis showed that the purified species was the monoiodotyrosine adduct of the peptide, and monoiodotyrosine–ChTX was demonstrated to block BK_{Ca} in excised outside-out patches from bovine aortic smooth muscle by a mechanism identical to that of native toxin (Fig. 5.4). However, the potency of this modified ChTX is reduced approximately 10-fold, and inhibition of channel activity requires the patch to be bathed in a medium of low ionic strength. These characteristics do not make it difficult to analyse toxin binding in intact cells or isolated membrane vesicles provided such studies are carried out at reduced ionic strength. It was found that separation of the monoiodotyrosine species from the other reaction products was critical for subsequent binding studies, since both the diiodotyrosine and monoiodohistidine toxin adducts have lost biological activity. This could account for some reports which have claimed that the binding activity of $[^{125}I]$ChTX is poor or non-existent (Harvey *et al.*, 1989; Luchesi *et al.*, 1989; Schweitz *et al.*, 1989a). It is also noteworthy that monoiodotyrosine–ChTX will interact differently with various species of K_{Ca}, since the affinity of $[^{125}I]$ChTX for the channel from rabbit skeletal muscle T-tubular membranes is reduced (M. L. Garcia & S. Fleischer, unpublished observations). Perhaps iodination of the toxin disrupts its tertiary structure, which in turn, interferes with the binding of ChTX to its target. Nevertheless, this radiolabelled probe has been very useful for the biochemical characterization of BK_{Ca} in smooth muscle, as well as for studying a different ChTX-sensitive voltage-dependent K-channel present in brain (Vazquez *et al.*, 1990) and T-lymphocytes (Deutsch *et al.*, 1991; Slaughter *et al.*, 1991).

Smooth muscle as a source of BK_{Ca}

Since smooth muscle is a rich source of BK_{Ca}, study of this channel has been facilitated by the isolation of a highly purified sarcolemmal membrane vesicle preparation from both bovine aorta (Slaughter *et al.*, 1989) and bovine trachea (Slaughter *et al.*, 1987). Marker enzyme studies clearly indicate that these membranes are of sarcolemmal origin (e.g. they are enriched in Na–Ca exchange, β-adrenoreceptor, Na, K–ATPase and L-type Ca-channel activities), and ChTX-sensitive BK_{Ca} have been observed following incorporation of these vesicles into planar lipid bilayers. When aortic membranes are incubated with $[^{125}I]$ChTX, radio-labelled toxin binds in a time- and concentration-dependent fashion to a single class of receptors (Fig. 5.5). These sites display a K_d of 100 pM and a B_{max} of 0.5 pmol/mg protein under defined experimental conditions (Vazquez *et al.*, 1989). Since this membrane preparation is an equal mixture of inside-out and outside-out vesicles, addition of small quantities of digitonin to permeabilize the membrane increases maximal binding by twofold, consistent with the idea that ChTX binds only at the external pore of BK_{Ca}. Toxin binding is a reversible bimolecular reaction and measurement of k_1 and k_{-1} values yields data similar to those determined in electrophysiological experiments, as well as allows calculation of a K_d that is identical to the one determined under equilibrium conditions. The other characteristics of binding are also consistent with the postulate that ChTX receptors in smooth muscle sarcolemma represent BK_{Ca}. Thus, the binding reaction is sensitive to metal ions which are known to bind at various loci along the ion conduction pathway of the channel, as well as to the ionic strength of the incubation medium. In addition, the quater-

nary ammonium ion TEA inhibits ChTX binding in an apparently competitive fashion, but similar agents like tetrabutylammonium ion (TBA),
which blocks K_V rather than BK_{Ca} activity, do not influence the interaction
of toxin with its receptor, as would be expected. Moreover, toxins which
have no effect on BK_{Ca} (e.g. noxiustoxin, leiurotoxin, α-dendrotoxin) do
not affect ChTX binding in smooth muscle, whilst other toxins which
inhibit BK_{Ca} (e.g. iberiotoxin, *see below*) block ChTX binding in this tissue
(Fig. 5.6). Therefore, [^{125}I]ChTX receptors in aortic sarcolemma display
the properties expected for sites associated with BK_{Ca}. Identical high
affinity sites exist in tracheal smooth muscle sarcolemmal membranes
(Slaughter *et al.*, 1988), whilst receptors with slightly different properties
are found in membrane vesicles prepared from porcine uterus (M. L.
Garcia, L. Toro & E. Stefani, unpublished observations). Taken together,
these data provide a convincing argument that [^{125}I]ChTX can be used to
monitor BK_{Ca} and to develop the molecular pharmacology of this channel
in smooth muscle.

Interaction of ChTX with K_V

A distinct class of receptor sites for ChTX which displays unique biochemical and pharmacological properties has been discovered in brain
synaptic plasma membrane vesicles (Schweitz *et al.*, 1989a; Vazquez *et al.*,
1990), as well as in human T-lymphocytes and related cell lines (Deutsch
et al., 1991; Slaughter *et al.*, 1991). The binding properties of these sites
indicate that they are associated with K_V. When cells, or vesicles isolated
from these sources are incubated with [^{125}I]ChTX under low ionic strength
conditions, there is a time- and concentration-dependent association of
toxin with the membrane. Equilibrium-binding analyses indicate that a
single class of receptors exists which displays a K_d of approximately
10–30 pM (Fig. 5.7). The receptor density in purified rat brain synaptic
plasma membranes is 0.3–0.5 pmol/mg protein, whilst there are approximately 500 sites per human T-lymphocyte. Toxin interaction is completely
reversible and the affinity for ChTX measured under equilibrium conditions is identical to that calculated based on the kinetics of toxin association and dissociation. Binding of [^{125}I]ChTX is modulated by metal ions

---

Fig. 5.4. (*Opposite*) Effect of monoiodotyrosine ChTX on BK_{Ca} activity in bovine
aorta. A single high conductance Ca^{2+}-activated K-channel was recorded in an outside-
out excized membrane patch from a bovine aortic smooth muscle cell. A, Control
recording; B, after addition of 10 nM I-ChTX; C, histograms representing channel
mean open time in either control (*upper*), or in the presence of I-ChTX (*lower*), are
shown and indicate that modified toxin has no affect on this parameter. A smaller
conductance channel which is not blocked by ChTX is also shown to indicate specificity in the action of iodinated toxin. (Reprinted with permission from Vazquez *et
al.* (1989) *Journal of Biological Chemistry* **264**, 20 902–20 909.)

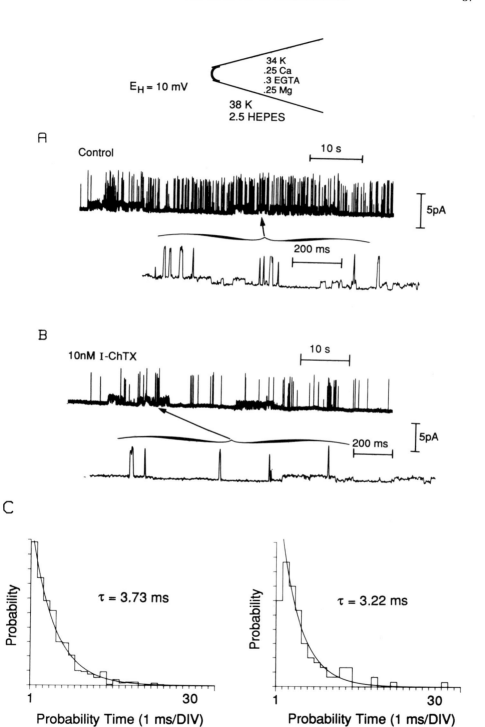

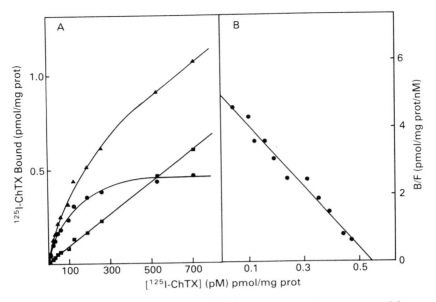

Fig. 5.5. Binding of monoiodotyrosine ChTX to sarcolemmal membrane vesicles from bovine aortic smooth muscle. A, Membranes were incubated with increasing concentrations of [^{125}I]ChTX, until equilibrium was achieved; ($\blacktriangle$) total binding ($\blacksquare$) non-specific binding determined in the presence of 10 nM ChTX, and ($\bullet$) specific binding are represented. B, Specific binding data from (A) are presented in the form of a Scatchard representation; K_d = 100 pM, B_{max} = 0.53 pM/mg protein. (Reprinted with permission from Vazquez *et al.* (1989) *Journal of Biological Chemistry* **264**, 20 902–20 909.)

which interact with K-channels, but the spectrum of activity is different from that determined with BK_{Ca}. Hence, some ions (e.g. Ba^{2+}) inhibit ChTX binding to both channels, whilst other ions (e.g. K^+, Na^+) block the interaction of ChTX with BK_{Ca} due to ionic strength effects, but cause stimulation of binding to K_V via an allosteric mechanism (Fig. 5.8). Interestingly, TEA has no effect on toxin binding in this system, whilst TBA displays inhibitory activity. Different toxins that are known inhibitors of K_V [e.g. noxiustoxin (NxTX), leiurotoxin and α-dendrotoxin (αDaTX)] block [^{125}I]ChTX binding, but other toxin inhibitors of BK_{Ca} [e.g. iberiotoxin (IbTX), *see below*] do not (Fig. 5.6). The inhibition of ChTX binding noted with various peptides results from allosteric interactions between separate binding sites for these agents and the ChTX receptor. Taken together, these data support the idea that [^{125}I]ChTX can be used to define regions on both BK_{Ca} and K_V and it is therefore useful as a biochemical probe for investigating different types of K-channel in a variety of target tissues. A comparison of the properties of ChTX binding to BK_{Ca} and K_V is shown in Table 5.1. Although BK_{Ca} are quite prevalent in neuronal tissue, there is no indication that [^{125}I]ChTX recognizes this

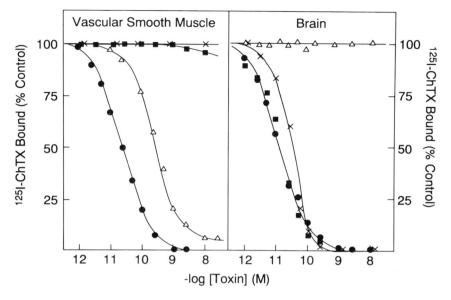

Fig. 5.6. Effect of different peptide toxins on ChTX binding to bovine aortic smooth muscle sarcolemmal and rat brain synaptic plasma membrane vesicles. Smooth muscle membranes (*left panel*) or brain membranes (*right panel*) were incubated with [^{125}I]ChTX in the absence, or presence, of increasing concentrations of either ChTX (●), NxTX (■), IbTX (△), or α-DaTX (×), until equilibrium was achieved. Inhibition of binding was assessed, in each case, relative to an untreated control.

site in the rat brain synaptic plasma membrane preparation that was investigated (Vazquez *et al.*, 1990). Perhaps either the site density of BK$_{Ca}$ in this preparation is low, or the neuronal high conductance BK$_{Ca}$ does not efficiently bind iodinated toxin.

Other blockers of BK$_{Ca}$ and K$_V$

Iberiotoxin

In an effort to identify other selective peptidyl modulators of BK$_{Ca}$ a wide variety of scorpion, spider and snake venoms were tested for their ability to influence ChTX binding to smooth muscle sarcolemma. Several venoms from different scorpion species have been discovered which display this property (Galvez *et al.*, 1990; Novick *et al.*, 1991). One such material is derived from the scorpion *Buthus tamulus*, and this extract potently blocks [^{125}I]ChTX binding to bovine aortic sarcolemmal membranes (Galvez *et al.*, 1990). This venom has been fractionated on a Mono S cation exchange FPLC (fast performance liquid chromatography) column and inhibitory activity is found in two well-separated regions. The less basic component has been purified to homogeneity by reversed phase HPLC and shown to

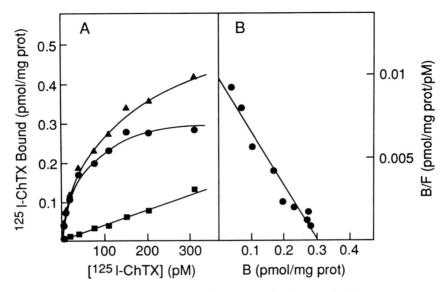

Fig. 5.7. Binding of monoiodotyrosine ChTX to rat brain synaptic plasma membrane vesicles. A, Brain membranes were incubated with increasing concentrations of [^{125}I]ChTX until equilibrium was achieved; (▲) total binding; (■) nonspecific binding determined in the presence of 10 nM ChTX, and (●) specific binding are represented. B, Specific binding data from (A) are presented in the form of a Scatchard representation; $K_d = 29$ pM, $B_{max} = 0.3$ pM/mg protein. (Reprinted with permission from Vazquez et al. (1990) *Journal of Biological Chemistry* **265**, 15 564–15 571.)

be a 4.3 kDa peptide. The primary structure of this peptide, IbTX, has been determined by sequence analysis (Fig. 5.9). It is 68% homologous with ChTX, but it has one less basic and four more acidic amino acid residues than the latter peptide, giving it an overall charge of +1. Interestingly, IbTX has a much different biological profile than ChTX. This peptide is a partial inhibitor of [^{125}I]ChTX binding to smooth muscle, and the extent of inhibition depends on the K$^+$ concentration of the incubation medium. A Scatchard analysis of these effects indicates that IbTX is a non-competitive inhibitor; it decreases the receptor density of ChTX, with no effect on toxin affinity. In addition, there are some differences in the blocking properties of both toxins as determined in single channel recordings of BK$_{Ca}$ reconstituted into planar lipid bilayers (Giangiacomo et al., 1991a; Candia et al., 1991). The association rate constant for IbTX is slower than that of ChTX, and channel block is long-lasting, due to decreased k_{-1}. Moreover, the ionic strength dependency of IbTX for blocking BK$_{Ca}$ is not as pronounced as that for ChTX. These results suggest that either ChTX and IbTX bind to different sites on the channel or that the kinetics of the interaction between IbTX and BK$_{Ca}$ are signifi-

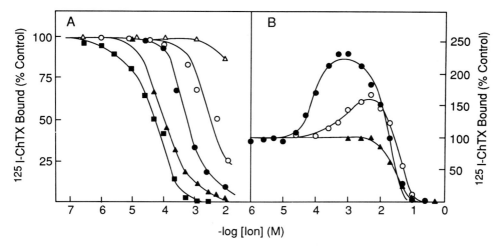

Fig. 5.8. Effects of ions on monoiodotyrosine ChTX binding to rat brain synaptic plasma membrane vesicles. Membrane vesicles were incubated with [^{125}I]ChTX in the absence, or presence, of increasing concentrations of : A, either BaCl$_2$ (■), CsCl (▲), CaCl$_2$ (●), TBA (○) or TEA (△); B, either KCl (●), NaCl (○) or LiCl (▲), at room temperature until equilibrium was achieved. Specific binding data in each case are presented relative to an untreated control. (Reprinted with permission from Vazquez *et al.* (1990) *Journal of Biological Chemistry* **265**, 15 564–15 571.)

Table 5.1. Comparison of [^{125}I]ChTX binding to BK$_{Ca}$- and K$_V$-channels.

	BK$_{Ca}$	K$_V$
K_d ([^{125}I]ChTX)	100 pm	30 pm
K_i (K$^+$)	17 μm	100 μm (K_S)
K_i (Ba^{2+})	12 μm	25 μm
K_i (Cs$^+$)	100 μm	50 μm
K_i (Na$^+$)	20 mm	1 mm (K_S)
K_i (TEA)	100 μm	No effect
K_i (TBA)	No effect	2.5 mm
K_i (ChTX)	10–20 pm	8–10 pm
K_i (IbTX)	250 pm	No effect
K_i (NxTX)	No effect	8 pm
K_i (αDaTX)	No effect	20 pm

Both binding reactions are sensitive to the ionic strength of the medium.
K_d values (dissociation constants) were determined from the slope of a linear transformation of data from saturation binding studies with [^{125}I]ChTX, while K_i and K_S values (inhibitory and stimulatory constants, respectively) were determined from competition experiments with iodinated toxin as described in Vazquez *et al.* (1989, 1990).

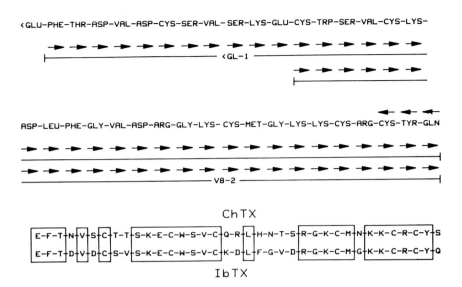

‹GLU—PHE—THR—ASP—VAL—ASP—CYS—SER—VAL— SER—LYS—GLU—CYS—TRP—SER—VAL—CYS—LYS—

‹GL–1

ASP—LEU—PHE—GLY—VAL—ASP—ARG—GLY—LYS— CYS—MET—GLY—LYS—LYS—CYS—ARG—CYS—TYR—GLN

V8–2

ChTX

| E-F-T | N | V | S | C | T-T | S-K-E-C-W-S-V-C | Q-R | L | H-N-T-S | R-G-K-C-M | N | K-K-C-R-C-Y | S |
| E-F-T | D | V | D | C | S-V | S-K-E-C-W-S-V-C | K-D | L | F-G-V-D | R-G-K-C-M | G | K-K-C-R-C-Y | Q |

IbTX

Fig. 5.9. Amino acid sequence determination of IbTX. A homogeneous preparation of IbTX was digested with various proteases; GL and V8 numbers refer to pyroglutaminase and *S. aureus* V8 protease-generated peptides, respectively. All residues identified by N-terminal sequence determination using Edman degradation techniques are denoted by single-headed arrows pointing to the right. Residues identified at the C-terminus by timed digestion with carboxypeptidase A are denoted by single-headed arrows pointing to the left. A comparison between the primary structures of IbTX and ChTX is also shown.

cantly different from those of ChTX, making IbTX appear to be a noncompetitive inhibitor under the conditions of the binding experiments.

The most interesting property of IbTX is that it is highly selective for BK_{Ca}. In voltage-clamp experiments with GH_3 cells, IbTX has no effect on Na-, Ca- (neither T- nor L-type), or A-type K-currents, although it completely abolishes currents due to BK_{Ca}. Furthermore, IbTX does not affect other K_V channels which are sensitive to inhibition by ChTX. Thus, IbTX does not block binding of $[^{125}I]$ChTX to K_V in either brain (Vazquez *et al.*, 1990) or lymphocytes (Deutsch *et al.*, 1991; Slaughter *et al.*, 1991), nor does it affect currents due to K_V in these preparations (M. L. Garcia, C. Deutsch & J. Reuben, unpublished observations). Iberiotoxin also has no effect on the current expressed after injecting the *Shaker* H4 clone into *Xenopus* oocytes. To date, the high conductance BK_{Ca} is the only target detected for IbTX, although this toxin has not been rigorously examined on all different types of K_{Ca}.

This finding potentially makes IbTX a unique tool with which to investigate the physiological role of BK_{Ca}. Unfortunately, all attempts so far to iodinate IbTX have resulted in material which is biologically inactive. Perhaps this situation can be rectified by producing radiolabelled toxin either through solid phase synthesis (Sugg *et al.*, 1990a), or by biosynthetic approaches. It is interesting to note that crude *B. tamulus* venom has been reported to block K_V in Jurkat cells, a human lymphoma cell line (Sands *et al.*, 1989). However, this activity is not associated with IbTX, but rather with the second more basic component of *B. tamulus* venom that inhibits [^{125}I]ChTX binding in aortic sarcolemmal membranes. This peptide has been purified to homogeneity using reversed phase HPLC and shown to block K_V in lymphocytes (M. L. Garcia & C. Deutsch, unpublished observations), although it has yet to be subjected to sequence analysis.

Limbatotoxin and margotoxin

Recently, another source of K-channel inhibitors has been discovered in venoms from several different New World scorpions of the genus *Centruroides* (Novick *et al.*, 1991). Using [^{125}I]ChTX binding to either BK_{Ca} in smooth muscle or K_V in brain as an assay, activities have been identified in *Centruroides limbatus, C. bi-color* and *C. margaritatus* venoms. In analogy with the purification procedures used for ChTX and IbTX, these activities have been fractionated using combined ion exchange FPLC and reversed phase HPLC techniques. Two peptides have been purified to homogeneity and their primary amino acid sequences were determined. One peptide, termed limbatotoxin (LiTX), isolated from *C. limbatus* displays extensive sequence homology with both ChTX and IbTX. Like IbTX, this toxin blocks [^{125}I]ChTX binding to BK_{Ca} but not to K_V. Furthermore, it is a potent inhibitor of BK_{Ca} as determined in single channel experiments, but it has no effect on K_V (i.e. the K_V3 clone) expressed in *Xenopus* oocytes (*see* Chapter 2 for further details of the K_V3 clones). Limbatotoxin displays a charge density between ChTX and IbTX (i.e. $+3$), has an acidic residue in its 24th position similar to IbTX, and Gly (present in IbTX) is substituted for Asn (present in ChTX) at the 30th position amino acid of the polypeptide. These two substitutions apparently confer IbTX-like behaviour onto LiTX. The other toxin, named margotoxin (MaTX), was purified from *C. margaritatus* venom. It does not affect either [^{125}I]ChTX binding to smooth muscle or BK_{Ca} in single channel recordings, but potently blocks [^{125}I]ChTX binding in brain and T-lymphocytes, as well as inhibits K_V (i.e. K_V3) expressed in the *Xenopus* system. A comparison between the primary structures of MaTX and ChTX indicates significant sequence homology in the C-terminal 12 residues, but the N-terminus of MaTX resembles more the sequence of NxTX isolated from *Centruroides noxius*, rather than the N-terminal sequence of ChTX (Fig. 5.10). This finding correlates with the observation that noxiustoxin is a selective inhibitor of K_V (Swanson *et al.*, 1990). Thus, two new toxins have been identified which may be useful for determining

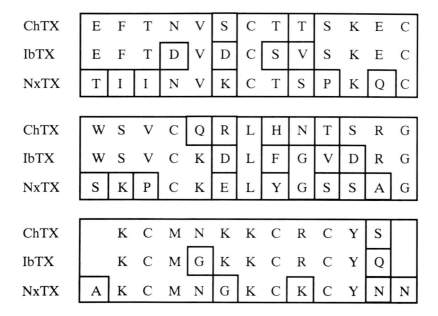

Fig. 5.10. Primary amino acid sequences and homologies between three different K-channel toxin inhibitors. The primary amino acid sequences of ChTX, IbTX and NxTX are compared; there are 68, 44 and 38% sequence homology between ChTX–IbTX, ChTX–NxTX and IbTX–NxTX, respectively.

the structural properties of receptor sites on BK_{Ca} and K_V, as well as for helping to elucidate which residues in a specific toxin molecule are important for its specificity and function. These agents also provide a battery of probes for defining the physiological role of a given ion channel in intact tissues. Similar purification studies with the venom from *C. bi-color* have led to the identification of another peptide which, like ChTX, recognizes both BK_{Ca} and K_V, but this toxin has yet to be subjected to primary structure determination.

Active sites on ChTX and IbTX

To determine which peptidyl-regions of ChTX and IbTX dictate the ChTX-like or IbTX-like behaviour observed for their interaction with BK_{Ca} and K_V, a synthetic strategy was employed (Sugg *et al.*, 1990a). Hybrid peptides containing the first 19 residues of one toxin spliced to the final 18 residues of the other toxin were synthesized and evaluated by combined receptor binding and electrophysiological techniques. The hybrid $IbTX_{1-19}ChTX_{20-37}$ blocks $[^{125}I]ChTX$ binding to both BK_{Ca} in smooth muscle sarcolemma and K_V in brain synaptic plasma membranes. It is approximately 50-fold less potent when compared with ChTX. A Scatchard analysis of the inhibition produced indicates that block of toxin binding is competitive in each case. On the other hand, when similar experiments were carried out with $ChTX_{1-19}IbTX_{20-37}$, this agent was found to be a non-competitive inhibitor of ChTX binding in aortic membranes, but it had no effect on $[^{125}I]ChTX$ binding in brain. Electrophysiological studies indicate that both hybrid toxins block BK_{Ca} single channel activity. However, $IbTX_{1-19}ChTX_{20-37}$ inhibits K_v expressed in *Xenopus* oocytes while $ChTX_{1-19}IbTX_{20-37}$ is without effect in this system. These data suggest that the C-terminal regions of each peptide are responsible for ChTX- or IbTX-like behaviour, and that residues 21–24 of IbTX are critically involved in its mechanism of action. These data are also consistent with the results obtained from studies with LiTX, another IbTX-like toxin (*see above*). Comparison of the nuclear magnetic resonance (NMR) solution structures of ChTX and IbTX is being used to confirm and extend these observations regarding the mechanism of action of the two toxins as blockers of BK_{Ca}.

Purification of BK_{Ca}/ChTX receptor

Purification strategy

The characterization of $[^{125}I]ChTX$ binding in smooth muscle sarcolemmal membranes has allowed identification of BK_{Ca} in that tissue. This accomplishment satisfies the initial two criteria necessary for purification of BK_{Ca}; namely, the discovery of a specific probe that can be used to follow the channel during purification procedures and the demonstration that toxin receptors are functionally associated with the channel. However, there are several other requirements which must be fulfilled in order to accomplish the purification of BK_{Ca}. Cross-linking procedures must be developed to identify the ChTX receptor in membrane vesicles. Furthermore, conventional purification techniques must be established and optimized to allow production of a homogeneous ChTX receptor preparation, and the purified protein must be reconstituted into phospholipid bilayers in order to demonstrate functional channel activity. These last three steps have recently been brought to fruition with the ChTX receptor from bovine aortic smooth muscle.

Cross-linking of ChTX to its receptor in aortic sarcolemmal membrane vesicles is problematic for two reasons. Typical cross-linking strategies rely on incorporation of a reactive functionality into a side chain of an appropriate amino acid; either an amino group, carboxyl group, or sulphydryl group. Unfortunately, this approach is impossible with ChTX because the ε-amino groups of all Lys residues are critically important for binding of toxin to the channel (Smith *et al.*, 1986), the C-terminal carboxyl group is buried within the peptide's tertiary structure (Sugg *et al.*, 1990b), and the reduced form of the toxin is inactive (Smith *et al.*, 1986).

Therefore, use of a bifunctional cross-linking reagent was considered as an alternative approach. Second, ChTX is a highly charged peptide so that levels of non-specific association with other membrane components are expected to be significant under low ionic strength conditions. However, using a bifunctional cross-linking reagent, and by prebinding ChTX to its receptor, followed by washing membranes in high ionic strength medium to eliminate low affinity non-specific interactions of toxin, these problems have now been overcome (Garcia-Calvo *et al.*, 1991b). Cross-linking experiments performed with sarcolemmal membranes in the presence of disuccinimidyl suberate and [^{125}I]ChTX indicate that toxin can be specifically incorporated into a protein that appears as a 35 kDa band upon sodium dodecylsulphate–polyacrylamide gel electrophoresis (SDS–PAGE). The migratory behaviour of this protein is not altered by carrying out the SDS–PAGE procedure in the presence of sulphydryl reducing reagents. Labelling of the 35 kDa protein is blocked in a concentration-dependent fashion by unlabelled ChTX, IbTX, TEA and K$^+$, the same profile that has been observed for inhibition of [^{125}I]ChTX association with sarcolemmal membranes in binding experiments. Non-specific labelling of other membrane proteins with [^{125}I]ChTX is minimal under the conditions employed in these studies. However, under particular experimental conditions, a band at 95 kDa has also been labelled (King *et al.*, 1988). Nevertheless, the pharmacological properties associated with covalent incorporation of toxin into this protein do not resemble those expected for an interaction with BK$_{Ca}$. Thus, the concentrations of either ChTX or IbTX needed to prevent labelling of the 95 kDa protein were several orders of magnitude higher than those required to block the binding reaction. In addition, the protection of labelling observed with TEA was later confirmed to be the result of a simple ionic strength effect which could be mimicked by Na$^+$. Therefore, the ChTX receptor in aortic smooth muscle appears to be associated exclusively with a 35 kDa protein.

Solubilization of the ChTX receptor

The ChTX receptor can be solubilized in functional form from either bovine aorta or trachea by extracting sarcolemmal membranes with selected detergents (Vazquez *et al.*, 1988; Garcia-Calvo *et al.*, 1991b). For example, treatment of vesicles with digitonin followed by high speed centrifugation results in the appearance of [^{125}I]ChTX binding activity in a soluble protein fraction. Similar results can be obtained with the detergent CHAPS. This ChTX receptor preparation is fully active based on the following criteria: [^{125}I]ChTX binds saturably and with the same high affinity as detected in intact membranes; ChTX binding is potently inhibited by IbTX and non-radiolabelled ChTX; ChTX binding is modulated by the ionic strength of the incubation medium; metal ions and TEA block the association of $[^{125}I]$ChTX with the same rank order and absolute potencies as determined in sarcolemmal membranes. When either the digitonin- or CHAPS- solubilized material was subjected to sucrose density gradient centrifugation and $[^{125}I]$ChTX binding activity was determined across the gradient, the solubilized receptor displayed a high apparent sedimentation coefficient (approximately 20 S). Given this result and the data from the $[^{125}I]$ChTX cross-linking experiments, the 35 kDa membrane protein previously identified may represent a subunit of a larger molecular weight complex. The solubilized ChTX receptor binds specifically to wheat germ agglutinin–Sepharose resin and can be eluted with N-acetylglucosamine. This result suggests that the receptor is a glycoprotein. Therefore, taken together, these findings provide the basis for purification of BK_{Ca} from smooth muscle.

Purification of the ChTX receptor

By following $[^{125}I]$ChTX binding, the ChTX receptor has been purified from aortic smooth muscle sarcolemma to apparent homogeneity (Garcia-Calvo *et al.*, 1991a). This was accomplished using a combination of conventional purification techniques. The ChTX receptor was solubilized from sarcolemmal membrane vesicles through a series of extractions with digitonin. The individual extracts which showed the highest specific activity of $[^{125}I]$ChTX binding were pooled and passed over a wheat germ lectin column. The ChTX binding activity was quantitatively adsorbed by this resin and then selectively eluted with N-acetylglucosamine. The receptor preparation was next subjected to two further fractionation procedures: ion exchange chromatography using a Mono Q resin and hydroxyl apatite chromatography. The resulting material that possessed binding activity was concentrated by adsorption onto wheat germ agglutinin–Sepharose resin, eluted with sugar, and then subjected to sucrose density gradient centrifugation. The material from this gradient displaying maximal $[^{125}I]$ChTX binding activity was reapplied to another sucrose density gradient and subjected to centrifugation once again. Upon the completion of these procedures, ChTX binding activity is purified approximately 1300-fold with respect to starting membrane material, and the total yield is about 5%. The final receptor preparation displays binding properties for $[^{125}I]$ChTX which are identical to those determined in intact sarcolemmal vesicles, indicating that the ChTX binding site has been faithfully preserved. Analysis by SDS–PAGE of those fractions from the second sucrose density gradient that display the highest levels of $[^{125}I]$ChTX binding activity indicates the presence of a single predominant protein which migrates as a 33 kDa band. Cross-linking of the resulting preparation with $[^{125}I]$ChTX followed by SDS–PAGE also reveals specific labelling of a

35 kDa protein since incorporation of radiolabelled toxin can be protected against by ChTX, IbTX, TEA and K^+. The apparent increase in molecular weight of this protein after the cross-linking procedure is not unexpected given the mass of the toxin. Since ChTX binding activity in the final preparation migrates at about 20 S upon sucrose density gradient centrifugation, it is suggested that BK_{Ca} is an oligomer of a 33 kDa subunit.

Reconstitution of the ChTX receptor

The purified ChTX receptor has been reconstituted into planar lipid bilayers and shown to possess BK_{Ca} activity (Giangiacomo *et al.*, 1991b). This was accomplished by first removing detergent and reconstituting receptor activity into phospholipid liposomes. These vesicles were then incorporated into artificial phospholipid bilayers, electrical recordings were made and BK_{Ca} activity was observed at the single channel level after this procedure. An analysis of the resulting single channel behaviour indicates that the purified BK_{Ca} is highly selective for K^+ over either Na^+ or Cl^-. The single channel conductance in symmetrical 150 mM KCl is 320 pS. Examination of the Ca and voltage dependency of the purified preparation indicates that Ca^{2+} shifts the voltage-dependency of the channel in the hyperpolarizing direction as is found with BK_{Ca} present in smooth muscle membranes. Importantly, purified BK_{Ca} is blocked by TEA and by ChTX with the same potency and inhibitory properties that are characteristic of the native channel. Thus, by these criteria the purified ChTX receptor is sufficient for generating BK_{Ca} with properties that are identical to those of channels present in intact cells. Given data previously obtained from reconstitution studies with other purified ion channels, it is remarkable that the final BK_{Ca} preparation maintains full functional activity after such extensive manipulation.

Future prospects

Final verification that the purified ChTX receptor represents BK_{Ca} and the subsequent characterization of the molecular structure of this channel awaits the cloning and expression of the protein. To this end, the purified receptor has been subjected to proteolysis with trypsin. Several tryptic peptides have been isolated and sequence analysis has been performed on these fragments. The resulting sequences are unique and have been used to generate probes in an attempt to clone BK_{Ca} from bovine aortic smooth muscle. These studies are currently underway.

Physiology of BK$_{Ca}$

Involvement in spontaneous myogenic activity

With the use of synthetic methodologies that allow production of significant quantities of ChTX, it has been possible to employ this peptide as a probe to investigate the physiological role of BK$_{Ca}$ in intact tissues. Many investigations have focused on smooth muscle because of the prevalence of this channel in that tissue, and studies have been performed with both spontaneously active and quiescent preparations. In an initial report where the effects of ChTX were monitored on a spontaneously contracting tissue, the rat portal vein, the toxin produced a concentration-dependent increase in contractility in the 1—100 nM range, with an EC$_{100}$ of 4 nM (Winquist *et al.*, 1989). TEA in a concentration range in which it selectively blocks BK$_{Ca}$ (i.e. 100 μM–1 mM) produced the same magnitude of contraction, while 4-aminopyridine or higher concentrations of TEA (i.e. those conditions where many different types of K-channel are blocked), caused more substantial contractures. Apamin, a blocker of SK$_{Ca}$ had no effect. These data suggest that a ChTX-sensitive BK$_{Ca}$ plays a role in repolarizing rat portal vein when it is depolarized, and, as expected, blocking this repolarization pathway will increase the magnitude of spontaneous contractions in that tissue.

Investigation of ChTX and other BK$_{Ca}$ inhibitors has been extended by monitoring the action of these agents on the spontaneous motility and tonus of various smooth muscles from the guinea-pig (Suarez-Kurtz *et al.*, 1991). Of the four tissues studied which display myogenic activity, bladder and taenia coli were contracted by ChTX, whilst portal vein and uterus were only moderately affected. Charybdotoxin in the 10–100 nM range produced a concentration-dependent increase in myogenic activity in the former two tissues, with bladder being most sensitive to blockade of BK$_{Ca}$. These effects of ChTX were mirrored by two other BK$_{Ca}$ inhibitors, IbTX and TEA. Both of these compounds increased the contractility of bladder, but not portal vein. Iberiotoxin was active at 10–100 nM, whilst 0.3–3.0 mM TEA was required to achieve the same effect. These are concentrations at which inhibition of BK$_{Ca}$ is pronounced. Two quiescent preparations were also investigated: aorta and trachea. Both ChTX and IbTX (10–100 nM) caused contracture of aortic rings. On the other hand, rat aorta is insensitive to ChTX which also does not affect indomethacin-treated guinea-pig trachea. However, trachea not exposed to indomethacin, and hence under spontaneous tone due to release of endogenous prostanoids, is contracted by exposure to ChTX (T. Jones, unpublished observations). Taken together, several conclusions can be made from these findings. The increased contractility of certain guinea-pig smooth muscles elicited by ChTX, IbTX and TEA is consistent with selective blockade of BK$_{Ca}$. In tissues displaying myogenic activity, such as bladder and taenia coli, BK_{Ca} drives repolarization after membrane depolarization. In quiescent tissue such as aorta, BK_{Ca} helps to maintain cellular resting potential. In other quiescent tissues exposed to spasmogens and having elevated levels of intracellular Ca^{2+} (e.g. trachea in the absence of a cyclooxygenase inhibitor), BK_{Ca} also appears to be active. Thus, within a given species, BK_{Ca} affects excitation–contraction (E–C) coupling responses in smooth muscle in a tissue-specific fashion. Considering the differences observed in the contribution of BK_{Ca} to E–C coupling in the same smooth muscle from different species (i.e. compare effects of ChTX on either the portal vein or aorta in guinea pig versus rat), the role of this channel in cellular electrical activity is also likely to be species-dependent.

Role of BK_{Ca} in response to the K-channel openers

There is some confusion in the literature as to whether or not a potential site of action of the K-channel openers currently in development is BK_{Ca}. Although our group has never observed any stimulatory effects of BRL 34915 (cromakalim), pinacidil or RP 49356 on BK_{Ca} in single channel recordings obtained from excised membrane patches of bovine aorta (J. Reuben, unpublished observations), others have claimed these agents can open this channel (Gelband et al., 1989; Hu et al., 1990; Bowen et al., 1991). To investigate this issue further, ChTX was used as a probe in two separate pharmacological studies to determine whether toxin could block the relaxant effects of K-channel openers in smooth muscle. In rat portal vein, ChTX (100 nM) did not block relaxation caused by cromakalim, minoxidil sulphate or diazoxide (Winquist et al., 1989). However, these responses were completely inhibited by glyburide, an inhibitor of ATP-sensitive K-channels in pancreatic β-cells and in cardiac muscle. Glyburide does not affect BK_{Ca} activity. Similar data were obtained with RP 49356 (G. Suarez-Kurtz, unpublished observations). Interestingly, ChTX appeared slightly to potentiate the relaxant properties of cromakalim, but not that of the other agonists. In another study employing carbachol contracted guinea-pig trachea, ChTX (60–180 nM) did not block the relaxant effect of either cromakalim or pinacidil, although glyburide did display this action (Jones et al., 1990). Again, ChTX appeared to potentiate slightly the ability of cromakalim to relax smooth muscle, but it had no significant effect on the profile of pinacidil. Perhaps this enhancement of cromakalim's action is due to toxin block of one K-conductance pathway, as well as an increase by agonist in a parallel pathway of overall higher conductance, allowing the cell's membrane potential to approach the equilibrium potential for K^+ more closely. As a net result, this would further enhance muscle relaxation. Some evidence has been presented that crude Leiurus quinquestriatus venom blocks stimulation of $^{86}Rb^+$-efflux from rat portal vein by cromakalim (Quast & Cook, 1988). Since many other K-channel blocking peptides are present in this venom besides ChTX, such an effect cannot be considered as evidence for involvement of BK_{Ca} in the mechanism of action of cromakalim. Moreover, crude *Leiurus* venom does not block relaxation of rat portal vein induced by cromakalim (R. Winquist, unpublished observations). Therefore, taken together, these pharmacological data imply that the target of K-channel openers cannot be BK_{Ca}. The precise site of action of the currently available openers in smooth muscle remains to be defined. For further discussion of this, *see* Chapters 14 and 15.

Role of BK_{Ca} in relaxations produced by β-adrenoceptor agonists

The effects of certain smooth muscle relaxants are blunted by ChTX. For example, in guinea-pig trachea contracted with carbachol, ChTX inhibits tissue relaxation induced by β-adrenoceptor agonists in a concentration-dependent fashion, whilst glyburide is without effect (Jones *et al.*, 1990). The concentration–response curves for relaxation produced by iso-proterenol (non-selective β-agonist) and salbutamol (β_2-selective agonist) were shifted 27-fold, or more than 40-fold, respectively, in the presence of 180 nM toxin. In addition, the inhibition of β-agonist action by ChTX is non-competitive. Such patterns do not appear to be related simply to the level of intracellular cAMP produced since relaxations induced by ami-nophylline, a phosphodiesterase inhibitor, or dibutyryl cAMP, a membrane permeant form of cAMP, are less effectively blocked by ChTX, and inhibition of those responses by toxin appears competitive. In any event, these results suggest that β_2-adrenoceptor selective agonists relax carbachol contracted trachea by activating BK_{Ca}. Part of this response may be related to cyclic adenosine monophosphate (cAMP) effects, whilst part could result from a direct interaction between the β-adrenergic receptor and BK_{Ca} via G-protein or some other form of coupling. It is interesting that angiotensin II receptors appear to be directly coupled to BK_{Ca} in pig coronary artery (Toro *et al.*, 1990).

Part of the interaction between β-adrenoreceptors and BK_{Ca} in trachea is most likely related to the recent observation (Kume *et al.*, 1989) that β-agonists can activate this channel through a cAMP-dependent protein kinase phosphorylation pathway. It had previously been shown that isoproterenol hyperpolarizes airways smooth muscle, and that this response can also be elicited by theophylline and dibutyryl cAMP, all of which suggest possible involvement of a cAMP-dependent phosphorylation mechanism (Honda *et al.*, 1986). Using whole-cell patch-clamp techniques to monitor BK_{Ca} in single-channel measurements of rabbit tracheal myocytes, bath application of isoproterenol markedly increased channel activity (Kume *et al.*, 1989). Addition of okadaic acid, a protein phosphatase inhibitor, to the bathing medium significantly enhanced and prolonged the effect of the β-adrenoceptor agonist. A similar increase in BK_{Ca} activity was induced by treating excized inside-out patches with protein kinase A and ATP. Okadaic acid was also found to enhance this latter effect. Thus, BK_{Ca} appears to be regulated by direct phosphorylation of the channel protein in trachea. Consistent with this notion is the observation that ChTX-sensitive BK_{Ca} channels from bovine tracheal sarcolemmal membrane vesicles reconstituted into bilayers can be activated by protein kinase A-dependent phosphorylation (K. Giangiacomo & O. McManus, unpublished observations). Such a mechanism may be related to the clinical efficacy of β-adrenoceptor agonists as airway smooth muscle relaxants in asthma. A similar cAMP-dependent phosphorylation mechanism has been reported to regulate BK_{Ca} in aortic smooth muscle (Sadoshima et al., 1988).

Role of BK_{Ca} in relaxations associated with an increase in cyclic guanosine monophosphate (cGMP)

Other smooth muscle relaxants also appear to modulate BK_{Ca} activity. Patch-clamp studies with single bovine aortic smooth muscle cells indicate that atrial natriuretic peptide, nitroprusside and adenosine can activate BK_{Ca} when recordings were made using cell-attached patches (Williams et al., 1988). Since all these agents have been shown to relax smooth muscle via elevation in cGMP levels, it follows that one of the mechanisms of action of this cyclic nucleotide might involve BK_{Ca}. Indeed, the membrane-permeant form of cGMP, dibutyryl cGMP, caused a similar increase in channel activity when applied extracellularly. Strikingly, when these experiments were repeated using excized inside-out patches, cGMP was found to activate single channel activity as expected, but GMP was a much more effective agent in this respect. Single channel analysis reveals that GMP (50 μM) will increase both the probability of channel opening, as well as the channel mean open time. Other nucleotides such as guanosine diphosphate and triphosphate and ATP were essentially ineffective in modulating BK_{Ca} in excized patches. In experiments which are the pharmacological correlate of these studies, ChTX was found to block sodium nitroprusside induced-relaxation of guinea-pig trachea by a non-competitive mechanism (Jones et al., 1990). These data are similar to the results obtained with β-adrenoceptor agonists. Taken together, these findings suggest that there is a nucleotide regulatory site associated with BK_{Ca} in smooth muscle, and that binding of GMP or cGMP to the site will result in channel activation. Such action would promote the relaxation of smooth muscle, in analogy to the pharmacological effects of K-channel openers. A summary of the pharmacological effects of ChTX in smooth muscle is shown in Table 5.2.

Table 5.2. Pharmacological properties of ChTX in smooth muscle.

Effect of ChTX on spontaneous motility and tonus
Guinea-pig
   Increases myogenic activity of bladder and taenia coli
   No significant effect on portal vein or uterus
   Contracts aorta
   No effect on indomethacin-treated trachea

Rat
   Increases myogenic activity of portal vein
   No effect on aorta or uterus

Rabbit
   Contracts iliac and basilar artery
   No effect on aorta

Interaction of ChTX with smooth muscle relaxants
No effect on relaxation induced by cromakalim, pinacidil, RP49356, minoxidil
sulphate, or diazoxide in a variety of smooth muscles from different species

Non-competitively antagonizes β_2-adrenoceptor agonist-induced relaxation of
carbachol contracted guinea-pig trachea

Blocks relaxation of guinea-pig trachea and rat portal vein induced by agents which
elevate cGMP

Miscellaneous roles of BK_{Ca}

In addition to the studies outlined above with smooth muscle, ChTX has
been used in pharmacological studies with other cell types. ChTX was
found to block mitogen activation of human T-lymphocytes and release of
the lymphokine interleukin-2 at nanomolar concentrations (Price *et al.*,
1989). However, this action appears due to inhibition of an inactivating
K_V, rather than to block of BK_{Ca}. This hypothesis has been confirmed by
demonstrating that NxTX, which also blocks K_V produces similar inhibition of mitogen-induced T-lymphocyte proliferation, whilst IbTX is
without effect in this paradigm (Slaughter *et al.*, 1991). Thus, ChTX is
useful as a probe of signal transduction mechanisms in non-electrically
excitable cells. In cultured canine airways epithelial cells, ChTX blocks a
low conductance K_{Ca} present on the basolateral membrane surface
(McCann *et al.*, 1990). This channel is distinct from the BK_{Ca}-channel
because it is insensitive to TEA, and it displays a lower affinity for ChTX.
Interestingly, under certain experimental conditions, ChTX inhibition of
the basolateral BK_{Ca} blocks secretion of Cl^- via channels located on the
apical membrane face by preventing the hyperpolarization that is coupled
to elevation of intracellular Ca^{2+} in these cells (McCann & Welsh, 1990).
These data suggest a hypothesis that agents which could open the epithelial
cell BK_{Ca} might have utility for controlling Cl^- secretion in pathophysio-

logies such as cystic fibrosis. Unfortunately, very few neuropharmacological studies have been performed with ChTX, or any of the other peptidyl inhibitors of K-channels. Such studies would be interesting because toxin probes exist not only for BK_{Ca}, but also for a ChTX-sensitive, K_V-channel ($K_V 3$ type) recently cloned from rat brain (Stühmer et al., 1989; Swanson et al., 1990).

Conclusions

Initially, BK_{Ca} in smooth muscle was characterized solely by using electrophysiological/biophysical techniques. With the discovery of high affinity peptidyl inhibitors of BK_{Ca}, it has been possible to analyse the channel biochemically, as well as to bring about its purification. These inhibitors have also been useful in initial efforts to characterize the physiological role of BK_{Ca} in intact tissues. Given that all ion channels possess receptors for many drugs, screening by ligand binding at one site on a channel should allow detection of agents that bind at relatively distal sites on the protein, and those which modulate the original receptor via allosteric coupling mechanisms. This procedure can be used to discover other novel peptidyl toxins, as well as small molecules that will affect BK_{Ca} activity. Using [^{125}I]ChTX binding, a number of new K-channel toxins have been discovered. These agents are not only useful for pharmacological and physiological studies with BK_{Ca}, but also can be employed to develop the molecular pharmacology of other types of K-channel, for which such determinations have not previously been possible.

Acknowledgements

The authors wish to thank Drs K. Giangiacomo, T. Jones, O. McManus, J. Reuben, G. Suarez-Kurtz and R. Winquist for sharing their data prior to publication.

References

Anderson, C. S., MacKinnon, R., Smith, C. & Miller, C. (1988) Charybdotoxin block of single Ca^{2+}-activated K^+ channels: effects of channel gating, voltage, and ionic strength. Journal of General Physiology **91**, 317–333.

Ashcroft, F. M., Ashcroft, S. J. H., Berggren, P. O., Betzholz, C., Rossman, P., Trube, G. & Welsh, M. (1988) Expression of K channels in Xenopus laevis oocytes injected with poly(A^+) mRNA from the insulin-secreting β cell line, HIT T15. FEBS Letters **239**, 185–189.

Benham, C. D., Bolton, T. B., Lang, R. J. & Takewaki, T. (1985) The mechanism of action of Ba^{2+} and TEA on single Ca^{2+}-activated K^+ channels in arterial and intestinal smooth muscle cell membranes. Pflügers Archiv **403**, 120–127.

Blatz, A. L. & Magleby, K. L. (1986) Single apamin-blocked Ca^{2+}-activated K^+ channels of small conductance in cultured rat skeletal muscle. Nature **323**, 718–720.

Blatz, A. L. & Magleby, K. L. (1987) Calcium-activated potassium channels. *Trends in Neurosciences* **10**, 463–467.

Bowen, S. M., Carl, A., Gelband, C. H., Sander, K. M. & Hume, J. R. (1991) Cromakalim and lemakalim activate a large conductance, calcium-activated potassium channel in canine colon cells. *Biophysical Journal* **59**, 79a.

Candia, S., Garcia, M. L. & Latorre, R. (1991) Iberiotoxin blockade of a large conductance Ca^{2+} activated K^+ channel from skeletal muscle. *Biophysical Journal* **59**, 213a.

Christie, M. J., Adelman, J.P., Douglass, J. & North, R. A. (1989) Expression of a cloned rat brain potassium channel in *Xenopus* oocytes. *Science* **244**, 221–224.

Deutsch, C., Price, M., Lee, S., King, V. F. & Garcia, M. L. (1991) Characterization of high affinity binding sites for charybdotoxin in human T-lymphocytes. *Journal of Biological Chemistry* **266**, 3668–3674.

Folander, K., Smith, J. S., Antanavage, J., Bennett, C., Stein, R. B. & Swanson, R. (1990) Cloning and expression of the delayed-rectifier I_{SK} channel from neonatal rat heart and diethylstilbestrol-primed rat uterus. *Proceedings of the National Academy of Sciences USA* **87**, 2975–2979.

Frech, G. C., VanDongen, A. M. J., Schuster, G., Brown, A. M. & Joho, R. M. (1989) A novel potassium channel with delayed rectifier properties isolated from rat brain by expression cloning. *Nature* **340**, 642–645.

Galvez, A., Gimenez-Gallego, G., Reuben, J. P., Roy-Contancin, L., Feigenbaum, P., Kaczorowski, G. J. & Garcia, M. L. (1990) Purification and characterization of a unique, potent, peptidyl probe for the high conductance calcium-activated potassium channel from venom of the scorpion *Buthus tamulus*. *Journal of Biological Chemistry* **265**, 11 083–11 090.

Garcia, M. L., Galvez, A., Garcia-Calvo, M., King, V. F., Vazquez, J. & Kaczorowski, G. J. (1991) Use of toxins to study potassium channels. *Journal of Bioenergetics and Biomembranes* **23**, 615–646.

Garcia-Calvo, M., Smith, M. M., Kaczorowski, G. J. & Garcia, M. L. (1991a) Purification of the charybdotoxin receptor from bovine aortic smooth muscle. *Biophysical Journal* **59**, 78a.

Garcia-Calvo, M., Vazquez, J., Smith, M., Kaczorowski, G. J. & Garcia, M. L. (1991b) Characterization of the solubilized charybdotoxin receptor from bovine aortic smooth muscle. *Biochemistry* **30**, 11 157–11 164.

Gelband, C. H., Lodge, N. J. & VanBreemen, C. (1989) A Ca^{2+}-activated K^+ channel from rabbit aorta: modulation by cromakalim. *European Journal of Pharmacology* **167**, 201–210.

Giangiacomo, K. M., Garcia, M. L. & McManus, O. B. (1991a) Mechanism of iberiotoxin block of the high conductance Ca^{2+}-activated K^+ channel from aortic smooth muscle. *Biophysical Journal* **59**, 79a.

Giangiacomo, K. M., Garcia-Calvo, M., Garcia, M.L. & McManus, O.B. (1991b) Functional reconstitution of the large-conductance Ca^{2+}-activated K^+ channel purified from bovine aortic smooth muscle. *Biophysical Journal* **59**, 214a.

Gimenez-Gallego, G., Navia, M. A., Reuben, J. P., Katz, G. M., Kaczorowski, G. J. & Garcia, M. L. (1988) Purification, sequence, and model structure of charybdotoxin, a potent selective inhibitor of calcium-activated potassium channels. *Proceedings of the National Academy of Sciences USA* **85**, 3329–3333.

Goh, J. W. & Pennefather, P. S. (1987) Pharmacological and physiological properties of the after-hyperpolarization current of bullfrog ganglion neurones. *Journal of Physiology* **394**, 315–330.

Guggino, S. E., Guggino, W. B., Green, N. & Sacktor, B. (1987) Blocking agents of

Ca^{2+}-activated K^+ channels in cultured medullary thick ascending limb cells. *American Journal of Physiology* **252**, C128–C137.

Habermann, E. (1972) Bee and wasp venom. *Science* **177**, 314–322.

Harvey, A. L., Marshall, D. L., DeAllie, F. A. & Strong, P. N. (1989) Interactions between dendrotoxin, a blocker of voltage-dependent potassium channels, and charybdotoxin, a blocker of calcium-activated potassium channels, at binding sites on neuronal membranes. *Biochemical and Biophysical Research Communications* **163**, 394–397.

Hermann, A. & Erxleben, C. (1987) Charybdotoxin selectively blocks small Ca^{2+}-activated K^+ channels in *Aplysia* neurones. *Journal of General Physiology* **91**, 27–47.

Honda, K., Satake, T., Takagi, K. & Tomita, T. (1986) Effects of relaxants on electrical and mechanical activities in the guinea pig tracheal muscle. *British Journal of Pharmacology* **87**, 665–671.

Hu, S., Kim, H. S., Okalie, P. & Weiss, G. B. (1990) Alterations by glyburide of effects of BRL 34915 and P 1060 on contraction, $^{86}Rb^+$ efflux, and the maxi-K^+ channel in rat portal vein. *Journal of Pharmacology and Experimental Therapeutics* **253**, 771–777J.

Hu, S. L., Yamamoto, Y. & Kao, C. Y. (1989) The Ca^{2+}-activated K^+ channel and its functional roles in smooth muscle cells of guinea pig taenia coli. *Journal of General Physiology* **94**, 833–847.

Inoue, R., Kitamura, K. & Kuriyama, H. (1985) Two Ca^{2+}-dependent K^+ channels classified by the application of tetraethylammonium distributed to smooth muscle membranes of the rabbit portal vein. *Pflügers Archiv* **405**, 173–179.

Jan, L. Y. & Jan, Y. N. (1990) How might the diversity of potassium channels be generated? *Trends in Neuroscience* **13**, 415–419.

Jones, T. R., Charette, L., Garcia, M. L. & Kaczorowski, G. J. (1990) Selective inhibition of relaxation of guinea pig trachea by charybdotoxin, a potent Ca^{2+}-activated K^+ channel inhibitor. *Journal of Pharmacology and Experimental Therapeutics* **255**, 697–706.

King, V. F., Kaczorowski, G. J. & Garcia, M. L. (1988) Cross-linking of charybdotoxin to sites in bovine aortic and tracheal smooth muscle sarcolemmal membrane vesicles. *Journal of Cell Biology* **107**, 143a.

Kitamura, K., Sakai, T., Kajioka, S. & Kuriyama, H. (1989) Activations of the Ca^{2+}-dependent K^+ channels by Ca^{2+} released from the sarcoplasmic reticulum of mammalian smooth muscles. *Biomedica et Biochemica Acta* **4B**, 364–369.

Klöckner, U., Trieschmann, U. & Isenberg, G. (1989) Pharmacological modulation of calcium and potassium channels in isolated vascular smooth muscle cells. *Arzneimittel-Forschung* **39**, 120–126.

Kume, H., Takai, A., Tokuno, H. & Tomita, T. (1989) Regulation of Ca^{2+}-dependent K^+ channel activity in tracheal myocytes by phosphorylation. *Nature* **341**, 152–154.

Lambert, P., Kuroda, M., Chino, N., Watanabe, T. X., Kimura, T. & Sakakibara, S. (1990) Solution synthesis of charybdotoxin (ChTX), a K^+ channel blocker. *Biochemical and Biophysical Research Communications* **170**, 684–690.

Latorre, R., Oberhauser, A. & Alvarez, O. (1989) Varieties of calcium-activated potassium channels. *Annual Review of Physiology* **51**, 385–399.

Lu, L., Montrose-Rafizadek, C. & Guggino, W. B. (1990) Ca^{2+}-activated K^+ channels from rabbit kidney medullary thick ascending limb cells expressed in *Xenopus* oocytes. *Journal of Biological Chemistry* **265**, 16190–16194.

Luchesi, K., Ravindran, A., Young, H. & Moczydlowski, E. (1989) Analysis of the blocking activity of charybdotoxin homologs and iodinated derivatives against Ca^2-activated K^+ channels. *Journal of Membrane Biology* **109**, 269–281.

McCann, J. D. & Welsh, M. J. (1986) Calcium-activated potassium channels in canine airway smooth muscle. *Journal of Physiology* **372**, 113-127.

McCann, J. D. & Welsh, M. J. (1990) Basolateral K$^+$ channels in airway epithelia II. Role of Cl$^-$ secretion and evidence for two types of K$^+$ channels. *American Journal of Physiology* **258**, L343-L348.

McCann, J. D., Matsuda, J., Garcia, M., Kaczorowski, G. & Welsh, M. J. (1990) Basolateral K$^+$ channels in airway epithelia I. Regulation by Ca^{2+} and block by charybdotoxin. *American Journal of Physiology* **258**, L334-L342.

McKinnon, D. (1989) Isolation of a cDNA clone coding for a putative second potassium channel indicates the existence of a gene family. *Journal of Biological Chemistry* **264**, 8230-8236.

MacKinnon, R. & Miller, C. (1988) Mechanism of charybdotoxin block of the high-conductance Ca^{2+}-activated K$^+$ channel. *Journal of General Physiology* **91**, 335-349.

MacKinnon, R. & Miller, C. (1989) Functional modification of a Ca^{2+}-activated K$^+$ channel by trimethyloxonium. *Biochemistry* **28**, 8087-8092.

MacKinnon, R., Heginbotham, L. & Abramson, T. (1990) Mapping the receptor site for charybdotoxin, a pore-blocking potassium channel inhibitor. *Neuron* **5**, 767-771.

MacKinnon, R., Latorre, R. & Miller, C. (1989) Role of surface electrostatics in the operation of a high conductance Ca^{2+}-activated K$^+$ channel. *Biochemistry* **28**, 8092-8099.

MacKinnon, R., Reinhart, P. H. & White, M. M. (1988) Charybdotoxin block of *Shaker* K$^+$ channels suggests that different types of K$^+$ channels share common structural features. *Neuron* **1**, 997-1001.

Massefski, W. Jr, Redfield, A. G., Hare, D. R. & Miller, C. (1990) Molecular structure of charybdotoxin, a pore directed inhibitor of potassium ion channels. *Science* **249**, 521-524.

Miller, C. (1988) Competition for block of a Ca^{2+}-activated K$^+$ channel by charybdotoxin and tetraethylammonium. *Neuron* **1**, 1003-1006.

Miller, C., Moczydlowski, E., Latorre, R. & Phillips, M. (1985) Charybdotoxin, a protein inhibitor of single Ca^{2+}-activated K$^+$ channels from skeletal muscle. *Nature* **313**, 316-318.

Novick, J., Leonard, R. J., King, V. F., Schmalhofer, W., Kaczorowski, G. J. & Garcia, M. L. (1991) Purification and characterization of two novel peptidyl toxins directed against K$^+$ channels from venom of New World scorpions. *Biophysical Journal* **59**, 78a.

Oliva, C., Folander, K. & Smith, J. S. (1991) Charybdotoxin is not a high affinity blocker of *Shaker* K$^+$ channels expressed in *Xenopus* oocytes. *Biophysical Journal* **59**, 450a.

Pennefather, P. S., Kelley, M. E. M., Goh, J. W., Chicchi, G. G., Cascieri, M. A., Garcia, M. L. & Kaczorowski, G. J. (1989) Effect of charybdotoxin and leiurotoxin I on calcium-activated K$^+$ currents of the bullfrog sympathetic ganglion neurones. *Canadian Federation of Biological Societies. Proceedings of the 32th Annual Meeting*, p. 95.

Petersen, O. H. & Maruyama, Y. (1984) Calcium-activated potassium channels and their role in secretion. *Nature* **307**, 693-696.

Pragnell, M., Snay, K. J., Trimmer, J. S., MacLusky, N. J., Naftolin, F., Kaczmarek, L. K. & Boyle, M. B. (1990) Estrogen induction of a small, putative K$^+$ channel mRNA in rat uterus. *Neuron* **4**, 807-812.

Price, M., Lee, S. C. & Deutsch, C. (1989) Charybdotoxin inhibits proliferation and interleukin 2 production in human peripheral blood lymphocytes. *Proceedings of the National Academy of Sciences USA* **86**, 10171-10175.

Quast, U. & Cook, N. S. (1988) *Leiurus quinquestriatus* venom inhibits BRL 34915 induced $^{86}Rb^+$ efflux from the rat portal vein. *Life Sciences* **42**, 805–810.

Reinhart, P. H., Chung, S. & Levitan, I. B. (1989) A family of calcium-dependent potassium channels from rat brain. *Neuron* **2**, 1031–1041.

Sadoshima, J., Akaike, N., Kanaide, H. & Nakamura, M. (1988) Cyclic AMP modulates Ca^{2+}-activated K^+ channels in cultured smooth muscle cells of rat aorta. *American Journal of Physiology* **255**, H754–H759.

Sands, S. B., Lewis, R. S. & Cahalan, M. D. (1989) Charybdotoxin blocks voltage-gated K^+ channels in human and murine T lymphocytes. *Journal of General Physiology* **93**, 1061–1074.

Schneider, M. J., Rogowski, R. S., Krueger, B. K. & Blaustein, M. P. (1989) Charybdotoxin blocks both Ca-activated K channels and Ca-independent voltage-gated K channels in rat brain synaptosomes. *FEBS Letters* **250**, 433–436.

Schwartz, W. & Passow, H. (1983) Ca^{2+}-activated K^+ channels in erythrocytes and excitable cells. *Annual Review of Physiology* **5**, 359–374.

Schweitz, H., Bidard, J. N., Maes, P. & Lazdunski, M. (1989a) Charybdotoxin is a new member of the K^+ channel toxin family that includes dendrotoxin I and mast cell degranulating peptide. *Biochemistry* **28**, 9708–9714.

Schweitz, H., Stansfeld, C. E., Bidard, J. N., Fagni, L., Maes, P. & Lazdunski, M. (1989b) Charybdotoxin blocks dendrotoxin-sensitive voltage-activated K^+ channels. *FEBS Letters* **250**, 519–522.

Singer, J. J. & Walsh, J. V. Jr (1986) Large-conductance Ca^{2+}-activated K^+ channels in freshly dissociated smooth muscle cells. *Membrane Biochemistry* **6**, 83–110.

Slaughter, R. S., Kaczorowski, G. J. & Garcia, M. L. (1988) Charybdotoxin binds with high affinity to a single class of sites in bovine tracheal smooth muscle sarcolemmal membrane vesicles. *Journal of Cell Biology* **107**, 143a.

Slaughter, R. S., Shevell, J. L., Felix, J. P., Garcia, M. L. & Kaczorowski, G. J. (1989) High levels of sodium–calcium exchange in vascular smooth muscle sarcolemmal membrane vesicles. *Biochemistry* **28**, 3995–4002.

Slaughter, R. S., Shevell, J. L., Felix, J. P., Lin, C. S., Sigal, N. H. & Kaczorowski, G. J. (1991) Inhibition by toxins of charybdotoxin binding to the voltage-gated potassium channel of lymphocytes: correlation with block of activation of human peripheral T-lymphocytes. *Biophysical Journal* **59**, 213a.

Slaughter, R. S., Welton, A. F. & Morgan, D. W. (1987) Sodium–calcium exchange in sarcolemmal vesicles from tracheal smooth muscle. *Biochimica et Biophysica Acta* **904**, 92–104.

Smith, C., Phillips, M. & Miller, C. (1986) Purification of charybdotoxin, a specific inhibitor of the high conductance Ca^{2+}-activated K^+ channel. *Journal of Biological Chemistry* **261**, 14 607–14 613.

Strong, P. N., Weir, S. N., Beech, D. J., Heistand, P. & Kochner, H. P. (1989) Effects of potassium channel toxins from *Leiurus quinquestriatus hebraeus* venom on responses to cromakalim in rabbit blood vessels. *British Journal of Pharmacology* **98**, 817–826.

Stühmer, W., Ruppersberg, J. P., Schroter, K. H., Sakmann, B., Stocker, M., Giese, K. P., Perschke, A., Baumann, A. & Pongs, O. (1989) Molecular basis of functional diversity of voltage-gated potassium channels in mammalian brain. *EMBO Journal* **8**, 3235–3244.

Suarez-Kurtz, G., Garcia, M. L. & Kaczorowski, G. J. (1991) Effects of charybdotoxin and iberiotoxin on the spontaneous motility and tonus of different guinea pig smooth muscle tissues. *Journal of Pharmacology and Experimental Therapeutics* **259**, 439–443.

Sugg, E. E., Garcia, M. L., Johnson, B. A., Kaczorowski, G. J., Patchett, A. A. &

Reuben, J. P. (1990a) Synthetic studies on the K^+ channel antagonist charybdotoxin. In Rivier, J. E. & Marshall, G. R. (eds) *Peptides: Chemistry, Structure and Biology.* Escom Sci. Pub., Leiden, pp. 1069–1070.

Sugg, E. E., Garcia, M. L., Reuben, J. P., Patchet, A. A. & Kaczorowski, G. J. (1990b) Synthesis and structural characterization of charybdotoxin, a potent peptidyl inhibitor of the high conductance Ca^{2+}-activated K^+ channel. *Journal of Biological Chemistry* **265**, 18 745–18 748.

Swanson, R., Marshall, J., Smith, J. S., Williams, J. B., Boyle, M. B., Folander, K., Luneau, C. J., Antanavage, J., Oliva, C., Buhrow, S. A., Bennett, C., Stein, R. B. & Kaczmarek, L. K. (1990) Cloning and expression of cDNA and genomic clones encoding three delayed rectifier potassium channels in rat brain. *Neuron* **4**, 929–939.

Takumi, T., Ohkubo, H. & Nakanishi, S. (1988) Cloning of a membrane protein that induces a slow voltage-gated potassium current. *Science* **242**, 1042–1045.

Temple, B. L., Jan, Y. N. & Jan, L. Y. (1988) Cloning of a probable potassium channel gene from mouse brain. *Nature* **332**, 837–839.

Toro, L., Amador, M. & Stefani, E. (1990) ANG II inhibits calcium-activated potassium channels from coronary smooth muscle in lipid bilayers. *American Journal of Physiology* **258**, H912–H915.

Valdivia, H. H., Smith, J. S., Martin, B. M., Coronado, R. & Possani, L. D. (1988) Charybdotoxin and noxiustoxin, two homologous peptide inhibitors of the K^+ (Ca^{2+}) channel. *FEBS Letters* **226**, 280–284.

Vazquez, J., Feigenbaum, P., Kaczorowski, G. J. & Garcia, M. L. (1988) Partial purification of the charybdotoxin receptor from bovine aortic and tracheal smooth muscle. *Journal of Cell Biology* **107**, 143a.

Vazquez, J., Feigenbaum, P., Katz, G. M., King, V. F., Reuben, J. P., Roy-Contancin, L., Slaughter, R. S., Kaczorowski, G. J. & Garcia, M. L. (1989) Characterization of high affinity binding sites for charybdotoxin in sarcolemmal membranes from bovine aortic smooth muscle. *Journal of Biological Chemistry* **264**, 20 902–20 909.

Vazquez, J., Feigenbaum, P., King, V. F., Kaczorowski, G. J. & Garcia, M. L. (1990) Characterization of high affinity binding sites for charybdotoxin in synaptic plasma membranes from rat brain. *Journal of Biological Chemistry* **265**, 15 564–15 571.

Villarroel, A., Alvarez, O., Oberhauser, A. & Latorre, R. (1988) Probing a Ca^{2+}-activated K^+ channel with quaternary ammonium ions. *Pflügers Archiv* **413**, 118–126.

Williams, D. L., Jr., Katz, G. M., Roy-Contancin, L. & Reuben, J. P. (1988) Guanosine 5′-monophosphate modulates gating of high conductance Ca^{2+}-activated K^+ channels in vascular smooth muscle cells. *Proceedings of the National Academy of Sciences USA* **85**, 9360–9364.

Winquist, R. J., Heaney, L. A., Wallace, A. A., Baskin, E. P., Stein, R. B., Garcia, M. L. & Kaczorowski, G. J. (1989) Glyburide blocks the relaxation responses to BRL 34915 (cromakalim), minoxidil sulfate and diazoxide in vascular smooth muscle. *Journal of Pharmacology and Experimental Therapeutics* **248**, 149–156.

Wolff, D., Cecchi, X., Spalvins, A. & Canessa, M. (1988) Charybdotoxin blocks with high affinity the Ca^{2+}-activated K^+ channel of HbA and HbS red cells: individual differences in the number of channels. *Journal of Membrane Biology* **106**, 243–252.

Chapter 6
The physiology and pharmacology of ATP-regulated potassium channels in insulin-secreting cells
M. J. Dunne

Introduction

Maintaining homeostatic blood glucose concentrations is a complex, integrated process primarily regulated by a single molecule — insulin. When the concentration of glucose in the plasma is high, insulin is released by the process of exocytosis from the β-cells of the pancreatic islets of Langerhans. It is now widely accepted that the key intracellular regulator of insulin secretion is an increase in the cytosolic concentrations of free Ca ions ($[Ca^{2+}]_i$), a rise that is totally dependent on the presence of Ca outside the cell (Wollheim & Sharp, 1981; Hoenig & Sharp, 1986).

It was first demonstrated in the late 1960s that when islets of Langerhans are challenged with a number of compounds known to elicit insulin secretion, including glucose and glyceraldehyde, marked changes are brought about in the electrical behaviour of the islet cells. In these experiments, using glass microelectrodes, Dean and Matthews (1968) were able to show that carbohydrate secretagogues caused both a depolarization of the cell membrane and the generation of spike potentials. Later Matthews and Sakamoto (1975) demonstrated that these voltage-gated spikes were caused by the inward movement of Ca^{2+}.

The link between carbohydrate metabolism and the initiation of the membrane depolarization was further demonstrated to be a decrease in the

110

Table 6.1. The properties of K_{ATP}-channels in insulin-secreting cells.

Tissue	Conductance (pS)	Configuration	K_iATP	Hill coefficient	Reference
Human	60–65 + 30	C/A K^+/Na^+			[1]
	58	I/O K^+/K^+	10 μM	1.2	[2]
Rat	85 + 30	C/A K^+/Na^+			[3]
adult	58	I/O K^+/K^+	26 μM	1	[4]
neonatal	54 + 21	I/O K^+/K^+	15 mM	1.2	[5, 6]
Mouse	50	C/A K^+/Na^+			[7]
	56	I/O K^+/K^+			[7]
		I/O K^+/K^+	18 μM	1.8	[8]
RINm5F	90 + 30	C/A K^+/Na^+			[3]
	50	C/A + I/O	50–70 μM	1.8	[9, 10]
		O/C	20–30 μM		[11]
HIT-T15	52	I/O K^+/K^+	60 μM		[12]
CRI-G1	56 + 28	I/O K^+/K^+	13 μM	1.2	[13]

Conductance measurements for the smaller of the two channels have been included wherever values are available. K_r values for 50% inhibition refer to the large channel; all values were obtained in the presence of 1–2 mM internal Mg^{2+}. Abbreviations refer to cell-attached (C/A), open-cell (O/C) and inside-out membrane patches (I/O). K^+ and Na^+ concentrations are each approximately 140 mM.
References: [1] Misler et al. (1989); [2] Ashcroft et al. (1987); [3] Findlay et al. (1985a); [4] Ashcroft & Kakei (1989); [5] Cook & Hales (1984); [6] Rorsman et al. (1989); [7] Rorsman & Trube (1985); [8] Ohno-Shosaku et al. (1987); [9] Ribalet et al. (1988); [10] Ribalet & Ciani (1987); [11] from Dunne et al. (1986, 1988a), Findlay et al. (1985a) and Dunne (1989b, 1990b); [12] Niki et al. (1989b); [13] Sturgess et al. (1986).

permeability of the membrane to K^+ (Sehlin & Taljedal, 1975; Henquin, 1978, 1980a). However, it was not until nearly 10 years later, through the use of the improved patch-clamp technique to study single channel currents that this conductance pathway was identified.

In intact, resting insulin-secreting cells, only one particular type of K-channel is operational—a channel that is closed when cells are challenged with carbohydrate secretagogues (Ashcroft et al., 1984; Rorsman & Trube, 1985; Dunne et al., 1986; Misler et al., 1986). Since this channel appears to be exactly the same as the one shown to be directly inhibited by intracellularly-applied adenosine 5'-triphosphate (ATP) (Cook & Hales, 1984), closure of such ATP-sensitive K-channels (K_{ATP}) in intact cells initiates the membrane depolarization. Patch-clamp experiments have been carried out on a number of insulin-secreting cell preparations, including human, rodent and clonal β-cells. Fortunately, it turns out that many of the properties of this channel in insulin-secreting cells (e.g. single channel conductance, sensitivity to ATP, etc.) show remarkably few species differences (see Table 6.1).

In this review the biophysical and pharmacological properties of K_{ATP}-channels in insulin-secreting cells will be examined. The physiological significance of these channels in the control of insulin secretion will also be described.

Biophysical properties

Two types of K_{ATP}-channel have been identified in insulin-secreting cells (Findlay *et al.*, 1985a). These channels appear to be controlled in a similar manner by both internally- and externally-applied molecules and they have somewhat similar biophysical characteristics — differing only in their unitary conductance (Findlay *et al.*, 1985a). This review will be restricted to the properties of the larger of these channels — the large K_{ATP}-channel.

The frequency of channel openings in intact cells is extremely low and typified by brief openings from one or two channels (Dunne *et al.*, 1986). However, when either a detergent, such as digitonin or saponin, is used to make holes in the plasma membrane (outside of the isolated patch area from which the recording is made), thereby equilibrating the cell interior with the bath solution ('open' or permeabilized cell) or when a patch of membrane is excised from the cell, many more channel open events become apparent, with much longer open times (Dunne *et al.*, 1986; Findlay & Dunne 1986a). Experiments of this type would tend to suggest that K_{ATP}-channels in intact cells are tonically inhibited by some endogenous factor, which is probably ATP (Dunne *et al.*, 1986; Findlay & Dunne, 1986a). Estimates of the number of K_{ATP}-channels per cell vary somewhat between 5000 and 10 000 (Dunne & Petersen, 1990; Rorsman & Trube, 1990), and although an average value of approximately 12 channels per patch has been reported (Dunne *et al.*, 1986), synchronous openings of upwards of 55 channels in individual patches have been seen (Dunne *et al.*, 1988b).

K_{ATP}-channels are highly selective for external K^+ relative to Na^+ [$P_{Na}/P_K = 0.007$ (Ashcroft *et al.*, 1989a)] which explains why in the presence of physiological solutions containing 140 mM Na^+, the zero-current transmembrane potential is invariably found to be close to the K-equilibrium potential. The channels will allow Rb^+ to pass through [$P_{Rb}/P_K = 0.73$: Ashcroft *et al.* (1989a)], but as with the Ca- and voltage-activated K-channel in exocrine cells (Gallacher *et al.*, 1984), the Rb-conductance is only a small fraction of the K conductance. Rubidium ions will therefore also act as permeable blockers of the channel (Ashcroft *et al.*, 1989a).

Current–voltage relationship plots obtained from either intact cells or excised patches in the presence of quasi-physiological cation gradients, suggest that the single channel current conductance is in the region of

50–90 pS for the larger K_{ATP}-channel and 20–30 pS for the smaller one (Table 6.1). K_{ATP} expresses a marked degree of inward current rectification and the current amplitude increases very little at potentials above $+20$ mV, thereby preferentially allowing K^+ to enter the cell while restricting its efflux (Ashcroft et al., 1984; Dunne et al., 1986; Arkhammar et al., 1987). Rectification probably results from the intracellular concentrations of either/both Mg^{2+} and Na^+ (Findlay, 1987). The permeability of the channel to internal Na^+ relative to K^+ has been estimated to be 0.39 (Ashcroft et al., 1989a).

Intracellular regulators of channel function

The frequency of K_{ATP} opening closure is relatively unaffected by changes in the membrane potential of the cell (Ashcroft et al., 1988) or by changes in the concentration of free $[Ca^{2+}]_i$ (Rorsman & Trube, 1985).

The effects of pH

Effects of changes in the intracellular pH (pH_i) on channel gating are interesting. In their original analysis on this subject both Cook and Hales (1984) and Misler and his collaborators (1986), reported that over the ranges 6.6–7.3, changes in pH_i had no effects on channel activity. However, in a re-evaluation of the effects of pH, Misler et al. (1989) have found that in the presence of cytosolic ATP, changes in pH_i do have marked effects on the channels. This is supported by three pieces of evidence: (i) the time-course of changes in K_{ATP} activity in cell-attached membrane patches exposed to the weak base NH_4Cl, resembled that of pH_i changes seen in other cells; (ii) in intact cells permeabilized to H^+ by nigericin, changes in external pH from 6.25 to 7.9 increased channel openings; and (iii) in excised patches exposed to low concentrations of ATP, increases in pH_i over a similar range activated channels. These data may therefore indicate that alterations in pH_i do not directly influence K_{ATP}, but rather that such changes are mediated through the availability of ATP^{4-} (see below). It is interesting, therefore, to compare the effects of pH_i on these channels with those of a similar K_{ATP}-channel found in cardiac and skeletal muscle cells. In these a decrease in pH_i has been found to inhibit channels in the absence of cytosolic ATP, but to open them in the presence of ATP (Lederer & Nicholls, 1989; Davies, 1990).

The effects of ATP

The principal action of ATP when added to the inside of the membrane is to evoke channel closure (Cook & Hales, 1984). This effect is concentration dependent, with K_i values, corresponding to half-maximal inhibition, between 10 and 70 μM (*see* Table 6.1). Estimates of the Hill coefficient for channel blockade vary from approximately 1 to 1.8 (Cook & Hales, 1984; Ohno-Shosaku *et al.*, 1987; Ribalet & Ciani, 1987), hence it is unclear whether several molecules of ATP are able to bind to the channel in a co-operative manner.

A major problem encountered when studying K_{ATP} is 'run-down' or the time-dependent loss of activity occurring during whole-cell recordings (Trube *et al.*, 1986), or whenever excised outside-out (Findlay *et al.*, 1985b), inside-out (Findlay *et al.*, 1985a,b; Ohno-Shosaku *et al.*, 1987) or open cells are formed (Dunne *et al.*, 1986; Findlay & Dunne, 1986a). Run-down of channels is extremely variable from experiment to experiment with near complete loss of channel openings occurring between tens of seconds and several minutes (Findlay *et al.*, 1985b; Findlay & Dunne, 1986a). The gradual loss of channel activity which occurs after separation of the membrane from the structural and biochemical environment of the intact cell, has also been observed for K_{ATP}-channels in cardiac (Kakei & Noma, 1984; Trube & Hescheler, 1984) and amphibian skeletal muscle cells (Spruce *et al.*, 1987), as well as for Ca-channels in a variety of tissues (Fenwick *et al.*, 1982; Cavalie *et al.*, 1983; Forscher & Oxford, 1985). In both cardiac (Kakei *et al.*, 1985) and insulin-secreting cells (Dunne *et al.*, 1986) the rate of channel run-down has been shown to be considerably reduced by using the open-cell recording configuration. This may suggest that de-activation of channels is, at least in part, mediated by cytoskeletal elements, possibly slowly-diffusible enzymes retained by the open cell. The mechanism of channel run-down has been studied in cardiac cells and appears to involve a Ca-dependent dephosphorylation process (Findlay, 1988). It is interesting to note that in permeabilized cells the apparent sensitivity of the channels to ATP is markedly altered. In one series of experiments on β-cells, 1 mM ATP was found to inhibit K_{ATP} completely in excised patches, whereas in open cells approximately 7% of the current was retained (Dunne *et al.*, 1986; *see* Fig. 6.1). Similarly in cardiac cells, K_i values of 0.1 mM ATP were obtained in patches, compared with 0.5 mM ATP in open cells (Kakei *et al.*, 1985).

Protein phosphorylation appears not to be involved in closing channels, since similar effects are also seen for a number of non- and partially-hydrolysable analogues of ATP (Ohno-Shosaku *et al.*, 1987; Dunne *et al.*, 1988a) and ATP is still an effective blocker of channels in the complete absence of internal Mg^{2+} (Ohno-Shosaku *et al.*, 1987; Dunne *et al.*, 1987; Ashcroft & Kakei, 1989). Indeed the effects of Mg^{2+}-free solutions on K_{ATP} are particularly interesting. In the absence of internal ATP (ATP_i), removing Mg^{2+} from the inner membrane causes an increase in channel activity (Dunne *et al.*, 1987). This activation is characterized by both an increase in the single channel conductance (Findlay, 1987; Ashcroft *et al.*, 1989a) and by an increase in the number of channel

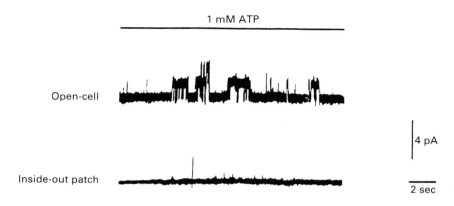

Fig. 6.1. Direct comparison of the effects of 1 mM ATP on K_{ATP} in an open cell (*upper panel*) and in an excised inside-out patch subsequently formed from the permeabilized cell (*lower panel*). (From Dunne *et al.*, 1986.)

openings (Dunne *et al.*, 1987; Findlay, 1987). In the presence of ATP_i, however, exactly the opposite occurs, with Mg^{2+} removal enhancing the potency of ATP (Dunne *et al.*, 1988a; Findlay, 1987; Ashcroft & Kakei, 1989). These findings suggest that it is the 'free' (non-Mg^{2+} bound) concentration of ATP, probably ATP^{4-} which determines the degree of K_{ATP} inhibition in pancreatic β-cells (Dunne *et al.*, 1987, 1988a; Ashcroft & Kakei, 1989). However, this is not the case in skeletal muscle where both the free acid and the Mg^{2+} salt of ATP are equally effective at blocking channels (Davies, 1990) or in cardiac cells where $MgATP^{2-}$ is more effective at blocking channels than free ATP (Findlay, 1988).

The inhibitory effects of ATP are further characterized by: (i) a decrease both in the mean open time of the channel and the number of open events per burst of activity (Ashcroft & Kakei, 1989); (ii) a lack of effect on the single channel conductance; and (iii) being independent of the holding potential applied to the membrane.

It has been suggested that a cyclic adenosine monophosphate (cAMP)-dependent protein kinase is closely associated with K_{ATP} and that the inhibitory effects of ATP on the channels can be explained by a decrease in protein kinase activity due to the ATP-dependent binding of an inhibitor protein to the enzyme; Ribalet *et al.*, 1989). The model goes further to explain how the stimulatory effects of ATP (*reviewed below*) result from kinase-mediated phosphorylation of the channel (Ribalet *et al.*, 1989). However, the hypothesis, which relies upon protein phosphorylation/dephosphorylation reactions, cannot readily explain how the inhibitory effects of ATP analogues are very rapidly and readily reversible (Ohno-Shosaku *et al.*, 1987; Dunne *et al.*, 1988a), nor how ATP can close channels in the absence of cytosolic Mg^{2+} (Dunne *et al.*, 1987; Ashcroft & Kakei, 1989).

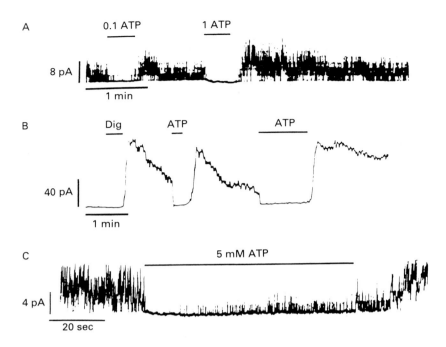

Fig. 6.2. Reactivation of K_{ATP}-channels by ATP. In B, cells were permeabilized using 10 μM digitonin (Dig). (Records A and B from Findlay & Dunne (1986a) and, C, from Dunne *et al.* (1986).)

Adenosine triphosphate also has a number of stimulatory effects on channels. First, ATP will effectively and dramatically reduce the rate of K_{ATP}-channel run-down. This effect is both concentration-dependent (*see* Fig. 6.2A), and influenced by the length of exposure to ATP (*see* Fig. 6.2B). Since this novel action of ATP, so-called 'refreshment' of channels, cannot be brought about either by non-hydrolysable analogues of ATP or by Mg^{2+}-free, ATP-containing solutions (Trube *et al.*, 1986; Findlay & Dunne, 1986a; Ohno-Shosaku *et al.*, 1987), the maintenance of the channels in an operational state, i.e. a state from which they are able to be activated, must involve at least one ATP-fuelled phosphorylation process (Findlay, 1987; Ashcroft & Kakei, 1989; Petersen, 1988). Second, at higher concentrations (e.g. 5 mM), ATP added to the inside of the membrane for extended periods of time results, after a period of complete channel inhibition, in a recovery of channel activity (*see* Fig. 6.2C). Finally, it has also been shown that at low concentrations (< 10 μM), ATP will open channels (Dunne *et al.*, 1988b; Ribalet *et al.*, 1989).

The effects of adenosine diphosphate (ADP)

As with ATP the overall effects of ADP on K_{ATP} are somewhat complicated.

In general, low concentrations, less than 0.5 mM, added to the inside of the membrane, open channels, whereas higher concentrations close channels (Dunne & Petersen, 1986a; Kakei *et al.*, 1986). The opening effects of ADP may involve protein phosphorylation since ADP-β-S, a non-hydrolysable analogue of ADP, only closes K_{ATP} (Dunne & Petersen, 1986a; Dunne *et al.*, 1988a).

These somewhat variable and unpredictable effects of ADP are also influenced by channel run-down (Dunne & Peterson, 1986a; Bokvist *et al.*, 1991), and may result from multiple ADP-binding sites on the channel. However in the presence of ATP, ADP invariably opens channels (Dunne & Petersen, 1986a; Kakei *et al.*, 1986; Dunne *et al.*, 1988a), even when the concentration of ADP is very low in comparison with that of ATP (Dunne *et al.*, 1988a). Interestingly, this action of ADP can also be mimicked by ADP-β-S and both molecules open K_{ATP} in the presence of either ATP-γ-S, AMP-PNP or AMP-PCP. This suggests that competitive interactions between the two molecules, rather than a protein phosphorylation-dependent process is important in determining the ability of channels to open (Dunne *et al.*, 1988a).

The effects of other nucleotides

The reduced and non-reduced forms of the pyridine nucleotides influence channel behaviour. High concentrations ($> 500\,\mu$M) evoke inhibition, whereas low concentrations ($< 500\,\mu$M) open channels, both directly and in the presence of ATP/ADP (Dunne *et al.*, 1988b). In Mg^{2+}-free solutions the stimulatory effects of the pyridine nucleotides are lost, while the inhibitory actions are retained (Dunne, 1989a). The intracellular concentrations of the pyridine nucleotides in unstimulated cells have been evaluated (see Dunne *et al.*, 1988b). Values of between 30 and 100 μM have been recorded for NADH, NADP and NADPH, whilst the concentration of NAD, on the other hand, is considerably higher, 200–350 μM. Since NAD was found to inhibit K_{ATP} in the presence of quasi-physiological ATP/ADP concentrations, this may indicate that in the intact cell, NAD could contribute to the tonic inhibition of K_{ATP}.

Regulation by G proteins

There are three major pieces of evidence to suggest that the activity of ATP-sensitive K-channels is regulated by a G protein(s) closely associated with the channel. First, guanosine triphosphate (GTP), guanosine diphosphate (GDP) and GTPγS evoke a reversible, concentration-dependent (10 μM–2 mM) increase in channel openings (Dunne & Petersen, 1986b), which requires the presence of Mg^{2+} (Findlay, 1987). Second, the aluminofluoride complex AlF_4^-, which is known to have effects on a number of G protein regulated systems (Bigay *et al.*, 1987), dose-dependently (1–10 mM) activates K_{ATP} (Dunne *et al.*, 1989). The effects of AlF_4^- are abolished when Al^{3+} is removed from the bathing solution by chelation with deferoxamine and enhanced when additional Al^{3+} is made available. Finally, the effects of a number of hormones and neurotransmitters which activate K_{ATP} and inhibit insulin secretion (*see below*), are lost whenever cells are pretreated for a number of hours with pertussis toxin (Dunne *et al.*, 1989; De Weille *et al.*, 1989).

Regulation by protein kinase C

Apart from the suggestion that K_{ATP}-channels are regulated by protein kinase A, the intricate control of these channels becomes even more complex when we consider that the channel is also influenced by a Ca- and phospholipid-dependent protein kinase C (Wollheim *et al.*, 1988).

Phorbol esters such as phorbol myristate acetate (PMA) which are potent activators of protein kinase C, can both induce secretion and potentiate glucose-induced insulin release from pancreatic β-cells (Virji *et al.*, 1978; Bozem *et al.*, 1987). Despite these effects, attempts to quantify the actions of PMA on the membrane potential have produced mixed results. In mouse islets of Langerhans, conventional microelectrode experiments indicate that phorbol esters have no effects on the membrane potential (Bozem *et al.*, 1987) and that PMA significantly modulates the glucose-induced electrical activity of the cells (Pace & Goldsmith, 1985). Patch-clamp experiments have apparently further complicated the issue. In intact cells, Wollheim and collaborators (1988) showed that PMA caused the closure of K_{ATP} and that this was associated with a depolarization of the membrane. However, exactly the opposite effect on K_{ATP} was recorded by Ribalet *et al.* (1988) and in a series of experiments carried out by De Weille *et al.* (1989), PMA-evoked channel activation was associated with a marked hyperpolarization of the membrane.

The experimental approaches used in each of these studies was somewhat different, namely, cell-attached membrane patches (Wollheim *et al.*, 1988) versus whole cells (De Weille *et al.*, 1989) and short-term (Wollheim *et al.*, 1988) versus long-term (Ribalet *et al.*, 1988) exposure of the membrane to PMA. Thus the effects of phorbol esters on K_{ATP} have recently been re-examined using open cells (Dunne *et al.*, 1990d). The results of these experiments suggested that when PMA was added directly to the inside of the plasma membrane for short periods, a marked inhibition of K_{ATP} resulted (Dunne *et al.*, 1990d), the time course of which was similar to that seen in intact cells (Wollheim *et al.*, 1988). When PMA was present for longer periods of time the inhibitory effects of the phorbol ester were transient, since channel closure was followed by a period of prolonged channel activation. The time course of these stimulatory effects was once again similar to that recorded in intact cells (Ribalet *et al.*, 1988). Furthermore, PMA was also found to open channels directly when it was added to the membrane 'late' in a particular experiment—in general 15 min after permeabilization had taken place (Dunne *et al.*, 1990d). Under these conditions extensive dialysis of the cell interior has taken place and the situation is somewhat analogous to the whole-cell experiments of De Weille and collaborators (1989), where PMA was also found to activate channels and hyperpolarize the membrane.

Clearly, the experimental approaches used and the length of incubation of the membrane with PMA can influence the results obtained. One interpretation of the fact that PMA can both open and close K_{ATP}-channels is that there is more than one form of protein kinase C associated with the channel. This is supported by the fact that cell-permeable diacyglycerols, such as didecomylglycerol (DC_{10}), can both activate (Dunne *et al.*, 1990d) and inhibit (Wollheim *et al.*, 1988) K_{ATP} under different experimental conditions. A somewhat analogous situation has been reported in cardiac cells in which phorbol esters were found to have novel biphasic effects on the gating of Ca-channels (Lacerda *et al.*, 1988).

Extracellular regulators of channel function

The effects of carbohydrate secretagogues

The action of 10 mM glucose on the membrane potential of a single isolated rat pancreatic β-cell is demonstrated in Fig. 6.3. The voltage recording was obtained using the whole-cell current-clamp mode of the patch-clamp technique. When challenged directly with glucose, added to the bathing solution, the cell underwent a marked depolarization, which led to the generation of Ca-spike potentials. This pattern of electrical activity is somewhat similar to that recorded from β-cells in intact islets of Langerhans using conventional microelectrode impalement techniques (Henquin & Meissner, 1984).

Adenosine triphosphate-regulated K-channels are the only operational K-channels seen under resting conditions in intact cells. It is now clear that K_{ATP}-channels play a key role in initiating the complex pattern of electrical activity shown in Fig. 6.3, since when the extracellular concentration of glucose, or of other nutrient secretagogues is raised, these channels close (Fig. 6.4). The resulting membrane depolarization opens voltage-gated Ca-channels, through which Ca^{2+} can enter the cell producing the 'upstroke' of the spike potential. At the point of opening of Ca-channels, the membrane potential will be about -20 mV, and this depolarization, coupled with the sharp increase in $[Ca^{2+}]_i$, will cause Ca- and voltage-activated K-channels (BK_{Ca}) to open. Opening of BK_{Ca}-channels will tend

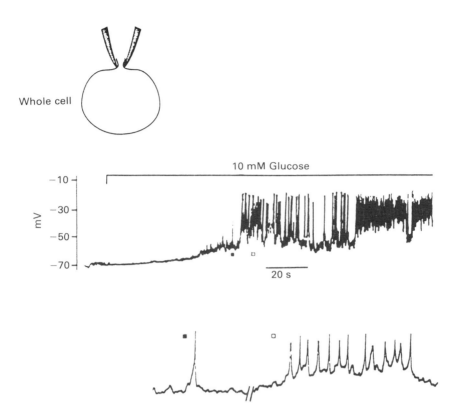

Fig. 6.3. Patch-clamp whole-cell voltage recording showing the effects of 10 mM glucose on the membrane potential of a cultured rat pancreatic β-cell. The trace begins 300 s after generating the recording configuration. Expanded time-base inserts come from the periods indicated by the solid and filled squares.

to repolarize the membrane, thereby closing the Ca^{2+} gate and producing the 'downstroke' of the spike potential. The delayed rectifier K-channel (K_V) also appears to contribute to the spike repolarization. The resulting closure of Ca-channels will cause the $[Ca^{2+}]_i$ to fall, which combined with a return towards the high resting negative membrane potential will tend to close both BK_{Ca} and K_V. As K_{ATP}-channels remain closed, a renewed depolarization of the membrane is generated, promoting opening of voltage-gated Ca-channels. A cycle of channel openings and closures has, therefore, been initiated which leads to the repetitive firing of Ca-spike potentials. The culmination of these changes in potential is the generation of finely controlled waves of Ca^{2+} influx (Grapengeisser *et al.*, 1988, 1989; Pralong *et al.*, 1990), which is the key internal regulator for the secretion of insulin by the process of exocytosis from the cell (Fig. 6.5). When the external concentration of glucose drops below the normal resting level, reopening of K_{ATP} and closure of other channels results and establishes

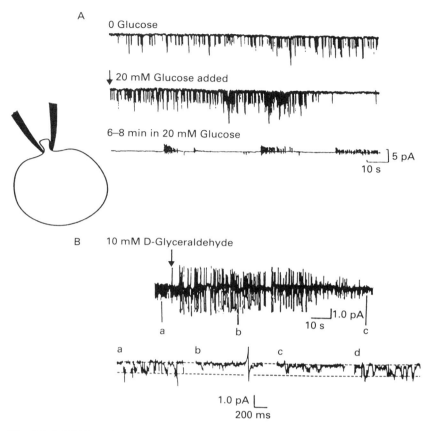

Fig. 6.4. Inhibition of K_{ATP}-channels in intact cells. (Record A modified from Rorsman & Trube (1990) with permission, and B from Dunne *et al.* (1986).)

once again the normal resting conditions. With external concentrations of glucose above threshold values (5–8 mM), there is a good correlation between the activity of K_{ATP} channels and the suprathreshold pattern of electrical activity (Cook *et al.*, 1988; Cook & Ikeuchi, 1989; Smith *et al.*, 1990a).

The link which couples metabolism to channel closure most likely involves changes in the concentrations of free ATP and ADP close to the cell membrane interior (Fig. 6.5) but the possible regulatory role of other small molecules, such as NAD(P)H/NAD(P), pH_i or the importance of protein kinase C-mediated channel phosphorylation cannot be excluded.

Considering that the intracellular concentration of ATP, estimated using a variety of techniques, is between 4 and 6 mM (Petersen & Findlay, 1987), how can K_{ATP} open in intact cells, when K_i values for ATP inhibition range between 10 and 70 μM (Table 6.1)? A number of explanations

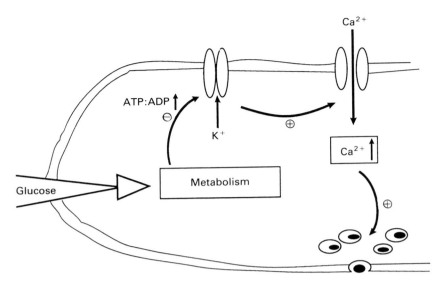

Fig. 6.5. The role of K_{ATP}-channels in the control of the cell membrane potential and the secretion of insulin in pancreatic β-cells.

have been offered to explain this discrepancy. These include the possibility that there are lower concentrations of ATP at the inner membrane than in the rest of the cell due possibly to sequestration of ATP into organelles, that ATP binds to macromolecules, or alternatively that cytosolic ATP gradients exist (as reviewed by Jones, 1986; Panten & Lenzen, 1988; Ashcroft, 1988). That $[ATP]_i$ is considerably lower at the membrane than in the cytosol is supported by the data of Niki *et al.* (1989a), who have shown that in HIT-T15 insulinoma β-cells the Na, K-ATPase can be inhibited by millimolar changes in ATP, even though the enzyme is saturated by much lower (micromolar) concentrations of ATP. However, despite these findings, probably the most important feature regarding the control of these channels in intact cells is that there are additional modulators of channel openings that are able to alter dramatically the sensitivity of membrane to ATP. The most effective regulator so far examined is ADP. Present in fairly high concentration in insulin-secreting cells, in comparison to other cell types (Petersen & Findlay, 1987), ADP is able to re-open ATP-inhibited channels (Dunne & Petersen, 1986a; Kakei *et al.*, 1986), even in the presence of excess ATP compared to ADP (e.g. 20:1) (Dunne *et al.*, 1988a). As well as ADP, AMP (Dunne, 1989a) and the pyridine nucleotides (Dunne *et al.*, 1988a) also reduce the ATP-sensitivity of channels, though to a much lesser extent.

   It has been estimated that due to the high sensitivity of K_{ATP}-channels to ATP, between 90 and 99% of the channels will be closed under normal resting conditions. Surprising since as glucose acts by closing K_{ATP} to evoke a membrane depolarization, it is convenient for the cell to have the majority of its K_{ATP} channels inhibited at rest ('spare channel hypothesis'; Cook et al. (1988)); any further channel inhibition will thus produce a large effect. Large numbers of channels provide the additional advantage of enabling the cell to respond with a high capacity for rapid inhibitory effects, for example in response to either galanin or somatostatin (see below).

The evidence in support of a role for K_{ATP} in mediating the glucose-dependent subthreshold depolarization is good. However, the relative involvement of other K-channels, such as BK_{Ca} or K_V in regulating the Ca^{2+}-spike potential is less well-defined. In whole cells, the generation of rapid $I_{BK(Ca)}$-currents and slowly activating $I_{K(V)}$-currents is dependent upon the internal Ca buffering capacity of the cell dialysing solution (Satin et al., 1990). When the buffering potential is low, $I_{BK(Ca)}$ predominates but when it is high, $I_{K(V)}$ prevails. A detailed analysis of the voltage noise associated with action potentials in intact cells has recently been carried out by Smith and collaborators (1990b). These data suggest that both $I_{BK(Ca)}$- and $I_{K(V)}$ contribute to the repolarization phase of the spike. This is further supported by the findings that tetraethylammonium (TEA), which is a more selective blocker of $I_{BK(Ca)}$ than $I_{K(V)}$ (Bokvist et al., 1990a,b), significantly augments the size and the duration of Ca-spike potentials in β-cells (Atwater et al., 1978; Findlay & Dunne, 1986b), and by the fact that in intact cells openings of an 8 pS channel (K_V) are associated with the spike (Smith et al., 1990b). At this stage, without the aid of more specific pharmacological tools it seems likely that both these channels aid in the repolarization of the spike potential.

In addition to the scheme of events outlined above and in Fig. 6.5, it has been shown that voltage-gated Ca-channels in these cells are influenced by carbohydrate metabolism (Velasco et al., 1988; Smith et al., 1990c), Glucose or glyceraldehyde metabolism increases the mean open time, decreases the longer of the two mean closed times and lowers the threshold for the voltage activation of L-type Ca-channels. As yet, the precise link which couples metabolism to channel opening is unknown, but it is possibly diacylglycerol (Velasco & Petersen, 1989). Since the effects of carbohydrate secretagogues on voltage-gated Ca-channels were only regularly observed at high concentrations, one possible physiological implication for this is that the activation of Ca-channels may in some way be involved in modulating the activity of cells at elevated concentrations of glucose. Between 5 and 8 mM glucose, the steady-state electrical activity of the membrane consists of oscillatory waves of depolarized plateau potentials with superimposed Ca-spikes ('slow waves'). At any one glucose concentration the slow waves are remarkably regular; however, as the concentration is increased (> 15 mM) the waves 'fuse' resulting in a sustained depolarization and continuous spiking, thereby potentiating the release of insulin (Meissner & Schmelz, 1974; Beigleman *et al.*, 1977). The precise ionic events mediating these changes in potential remain unknown.

Finally, it must be emphasized that simple closure of a large fraction of K_{ATP}- channels would not alone cause the cell membrane to depolarize. This can only be achieved against a background inward current (Petersen & Findlay, 1987; Dunne & Petersen, 1990, 1991). Such a current could be carried by either Na^+ or Cl^- or indeed by both ions. The functional significance of voltage-dependent Na-channels in β-cells is, however, a matter of controversy. Tetrodotoxin (TTX) partially inhibits glucose-induced insulin release, although to a lesser extent than the complete removal of Na^+ (Lambert *et al.*, 1974; Donatsch *et al.*, 1977; Hiriart & Matteson, 1988). In mouse β-cells it appears that voltage-dependent Na^+-channels are completely inactive at potentials more positive than $-80\,mV$, suggesting that they have no significant role to play in stimulus-secretion coupling (Plant, 1988). This, however, is apparently not the case in rat β-cells, as Hiriart and Matteson (1988) have demonstrated that channels were only inactivated at potentials less negative than $-40\,mV$. Voltage-activated Na-channels have also been described in RINm5F cells (Rorsman *et al.*, 1986) and TTX strongly influences the electrical activity and $[Ca^{2+}]_i$ in these cells (Dunne *et al.*, 1990e). Apart from Na^+, there is also evidence for a possible role for Cl^- in determining the membrane depolarization and/or maintaining the membrane potential in the presence of glucose. Studies of radiolabelled Cl^- fluxes have suggested the existence of voltage-dependent Cl^- channels (Sehlin, 1987) and substituting Cl^- by less permeant anions inhibits insulin release (Somers *et al.*, 1980; Sehlin & Meissner, 1988). If Cl^- were to be accumulated by the $Na^+-K^+-2Cl^-$ co-transport mechanism, the opening of Cl^- channels and efflux of Cl^- would provide the required inward current.

The effects of hormones and neurotransmitters

Galanin is a 29-amino acid polypeptide that has been known for a number of years to abolish insulin secretion under a number of experimental conditions, both *in vivo* and in the isolated perfused pancreas (Dunning *et al.*, 1986; Ahren *et al.*, 1987; Dunning & Taborsky, 1988; Drews *et al.*, 1990). At least part of these inhibitory effects involves actions of the peptide on K_{ATP}. Electrophysiological investigations of galanin have demonstrated that the polypeptide is able to hyperpolarize the membrane and thereby terminate the cells' electrical activity (De Weille *et al.*, 1988). These actions can be directly attributed to an increase in the open frequency of K_{ATP} (De Weille *et al.*, 1988; Dunne *et al.*, 1989). The actions of the peptide were, however, lost in cells pretreated for a number of hours with pertussis toxin (PTX). In addition activation of a G protein by AlF_4^- was found to mimic the actions of galanin which led to the conclusion that the effects of the hyperglycaemia-inducing neuropeptide were mediated though the activation of a PTX-sensitive G protein closely associated with the channel (Dunne *et al.*, 1989). A similar G protein also appears to be involved in mediating the actions of another inhibitory hormone, somatostatin, which hyperpolarizes the membrane and opens K_{ATP} in the absence of PTX (De Weille *et al.*, 1989).

A combination of patch-clamp recordings and measurement of single cell $[Ca^{2+}]_i$ has recently been used to investigate the effects of the hypogly-caemia-inducing hormone vasopressin (Martin *et al.*, 1989). In these experiments it was found that the peptide: (i) depolarized the membrane; (ii) evoked Ca-spike potentials; and (iii) elevated $[Ca^{2+}]_i$. These effects were initiated by vasopressin-induced closure of K_{ATP}. Channel inhibition appears to involve a receptor-mediated event since vasopressin had no effects on the frequency of channel openings or closures either when applied to the inside of an isolated plasma membrane patch or when added to the bath in experiments using cell-attached membrane patches (Martin *et al.*, 1989). The link between vasopressin receptor activation and the closure of K_{ATP} has yet to be determined, but it may involve the action of a protein kinase C closely associated with the channel.

Extracellular ATP, which can be considered as a neurotransmitter, stimulates insulin secretion both *in vivo* and *in vitro* (Loubantieres-Marni *et al.*, 1979; Blachier & Malaisse, 1988; Arkhammar *et al.*, 1990). The effects of ATP are thought to be mediated by the P_{2Y} purinoceptor (Bertrand *et al.*, 1989). A physiological role for external ATP in the regulation of insulin release is suggested by the fact that islets of Langer-hans are richly innervated with both sympathetic and parasympathetic fibres (Miller, 1981). In addition the ATP concentration of the secretory granule is high, which may indicate that the nucleotide plays a role in the autoregulation of hormone secretion (Li *et al.*, 1991). At relatively lower concentrations than required to close K_{ATP} from the inside of the membrane, externally applied ATP depolarizes the cell membrane, ini-tiates Ca-action potentials and elevates $[Ca^{2+}]_i$ (Arkhammar *et al.*, 1990; Dunne *et al.*, 1990c; Li *et al.*, 1991). In excised outside-out membrane patches these effects were shown to be initiated by ATP evoking the closure of K_{ATP}-channels (Dunne *et al.*, 1990c; Li *et al.*, 1991), suggesting that the purinergic receptor is either part of or closely associated with the channel (Fig. 6.6).

The pharmacology of K_{ATP}-channels

The K_{ATP}-channels have a very prominent role to play in regulating the actions of carbohydrate secretagogues, hormones and transmitters in insulin-secreting cells. It is not thus surprising that the pharmacology of

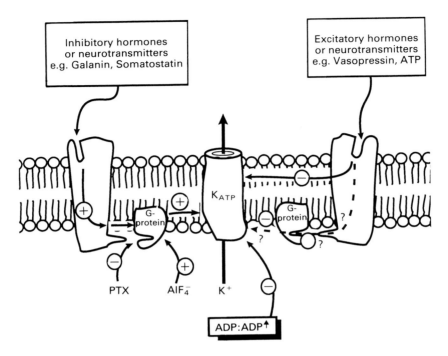

Fig. 6.6. Summary of the effects of inhibitory and stimulatory hormones and neurotransmitters on K_{ATP}-channels in pancreatic β-cells.

these channels is of particular importance in the treatment of insulin and/or glucose regulation disorders (Petersen & Dunne, 1989; Dunne & Petersen, 1990, 1991).

There is currently a great deal of interest in all forms of K-channel modulators, especially the K-channel openers. These compounds constitute a new class of drugs that are able to relax cardiac and vascular smooth muscle cells by opening glibenclamide-sensitive K-channels (Escande *et al.*, 1988, 1989; Standen *et al.*, 1989). They are currently of therapeutic interest due to their possible use as effective vasodilators and antihypertensive compounds. Among the best known of these are cromakalim (BRL 34915), pinacidil, RP 49356 and nicorandil (for detailed reviews see Cook, 1988; Quast & Cook, 1989; Edwards & Weston, 1990a,b). There is now both direct and indirect evidence from a number of studies to suggest that each of these drugs will activate K_{ATP}-channels in insulin-secreting cells.

The effects of K channel blockers

Sulphonylurea compounds, such as glibenclamide and tolbutamide constitute a class of hypoglycaemia-inducing drugs that have been used for a number of years to treat type II or non-insulin-dependent diabetes (reviewed by Hellman & Taljedal, 1975). It has been shown that the drugs decrease the K-permeability of the β-cell membrane (Henquin, 1980b; Gylfe et al., 1984), which leads to a depolarization of the cell, an enhanced Ca^{2+} influx and the release of insulin (Gylfe et al., 1984; Henquin & Meissner, 1982). Patch-clamp studies have now shown that these effects are mediated by the sulphonylureas which specifically close K_{ATP} (Sturgess et al., 1985; Ohno-Shosaku et al., 1987; Dunne et al., 1987; Zunkler et al., 1988a; Ashcroft et al., 1989b; Dunne, 1990a).

Not all the sulphonylureas currently used in the treatment of diabetes are equally effective, since the concentration for half-maximal inhibition of K_{ATP} lies over 3 orders of magnitude for tolbutamide ($K_i = 17\,\mu M$), meglitinide ($2.1\,\mu M$), glipizide ($6.4\,\mu M$) and glibenclamide (4–$20\,nM$) (Zunkler et al., 1988a; Ashcroft et al., 1989b; Sturgess et al., 1988). Sulphonylureas are effective from either side of the plasma membrane, closing channels in whole cells as well as excised inside-out, outside-out and cell-attached membrane patches. Inhibition of channels is not dependent upon the availability of Mg^{2+} (Dunne et al., 1987), but is enhanced by cytosolic ADP (Zunkler et al., 1988b), suggesting that the effects of the drug are not direct. Glibenclamide is a more potent inhibitor of K_{ATP} than either TTX or saxitoxin are of the voltage-gated Na^+-channel, and this has successfully helped in the biochemical identification of sulphonylurea receptors. Receptor occupancy by the sulphonylureas was first shown to be closely associated with channel blockade by Schmid-Antomarchi and collaborators (1987). Once suitable corrections have been made for albumin binding to the drug (Aguilar-Bryan et al., 1990), then the specificity and density of sulphonylurea-binding sites (Niki et al., 1989b; Schmid-Antomarchi et al., 1987) correlate very well with the estimated number of K_{ATP}-channels per cell (Dunne & Petersen, 1990; Rorsman & Trube, 1990), the efficacy of glibenclamide inhibition of K_{ATP}-channels and the ability of the sulphonylureas to elicit insulin secretion. This may indicate that the receptor — an ADP-binding protein (Niki et al. 1990), is located either on the channel or on part of its related control unit(s) (see Chapter 4, Fig. 4.10).

Gylfe and collaborators (1984) originally suggested that the drugs only act from the outside of the plasma membrane. However, this is not consistent with the findings of Trube et al. (1986), who demonstrated, using patch-clamp experiments, that tolbutamide added to the bathing solution closed channels in cell-attached patches. Since direct access to channels under the recording electrode in these experiments is occluded by the pipette, these data show that the receptor can be reached from inside of the membrane or alternatively by lateral diffusion in the membrane lipids. This conclusion is also reached by Zunkler et al. (1989) who showed that channels are inhibited by the undissociated forms of tolbutamide and its related compounds.

The affinity of glibenclamide for K_{ATP} is such that the drug was first used in the purification and isolation of the channel protein from pig brain, a protein of approximately 150 kDa (Bernadi *et al.*, 1988). A biologically active derivative of glibenclamide (5-indo-2-hydroxyglibenclamide) has recently been used to partially purify a similar protein (140 kDa) from the membranes of HIT-T15 insulinoma cells (Aguilar-Bryan *et al.*, 1990). However, despite these findings no sequence data have yet been reported nor has the protein been functionally reconstituted and shown to possess iontophoretic activity. It is interesting to note therefore, that in ventromedial hypothalamic neurones K_{ATP}-channels are unaffected by tolbutamide in excised inside-out membrane patches but are blocked by the drug in cell-attached experiments (Ashford *et al.*, 1990). One very important implication of these data is that the sulphonylurea receptor, at least in parts of the CNS, is not directly coupled to K_{ATP}, but merely associated with it.

It has been known for a number of years that certain α-adrenoceptor antagonists, such as phentolamine (α_1 and α_2) and efaroxan (α_2) are able to initiate insulin secretion from β-cells by a mechanism that does not solely involve binding of the compound to the α-adrenoceptor (Malaisse *et al.*, 1967; Schulz & Hasselblatt, 1989; Chan & Morgan, 1990). Furthermore, both phentolamine and efaroxan antagonize the diazoxide-induced inhibition of secretion and diazoxide-enhanced rate of $^{86}Rb^+$ efflux from preloaded islets (Henquin *et al.*, 1982; Dunne *et al.*, 1990b; Chan *et al.*, 1991). This can be explained by the fact that both phentolamine and efaroxan inhibit K_{ATP}-channels (Plant & Henquin, 1990; Dunne *et al.*, 1990b; Chan *et al.*, 1991; Dunne, 1991). Concentration–response relationships from excised patches suggest that 50% blockade of K_{ATP} can be achieved by approximately 12 μM efaroxan and 0.7 μM phentolamine (Chan *et al.*, 1991; Dunne, 1991). These compounds are therefore as effective as tolbutamide in blocking K_{ATP}. K_{ATP} can also be blocked by the other α_2-adrenoceptor antagonists, yohimbine (Plant & Henquin, 1990; Dunne, 1991), antazoline and tolazoline (Dunne, 1991). With the exception of yohimbine, the common structural feature of the effective α-adrenoceptor antagonists is the presence of an imidazoline group. Imidazoline-based compounds bind to sites in the plasma membrane other than the adrenoceptor (Michel & Insel, 1989) and it is now clear because of the close correlation between channel blockade and the initiation of secretion that one of these preferred binding sites is the K_{ATP}. By analogy with the effects of the sulphonylureas on K_{ATP}-channels in insulin-secreting cells (Ashcroft & Ashcroft, 1990), it is not yet clear from these preliminary studies whether the binding site, an 'imidazoline receptor', is on the K_{ATP}-channel or on a separate protein. The substituted imidazoline idazoxan, has little effect at low concentrations on insulin secretion in the absence of an adrenoceptor agonist (Ostenson *et al.*, 1988; Chan & Morgan, 1990) but at higher concentrations ($> 100\,\mu$M) partially reverses the diazoxide-induced inhibition of insulin secretion (Chan & Morgan, 1990) and blocks K_{ATP} (Chan *et al.*, 1991). If the relative affinities of both efaroxan and idazoxan for the imidazoline receptor are compared with the effects of these drugs on K_{ATP} and insulin secretion, there is a very obvious negative correlation. Both efaroxan and phentolamine have a low affinity for the imidazoline receptor (Langin & Lafontan, 1989) but they are capable of closing K_{ATP} and initiating insulin secretion. In contrast idazoxan has a very high affinity for the receptor but exerts relatively minor effects on K_{ATP} and insulin secretion over the same concentration range.

One major implication of the fact that α-adrenoceptor antagonists are also able to block K_{ATP} (phentolamine and yohimbine have relatively little effect on K_V and BK_{Ca} channels; Plant & Henquin, 1990) is that the results of many *in vitro* and *in vivo* studies using these compounds as specific blockers of adrenoceptors, clearly require re-interpretation. These recent findings do, however, provide an alternative strategy to the sulphonylurea-based drugs upon which to base future therapeutic treatment of diabetes mellitus. Such an approach would be feasible if it were possible to isolate the α-adrenoceptor blocking actions of compounds like phentolamine and efaroxan from their effects on K_{ATP}-channels.

K_{ATP}-channels are also closed by a number of more conventional K-channel blockers such as quinine (Findlay *et al.*, 1985b) ($K_d = 40\,\mu$M), aminoacridine ($100\,\mu$M) and 4-aminopyridine ($100\,\mu$M) (Cook & Hales, 1984). Tetraethylammonium at relatively low concentrations (< 2 mM) which completely blocks the BK_{Ca}-channel, has no effects on the K_{ATP}-channels (Findlay *et al.*, 1985b). Half-maximal inhibition of K_{ATP}-channels by TEA (applied to the outside of the plasma membrane) has been estimated to be 22 mM (Bokvist *et al.*, 1990a).

A number of other compounds has also been found to block K_{ATP}-channels including the plant extract ligustrazine (Peers *et al.*, 1990), the alkaloid sparteine, the dopaminergic agonist amantadine (Ashcroft & Ashcroft, 1990) and the local anaesthetics pentobarbitone, thiopentone, secobarbitone and phenobarbitone (Kozlowski & Ashford, 1991).

The effects of K-channel openers

Although structurally related to the sulphonylureas, the compound diazoxide has been used to treat certain forms of insulinoma of the pancreas (Altsuzler *et al.*, 1977) due to its ability to inhibit insulin secretion

(Henquin *et al.*, 1982). This inhibition is brought about by a repolarization of the cell membrane (Henquin & Meissner 1982), which results in a lowering of $[Ca^{2+}]_i$ (Dunne *et al.*, 1990f); effects that are principally initiated by the specific activation of K_{ATP} (Trube *et al.*, 1986; Dunne *et al.*, 1987; Dunne, 1989b; Kozlowski *et al.*, 1989; Dunne *et al.*, 1990f). Opening of these channels requires the presence of soluble cytosolic molecules, since the effects of the drug are only ever consistently observed in the presence of intracellular ATP ($[ATP]_i$) (Dunne *et al.*, 1987). Although ATP is required for the action of diazoxide, comparison of the half-maximal effective concentrations of the drug in the presence of 0.3 mM (20 μM) and 1 mM ATP (102 μM) (Kozlowski *et al.*, 1989), shows that ATP competes with diazoxide for control of channel openings (Dunne *et al.*, 1987). Phosphorylation, either of the channel or of a related control unit, also appears to be required in order for diazoxide to open channels, as the sulphonamide cannot open channels in the presence of either ATP-γ-S, AMP-PNP, AMP-PCP (Dunne, 1989b) or in the complete absence of the Mg–ATP complex (Kozlowski *et al.*, 1989).

In cells continually perfused with glucose, Dunne and collaborators (1990f) have recently shown that cromakalim will abolish the carbohydrate-induced depolarization of the cell membrane, prevent the generation of Ca-spike potentials and lower secretagogue-induced increases in $[Ca^{2+}]_i$. These effects, which result in the inhibition of insulin secretion (Garrino *et al.*, 1989) are due to the activation of K_{ATP} (Dunne *et al.*, 1990a). Pinacidil and nicorandil enhance $^{86}Rb^+$-efflux (Garrino *et al.*, 1989; Lebrun *et al.*, 1989) and inhibit insulin secretion (Garrino *et al.*, 1989) and pinacidil, RP 49356 and nicorandil have each been found to reverse the effects of glucose on the membrane potential by specifically opening K_{ATP}-channels (Dunne, 1990b).

There are a number of similarities between the effects of the novel K-channel openers and those of diazoxide in insulin-secreting cells. First, each of the compounds is effective from either side of the plasma membrane and does not affect single channel current conductance (Dunne *et al.*, 1990a,f). Second, cytosolic ATP ($[ATP]_i$) is always required for the drugs to operate effectively (Dunne, 1990b; Dunne *et al.*, 1990a). Indeed, in the complete absence of $[ATP]_i$, pinacidil, RP 49356 and nicorandil were each found to close K_{ATP} (Dunne, 1990b). Third, competitive inter-actions between each of the compounds and ATP have been found (Dunne, 1990b; Dunne *et al.*, 1990a). A similar effect is also seen in cardiac myocytes with RP 49356 (Thuringer & Escande, 1989), pinacidil (Arena & Kass, 1989; Tseng & Hoffman, 1990; Fan *et al.*, 1990) and nicorandil (Hiraokoa & Fan, 1989). In pancreatic β-cells, cromakalim, pinacidil, RP 49356 and nicorandil will all open K_{ATP} in the presence of cytosolic ATP and ADP, but have no effect on these channels in the presence of ATP analogues (Dunne, 1990b; Dunne *et al.*, 1990a). Finally,

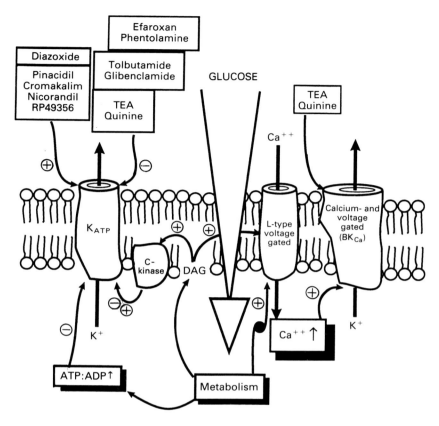

Fig. 6.7. Summary of the effects of K-channel openers and blockers on K_{ATP}-channels in insulin-secreting cells.

the sulphonylurea tolbutamide abolishes the effects of each of the openers on the membrane potential and $I_{K(ATP)}$ (Dunne *et al.*, 1987, 1990a,f; Dunne, 1990b; Fig. 6.7).

For all the similarities between diazoxide and the novel K-channel openers, the effects of cromakalim, pinacidil, RP 49356 and nicorandil are far less impressive than those of the sulphonamide. In the presence of 0.1 mM ATP, diazoxide was twice as effective at opening channels than the same concentration of either cromakalim (Dunne *et al.*, 1990a), pinacidil or RP 49356 (Dunne, 1990b),whereas in the presence of 0.5 mM ATP, the degree of channel activation brought about by 100 μM diazoxide could only be matched by 800 μM cromakalim (Dunne *et al.*, 1990a). In concentrations below 100 μM, the effects of all four compounds were weak and insignificant (Kozlowski *et al.*, 1989; Dunne, 1990b; Dunne *et al.*, 1990e), which is in sharp contrast to the actions of diazoxide, an effective opener of K-channels in insulin-secreting cells at concentrations below 20 μM (Dunne *et al.*, 1987, 1990a,f).

The apparent insensitivity of K_{ATP} in insulin-secreting cells to cromakalim, pinacidil, RP 49356 and nicorandil may have important pharmacological implications. The data gathered so far tend to suggest that these drugs are unlikely to replace diazoxide as effective oral hyperglycaemia-inducing compounds. If we consider that: (i) in a number of preparations vasorelaxant effects of the drugs have been regularly observed at concentrations below 10 μM (for reviews see Cook, 1988; Quast & Cook, 1989; Hamilton & Weston, 1989; Edwards & Weston, 1990a,b); and (ii) both cromakalim and RP 49356 have been shown to be openers of similar channels in smooth muscle* (Standen *et al.*, 1989) and cardiac cells (Thuringer & Escande, 1989) then these compounds will exert very little effect on the β-cell electrical activity. This indicates that at the therapeutically required doses of cromakalim, pinacidil, RP 49356, nicorandil as well as other similar compounds, smooth muscle relaxation could be achieved without influencing the secretion of insulin.

The observations that the β-cell and cardiac K_{ATP}-channels have a low affinity for cromakalim, whereas similar channels in smooth muscle cells have a relatively high affinity may indicate that there is a degree of diversity in the structure and regulation of ATP-sensitive K-channel subtypes. There is additional support for this. Firstly, Faivre and Findlay (1989) have shown that diazoxide, an opener of the β-cell and smooth muscle K_{ATP}-channel (Standen *et al.*, 1989), inhibits similar channels in ventricular muscle cells. Second, the cromakalim analogue SDZ PCO-400 blocks the β-cell K_{ATP}-channel (M. J. Dunne, unpublished observations). Thirdly, it has been shown that in cardiac ventricular myocytes neither cromakalim (Escande *et al.*, 1988) nor its related compound SR 44866 (Findlay *et al.*, 1989) requires cytosolic ATP to open K_{ATP}, whereas their effects on the β-cell channel are strictly dependent upon the presence of the nucleotide. The mechanisms through which K-channel openers act have only been examined in detail in insulin-secreting cells; the results of similar experiments with cardiac and smooth muscle cells will be interesting.

Conclusions

Although there can be little doubt that the closure of K_{ATP} initiates the membrane depolarization in response to carbohydrate metabolism, the mechanism by which channel inhibition is brought about is far from

---

*For an overview of the possible target K-channels for the K-channel openers in smooth muscle, *see* Chapters 7 and 14.

proven. Several hypothetical routes through which these topologically distinct events can be coupled have been reviewed, and although possible, their precise role(s) in stimulus-secretion coupling is by no means certain. Alternative mechanisms to explain the control of the various channel openings and closures may well be proposed in the future, and the ideas presented in this article re-evaluated. Significantly, the advancement of current technology to detect changes in internal free nucleotide concentrations at high resolution will either authenticate or dismiss the role(s) of the various nucleotides in stimulus-secretion coupling.

It must be stressed that the majority of patch-clamp experiments carried out to date have only addressed themselves to the events that mediate the initial or subthreshold depolarization of the membrane. Under steady-state conditions of carbohydrate stimulation, membrane potential fluctuations are complex, consisting of oscillatory waves of depolarization and repolarization, generating repetitive plateaus with superimposed Ca-spike potentials. The ionic events responsible for these changes and the cellular processes responsible for controlling them, remain largely unaddressed and unanswered.

There have been a number of studies in which the actions of hormones and neurotransmitters on K_{ATP} have been investigated. In addition it has recently been shown that adrenaline will activate a small conductance, sulphonylurea-insensitive K-channel in insulin-secreting cells (Rorsman et al., 1991). Although the involvement of G proteins has been implicated, the precise identity of the cellular events which couple receptor activation to the closure or opening of K_{ATP} has yet to be elucidated (see Chapter 4).

Finally, since the K_{ATP}-channels so far identified appear to be very similar in a number of insulin-secreting cell preparations (Table 6.1) investigations of ion channels in diabetic systems, including animal and human tissues are of obvious importance. Fetal rat β-cells have a similar aetiology to the clinical condition of human non-insulin-dependent diabetes mellitus (NIDDM) since they express deficient insulin secretion in response to glucose. The K_{ATP}-channels in these cells are not closed during carbohydrate stimulation, despite the fact that the channels are otherwise similar to those of adult cells (Rorsman et al., 1989). The fetal K_{ATP}-channels are, however, closed by the sulphonylurea tolbutamide, which may indicate that a regulatory dysfunction rather than a defect in the channel protein characterizes the diseased state of NIDDM (Rorsman et al., 1989, 1990). It would not be surprising if defects in either the channel protein, glucose metabolism or an impairment of the link which couples metabolism to K_{ATP} closure, may prevail in other forms of glucose and/or insulin regulation disorders.

Acknowledgements

I would like to thank Liz Harding and Jon Jagger for reading and correcting this manuscript, the Wellcome Trust, and the Yorkshire Cancer Research Campaign, the British Diabetic Association, The Royal Society, the Smith Kline Foundation, The Nuffield Foundation, Nordisk UK and the University of Sheffield for their generous financial support.

References

Aguilar-Bryan, L., Nelson, D. A., Vu, Q. A., Humphrey, M. B. & Boyd, A. E. III (1990) Photoaffinity labeling and partial purification of the β-cell sulfonylurea receptor using a novel, biologically active glyburide analog. *Journal of Biological Chemistry* **265**, 8218–8224.

Ahren, B., Rorsman, P. & Berggren, P-O. (1987) Galanin and the endocrine pancreas. *FEBS Letters* **229**, 233–237.

Altszuler, N., Hampshire, J. & Morarv, E. (1977) On the mechanism of diazoxide-induced hyperpolarisation. *Diabetes* **26**, 931–935.

Arena, J. P. & Kass, R. S. (1989) Activation of ATP-sensitive K^+ channels in heart cells by pinacidil: dependence on ATP. *American Journal of Physiology* **257**, H2092–H2096.

Arkhammar, P., Hallberg, A., Kindmak, H., Nilsson, T., Rorsman, P. & Berggren, P-O. (1990) Extracellular ATP increases cytoplasmic free Ca^{2+} concentration in clonal insulin-producing RINm5F cells. *Biochemical Journal* **265**, 203–211.

Arkhammar, P., Nilsson, T., Rorsman, P. & Berggren, P-O. (1987) Inhibition of ATP-sensitive K^+ channels precedes depolarization-induced increase in cytoplasmic free Ca^{2+} concentration in pancreatic β-cells. *Journal of Biological Chemistry* **262**, 5448–5454.

Ashcroft, F. M. (1988) Adenosine 5′-triphosphate-sensitive potassium channels. *Annual Review of Neuroscience* **11**, 97–118.

Ashcroft, F. M. & Kakei, M. (1989) ATP-sensitive K^+ channels in rat pancreatic β-cells: modulation by ATP and Mg^{2+} ions. *Journal of Physiology* **416**, 349–367.

Ashcroft, F. M., Ashcroft, S. J. H. & Harrison, D. E. (1988) Properties of single potassium channels modulated by glucose in rat pancreatic β-cells. *Journal of Physiology* **400**, 501–527.

Ashcroft, F. M., Harrison, D. E. & Ashcroft, S. J. H. (1984) Glucose induces closure of single potassium channels in isolated rat pancreatic β-cells. *Nature* **312**, 446–448.

Ashcroft, F. M., Kakei, M., Gibson, J. S., Gray, D. W. & Sutton, R. (1989b) The ATP-and tolbutamide-sensitivity of the ATP-sensitive K^+ channel from human pancreatic β-cells. *Diabetologia* **32**, 591–598.

Ashcroft, F. M., Kakei, M. & Kelly, R. P. (1989a) Rubidium and sodium permeability of the ATP-sensitive K^+ channel in single rat pancreatic β-cells. *Journal of Physiology* **408**, 413–430.

Ashcroft, F. M., Kakei, M., Kelly, R. P. & Sutton, R. (1987) ATP-sensitive K^+ channels in human isolated pancreatic β-cells. *FEBS Letters* **215**, 9–12.

Ashcroft, S. J. H. & Ashcroft, F. M. (1990) Properties and functions of ATP-sensitive k^+ channels. *Cellular Signalling* **2**, 117–214.

Ashford, M. L. J., Boden, P. R. & Treherne, J. M. (1990) Tolbutamide excites rat glucoreceptive ventromedial hypothalamic neurones by indirect inhibition of ATP-K$^+$ channels. *British Journal of Pharmacology* **101**, 531–538.

Atwater, I., Ribalet, B. & Rojas, E. (1978) Mouse pancreatic β-cells: tetraethylammonium blockage of the potassium permeability induced by depolarization. *Journal of Physiology* **288**, 561–574.

Beigleman, P. M., Ribalet, B. & Atwater, I. (1977) Electrical activity of mouse pancreatic β-cells. II. Effects of glucose and arginine. *Journal of Physiology* **73**, 201–217.

Bernadi, H., Fosset, M. & Lazdunski, M. (1988) Characterization, purification and affinity labeling of the brain ^{3}H-glibenclamide-binding protein, a putative neuronal ATP-regulated K$^+$ channel. *Proceedings of the National Academy of Sciences USA* **85**, 9816–9820.

Bertrand, G., Gross, J., Chapal, J. & Loubantieres, M-M. (1989) Difference in the potentiating effect of adenosine triphosphate and the α,β-methylene ATP on the biphasic insulin response to glucose. *British Journal of Pharmacology* **98**, 998–1004.

Bigay, J., Deterre, P., Pfister, C. & Chabre, M. (1987) Fluoride complexes of aluminium or beryllium act on G-proteins as reversibly bound analogues of the γ-phosphate of GTP. *EMBO Journal* **6**, 2907–2913.

Blachier, F. & Malaisse, W. J. (1988) Effect of exogenous ATP upon inositol phosphate production, cationic fluxes and insulin release in pancreatic islet cells. *Biochimica et Biophysica Acta* **970**, 222–279.

Bokvist, K., Ammala, C., Ashcroft, F. M., Berggren, P.-O., Lasson, O. & Rorsman, P. (1991) Separate processes mediate nucleotide-induced inhibition and stimulation of the ATP-regulated K$^+$-channel in mouse pancreatic β-cells. *Proceedings of the Royal Society (Series B)* **243**, 139–144.

Bokvist, K., Rorsman, P. & Smith, P. A. (1990a) Block of ATP-regulated and Ca^{2+}-activated K$^+$ channels in mouse pancreatic β-cells by external tetraethylammonium and quinine. *Journal of Physiology* **423**, 327–347.

Bokvist, K., Rorsman, P. & Smith, P. A. (1990b) Effect of external tetraethylammonium ions and quinine on delayed rectifying K$^+$ channels in mouse pancreatic β-cells. *Journal of Physiology* **423**, 311–325.

Bozem, M., Nenquin, M. & Henquin, J. C. (1987) The ionic, electrical and secretory effects of protein kinase C activation in mouse pancreatic β-cells: studies with phorbol ester. *Endocrinology* **121**, 1025–1033.

Cavalie, A., Ochi, R., Pelzer, D. & Trautwein, W. (1983) Elementary currents through Ca^{2+} channels in guinea pig myocytes. *Pflügers Archiv* **398**, 284–297.

Chan, S. L. F. & Morgan, N. G. (1990) Stimulation of insulin secretion by efaroxan may involve interaction with potassium channels. *European Journal of Pharmacology* **176**, 97–101.

Chan, S. L. F., Dunne, M. J., Stillings, M. R. & Morgan, N. G. (1991) The α_2-antagonist efaroxan modulates K$_{ATP}$ channels in insulin-secreting cells. *European Journal of Pharmacology* **204**, 41–48.

Cook, D. L. & Hales, C. N. (1984) Intracellular ATP directly blocks K$^+$ channels in pancreatic β-cells. *Nature* **311**, 271–273.

Cook, D. L. & Ikeuchi, M. (1989) Tolbutamide as mimic of glucose on β-cell electrical activity. *Diabetes* **38**, 416–421.

Cook, D. L., Satin, L. S., Ashford, M. L. J. & Hales, C. N. (1988) ATP-sensitive K$^+$ channels in pancreatic β-cells. *Diabetes* **37**, 495–498.

Cook, N. S. (1988) The pharmacology of potassium channels and their therapeutic potential. *Trends in Pharmacological Sciences* **9**, 21–28.

Davies, N. W. (1990) Modulation of ATP-sensitive K$^+$ channels in skeletal muscle by intracellular protons. *Nature* **343**, 375–377.

Dean, P. M. & Matthews, E. K. (1968) Electrical activity in pancreatic islet cells. *Nature* **219**, 389–390.

De Weille, J., Schmid-Antomarchi, H., Fosset, M. & Lazdunski, M. (1988) ATP-sensitive K$^+$ channels that are blocked by hypoglycemia-inducing sulphonylureas in insulin-secreting cells are activated by galanin, a hyperglycemia-inducing hormone. *Proceedings of the National Academy of Sciences USA* **85**, 1312–1316.

De Weille, J. R., Schmid-Antomarchi, H., Fosset, M. & Lazdunski, M. (1989) Regulation of ATP-sensitive K$^+$ channel in insulinoma cells: Activation by somatostatin and protein kinase C and the role of cAMP. *Proceedings of the National Academy of Sciences USA* **86**, 2971–2975.

Donatsch, P., Lowe, D. A., Richardson, B. P. & Taylor, P. (1977) The functional significance of sodium channels in pancreatic beta-cell membranes. *Journal of Physiology* **267**, 357–376.

Drews, G., Debuyser, A., Nenquin, M. & Henquin, J. C. (1990) Galanin and epinephrine act on distinct receptors to inhibit insulin release by the same mechanisms including an increase in K$^+$ permeability of the β-cell membrane. *Endocrinology* **126**, 1646–1653.

Dunne, M. J. (1989a) Ion Channels in Insulin-Secreting Cells, PhD Thesis, Liverpool University, England.

Dunne, M. J. (1989b) Protein phosphorylation is required for diazoxide to open ATP-sensitive potassium channels in insulin (RINm5F) secreting cells. *FEBS Letters* **250**, 262–266.

Dunne, M. J. (1990a) Nutrient and pharmacological stimulation of insulin-secreting cells; marked differences in the onset of electrical activity. *Experimental Physiology* **75**, 771–777.

Dunne, M. J. (1990b) Effects of pinacidil, RP 49356 and nicorandil on ATP-sensitive potassium channels in insulin-secreting cells, *British Journal of Pharmacology* **99**, 487–492.

Dunne, M. J. (1991) Block of ATP-regulated potassium channels by phentolamine and other α-adrenoceptor antagonists. *British Journal of Pharmacology* **103**, 1847–1850.

Dunne, M. J. & Petersen, O. H. (1986a) Intracellular ADP activates K$^+$ channels that are inhibited by ATP in an insulin-secreting cell line. *FEBS Letters* **208**, 59–62.

Dunne, M. J. & Petersen, O. H. (1986b) GTP and GDP activation of K$^+$ channels that are inhibited by ATP. *Pflügers Archiv* **407**, 564–565.

Dunne, M. J. & Petersen, O. H. (1990) Ion channels in insulin-secreting cells; their role in stimulus-secretion coupling. In Young, J.A. & Wong, P.Y.D. (eds), *Epithelial Secretion of Water and Electrolytes*. Berlin, Springer-Verlag, pp. 277–291.

Dunne, M. J. & Petersen, O. H. (1991) Potassium selective ion channels in insulin-secreting cells: physiology, pharmacology and their role in stimulus-secretion coupling. *Biochimica et Biophysica Acta* **1071**, 67–82.

Dunne, M. J., Aspinall, R. J. & Petersen, O. H. (1990a) The effects of chromakalim on ATP-sensitive potassium channels in insulin-secreting cells. *British Journal of Pharmacology* **99**, 169–175.

Dunne, M. J., Bullett, M. J., Li, G., Wollheim, C. B. & Petersen, O.H. (1989) Galanin activates nucleotide-dependent K$^+$ channels in insulin-secreting cells via a pertussis toxin-sensitive G-protein. *EMBO Journal* **8**, 412–420.

Dunne, M. J., Chan, S. L. F., Morgan, N. G. & Stillings, M. R. (1990b) Block of ATP-sensitive potassium channels in isolated islets of Langerhans and clonal insulin secreting cells by α_2-adrenergic antagonists. *Journal of Physiology* **434**, 34P.

Dunne, M. J., Findlay, I. & Petersen, O. H. (1988b) The effects of pyridine nucleotides on the gating of ATP-sensitive K$^+$ channels in insulin-secreting cells. *Journal of Membrane Biology* **102**, 205–216.

Dunne, M. J., Findlay, I., Petersen, O. H. & Wollheim, C. B. (1986) ATP-sensitive K$^+$ channels in an insulin-secreting cell-line are inhibited by D-glyceraldehyde and activated by membrane permeabilization, *Journal of Membrane Biology* **93**, 271–279.

Dunne, M. J., Illot, M. C. & Petersen, O. H. (1987) Interactions of diazoxide, tolbutamide and ATP^{4-} on nucleotide-dependent K$^+$ channels in an insulin-secreting cell line. *Journal of Membrane Biology* **99**, 215–224.

Dunne, M. J., Li, G-D., Milani, D., Wollheim, C. B. & Petersen, O. H. (1990c) Externally applied ATP closes ATP-sensitive K$^+$ channels, increases cytosolic Ca^{2+} and evokes the secretion of insulin from clonal pancreatic β-cells. *Journal of Physiology* **430**, 124P.

Dunne, M. J., Tucker, L. M. & Petersen, O. H. (1990d) Activators of protein kinase C have novel effects on ATP-sensitive potassium channels in insulin-secreting cell. *Journal of Physiology* **429**, 93P.

Dunne, M. J., West-Jordan, J., Abraham, R. J., Edwards, R. T. H. & Petersen, O. H. (1988a) The gating of nucleotide dependent K$^+$ channels in insulin-secreting cells can be modulated by changes in the ratio of ATP^{4-}/ADP^{3-} and by non-hydrolyzable analogues of ATP and ADP. *Journal of Membrane Biology* **104**, 165–172.

Dunne, M. J., Yule, D. I., Gallacher, D. V. & Petersen, O. H. (1990e) The stimulant-evoked depolarisation and increase in [Ca^{2+}]$_i$ in insulin-secreting cells is dependent on external Na$^+$. *Journal of Membrane Biology* **113**, 131–138.

Dunne, M. J., Yule, D. I., Gallacher, D. V. & Petersen, O. H. (1990f) A comparative study of the effects of cromakalim (BRL 34915) and diazoxide on membrane potential, [Ca^{2+}]$_i$ and ATP-sensitive potassium currents in insulin-secreting cells. *Journal of Membrane Biology* **114**, 54–61.

Dunning, B. E., Ahrem, B., Veith, R. C., Bottcher, G., Sandler, F. & Taborsky (1986) Galanin: a novel pancreatic neuropeptide. *American Journal of Physiology* **215**, E127–E132.

Dunning, B. E. & Taborsky, G. T. (1988) Galanin—a novel sympathetic neurotransmitter in endocrine pancreas. *Diabetes* **37**, 1157–1162.

Edwards, G. & Weston, A. H. (1990a) Potassium channel openers and vascular smooth muscle relaxation. *Pharmacology and Therapeutics* **48**, 237–258.

Edwards, G. & Weston, A. H. (1990b) Structure–activity relationships of K$^+$ channel openers. *Trends in Pharmacological Sciences* **11**, 417–423.

Escande, D., Thuringer, D., Le Guern, S. & Cavero, I. (1988) The potassium channel opener cromakalim (BRL 34915) activates ATP-dependent K$^+$ channels in isolated cardiac myocytes. *Biochemical and Biophysical Research Communications* **154**, 620–625.

Escande, D., Thuringer, D., Le Guern, S., Courtiex, J., Laville, M. & Cavero, I. (1989) Potassium channel openers act through an activation of ATP-sensitive K$^+$ channels in guinea-pig cardiac myocytes. *Pflügers Archiv* **414**, 669–675.

Faivre, J-J. & Findlay, I. (1989) Effects of tolbutamide, glibenclamide and diazoxide upon action potentials recorded from rat ventricular muscle. *Biochimica et Biophysica Acta* **984**, 1–5.

Fan, Z., Nakayama, K. & Hiraoka, M. (1990) Pinacidil activates the ATP-sensitive K$^+$ channel in inside-out and cell-attached patch membrane of guinea-pig ventricular myocytes. *Pflügers Archiv* **415**, 387–394.

Fenwick, E. M., Marty, A. & Neher, E. (1982) Sodium and calcium channels in bovine chromaffin cells. *Journal of Physiology* **331**, 599–635.

Findlay, I. (1987) The effects of magnesium upon adenosine triphosphate-regulated potassium channel in a rat insulin-secreting cell line. *Journal of Physiology* **391**, 611–629.

Findlay, I. (1988) Calcium-dependent inactivation of the ATP-sensitive K$^+$ channel of ventricular myocytes. *Biochimica et Biophysica Acta* **943**, 297–304.

Findlay, I. & Dunne, M. J. (1986a) ATP maintains ATP-inhibited K$^+$ channels in an operational state. *Pflügers Archiv* **407**, 238–240.

Findlay, I. & Dunne, M. J. (1986b) Voltage-gated Ca^{2+} currents in insulin-secreting cells. In Atwater, I., Rojas, E. & Soria, B. (eds), *Biophysics of the Pancreatic B-Cell*, New York: Plenum Press, pp. 177–189.

Findlay, I., Deroubaix, E., Guiradudou, P. & Coraboeuf, E. (1989) Effects of activation of ATP-sensitive K$^+$ channels in mammalian ventricular myocytes. *American Journal of Physiology* **257**, H1551–H1559.

Findlay, I., Dunne, M. J. & Petersen, O. H. (1985a) ATP-sensitive inward rectifier and voltage- and calcium-activated K$^+$ channels in cultured pancreatic islet cells. *Journal of Membrane Biology* **88**, 165–172.

Findlay, L., Dunne, M.J., Ullrich, S., Wollheim, C. B. & Petersen, O. H. (1985b) Quinine inhibits Ca^{2+}-independent K$^+$ channels whereas tetraethylammonium inhibits Ca^{2+}-activated K$^+$ channels in insulin-secreting cells. *FEBS Letters* **185**, 4–8.

Forscher, P. & Oxford, G. S. (1985) Modulation of calcium currents by noradrenaline in internally dialysed avian sensory neurones. *Journal of General Physiology* **85**, 743–763.

Gallacher, D. V., Maruyama, Y. & Petersen, O. H. (1984) Patch-clamp study of rubidium and potassium conductances in single cation channel from mammalian exocrine acini. *Pflügers Archiv* **401**, 361–367.

Garrino, M. G., Plant, T. D. & Hergin, J. C. (1989) Effects of putative activators of K$^+$ channels in mouse pancreatic β-cells. *British Journal of Pharmacology* **98**, 957–965.

Grapengeisser, E., Gylfe, E. & Hellman, B. (1988) Glucose-induced oscillations of cytoplasmic Ca^{2+} in the pancreatic β-cell. *Biochemical and Biophysical Research Communications* **151**, 1299–1304.

Grapengeisser, E., Gylfe, E. & Hellman, B. (1989) Three types of cytoplasmic Ca^{2+} oscillations in stimulated pancreatic β-cells. *Archives of Biochemistry and Biophysics* **268**, 404–407.

Gylfe, E., Hellman, B., Sehlin, J. & Taljedal, I-B. (1984) Interaction of sulphonylurea with the pancreatic β-cell. *Experientia* **40**, 1126–1134.

Hamilton, T. C. & Weston, A. H. (1989) Cromakalim, nicorandil and pinacidil: novel drugs which open potassium channels in smooth muscle. *General Pharmacology* **20**, 1–9.

Hellman, B. & Taljedal, I-B. (1975) Effects of sulphonylurea derivatives on pancreatic β-cells. In Hasselblatt, A. & Bruchhausen, F. (eds), *Handbook of Experimental of Physiology vol XXXII*. Springer-Verlag, Berlin, pp. 175–194.

Henquin, J. C. (1978) D-glucose inhibits potassium efflux from pancreatic islet cells. *Nature* **271**, 271–272.

Henquin, J. C. (1980a) Metabolic control of potassium permeability in pancreatic islet cells. *Journal of Biological Chemistry* **186**, 541–550.

Henquin, J. C. (1980b) Tolbutamide stimulation and inhibition of insulin release: studies of the underlying ionic mechanism in isolated rat islets. *Diabetologia* **18**, 151–160.

Henquin, J. C. & Meissner, H. P. (1982) Opposite effects of tolbutamide and diazoxide on ^{86}Rb fluxes and membrane potential in mouse pancreatic β-cells. *Biochemical Pharmacology* **31**, 1407–1413.

Henquin, J. C. & Meissner, H. P. (1984) Significance of ionic fluxes and changes in membrane potential for stimulus-secretion coupling in pancreatic β-cells. *Experentia* **40**, 1043–1054.

Henquin, J. C., Charles, S., Nenquin, M., Mathot, F. & Tamagawa, T. (1982) Diazoxide and D600 inhibition of insulin release. Different mechanisms explain the specificity for different stimuli. *Diabetes* **31**, 776–783.

Hiraoka, M. & Fan, Z. (1989) Activation of ATP-sensitive outward K^+ current by nicorandil (2-nicotinamidoethyl nitrate) in isolated ventricular myocytes. *Journal of Pharmacology and Thereputics* **250**, 278–285.

Hiriart, M. & Matteson, D. R. (1988) Na channels and two types of Ca channels in rat pancreatic B cells identified with the reverse hemolytic plaque assay. *Journal of General Physiology* **91**, 617–639.

Hoenig, M. & Sharp, G. W. G. (1986) Glucose induces insulin release and a rise in cytosolic calcium concentration in a transplantable rat insulinoma. *Endocrinology* **119**, 2502–2507.

Jones, D. P. (1986) Intracellular diffusion gradients of O_2 and ATP. *American Journal of Physiology* **250**, C663–C675.

Kakei, M. & Noma, A. (1984) Adenosine-5′-triphosphate-sensitive single potassium channels in the atrioventricular node cell of rabbit heart. *Journal of Physiology* **352**, 265–284.

Kakei, M., Kelly, R. P., Ashcroft, F. M. & Ashcroft, S. H. (1986) The ATP-sensitivity of K^+ channels in rat pancreatic B-cells. *FEBS Letters* **208**, 63–66.

Kakei, M., Noma, A. & Shibasaki, I. (1985) Properties of adenosine triphosphate-regulated potassium channels in guinea-pig ventricular cells. *Journal of Physiology* **363**, 441–462.

Kozlowski, R. Z. & Ashford, M. L. J. (1991) Barbiturates inhibit ATP-K^+ channels and voltage activated currents in CRI-G1 insulin-secreting cells. *British Journal of Pharmacology* **103**, 2021–2029.

Kozlowski, R. Z., Hales, C. N. & Ashford, M. L. J. (1989) Dual effects of diazoxide on ATP-K^+ currents recorded from an insulin-secreting cell line. *British Journal of Pharmacology* **97**, 1039–1050.

Lacerda, A. E., Rampe, D. & Brown, A. M. (1988) Effects of protein kinase C activators on cardiac Ca^{2+} channels. *Nature* **335**, 249–251.

Lambert, A. E., Henquin, J. C. & Orci, L. (1974) Role of beta cell membrane in insulin secretion. *Excerpta Medica, International Congress Series* **312**, 79–94.

Langin, D. & Lafontan, M. (1989) [^{3}H] idazoxan binding at non α_2-adrenoceptors in rabbit adipocyte membranes, *European Journal of Pharmacology* **159**, 199–203.

Lebrun, P., Devreux, V., Hermann, M. & Herchuelz, A. (1989) Pinacidil inhibits insulin release by increasing K^+ outflow from pancreatic β-cells. *European Journal of Pharmacology* **156**, 283–286.

Lederer, W. J. & Nicholls, C. G. (1989) Nucleotide modulation of the activity of rat heart ATP-sensitive K^+ channel in isolated membrane patches. *Journal of Physiology* **419**, 193–211.

Li, G-D., Milani, D., Dunne, M. J., Pralong, W-F., Theler, J.-M., Petersen, O. H. & Wollheim, C. B. (1991) Extracellular ATP causes Ca^{2+}-dependent and independent insulin secretion in RINm5F cells. *Journal of Biological Chemistry* **266**, 3449–3457.

Loubantieres-Marni, M-M., Chapal, J., Lignon, F. & Valette, G. (1979) Structural specificity of nucleotides for insulin secretory action from isolated perfused rat pancreas. *European Journal of Pharmacology* **59**, 277–286.

Malaisse, W. J., Malaisse-Lagae, F., Wright, P. H. & Ashmore, J. (1967) Effects of adrenergic and cholinergic agents upon insulin-secretion *in vivo*. *Endocrinology* **80**, 975–978.

Martin, S. C., Yule, D. I., Dunne, M. J., Gallacher, D. V. & Petersen, O. H. (1989)

Vasopressin directly closes ATP-sensitive potassium channels evoking membrane depolarization and an increase in the free intracellular Ca^{2+} concentration in insulin-secreting cells. *EMBO Journal* **8**, 3595–3599.

Meissner, H. P. & Schmelz, H. (1974) Membrane potential of β-cells in pancreatic islets. *Pflügers Archiv* **351**, 195–206.

Matthews, E. K. & Sakamoto, Y. (1975) Electrical characteristics of pancreatic islet cells. *Journal of Physiology* **246**, 421–437.

Michel, M. C. & Insel, P. A. (1989) Are there multiple imidazoline binding sites? *Trends in Pharmacological Sciences* **10**, 342–344.

Miller, R. E. (1981) Pancreatic neuroendocrinology; peripheral neural mechanisms in the regulation of the islets of Langerhans, *Endocrine Reviews* **2**, 471–498.

Misler, S., Falke, L. C., Gillis, K. & McDaniel, M. L. (1986) A metabolite regulated potassium channel in rat pancreatic B-cells. *Proceedings of the National Academy of Sciences USA* **83**, 7119–7123.

Misler, S., Gillis, K. & Tabcharni, J. (1989) Modulation of gating of a metabolically regulated ATP-dependent K^+ channel by intracellular pH in β-cells of the pancreatic islets. *Journal of Membrane Biology* **109**, 135–143.

Niki, I., Ashcroft, F. M. & Ashcroft, S. J. H. (1989a) The dependence on intracellular ATP concentration of ATP-sensitive K^+ channels and of a Na,K-ATPase in intact HIT-T15 β-cells. *FEBS Letters* **257**, 361–364.

Niki, I., Kelly, R. P., Ashcroft, S. J. H. & Ashcroft, F. M. (1989b) ATP-sensitive K^+ channel in HIT-T15 β-cells studied by patch-clamp methods, ^{86}Rb efflux and gliben-clamide binding. *Pflügers Archiv* **415**, 47–55.

Niki, I., Nicks, J. L. & Ashcroft, S. J. H. (1990) The β-cell glibenclamide receptor is an ADP-binding protein. *Biochemical Journal* **268**, 713–718.

Ohno-Shosaku, T., Zunkler, B. J. & Trube, G. (1987) Dual effects of ATP on K^+ currents in mouse pancreatic B-cells. *Pflügers Archiv* **408**, 133–138.

Ostenson, C. G., Pigon, J., Doxley, J. C. & Efendic, S. (1988) α_2-adrenoceptor blockade does not enhance glucose-induced insulin release in normal subjects or patients with non-insulin dependent diabetes. *Journal of Clinical Endocrinology and Metabolism* **67**, 1054–1059.

Pace, C. S. & Goldsmith, K. T. (1985) Action of a phorbol ester on β-cells, potentiation of stimulant-induced electrical activity. *American Journal of Physiology* **248**, C527–C534.

Panten, U. & Lenzen, S. (1988) Alterations in energy metabolism of secretory cells. In Ackermann, J. W. N. (ed.), *The Energetics of Secretion Responses*, CRC, Boca Raton, Florida, pp. 88–95.

Peers, C., Smith, P. A. & Nye, P. C. G. (1990) Ligustrazine selectively blocks ATP-sensitive K^+ channels in mouse pancreatic β-cells *FEBS Letters* **261**, 5–7.

Petersen, O. H. (1988) Control of potassium channels in insulin-secreting cells. *ISI Atlas of Science (Biochemistry)* **1**, 144–149.

Petersen, O. H. & Dunne, M. J. (1989) Regulation of K^+ channels plays a crucial role in the control of insulin secretion. *Pflügers Archiv* **414**, S115–S120.

Petersen, O. H. & Findlay, I. (1987) Electrophysiology of the pancreas. *Physiological Reviews* **67**, 1054–1116.

Plant, T. D. (1988) Na^+ currents in cultured mouse pancreatic B-cells. *Pflügers Archiv* **411**, 429–435.

Plant, T. D. & Henquin, J. C. (1990) Phentolamine and yohimbine inhibit ATP-sensitive K^+ channels in mouse pancreatic β-cells. *British Journal of Pharmacology* **101**, 115–120.

Pralong, W. F., Bartley, C. & Wollheim, C. B. (1990) Single islet β-cell stimulation by nutrients: relationship between pyridine nucleotides, cytosolic Ca^{2+} and secretion. *EMBO Journal* **9**, 53–60.

Quast, U. & Cook, N. S. (1989) Moving together: K^+ channel openers and ATP-sensitive K^+ channels. *Trends in Pharmacological Sciences* **10**, 431–435.

Ribalet, B. & Ciani, S. (1987) Regulation by cell metabolism and adenine nucleotides of a K^+ channel in insulin-secreting β-cells. *Proceedings of the National Academy of Sciences USA* **84**, 1721–1725.

Ribalet, B., Ciani, S. & Eddlestone, G. T. (1989) ATP mediates both activation and inhibition of K(ATP) channel activity via cAMP-dependent protein kinase in insulin-secreting cell lines. *Journal of General Physiology* **94**, 693–717.

Ribalet, B., Eddlestone, G. T. & Ciani, S. (1988) Metabolic regulation of the K(ATP) and a maxi-K(V) channel in the insulin-secreting RINm5F cell. *Journal of General Physiology* **92**, 219–237.

Rorsman, P. & Trube, G. (1985) Glucose dependent K^+ channels in pancreatic β-cells are regulated by intracellular ATP. *Pflügers Archiv* **405**, 305–309.

Rorsman, P. & Trube, G. (1990) Biophysics and physiology of ATP-regulated K^+ channel (K_{ATP}) channel. In Cook, N. S. (ed.), *Potassium Channels*. J. Wiley & Sons, New York, pp. 96–116.

Rorsman, P., Arkhammar, P. & Berggren, P-O. (1986) Voltage-activated Na^+ currents and their suppression by phorbol ester in clonal insulin-producing RINm5F cells. *American Journal of Physiology* **251**, C912–919.

Rorsman, P., Arkhammar, P., Bokvist, K., Hellerstrom, C., Nilsson, T., Welsh, M., Welsh, N. & Berggren, P-O. (1989) Failure of glucose to elicit a normal secretory response in fetal pancreatic β-cells results from glucose insensitivity of the ATP-regulated K^+ channel. *Proceedings of the National Academy of Sciences USA* **86**, 4505–4509.

Rorsman, P., Berggren, P-O., Bokvist, K. & Efandic, S. (1990) ATP-regulated K^+ channel and diabetes mellitus. *News in Physiological Sciences* **5**, 143–147.

Rorsman, P., Bokvist, K., Ammala, C., Arkhammar, P., Berggren, P-O., Larsson, O. & Wahlander, K. (1991) Activation of a low conductance G protein-dependent K^+ channel in mouse pancreatic β-cells. *Nature* **349**, 77–79.

Satin, L. S., Hopkins, W. F., Fatherazi, S. & Cook, D. L. (1990) Expression of rapid, low threshold K current in insulin-secreting cell is dependent on intracellular calcium buffering. *Journal of Membrane Biology* **112**, 213–222.

Schmid-Antomarchi, H., De Weille, J., Fosset, M. & Lazdunsk, M. (1987) The receptor for the antidiabetic sulphonylurea controls the activity of the ATP-regulated K^+ channels in insulin-secreting cells. *Journal of Biological Chemistry* **262**, 15 840–15 844.

Schulz, A. & Hasselblatt, A. (1989) An insulin-secreting property of imidazoline derivatives is not limited to compounds that block α-adrenoceptors. *Naunyn-Schmiedeberg's Archives of Pharmacology* **340**, 321–327.

Sehlin, J. (1987) Evidence for voltage-dependent Cl^- permeability in mouse pancreatic β-cells. *Bioscience Reports* **7**, 67–72.

Sehlin, J. & Meissner, H. P. (1988) Effects of Cl^- deficiency on the membrane potential in mouse pancreatic β-cells. *Biochimica et Biophysica Acta* **938**, 309–318.

Sehlin, J. & Taljedal, I-P. (1975) Glucose-induced decrease in Rb^+ permeability in pancreatic β-cells. *Nature* **253**, 635–636.

Smith, P. A., Ashcroft, F. M. & Rorsman, P. (1990a) Simultaneous recording of glucose dependent electrical activity and ATP-regulated K^+ currents in mouse pancreatic β-cells. *FEBS Letters* **261**, 187–191.

Smith, P. A., Bokvist, K., Arkhammar, P., Berggren, P-O. & Rorsman, P. (1990b) Delayed rectifier and calcium-activated K^+ channels and their significance for action potential repolarization in mouse pancreatic β-cells. *Journal of General Physiology* **95**, 1041–1059.

Smith, P. A., Rorsman, P. & Ashcroft, F. M. (1990c) Modulation of dihydropyridine-sensitive Ca^{2+} channels by glucose in mouse pancreatic β-cells. *Nature* **342**, 550–553.

Somers, G., Sener, A., Devis, G. & Malaisse, W. J. (1980) The stimulus-secretion coupling of glucose-induced insulin release. The anion-osmotic hypothesis for exocytosis. *Pflügers Archiv* **308**, 249–253.

Spruce, A. E., Standen, N. B. & Stanfield, P. R. (1987) Voltage-dependent ATP-sensitive potassium channels of skeletal muscle membranes. *Journal of Physiology* **382**, 213–236.

Standen, N. B., Quale, J. M., Davies, N. W., Brayden, J. E., Huang, Y. & Nelson, M. T. (1989) Hyperpolarizing vasodilators activate ATP-sensitive K^+ channels in arterial smooth muscle cells. *Science* **245**, 177–180.

Sturgess, N. C., Ashford, M. L. J., Carrington, C. A. & Hales, C.N. (1986) Single channel current recordings of potassium channels in an insulin-secreting cell line. *Endocrinology* **109**, 201–207.

Sturgess, N. C., Ashford, M. L. J., Cook, D. L. & Hales, C. N. (1985) The sulphonylurea receptor may be an ATP-sensitive potassium channel. *Lancet* **ii**, 474–475.

Sturgess, N. C., Kozlowoski, R. Z., Carrington, C. A., Hales, C. N. & Ashford, M. L. J. (1988) Effects of sulphonylureas and diazoxide on insulin secretion and nucleotide-sensitive channels in an insulin-secreting cell line. *British Journal of Pharmacology* **95**, 83–94.

Thuringer, D. & Escande, D. (1989) Apparent competition between ATP and the potassium channel opener RP 49356 on ATP-sensitive K^+ channel of cardiac myocytes. *Molecular Pharmacology* **36**, 897–902.

Trube, G. & Hescheler, J. (1984) Inward-rectifying channels in isolated patches of the heart cell membrane: ATP-dependence and comparison with cell-attached patches. *Pflügers Archiv* **401**, 178–184.

Trube, G., Rorsman, P. & Ohno-Shosaku, T. (1986) Opposite effects of tolbutamide and diazoxide on the ATP-dependent K^+ channel in mouse pancreatic B-cells. *Pflügers Archiv* **407**, 493–499.

Tseng, G-N. & Hoffman, B. F. (1990) Actions of pinacidil on membrane currents in canine ventricular myocytes and their modulation by intracellular ATP and cAMP. *Pflügers Archiv* **415**, 414–424.

Velasco, J. M. & Petersen, O. H. (1989) The effects of a cell-permeable diacylglycerol analogue on single Ca^{2+} (Ba^{2+}) channel currents in the insulin-secreting cell line RINm5F. *Quarterly Journal of Experimental Physiology* **74**, 367–370.

Velasco, J. M., Petersen, J. U. H. & Petersen, O. H. (1988) Single-channel Ba^{2+} currents in insulin-secreting cell are activated by glyceraldehyde stimulation. *FEBS Letters* **231**, 366–370.

Virji, M. A. G., Staffs, M. W. & Estensen, R. D. (1978) Phorbol myristate acetate: effect of a tumor promotor on insulin release from isolated rat islets of Langerhans. *Endocrinology* **102**, 706–711.

Wollheim, C. B. & Sharp, G. W. G. (1981) Regulation of insulin release by calcium. *Physiological Reviews* **61**, 914–973.

Wollheim, C. B., Dunne, M. J., Peter-Reisch, B., Bruzzone, R., Pozzan, T. & Petersen, O. H. (1988) Activators of protein kinase C depolarise insulin-secreting cells by closing K^+ channels. *EMBO Journal* **7**, 2443–2449.

Zunkler, B. J., Lenzen, S., Manner, K., Panten, U. & Trube, G. (1988a) Concentration-dependent effects of tolbutamide, meglitinide, glipizide, glibenclamide and diazoxide on ATP-regulated K^+ currents in pancreatic β-cells. *Naunyn-Schmiedeberg's Archives of Pharmacology* **337**, 225–230.

Zunkler, B. J., Lins, S., Ohno-Shosaku, T., Trube, G. & Panten, U. (1988b) Cytosolic ADP enhances the sensitivity to tolbutamide of ATP-dependent K$^+$ channels from pancreatic β-cells. *FEBS Letters* **239**, 241–244.

Zunkler, B. J., Trube, G. & Panten, U. (1989) How do sulphonylureas approach their receptor in the B-cell plasma membrane? *Naunyn-Schmiedeberg's Archives of Pharmacology* **340**, 328–332.

Chapter 7
Smooth muscle potassium channels: their electrophysiology and function

T. B. Bolton and D. J. Beech

Introduction

Tension in smooth muscles is controlled by electrical changes in the membrane and by other, intracellular, mechanisms involving second messenger systems. The only function of electrical changes which has so far been established is to control the entry of Ca^{2+} into the cells down its electrochemical gradient by gating potential-sensitive Ca-channels in the membrane; from this may follow secondary effects such as Ca^{2+}-induced Ca^{2+} release from stores. The ability of an action potential to propagate is also very important in co-ordinating contraction of large numbers of smooth muscle cells. In smooth muscles which are highly excitable and freely discharge action potentials, tension seems to be determined largely, if not exclusively, by the frequency of action potential discharge and also probably the extent to which an action potential can propagate through the muscle. Neurotransmitters, hormones and drugs exert their effects through a final common path, which is the frequency and perhaps pattern of action potential discharge (Bülbring 1955; Bülbring & Kuriyama, 1963). Other mechanisms, such as variations in spike size upon receptor activation, may play some role but this seems minor; a role of second messengers in modulating primary tension generated by action potential discharge in highly excitable smooth muscles is suspected but their importance for regulation of tension in the *in vivo* muscle has yet to be established.

The situation in less-excitable smooth muscles is very different: second messenger systems seem to be of great importance in determining tension;

electrical changes correspondingly less so. The smooth muscle of some large blood vessels generally does not discharge action potentials either spontaneously or when stimulated electrically. Noradrenaline will contract such muscle at concentrations which are without significant effect on membrane potential; higher concentrations, however, depolarize the muscle and may in some arterial muscles cause action potential or slow wave discharge. A number of visceral muscles (which include tracheal, parts of the stomach and the anococcygeus muscle) are of intermediate but relatively low excitability; tension generation in these seems to depend dually on voltage-gated Ca^{2+} entry and on second messenger systems.

Potassium channels are membrane-spanning proteins that form pores between the intracellular and extracellular media. These pores are highly selective for K^+ compared with other physiological ions and have a permeability sequence that is well-conserved throughout the K-channel family (Hille, 1984). Such conservation of selectivity may originate from a common pore structure typified by the H5 amino acid region of the cloned A-type K-channel (K_A) from *Drosophila* (Yool & Schwarz, 1991). The pore of the K-channels is, however, one of the few common features, for in other respects these proteins are highly diverse. Most notably they are diverse in their unitary conductance and in their sensitivity to cellular factors that 'gate' the flow of current through the pore (i.e. open the channel). In K_A-channels from fruit fly or rat brain, functional diversity seems to arise by different combinations of several (perhaps four) different subunits assembled as heteromultimers; these subunits may arise by alternative splicing of messenger RNA from the same gene locus (Schwartz *et al.*, 1988; Isacoff *et al.*, 1990; Ruppersberg *et al.*, 1990). It is believed that voltage sensitivity is conferred on K_A-channels from the fruit fly by the presence of an S4 sequence (Papazian *et al.*, 1991), which is also found in Na- and Ca-channels.

Interest in smooth muscle K-channels and in the currents which they carry has been stimulated by the realization that a variety of drugs can increase their open probability. The effect of this is to hyperpolarize the membrane, moving it closer to the K-equilibrium potential. In highly excitable muscles this tends to inhibit spike discharge and relax existing tension in the muscle. In less-excitable muscles, voltage-gated Ca^{2+} entry still plays an important role in determining the level of tension in the muscle, i.e. tone, and hyperpolarization reduces both this and so tension also. Whether K-channel opening drugs have other modes of action is clear in some cases (nicorandil) and uncertain in others (cromakalim).

A number of investigations of compounds such as tetraethylammonium (TEA), 4-aminopyridine (4-AP), procaine, quinine, quinidine, etc. which block K-channels have been made on the electrical activity of smooth muscles. The selectivity or otherwise of these drugs for the various K-channel types is only now becoming apparent from single-channel studies. Tetraethylammonium, although blocking a variety of K-channels at concentrations above 5 mM, seems to affect only large Ca^{2+}-activated K-channels (BK_{Ca}) to a significant extent at concentrations below this (e.g. Beech & Bolton, 1989a). In smooth muscle of the taenia caeci for example, TEA (3–5 mM) was described as having no effect on the resting membrane potential, but was able to reduce the marked rectification of the membrane; spike size was increased without effect on rate of rise and duration was also increased by slowing of the rate of repolarization (Ito et al., 1970). It could be inferred that by blocking BK_{Ca}-channels TEA has revealed a role for these channels in the repolarization phase of the spike and in rectification of the membrane; however, such channels do not appear to contribute to the resting membrane potential and open only after the inward current in this muscle has developed. Above 5 mM, TEA affects most K-channels to some extent and its effects on electrical activity may represent multiple sites of action. Charybdotoxin and iberiotoxin, peptides from scorpion venom, may be more specific blockers of these BK_{Ca}-channels (see Chapters 5 and 11 for a full discussion of this point). Apamin, a toxin from bee venom, may block only small Ca^{2+}-activated K-channels ($SK_{Ca(Ap)}$, see later); Fujii et al. (1990) showed that apamin blocks the after-hyperpolarization of the spike in guinea-pig bladder. Other K-channel blockers do not offer such possibilities for distinguishing between particular classes of K-channel. Quinine and quinidine are rather non-specific blockers (e.g. Beech & Bolton, 1989a), blocking the after-hyperpolarization of the spike and depolarizing the circular muscle of the small intestine. Voltage-clamp experiments on single cells from the same muscle revealed an action on both the early peak in the outward current (probably carried by BK_{Ca}) and on the steady-state outward current after 200 ms (probably carried by delayed rectifier channels proper) (K_V, Nakao et al., 1986). 4-Aminopyridine blocks both K_V- and K_A-channels (Beech & Bolton, 1989a,c), and may interfere with Ca^{2+} cycling in intracellular stores (Beech & Bolton, 1989a).

When single smooth muscle cells are subjected to a step depolarization under voltage-clamp, an outward current develops. The peak size of this current usually exceeds the size of the current needed to command the potential by an equal amount in the hyperpolarizing direction, i.e. the membrane rectifies. Since the outward current which gives rise to this rectification develops after a short delay and more slowly than the voltage-dependent inward current, the current is referred to as the delayed rectifier. In most smooth muscles the delayed rectifier can be explained principally by the existence of two types of K-current present in varying proportions in different smooth muscle cell types: current carried by BK_{Ca}-channels and by small Ca^{2+}-insensitive, voltage-gated K-channels (K_V). Although both of these K-channel types underlie delayed rectification in smooth muscle we will refer to the latter, Ca^{2+}-insensitive, type as delayed rectifier channels proper. This distinction follows the precedent of Rudy (1988) where the Ca^{2+}-insensitive, voltage-gated, non-A-type K-channels have been dubbed 'delayed rectifiers' despite the observation that other types of K-channel may also generate delayed rectification. In visceral smooth muscle cells (colon, stomach, ureter, bladder) the current carried by K_V ($I_{K(V)}$) may be small. In certain arterial cells, however, in experiments where internal Ca was strongly buffered (4 mM or more EGTA), a strong outward current can be seen; this current is frequently sensitive to blockade by 4-AP (1–5 mM) (e.g. Okabe $et\ al.$, 1987), a blocker that in this concentration range does not affect BK_{Ca}-channels. Current carried by BK_{Ca}- and by K_V-channels seems to be the major contributor to the repolarization phase of the action potential and perhaps also of the slow wave where this occurs in smooth muscles.

Types of K-channel in smooth muscle

Large Ca^{2+}-activated K-channels (BK_{Ca})

When recording from smooth muscle membrane patches with a physiological K^+-gradient, the dominant events are unitary K^+-currents through single ionic channels that have a large conductance (100–150 pS). These K-channels are activated by raised $[Ca^{2+}]_i$ (Table 7.1) and are presumably a major mechanism for limiting excitability when $[Ca^{2+}]_i$ rises in response to a neurotransmitter, hormone or depolarizing stimulus. They are present at high density in intestinal, vascular, tracheal and uterine muscles and much is known about their elementary properties.

Single channel recordings

Several biophysical properties of BK_{Ca} have been described. The permeability sequence is Tl^+ (1.4) > K^+ (1.0) > Rb^+ (0.5–0.7) > NH_4^+ (0.14–0.5), while Na^+, Li^+, Cs^+ and TEA^+ may be considered impermeant (Table 7.1). The single channel current–voltage relationship is linear when the K^+-gradient is symmetrical, but mild outward rectification occurs when the K^+-concentration is higher on the inside relative to the outside. Rectification of this magnitude may be described by the Goldman–Hodgkin–Katz equation and the channel conductance specified as the slope or chord conductance at a particular voltage, often 0 mV. Block by internal Na^+ (> 1 mM) or Cs^+ is voltage-dependent, causing rectification by reducing mostly current at positive voltages (Singer & Walsh, 1984; Benham $et\ al.$, 1986; Cecchi $et\ al.$, 1987; Hu $et\ al.$, 1989b). Internal TEA^+ blocks BK_{Ca}-channels in a similar voltage-dependent manner in tracheal muscle (McCann & Welsh, 1986), but for BK_{Ca}-channels from arterial (Benham $et\ al.$, 1985b) or intestinal (Hu $et\ al.$, 1989b)

Table 7.1. BK$_{Ca}$-channels in smooth muscle.

Muscle type	g pS (K_i:K_o) (mM)	Permeability	External block	Internal block	[Ca^{2+}]$_i$ for opening at -40 mV (in μM)	Voltage for opening [Ca^{2+}]$_i$ = 0.1 μM	Reference
Rabbit jejunum	198 (126:126)	Tl > K > Rb ≫ Na=Cs	Cs	Ba	0.1–1	+ve of -20 mV	Benham et al. (1985b, 1986); Bolton et al. (1985)
Bufo marinus stomach	222 (120:120)	–	–	Na	1–10	+ve of $+50$ mV	Singer & Walsh (1984, 1987)
Guinea-pig taenia caeci	[147 (135:5.4)]	K > Rb > NH$_4$ ≫ Na=Li=Cs	TEA	Na, Cs, TEA	0.1–1	+ve of -20 mV	Hu et al. (1989a,b)
Dog colon	206 (140:140)	K > Rb ≫ Na=Li	TEA	–	0.5–1	+ve of $+50$ mV	Carl & Sanders (1989)
Rabbit intestine (bilayer)	230 (100:100)	K > Rb ≫ Na=Li=Cs	–	Cs, Na, Li, Ca	2–1000	+ve of $+50$ mV	Cecchi et al. (1986)
Rabbit portal vein	273 (142:142)	–	TEA, ChTX, Qd, Qn	TEA	–	+ve of 0 mV	Inoue et al. (1985); Beech & Bolton (1989a); Strong et al. (1989)
Guinea-pig mesenteric artery	183 (126:126)	–	–	TEA, Ba, procaine	0.2–1	+ve of -40 mV	Benham et al. (1985b, 1986)

Tissue	g	Selectivity					Reference
Rat aorta	135 (142:142)	K > Rb ≫ Na	TEA	Ba	0.1–1	+ve of −10 mV	Sadoshima et al. (1988a)
Human aorta	250 (140:140)	—	Qn	Qn	—	—	Bregestovski et al. (1986)
Rat pancreatic arterioles	276 (145:145)	K ≫ Na	—	Na, Cs, Ba	>0.1	+ve of +40 mV	Stuenkel (1989)
Rabbit aorta (bilayer)	232 (250:250)	K > Rb > NH$_4$ ≫ Na=Cs	—	—	—	—	Gelband & van Breemen (1989)
Rabbit trachea	187 (130:130)	—	—	Decreased pH	1–10	—	Kume et al. (1990)
Dog trachea	266 (135:135)	—	Ba, TEA, Cs	TEA, TMA, Cs, Ba, haloperidol	—	+ve at +20 mV	McCann & Welsh (1986, 1987)
Rat pregnant uterus	204 (130:130)	—	—	W-7, W-5, trifluoperazine	—	—	Kihira et al. (1990)
Rat or pig myometrium	[260 (60:260)]	—	—	Mg	>1	+ve of +50 mV	Toro et al. (1990b)

ChTX, charybdotoxin; g, conductance; TMA, tetramethylammonium; Qd, quinidine; Qn, quinine; W-5, N-(6-aminohexyl)-1-naphthalenesulphonamide; W-7, N-(6-aminohexyl)-5-chloro-1-naphthalenesulphonamide.

muscles the block seems most voltage-independent. Large Ca^{2+}-activated K-channels are blocked by other substances (Table 7.1), many of which are non-selective. The distinguishing pharmacology of the BK_{Ca}-channel is the block by external charybdotoxin (Strong *et al.*, 1989) or 0.1–1 mM external TEA^+ (Table 7.1) and no effect of 4-AP (Beech & Bolton, 1989a; Carl & Sanders, 1989), apamin (Beech & Bolton, 1989b) or glibenclamide (Langton *et al.*, 1991).

Large Ca^{2+}-activated K-channels are activated when $[Ca^{2+}]_i$ rises. An important feature of their Ca^{2+}-activation is that it is voltage-dependent. At the resting membrane potential, 1 µM $[Ca^{2+}]_i$ may be required for activation, but at the peak of a spike, values as low as 1 nM may suffice (Benham *et al.*, 1986; Hu *et al.*, 1989a), suggesting that BK_{Ca}-channels will open during the spike even if $[Ca^{2+}]_i$ remains at the resting level of about 130 nM (from Aaronson & Benham, 1989). That BK_{Ca}-channels will open on depolarization without a rise in $[Ca^{2+}]_i$ is supported by cell-attached patch (Coleman & Parkington, 1987), whole-cell (Beech & Bolton, 1989b) and excised patch (Hu *et al.*, 1989a) experiments.

The absolute values of $[Ca^{2+}]_i$ required for BK_{Ca} activation seem to vary between smooth muscle types (Table 7.1). This variation could, however, reflect difficulties in measuring the Ca^{2+}-sensitivity of the channels. First, the estimate of free Ca^{2+} in the EGTA test solution depends on the values taken, for example, for the dissociation constant of EGTA, the concentration of Mg^{2+}, contaminating Ca^{2+} and the final pH of the solution. Second, the metabolic status of the inside-out patch (adenosine triphosphate (ATP), guanosine triphosphate (GTP) or cyclic nucleotides have rarely been included in the solution applied to the intracellular side of the membrane) may affect the Ca^{2+}-sensitivity of the BK_{Ca}-channel. For example (*see also below*), it has been shown for aortic muscle that phosphorylation by cyclic adenosine monophosphate (cAMP)-dependent protein kinase increases the sensitivity of BK_{Ca}-channels to $[Ca^{2+}]_i$ (Sadoshima *et al.*, 1988b).

Depolarization increases the probability of opening (P_o) of BK_{Ca}-channels mostly by decreasing the mean closed time. For example, in patches from the toad stomach, the mean closed time of BK_{Ca} decreases 140-fold from 700 to 5 ms when the holding potential is changed from -20 to $+40$ mV, but the mean open time increases less than three-fold from 13 to 30 ms for the same voltage shift (Singer & Walsh, 1987; $[Ca^{2+}]_i = 1$ µM; room temperature). Raised $[Ca^{2+}]_i$ has a similar effect (Benham *et al.*, 1986; Singer & Walsh, 1987; Sadoshima *et al.*, 1988a; Carl & Sanders, 1989; Hu *et al.*, 1989a), which may suggest that the voltage dependence of BK_{Ca}-channels results from voltage-dependent binding of Ca^{2+}. It is not known if Ca^{2+} binds directly to BK_{Ca} although smooth muscle BK_{Ca}-channels retain Ca^{2+}-sensitivity for long periods in excised patches and after incorporation into lipid bilayers. Furthermore, calmodulin is not involved (McCann & Welsh, 1987; Kihira et al., 1990).

The number of exponentials required to describe open- or closed-time distributions for a channel gives some indication of the minimum number of conformational states the protein enters. Smooth muscle BK_{Ca}-channels appear to enter one (Sadoshima et al., 1988a; Hu et al., 1989a) or two (Benham et al., 1986; Carl & Sanders, 1989; Kihira et al., 1990) open states and two (Sadoshima et al., 1988a; Hu et al., 1989a), three (Carl & Sanders, 1989; Kihira et al., 1990) or even four (Benham et al., 1986) closed states. Large Ca^{2+}-activated K-channels open for much longer times in adult than in fetal aorta: the open time distribution for BK_{Ca}-channels from fetal aorta was fitted by a single exponential with a time constant of 2.3 ms but in the adult, the short time constant was similar (2.7 ms) but an additional exponential was found with a longer time constant of 37 ms (Bregestovski et al., 1988). Subconductance levels occur occasionally in smooth muscle BK_{Ca}-channels, indicating further open states. The most common subconductance level seems to be two-thirds of the fully open state, but levels of one-half or one-third have also been reported (Berger et al., 1984; Bregestovski et al., 1985; Benham et al., 1986; Singer & Walsh, 1987).

Large Ca^{2+}-activated K-channels are affected by factors in addition to $[Ca^{2+}]_i$ and membrane potential. Using cell-attached patches from aortic muscle, Sadoshima et al. (1988b) have shown that bath-applied isoprenaline, forskolin or dibutyryl cAMP increase the P_o of BK_{Ca}-channels. Cyclic AMP-dependent protein kinase, bath-applied to inside-out patches, also increased P_o. Kume et al. (1989) have found a similar phenomenon for tracheal muscle. Bath-applied isoprenaline or okadaic acid (a phosphatase inhibitor) increased P_o in cell-attached patches. Using inside-out patches, Kume et al. (1989) observed that P_o was increased when either protein kinase A (with cAMP and ATP) or the catalytic subunit of protein kinase A (with ATP but not cAMP) were bath-applied (Fig. 7.1). In addition, Toro et al. (1990b) have shown that myometrial BK_{Ca}-channels incorporated into bilayers can be activated by GTPγS (with Mg^{2+}) in the presence of adenyl imidodiphosphate (an ATP analogue that does not support phosphorylation), suggesting that BK_{Ca}-channels might be activated directly by a G protein. Large Ca^{2+}-activated K-channel activity may be inhibited by angiotensin II in coronary artery muscle (Toro et al., 1990a) or by acetylcholine in colonic muscle (Cole et al., 1989), but the signal transduction mechanisms have not been elucidated. Sodium nitroprusside is reported to stimulate BK_{Ca}-channels in cell-attached patches from cultured aortic muscle (Williams et al., 1988). The authors propose that this effect might result from stimulation of BK_{Ca}-channels not by cyclic guanosine monophosphate (GMP) but by intracellular guanosine 5'-monophosphate. Large Ca^{2+}-activated K-channels are also particularly

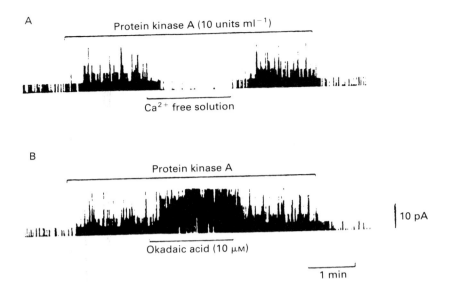

Fig. 7.1. Regulation of BK_{Ca}-channel activity by phosphorylation in tracheal smooth muscle. Current recording was from an inside-out patch (holding potential, 0 mV; $[Ca^{2+}]_i$, 0.1 μM) and protein kinase A (with 0.1 mM cAMP and 0.3 mM ATP) and okadaic acid were bath-applied. The Ca-free solution contained no added $CaCl_2$ ([EGTA] = 5 mM). $[K^+]_i$ = 80 mM and $[K^+]_o$ = 5.9 mM (With permission from Kume *et al.*, 1989.)

sensitive to intracellular pH (pH_i). Using inside-out patches from tracheal muscle, Kume *et al.* (1990) showed that P_o dropped from 0.9 to almost zero when pH_i was reduced from 7.4 to 7.0 ($[Ca^{2+}]_i$ = 1 μM) and for a pH_i drop of half a unit the channels became about eight times less sensitive to $[Ca^{2+}]_i$. Therefore, acidosis should reduce any effect BK_{Ca}-channels have on the membrane potential, promoting depolarization. Finally, it has been reported that in rabbit tracheal (Groschner *et al.*, 1991) and aortic smooth muscles (Gelband *et al.*, 1990), and in porcine coronary artery (Silberberg & van Breemen, 1990) ATP (0.5–2 mM) reduced the P_o of BK_{Ca}-channels. This result, however, is not observed by others working on calf aorta (Williams *et al.*, 1988), rat portal vein (Hu *et al.*, 1990) and rabbit mesenteric artery (Langton *et al.*, 1991).

Single cell recordings

Calcium-inward current causes the depolarizing phase of the spike in most smooth muscles. This Ca^{2+}-influx raises $[Ca^{2+}]_i$ (Aaronson & Benham, 1989) and so Ca^{2+}-activated K (K_{Ca})-channels may open. The majority of such channels are of the BK_{Ca} type. 'Small' conductance TEA^+-resistant K_{Ca}-channels (Inoue *et al.*, 1985) or apamin-sensitive K-channels (Fujii *et al.*, 1990) may contribute to the Ca^{2+}-activated K-current ($I_{K(Ca)}$) in some cells and under certain conditions although definite evidence is lacking.

Calcium-activated K-currents in a smooth muscle cell have been identified by investigating the dependence of the current on Ca^{2+}-influx or intracellular Ca^{2+} release. In studying this dependence, however, it should be borne in mind that many of the methods used may give misleading results. Calcium-influx through voltage-gated Ca-channels can be blocked by Ca antagonist drugs but verapamil, nicardipine and diltiazem also block smooth muscle K-channels independently of Ca^{2+}-influx (Terada *et al.*, 1987). Calcium-influx can be reduced by changing to a low Ca^{2+} medium (with or without a substituting divalent cation) but alterations in the external divalent cation type or concentration cause apparent shifts in the voltage-dependent gating of some ionic channels in smooth muscle (Beech & Bolton, 1989c) and other tissues (reviewed by Hille, 1984). Application of caffeine, ryanodine and some neurotransmitters can indicate a dependence on Ca^{2+} release from intracellular stores (Benham & Bolton, 1986; Ohya *et al.*, 1987a; Bolton & Lim, 1989). Cole *et al.* (1989), however, suggest that inhibition of transient K-current by acetylcholine in intestinal muscle (Benham & Bolton, 1986) could be by a 'direct' modulation of K-channels by muscarinic receptors and not an effect linked to Ca^{2+} release. Caffeine has many actions, including block of K-channels (Noack *et al.*, 1990) and Ca-channels (Imaizumi *et al.*, 1989; Hughes *et al.*, 1990).

An alternative method for identifying $I_{K(Ca)}$-current is that used by Meech and Standen (1975) for *Helix aspersa* neurones. They made use of the 'U-shaped' current–voltage relationship of voltage-dependent Ca-current. The Ca-channels are activated by depolarization but inward Ca^{2+}-flux declines at positive potentials as the membrane potential approaches the Ca^{2+}-reversal potential (for smooth muscle, see Yamamoto *et al.*, 1989a). Thus maximum Ca^{2+}-inward current occurs near $-10\,mV$ and there is no net inward current at $+40\,mV$ or more positive voltages (Aaronson *et al.*, 1988). If K-channels are dependent on $[Ca^{2+}]_i$ then their current–voltage relationship should follow that of Ca^{2+} entry, resembling an inverted 'U-shape' with a maximum at about $-10\,mV$. It might be expected that this phenomenon would be observed in many smooth muscles, but in fact it has been readily seen only by Walsh and Singer (1981), using a microelectrode voltage-clamp, and by Klöckner and Isenberg (1985b), using a whole-cell clamp with minimal Ca^{2+}-buffering capacity in the pipette solution. Yamamoto *et al.* (1989b), using a whole-cell clamp, only rarely observed a distinct inverted 'U-shape', and usually needed to subtract the Ca^{2+}-current as estimated from another cell loaded with Cs^+ to block K^+-currents. The common lack of an inverted 'U-shape' in smooth muscle suggests either some interference from the pipette solution or that most smooth muscles have an insufficient Ca^{2+}-current density to activate the BK_{Ca}-channels. Care should be taken in interpreting a mild inverted 'U-shape' because a similar pattern can be obtained under circumstances when activation of K_V-channels reaches a maximum (Beech & Bolton, 1989b; Yamamoto *et al.*, 1989b).

What are the characteristics of the $I_{K(Ca)}$ in whole tissues and in single cells? Weigel *et al.* (1979) showed that depolarization of intestinal muscle caused a rapid Ca-inward current followed by a large, slowly rising and then declining outward K-current (duration, 0.5–2 s). This transient K-current was Ca^{2+}-activated. However, the double sucrose-gap does not clamp smooth muscle adequately and may have given time-courses for currents that are more a reflection of clamp deficiencies than of the gating kinetics of underlying ionic channels. Nevertheless, Walsh and Singer (1981, 1987) have used a two microelectrode method to voltage-clamp isolated muscle cells from toad stomach and also find a rapid Ca-inward current followed by a large, slowly declining K-current lasting 3 s.

The whole-cell patch-clamp recording method provides good temporal and spatial control of the smooth muscle cell membrane potential (Klöckner & Isenberg, 1985a; Yamamoto *et al.*, 1989a) and also allows control over intracellular ionic concentrations. This method often reveals an $I_{K(Ca)}$ with a faster time-course, mostly because of the oscillatory or spontaneous transient outward current (STOC). A STOC is believed to result from a sudden transient release of Ca^{2+} from inositol triphosphate (IP_3)-sensitive Ca^{2+}-stores which raises the internal Ca^{2+}-concentration causing an outward current lasting about 100 ms (Benham & Bolton, 1986; Ohya *et al.*, 1987a; Komori & Bolton, 1990). When studying STOCs it is important to note that they depend on the metabolic and Ca^{2+} status of the cell, which is affected to a variable extent by the solution in the patch pipette. The channels underlying STOCs are not the small conductance Ca^{2+}-activated K-channels (SK_{Ca}) described by Inoue *et al.* (1985) but are BK_{Ca}-channels because they are blocked by external TEA (4 mM) or charybdotoxin (0.1 mM) (Beech & Bolton, 1989a,b; Strong *et al.*, 1989; Muraki *et al.*, 1990).

The STOC frequency is enhanced by depolarization (Benham & Bolton, 1986; Ohya *et al.*, 1987a; Désilets *et al.*, 1989; Hisada *et al.*, 1990) and STOCs may cluster at the beginning of a depolarizing step (Hisada *et al.*, 1990) or a single large initial STOC may be evoked (Benham & Bolton, 1986; Ohya *et al.*, 1987a,b). This transient Ca^{2+}-activated K-current is brief (< 200 ms) and is blocked by 1 mM external TEA (Ohya *et al.*, 1987a). Higher EGTA (1–3 mM) or buffering Ca^{2+} with an EGTA-Ca^{2+} mixture to 0.1–1 μM in the patch pipette solution may increase the duration of the $I_{K(Ca)}$ (Mitra & Morad, 1985; Klöckner & Isenberg, 1985b; Ohya *et al.*, 1987a).

The actions of 'low' concentrations of TEA (< 5 mM) on electrical activity may indicate the contribution of BK_{Ca}-channels to the spike and to the resting potential. In freely-spiking smooth muscles, 5 mM TEA or less increases the frequency of spike discharge (Suzuki et al., 1963) and increases spike size and duration (Ito et al., 1970; Osa, 1974); rate of repolarization is slowed and any plateau component is enhanced (Szurszewski, 1978). Spike after-hyperpolarization is blocked (Bauer & Kuriyama, 1982). Conspicuous increases in the rate of rise of the spike are usually seen only in non-spiking smooth muscles where excitability is low; these may generate spikes freely in TEA (e.g. Fujiwara & Kuriyama, 1983). These effects of TEA suggest that BK_{Ca}-channels open mostly when $[Ca^{2+}]_i$ rises after Ca^{2+} entry during the upstroke of the spike in highly excitable smooth muscles; in those of low excitability their early opening may prevent development of regenerative spikes. As to the resting potential, 5 mM TEA or less often does not affect it (Suzuki et al., 1963; Ito et al., 1970; Osa, 1974; Szurszewski, 1978; Bauer & Kuriyama, 1982; Suzuki & Kasuya, 1986; Fujii et al., 1990; but see Creed & Kuriyama, 1971; Small, 1982; Trieschmann & Isenberg, 1989), suggesting that BK_{Ca}-channels are not involved. There are a large number of papers which describe the actions of TEA at concentrations of 10 mM or above (e.g. Stanfield, 1983), which probably involve several K-channel types in the observed modified electrical discharge.

Apamin-sensitive K-channels ($SK_{Ca(Ap)}$)*

Vladimirova and Shuba (1978) showed that apamin, a bee venom toxin, blocks the hyperpolarizing actions of external ATP or non-adrenergic non-cholinergic inhibitory ($NANC_i$) nerve stimulation in the guinea-pig stomach or taenia caeci. Apamin also increases spike frequency and blocks $NANC_i$ junction potentials in the guinea-pig ileum (Fig. 7.2), and blocks adrenaline-induced hyperpolarization in the guinea-pig taenia caeci (Maas et al., 1980) and ATP-induced hyperpolarization in the guinea-pig ileum (Yamanaka et al., 1985) and gall bladder (Ishikawa et al., 1983). Apamin, which is active on the guinea-pig taenia caeci, does not block hyperpolarizations in response to ATP or $NANC_i$ nerve stimulation in the guinea-pig trachealis (Zacour et al., 1987). The increase in ^{86}Rb-efflux stimulated by α-adrenoceptor agonists in the taenia caeci was blocked by apamin and also by quaternary neuromuscular blockers such as atracurium (Gater et al., 1985).

Banks et al. (1979) linked the action of apamin to the block of a K-channel. They showed that apamin inhibits Ca-dependent K-

---

*The designation $SK_{Ca(Ap)}$ has been used to distinguish this smooth muscle channel from the SK_{Ca}-channel described in portal vein by Inoue et al. (1985) and from which $SK_{Ca(Ap)}$ appears to differ. For further details on the properties of apamin, see Chapter 11.

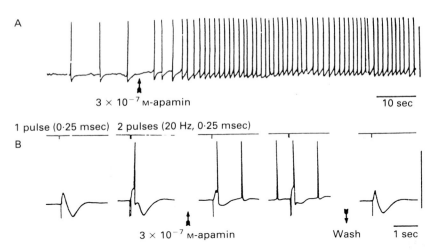

Fig. 7.2. Actions of apamin in the longitudinal smooth muscle of the guinea-pig ileum. A, Increased frequency of spontaneous spikes. B, Block of NANC$_i$ (but not excitatory) junction potentials (elicited by field stimulation). Membrane potential was recorded using a conventional glass capillary microelectrode filled with 3 M KCl and the tissue was pretreated for 20 min with atropine (1 μM) and guanethidine (10 μM). Both vertical calibration bars are 50 mV. (With permission from Bauer & Kuriyama, 1982.)

permeability in hepatocytes and proposed this as the mode of action of apamin in the guinea-pig taenia caeci. This view is consistent with the finding that ATP- and adrenaline-induced hyperpolarizations in the guinea-pig taenia caeci are Ca-dependent (Den Hertog, 1981, 1982). In addition, apamin abolishes the after-hyperpolarization of the spike in guinea-pig bladder (Fujii *et al.*, 1990), and perhaps also in the guinea-pig ileum (Fig. 7.2A). It depolarizes the taenia caeci by 3 mV and increases the amplitude and decay time of the spike (Maas *et al.*, 1980). Apamin potentiates spontaneous contractions and blocks α-adrenoceptor agonist- or bradykinin-induced inhibition of physalaemin contractions in the rabbit duodenum (Gater *et al.*, 1985) and potentiates histamine-, acetyl-choline- and ATP-induced contractions in the guinea-pig vas deferens (Fedan *et al.*, 1984). Overall the results are consistent with the hypothesis that apamin blocks a K_{Ca}-channel in smooth muscle.

The apamin-sensitive K-channel has not been identified at the whole-cell or single channel level in smooth muscle. The SK_{Ca}-channel found in patches from portal vein muscle (Inoue *et al.*, 1985) is unlikely to be the same as $SK_{Ca(Ap)}$ because SK_{Ca} is voltage-dependent and insensitive to $[Ca^{2+}]_i$ at negative membrane potentials (apamin was not tested). To look further at $SK_{Ca(Ap)}$ we must refer to the work of Blatz and Magleby (1986) on skeletal muscle and Capiod and Ogden (1989) on liver cells. With a quasi-physiological K^+-gradient the conductance of $SK_{Ca(Ap)}$ in liver cells was found to be 6 pS, about 20 times smaller than the BK_{Ca}-channel. The channel in skeletal muscle was voltage-independent and activated by raised $[Ca^{2+}]_i$ (> 10 nM), even at negative membrane potentials (tested between -90 and 40 mV). It was inhibited by external apamin but not by 5 mM external TEA (Blatz & Magleby, 1986). Note that more than 15 mM external TEA is required to block the apamin-sensitive inhibitory junction potential in guinea-pig ileum (Bauer & Kuriyama, 1982).

Delayed rectifier K-channels (K_V)

Delayed rectifier K-channels proper (K_V) are probably responsible for a large part of the voltage-activated K-current in smooth muscle. The term 'delayed rectifier' was used originally by Hodgkin and Huxley (1952) to identify that K-current in the squid axon which assists in the repolarization of the spike. As described in the Introduction, we will use the term 'delayed rectifier proper' to refer to voltage-activated K-channels that are not activated by internal Ca^{2+} in its physiological range (> 100 nM) and which are not A-channels; strictly the M-channel (K_M) should be included (*see later*). The word 'proper' is included to distinguish this category of K-channel from the Ca^{2+}-activated K-channels mentioned above and the other K-channels which may also contribute to the phenomenon of delayed rectification. In cells other than smooth muscle, delayed rectifiers proper are diverse and may or may not inactivate (Rudy, 1988). To demonstrate K_V, contaminating $I_{K(Ca)}$-currents must be substantially eliminated. Fairly stringent conditions are needed for this: Ca^{2+}-buffering in the cell should exceed 4 mM EGTA or equivalent; in some cases, in addition, the external solution should be Ca^{2+}-free (with EGTA or equivalent chelator because 10 μM or more Ca^{2+} may be present as a contaminant of 'Ca^{2+}-free' solutions). Some contribution from K_{Ca}-channels at positive potentials may occur, if 1 mM or more external Ca^{2+} is present, despite the presence of an inorganic Ca^{2+}-entry blocker (Co^{2+}, Mn^{2+}, Cd^{2+}) since 10 channels open out of the cell complement of about 10 000 ($P_o = 0.001$) may generate 100 pA of outward current. Figure 7.3 shows current through both K_V- and BK_{Ca}-channels, which were only slightly affected when extracellular Ca^{2+} was removed and when Cd^{2+} was applied at a concentration sufficient to block Ca-channels completely. The smooth current at 0 mV is the delayed rectifier, which is reduced by 4-AP (Fig. 7.3B), and the noisy current at $+80$ mV (largely unaffected by 4-AP) is that through BK_{Ca}-channels. In this whole-cell recording it can be seen that at strong positive potentials there is substantial contribution from BK_{Ca}-channels even with 0.8 mM EGTA in the pipette and zero Ca^{2+} in the bath.

Delayed rectifiers proper have been characterized in only a few smooth muscle types. In rabbit portal vein muscle cells (Beech & Bolton, 1989b), $I_{K(V)}$ was activated by stepping positive to -40 mV in a zero Ca^{2+}-medium

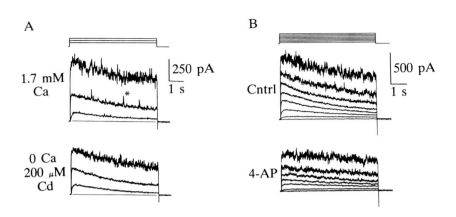

Fig. 7.3. Delayed rectifier (K_V) proper and contamination by BK_{Ca}-channel current in isolated smooth muscle cells from the rabbit portal vein. Recording was by whole-cell voltage-clamp (holding potential, -70 mV; [EGTA]$_i$ = 0.8 mM). A, The test voltage steps were to 0, $+40$ and $+80$ mV. The asterisk (∗) labels a STOC. (With permission from Beech & Bolton, 1989b.) B, Block of K_V by bath-applied 4-AP (5 mM). The test voltage steps were -50 to $+90$ mV in 20 mV increments. (D. J. Beech & T. B. Bolton, unpublished data.)

(with Cd^{2+}). It reached a peak after about 100 ms at 0 mV (20–23°C) and inactivated incompletely over many seconds. Steady-state inactivation was 50% complete at -30 mV. There was a 'delay' before activation, which for a test potential of 0 mV could be described well by a fourth order single exponential. The current was carried mostly by K^+ and the channels were blocked by bath-applied 4-AP (Fig. 7.3B), which often blocks delayed rectifiers (Rudy, 1988), or by phencyclidine. Apamin (100 nM), charybdotoxin (100 nM) or less than 4 mM TEA had little or no effect on the current (Beech & Bolton, 1989a). The single channel chord conductance was small, about 5 pS with a quasi-physiological K^+-gradient. In guinea-pig taenia caeci cells (Yamamoto *et al.*, 1989b), $I_{K(V)}$ was activated by stepping positive to -20 mV in a 5 mM Co^{2+}- and 3 mM Ca^{2+}-containing medium. It reached a peak after about 10 ms at 0 mV (33°C) and then inactivated partially within about 4 s. Steady-state inactivation was 50% complete at -51 mV. The channels activated after a 'delay' and were permeable mostly to K^+.

Delayed rectifier K-channels are probably present in vascular (Okabe *et al.*, 1987; Toro & Stefani, 1987; Bkaily *et al.*, 1988; Beech & Bolton, 1989b; Hume & Leblanc, 1989; Wilde & Lee, 1989; Noack *et al.*, 1990), intestinal (Nakao *et al.*, 1986; Ohya *et al.*, 1986; Buryi *et al.*, 1987; Ohya *et al.*, 1987a; Terada *et al.*, 1987; Walsh & Singer, 1987; Cole & Sanders, 1989; Yamamoto *et al.*, 1989b), vas deferens (Nakazawa *et al.*, 1987), uterine (Mironneau & Savineau, 1980; Toro *et al.*, 1990c) and tracheal smooth muscles (Hisada *et al.*, 1990; Muraki *et al.*, 1990). The K-channels underlying $I_{K(V)}$ in smooth muscle are quite likely to be a heterogeneous population. In vascular and tracheal muscles, $I_{K(V)}$ is inhibited by 4-AP and activates at potentials positive to $-40\,mV$ (Okabe et al., 1987; Beech & Bolton, 1989a,b; Hisada et al., 1990; Muraki et al., 1990; Noack et al., 1990). In small intestine and taenia caeci, $I_{K(V)}$ seems to be insensitive to 4-AP and activates positive to $-20\,mV$ (Ohya et al.,1986; Ohya et al., 1987a; Terada et al., 1987; Imaizumi et al., 1989). In ureter, apart from the A-current, the K-current not carried by BK_{Ca}-channels is very small (Imaizumi et al., 1989; Lang, 1989). There are indications that more than one K_V-channel type carry the $I_{K(V)}$-currents. This is to be anticipated from work on the node of Ranvier (Dubois, 1981) and on pheochromocytoma cells (Hoshi & Aldrich, 1988). In the smooth muscle of portal vein, there are often two phases of inactivation: 4-AP does not block $I_{K(V)}$ completely and two distinct single channel currents are evident in outside-out patches (Beech & Bolton, 1989b; see also Yamamoto et al., 1989b).

There is some uncertainty whether in some conditions (particularly if $[Ca^{2+}]_o$ is high) BK_{Ca}-channels may make a contribution even when a Ca^{2+}-entry blocker is present in the external solution and/or moderate Ca^{2+} buffering with EGTA is used in the pipette solution. In single cells of taenia caeci in a $3\,mM\ Ca^{2+}/5\,mM\ Co^{2+}$-containing solution with $1\,mM$ EGTA in the patch pipette, outward current was noisy which is suggestive of a contribution from BK_{Ca}-channels (Yamamoto et al., 1989b). In single cells of small intestine in a nominally Ca^{2+}-free, $2.5\,mM\ Mn^{2+}$ bathing solution with $4\,mM$ EGTA internal buffering, an outward current sensitive to $2\,mM$ TEA externally was seen (Terada et al., 1987). It is difficult to believe that the TEA-sensitive component was a K-current through BK_{Ca}-channels in this latter case. If this result can be confirmed it would seem that the delayed rectifier proper is considerably more sensitive to block by TEA in the small intestine than in arteries or veins. Likewise, in tracheal smooth muscle cells (Hisada et al., 1990) $[Ca^{2+}]_i$ was buffered to $10\,nM$ by a $5\,mM\ EGTA/Ca^{2+}$ mixture; when $1.8\,mM\ Ca^{2+}$ was present externally, clear evidence of BK_{Ca}-channel opening was seen. In nominally Ca^{2+}-free solution, a declining outward current was seen. This disappeared if $[Ca^{2+}]_i$ was buffered below $1\,nM$ with $5\,mM$ EGTA (Hisada et al., 1990); it seems plausible that the declining outward current, although requiring internal Ca^{2+}, was not through BK_{Ca}-channels but was through K_V-channels proper which require Ca^{2+} for normal gating (Begenisich, 1988).

Slow, potential-sensitive K-channels ($K_{V(S)}$)

In muscle cells of the rabbit jejunum and guinea-pig mesenteric artery there are some K-channels which activate slowly (1–10 s) on application of a square depolarizing step and deactivate slowly on hyperpolarization (Benham & Bolton, 1983; Bolton et al., 1985). The channels were identified at the single channel level in inside-out patches. They activated when the patch was depolarized of -40 mV, were not sensitive to $[Ca^{2+}]_i$, had a conductance of 50–60 pS ($[K^+]_o = 2.5$–6 mM; $[K^+]_i = 126$ mM), and were blocked completely by 10 mM internal TEA. The properties of this slow K-channel are such that it could be considered within the delayed rectifier category.*

A similar K-channel can be expressed in *Xenopus* oocytes by the injection of messenger RNA from oestrogen-treated rat myometrium (Boyle *et al.*, 1987a,b). Recordings from the whole oocyte with a two microelectrode voltage-clamp showed that the slow potential-sensitive K-current $I_{K(VS)}$ was activated from a holding potential of -40 mV and that activation and deactivation took many seconds; the current was not Ca^{2+}-dependent. The current was blocked by Ba^{2+}, La^{3+} or the anti-arrhythmic, clofilium (Folander *et al.*, 1990). Caution should, however, be used in the interpretation of these data because $I_{K(VS)}$ has not been observed in electrophysiological recordings from myometrial smooth muscle cells.

Benham and Bolton (1983) suggested that the $K_{V(S)}$-channel may contribute to slow-wave activity in the jejunum, causing slow repolarization. The role of such channels in the myometrium is not clear but the increased presence of its messenger RNA species during the oestrus cycle and at the end of pregnancy (Boyle *et al.*, 1987b) suggests that it may be important for maintaining quiescence of the uterus.

Muscarinic (M) receptor-inactivated K-channels (K_M)

The current carried by this channel (M-current, $I_{K(M)}$) is a non-inactivating, time- and voltage-dependent K-current that is suppressed by acetylcholine acting at muscarinic receptors; it is not Ca^{2+}-activated. The K_M is usually categorized separately from the delayed rectifiers proper (Rudy, 1988) even though it has many similar features.

After the initial description of $I_{K(M)}$ in bullfrog sympathetic neurones (Brown & Adams, 1980), Sims *et al.* (1985) found a very similar K-current in smooth muscle cells from the stomach of the toad, *Bufo marinus*. The smooth muscle $I_{K(M)}$ is maximally activated at -20 mV and mostly switched off at -70 mV. It is suppressed by muscarinic agonists, not dependent on external Ca^{2+}, and blocked by 5 mM external Ba^{2+} (Sims *et al.*, 1985). The $I_{K(M)}$ switches on slowly at -35 mV and off slowly at -65 mV (1–2 s). It is suppressed by substance P (or physalaemin) and this modulation is not additive with that of acetylcholine (Sims *et al.*, 1986). Isoprenaline augments $I_{K(M)}$, apparently by raising intracellular cyclic

---

*It seems reasonable to give this channel the nomenclature 'slow delayed rectifier', and to designate it and its current as $K_{V(S)}$ and $I_{K(VS)}$, respectively.

AMP (Sims *et al.*, 1988). The coupling pathway between muscarinic or substance P receptors and K_M-channels is not known. Because $I_{K(M)}$ is present at the resting potential and is non-inactivating it contributes a constant inhibitory influence on the membrane potential. Therefore, modulation of $I_{K(M)}$ is an important mechanism for contraction by acetylcholine or substance P and relaxation by noradrenaline in these amphibian stomach smooth muscle cells. This current has not been identified in any mammalian smooth muscle type. Acetylcholine depolarizes mammalian smooth muscles by opening non-selective cationic channels (Bolton, 1972; Benham *et al.*, 1985a; Vogalis & Sanders, 1990). Different K-channels are thought to provide the resting K-permeability of the mammalian smooth muscle membrane (Inoue *et al.*, 1986; Hu *et al.*, 1989a., Stuenkel, 1989; Nelson *et al.*, 1990; *see also* Chapter 1).

A-type K-channels

Like the delayed rectifier proper, A-type K-current ($I_{K(A)}$) (Hagiwara *et al.*, 1961; Connor & Stevens, 1971a) is activated by depolarization and is not Ca^{2+}-activated (reviewed by Rogawski, 1985; Rudy, 1988). In neurones, $I_{K(A)}$ is distinguished from the delayed rectifier proper because it can be activated only from very negative voltages and it inactivates rapidly, making a transient appearance. The $I_{K(A)}$ is blocked readily and reversibly by 4-AP but not by external TEA. An important function of this current in neurones is probably to retard depolarization after the after-hyperpolarization of the spike (Connor & Stevens, 1971b). However, if the resting potential is very negative then $I_{K(A)}$ will attenuate the spike and cause fast repolarization (Belluzzi *et al.*, 1985). In rat ventricular cells (Josephson *et al.*, 1984) a current termed I_{EO} was described which resembles $I_{K(A)}$ in that it was transient and blocked by 4-AP. However, I_{EO} was available for activation at quite depolarized potentials and thus in this case also may act mostly to reduce the rate of depolarization.

Potassium current in the A-type category exists in smooth muscle cells of the body wall of *Beroe ovata* (Bilbaut *et al.*, 1988), rabbit portal vein (Beech & Bolton, 1989c) and guinea-pig ureter (Lang, 1989; Imaizumi *et al.*, 1989). It may also occur in smooth muscle from the rabbit colon (Bielefeld *et al.*, 1990), toad stomach (Walsh & Singer, 1987) and guinea-pig myometrium (Vassort, 1975). A very prominant A-like current has been briefly described in rat portal vein (Noack *et al.*, 1992).

In rabbit portal vein muscle, $I_{K(A)}$ resembles neuronal A-current very closely (Beech & Bolton, 1989c). $I_{K(A)}$ is blocked readily and reversibly by bath-applied 4-AP but not by TEA, toxin-I (from *Dendroaspis polylepis*) or charybdotoxin. It is not Ca^{2+}-activated but activates rapidly on depolarization to positive of $-60\,mV$ and steady-state inactivation is 50% complete at $-79\,mV$ (Fig. 7.4). The kinetics of its inactivation are fast and

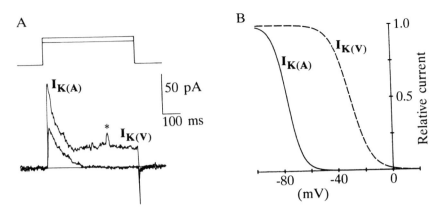

Fig. 7.4. A-current ($I_{K(A)}$) in an isolated smooth muscle cell from the rabbit portal vein. Recording was by whole-cell voltage-clamp. A, The test step to $-45\,mV$ from the holding potential of $-90\,mV$ elicited a transient outward current, $I_{K(A)}$. Depolarizing more (to $-35\,mV$) elicited a larger $I_{K(A)}$ and also delayed rectifier current proper $I_{K(V)}$. The asterisk (*) labels a STOC. B, Steady-state inactivation curve for $I_{K(A)}$ compared with that for $I_{K(V)}$. (Adapted with permission from Beech & Bolton, 1989b,c.)

can be described by a single exponential. At a test potential of $-40\,mV$ the time constant of this exponential is about 120 ms (20–23°C). The time constants become shorter with depolarization between -45 and $-15\,mV$. The channels recover completely from inactivation after about 0.5 s at $-100\,mV$. In guinea-pig ureter muscle, $I_{K(A)}$ is also blocked by 4-AP; it has a transient time-course and is carried by K^+, but 50% steady-state inactivation occurs at about 15 mV less negative, at about $-65\,mV$ (Lang, 1989; Imaizumi et al., 1990). The single channel current carried by K_A channels has been identified for the ureter muscle cells and the channel conductance estimated to be 14 pS (Imaizumi et al., 1990). The channels were observed in only four of 210 patches, suggesting paucity or intense clustering.

Divalent cations have a strong influence on the voltage dependence of $I_{K(A)}$ in neurones (Mayer & Sugiyama, 1988) and in smooth muscle (Beech & Bolton, 1989c; Imaizumi et al., 1990). Increasing the external divalent cation concentration changes $I_{K(A)}$ so that it operates in a more depolarized voltage range: Cd^{2+} is particularly potent in this respect. The effect can be described in part if divalent ions are considered to shield negative surface charges on the membrane lipids, but some direct interaction with the K_A-channels is also likely. This effect of divalent cations presents a problem when determining the voltage range in which $I_{K(A)}$ operates because Ca^{2+} substitutes are often used to block contaminating inward current.

The function of $I_{K(A)}$ in smooth muscle is uncertain. In the case of portal vein muscle, microelectrode recordings measure a resting potential of about $-50\,mV$ or more depolarized (Somlyo et al., 1969; Ito & Kuriyama, 1971; Kuriyama et al., 1971; Karashima & Takata, 1979; Hara et al., 1980; Takata, 1980; Hotta & Yamamoto, 1983; Nanjo, 1984), and so $I_{K(A)}$ should always remain inactive (see Fig. 7.4B). This may not be so, however, as the reduced-dialysis whole-cell recording of Hume and Leblanc (1989) show that some portal vein muscle cells rest negative of $-60\,mV$ and even hyperpolarize more after the spike, and the microelectrode recordings of Hamilton et al. (1986) show resting potentials at $-60\,mV$. Thus, $I_{K(A)}$ could be activated in some cells (perhaps 'pacemakers') with large resting potentials and rhythm in their firing pattern. Indeed, smooth muscle spike frequency increases with depolarization and in neurones this is explained by activity of $I_{K(A)}$ (Hille, 1984). Furthermore, 4-AP increases spike frequency in the portal vein (Hara et al., 1980), suggesting that $I_{K(A)}$ might be functional in the intact tissue. It is also possible that neurotransmitters, hormones or intracellular factors shift the activation of $I_{K(A)}$ into the range of the resting potential as occurs with I_f-type current in the heart.* Alternatively, $I_{K(A)}$ may act to slow the decline of inhibitory junction potentials. Another possibility is that K_A-channels are coexpressed with closely-related K-channels, for example delayed rectifier K_V-channels proper, not because they are required for the function of that smooth muscle but simply because the cell has no need to exclude them. In this case the K_A-channel would have no function.

ATP-sensitive K-channels (K_{ATP})

Adenosine triphosphate-sensitive K-channels (K_{ATP}-channels) were first identified in cardiac muscle (Noma, 1983), but are also present in pancreatic β-cells, skeletal muscle and neurones (reviewed by Ashcroft, 1988; Miller, 1990). Activation of these would be expected when intracellular ATP decreases, providing a link between metabolism and electrical activity. The ATP effect seems not to reflect a phosphorylation (Cook & Hales, 1984) and the channels do not have a pronounced dependence on membrane potential or Ca^{2+}.

It has been suggested that the K_{ATP}-channel is the site of action of K-channel openers such as cromakalim, nicorandil and pinacidil (Standen et al., 1989) but there are a number of difficulties with this proposal. We have been unable to detect single K_{ATP} channels or ATP-sensitive K-currents ($I_{K(ATP)}$ in single cells of rabbit portal vein (Nakao & Bolton, 1991, see also Hu et al., 1990) and published records on these cells by others (Kajioka et al., 1990) show unconvincing effects of ATP on the P_o of small conductance channels. However, in portal vein cromakalim will produce

*For further details on I_f, see Chapters 8 and 12.

substantial outward current which is blocked by 0.1–3 μM glibenclamide (Nakao & Bolton, 1991) (*see* Chapter 14, Fig. 14.3). This concentration is less than that (20 μM) used to partially reverse the effects of cromakalim on K-channel opening in rabbit mesenteric artery (Standen *et al.*, 1989); 20 μM is more than two orders of magnitude larger than that needed to block K_{ATP}-channels in pancreatic β-cells (Ashcroft, 1988).*

Adenosine triphosphate (1 mM) had a conspicuous inhibitory effect on K-channel opening in rabbit mesenteric artery cell-membrane patches (Standen *et al.*, 1989). Channel conductance was 135 pS (60 mM K_o: 120 mM K_i). This is very similar to that of the BK_{Ca}-channel, but unlike the latter the reported K_{ATP} was insensitive to Ca on the internal surface of the membrane and to external charybdotoxin (0.1 μM). Opening of the channel in the presence of ATP and cromakalim was severely inhibited by 20 μM glibenclamide. Much lower concentrations of glibenclamide (0.1–0.25 μM) were shown to inhibit relaxations to diazoxide, cromakalim and pinacidil of mesenteric artery strips and 10 μM glibenclamide inhibited vasoactive intestinal peptide (VIP)- or acetylcholine-induced hyperpolarization. On the basis of antagonism by glibenclamide the ATP-sensitive channel was also implicated in the effects on this artery of calcitonin gene-related peptide which opened K-channels insensitive to 0.1 μM charybdotoxin on the external surface. These had a slope conductance at 0 mV of 20 pS (Nelson *et al.*, 1990) and were inhibited by 15 or 30 μM glibenclamide.

It seems that large (135 pS) or medium (20 pS) conductance ATP-sensitive channels which are not BK_{Ca}-channels may occur in some vascular smooth muscle. However, in other vascular muscles where cromakalim produces an outward current and hyperpolarization, ATP-sensitive channels are difficult to demonstrate. There is also a disconcerting difference (cf. smooth muscle and β-cells) in the sensitivity of various ATP-regulated K-channels to glibenclamide (and to cromakalim, Ashford *et al.*, 1988; Garrino *et al.*, 1989). At present it is difficult to believe that K-channel openers act in all smooth muscles on a single variety of K_{ATP}-channels which are also inhibited by glibenclamide. Also, in intestinal smooth muscle, cromakalim is an effective relaxant and yet several reports are not consistent with the presence of ATP-sensitive channels in these cells. In the guinea-pig taenia caeci, a decrease in extracellular glucose causes depolarization and it is the readmission of glucose that causes hyperpolarization (Axelsson *et al.*, 1965). This is the opposite to that expected for a system expressing K_{ATP}-channels (pancreatic β-cells; Dean & Matthews, 1970). Also in rabbit ileum muscle cells, intracellular perfusion of ATP (> 0.3 mM) had no effect on resting input resistance although it strongly increased the voltage-gated Ca^{2+}-current (Ohya

---

*See Chapter 6 for further details of the glibenclamide sensitivity of K_{ATP} in the β-cell.

et al., 1987b). Nevertheless, single channel and whole-cell recordings will tell us more about the existence of K_{ATP}-channels in smooth muscle. At present we have only a few details about the single channel characteristics of K_{ATP} and know nothing of the $I_{K(ATP)}$ in the whole-cell.

Inward rectifier K-channels (K_{IR})

Inward (or anomalous) rectifier channels (K_{IR}) pass more current with hyperpolarization than with depolarization (Hagiwara & Takahashi, 1974; reviewed by Hille, 1984). In addition, as $[K^+]_o$ is raised, the channels conduct at less hyperpolarized potentials, passing current mostly negative of the K-equilibrium potential (E_K). The mechanism for the voltage dependence is not known for all inward rectifiers, but in ventricular cells it is largely because the channels are blocked by $[Mg^{2+}]_i$ in a voltage-dependent manner (Matsuda *et al.*, 1987). Raised $[K^+]_o$ thus shifts the voltage range over which the K_{IR}-channels rectify because K^+ moving in through the channels 'pushes' Mg^{2+} away. Although the channels are called 'inward rectifiers', under physiological conditions they probably only pass outward K^+-current and serve to stabilize the membrane potential. The inward rectifier is distinct from another current activated by hyperpolarization, I_h. This is a mixed cation current (partly K^+) with slow kinetics and which, unlike $I_{K(IR)}$, is not blocked by external Ba^{2+}. The I_h is present in smooth muscle cells from the rabbit jejunum (Benham *et al.*, 1987); I_h may be similar to I_F (*see* Chapters 8 and 12).

The $I_{K(IR)}$ has only been described in arteriolar smooth muscle. Working on guinea-pig ileum submucosal arterioles, Edwards and Hirst (1988) found a K^+-current that was activated at voltages negative to $-60\,mV$. The current showed no obvious time dependence, was K^+-selective and blocked completely by 1 mM external Ba^{2+}. Consistent with $I_{K(IR)}$ being an inward rectifier, its conducting range shifted to less negative voltages as $[K^+]_o$ was raised (Fig. 7.5). Edwards and Hirst (1988) proposed that the inward rectifier contributes strongly to the resting potential because it remains partially conducting positive to E_K.

The $I_{K(IR)}$ may also be present in smooth muscle of the urinary bladder (fig. 11 in Klöckner & Isenberg, 1985b) but it does not seem to exist in most smooth muscles (Walsh & Singer, 1981; Sims *et al.*, 1985; Nakao *et al.*, 1986; Beech & Bolton, 1989c; Cole & Sanders, 1989; Hume & Leblanc, 1989; Imaizumi *et al.*, 1989; Lang, 1989; Wilde & Lee, 1989). However, the use of whole-cell recording for many smooth muscle studies (a switching microelectrode voltage-clamp was used by Edwards & Hirst, 1988) may mean that the inward rectifier is lost as a result of uncontrolled cell dialysis, which may for example reduce $[Mg^{2+}]_i$. Nevertheless, the lack of inward rectification in the reduced-dialysis whole-cell recordings of Hume & Leblanc (1989) and microelectrode recordings of Walsh and

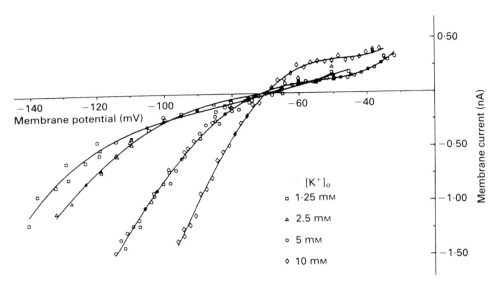

Fig. 7.5. Dependence of inward rectification in a submucosal arteriole on the external K^+-concentration. Cells were impaled with a single 80–120 MΩ microelectrode containing 0.5 M KCl and membrane voltage controlled by a switching clamp. The holding potential was − 70 mV. (With permission from Edwards & Hirst, 1988.)

Singer (1981) and Sims *et al.* (1985) argues for the view that inward rectification is restricted to some specialized smooth muscle types.

Hu *et al.* (1989a) report that BK_{Ca}-channels can generate a different form of inward rectification in cells of the guinea-pig taenia caeci. The BK_{Ca}-channels show a minimum activation at about − 30 mV but then activate not only with depolarization but also with hyperpolarizations up to − 50 mV. This correlates with a U-shaped mean closed time against voltage curve, which is also evident in the results of Benham *et al.* (1986) and Carl and Sanders (1989). Anomalous behaviour like this may be an example of how other smooth muscles use K-channels to control the resting potential. In addition, we should note that other K-channels can be blocked by $[Mg^{2+}]_i$ and thus generate inward rectification that is similar to that of the inward rectifier proper. One K-channel in particular which might behave like this is the K_{ATP}-channel (*see above*), which is blocked by $[Mg^{2+}]_i$ in a voltage-dependent manner in ventricular cells (Horie *et al.*, 1987). It is conceivable that the K-channels underlying the inward rectifier in guinea-pig arteriolar smooth muscle (Edwards & Hirst, 1988) are in fact K_{ATP}-channels.

Potassium channels dependent on external Ca^{2+} (K_{Ca_o})

In excised patches from rabbit portal vein muscle, Inoue *et al.* (1986)

observed a voltage-independent K-channel that was sensitive to the external Ca^{2+} concentration in the range 0.01–3 μM. With a symmetrical 142 mM K^+-gradient this 'K_M' channel ('M' for medium)* had a conductance of 180 pS and was inhibited only 50% by 10 mM external TEA, showing that it is not the BK_{Ca}-channel: BK_{Ca}-channels do not seem to require external Ca^{2+} (Singer & Walsh, 1987; Hu et al., 1989a; see also Marty, 1981). The channel was also activated by internal Ca^{2+}, but at high concentrations ($> 35\mu$M). A similar channel may exist in smooth muscle cells from the coronary artery (Inoue et al., 1989). The K_{Ca_o}-channel opens at the resting potential and so may contribute to the resting K-permeability of the smooth muscle cell.

It is possible that $I_{K(Ca_o)}$ contributes to the leakage current seen in whole-cell recordings. In rabbit portal vein muscle cells, Hume and Leblanc (1989) showed that after 20 min exposure to nominally Ca^{2+}-free bath solution the time-independent leak current was reduced by about 80%. The leak current was also reduced by 20 mM external TEA, suggesting it was a K-current. In dog coronary artery muscle cells, Wilde and Lee (1989) observed that the time-independent leak current was abolished when external Ca^{2+} was reduced from 10 μM to essentially zero (1 mM EGTA with no added Ca^{2+}). The records of Mitra and Morad (1985) show a decrease in leak current in guinea-pig gastric smooth muscle cells when the bath solution was changed to a Ca^{2+}-free medium. However, all of these whole-cell currents were enhanced by depolarization, which contrasts with the single channel data on K_{Ca_o}.

A fatty acid-activated K-channel (K_{FA})

Arachidonic, myristic, linoelaidic, linolenic, palmitoleic and eicosatetraynoic acids (20–100 μM) all activate a small K-channel in outside-out patches from smooth muscle cells of toad stomach (Fig. 7.6) (Ordway et al., 1989; reviewed by Ordway et al., 1991). The channel has a conductance of 23 pS ($[K^+]_i$ 130 mM, $[K^+]_o$ 20 mM). Potassium current is also activated in the whole cell by the same fatty acids. Ordway et al. (1989) argue that it is the fatty acids themselves (and not their metabolites) which activate the K-channel directly because palmitoleic, linoelaidic, and myristic acids are not substrates for cyclo- or lipoxygenases and eicosatetraynoic acid blocks cyclo- and lipoxygenase and cytochrome P450. The K_{FA} is active in the absence of Ca^{2+} or nucleotides and shows no pronounced voltage dependence. It is not clear yet whether this is a K-channel already identified by other means, although the channel conductance does not correspond to any other example from smooth muscle (Table 7.2). The

---

*The designation K_M is more appropriate for muscarinic receptor-inactivated K-channels. The nomenclature K_{Ca_o} for the channel and $I_{K(Ca_o)}$ for the associated current will be adopted in this volume.

Table 7.2. Types of K-channel in smooth muscle cells.

Type	Channel conductance	Factors affecting opening	Blockers	Roles	Smooth muscle types
BK_{Ca}	100–150 pS	Activated by raised $[Ca^{2+}]_i$ and/or depolarization; Opened by phosphorylation; Inhibited by intracellular acidosis	TEA_o (1 mM), Charybdotoxin$_o$	Limit excitability if $[Ca^{2+}]_i$ rises; Decrease spike amplitude; Cause spike after-hyperpolarization?	All (*see* Table 7.1)
$SK_{Ca(Ap)}$	6–12 ps?	Activated by raised $[Ca^{2+}]_i$? (not shown for smooth muscle); Opened by activation of receptors for ATP or noradrenaline	Apamin$_o$, Atracurium	Generate inhibitory junction potentials?; Cause spike after-hyperpolarization?	Intestine, bladder, (vas deferens)
K_V	5 pS	Activated by depolarization from rest; Inactivated by sustained depolarization	4-AP, Phencyclidine	Assist repolarization phase of spike; Inhibit spike generation	Most
$K_{V(s)}$	50 pS	Activated by prolonged depolarization	–	Cause slow wave repolarization?; Inhibit excitability	Intestine, artery, (uterus?)
K_M	–	Activated by depolarization with no inactivation	Ba^{2+}	Resting K-permeability	Intestine (toad)
K_A	14 pS	Activated by depolarization from potentials negative of resting potential; Inactivated rapidly on depolarization	4-AP, Phencyclidine	Regulate spike frequency?	Portal vein, ureter, ctenophore body wall

K_{ATP}	*See relevant section*	Opened by decreased $[ATP]_i$; K-channel openers?	Glibenclamide?	Cause hyperpolarization during hypoxia?	Mesenteric artery
K_{IR}	–	Hyperpolarization increases conductance	Ba^{2+}	Resting K-permeability	Submucous arterioles
K_{Ca_o}	90 pS	Switched off when $[Ca^{2+}]_o$ decreases	–	Resting K-permeability	Portal vein (artery, uterus?)
K_{FA}	23 pS	Activated by various fatty acids	–	Increase resting K-permeability	Intestine (toad)

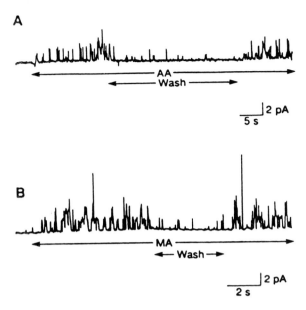

Fig. 7.6. A fatty acid activated K-channel (K_{FA}) in an outside-out patch excised from a single toad stomach smooth muscle cell. The pipette K^+-concentration was 130 mM. A, Application and wash-out of arachidonic acid (AA; 40 μM). The holding potential was +40 mV and $[K]_o$ was 3 mM. B, Application and wash-out of myristic acid (MA; 40 μM), which is not a substrate for cyclo- or lipoxygenases. The holding potential was +50 mV and $[K]_o$ was 20 mM. (With permission from Ordway *et al.* (1989). Copyright 1989 by the AASS.)

K_{FA}-channels have not been reported for other smooth muscle types. 2-Decenoic acid (1 mM) has been observed to increase P_o of BK_{Ca}-channels 10-fold and convert Mg^{2+} to an activator of the channel when acting from the inside (Bregestovski *et al.*, 1989).

5,8,11,14,17-Eicosapentanoic acid dilates cat coronary arteries independently of the endothelium (Yanagisawa & Lefer, 1987), and pulmonary, femoral and saphenous veins of the dog are all relaxed by arachidonic acid, also in the absence of endothelium (De Mey & Vanhoutte, 1982). The mechanisms of action of these fatty acids is unknown, but their actions could be explained by the opening of K-channels. It must also be borne in mind, however, that such hydrophobic compounds can alter the fluidity of the membrane, perhaps affecting membrane protein activity (Rimon *et al.*, 1978). Cholesterol levels in the membrane affect the kinetics of opening of BK_{Ca}-channels (Bolotina *et al.*, 1989).

Conclusions

With the exception of the Na-activated K-channel (K_{Na}) (reviewed by Martin & Dryer, 1989), all the major categories of K-channel have been identified in one smooth muscle or another. Table 7.2 summarizes the data on smooth muscle K-channels, indicating which smooth muscles have which K-channels and suggesting roles that the various K-channels might play. However, although it is clear for some smooth muscles that a K-channel type is either absent or of minor significance, in most cases we do not yet know what is the true complement of K-channels in each smooth muscle cell. It is still unclear which type(s) of K-channel is responsible for the resting membrane potential of smooth muscle cells — K_{Ca_0} (Inoue et al., 1986), K_{Ca} (Hu et al., 1989a) and K_{IR} (Edwards & Hirst, 1988) — have all been suggested to make a contribution (see also Chapter 1). In addition, there are not only many categories of K-channel but also a plethora of variations on these themes depending on the smooth muscle and perhaps on the experimental conditions. Different conditions may generate apparent variety because many of the K-channels are probably intimately dependent on their environment. We are only just learning about the effects of the intracellular milieu and of second messengers on K-channels, mostly through the investigation of the modulatory actions of neurotransmitters and hormones.

The amount of data on smooth muscle K-channels will increase further with the continued use of the patch-clamp method, the development of the nystatin-perforated whole cell and patch, the use of toxins and drugs that distinguish K-channel types, and the application of molecular cloning and developmental biology techniques to smooth muscle. These new data will both enhance our understanding of the classification and elementary properties of smooth muscle K-channels and also clarify the contribution which individual K-channels make to the wide array of smooth muscle electrical activity.

Acknowledgements

Work by the authors mentioned in this review was supported by the Medical Research Council. D.J.B. is supported by the Wellcome Trust.

References

Aaronson, P. I. & Benham, C. D. (1989) Alterations in $[Ca^{2+}]_i$ mediated by sodium–calcium exchange in smooth muscle cells isolated from guinea-pig ureter. Journal of Physiology **416**, 1–18.

Aaronson, P. I., Bolton, T. B., Lang, R. J. & MacKenzie, I. (1988) Calcium currents in single isolated smooth muscle cells from the rabbit ear artery in normal-calcium and high-barium solutions. Journal of Physiology **405**, 57–75.

Ashcroft, F. M. (1988) Adenosine 5′-triphosphate-sensitive potassium channels. Annual Review Neuroscience **11**, 97–118.

Ashford, M. L. J., Hales, C. & Kozlowski, R. Z. (1988) Diazoxide, but not BRL 34915, activates ATP-sensitive potassium channels in a rat insulinoma cell line. Journal of Physiology **409**, 53P.

Axelsson, J., Hogberg, S. G. R. & Timms, A. R. (1965) The effect of removing and readmitting glucose on the electrical and mechanical activity and glucose and glycogen content of intestinal smooth muscle from the taenia coli of the guinea-pig. *Acta Physiologica Scandinavica* **64**, 28–42.

Banks, B. E. C., Brown, C., Burgess, G. M., Burnstock, G., Claret, M., Cocks, T. M. & Jenkinson, D. H. (1979) Apamin blocks certain neurotransmitter-induced increases in potassium permeability. *Nature* **282**, 415–417.

Bauer, V. & Kuriyama, H. (1982) The nature of non-cholinergic, non-adrenergic transmission in longitudinal and circular muscles of the guinea-pig ileum. *Journal of Physiology* **332**, 375–391.

Beech, D. J. & Bolton, T. B. (1989a) Properties of the cromakalim-induced potassium conductance in smooth muscle cells isolated from the rabbit portal vein. *British Journal of Pharmacology* **98**, 851–864.

Beech, D. J. & Bolton, T. B. (1989b) Two components of potassium current activated by depolarization of single smooth muscle cells from the rabbit portal vein. *Journal of Physiology* **418**, 293–309.

Beech, D. J. & Bolton, T. B. (1989c) A voltage-dependent outward current with fast kinetics in single smooth muscle cells isolated from the rabbit portal vein. *Journal of Physiology* **412**, 397–414.

Begenisch, T. (1988) The role of divalent cations in potassium channels. *Trends in Neuroscience* **11(6)**, 270–273.

Belluzzi, O., Sacchi, O. & Wanke, E. (1985) A fast transient outward current in the rat sympathetic neurone studied under voltage-clamp. *Journal of Physiology* **358**, 91–108.

Benham, C. D. & Bolton, T. B. (1983) Patch-clamp studies of slow potential-sensitive potassium channels in longitudinal smooth muscle cells of rabbit jejunum. *Journal of Physiology* **340**, 469–486.

Benham, C. D. & Bolton, T. B. (1986) Spontaneous transient outward currents in single visceral and vascular smooth muscle cells of the rabbit. *Journal of Physiology* **381**, 385–406.

Benham, C. D., Bolton, T. B., Denbigh, J. S. & Lang, R. J. (1987) Inward rectification in freshly isolated single smooth muscle cells of the rabbit jejunum. *Journal of Physiology* **383**, 461–476.

Benham, C. D., Bolton, T. B. & Lang, R. J. (1985a) Acetylcholine activates an inward current in single mammalian smooth muscle cells. *Nature* **316**, 345–347.

Benham, C. D., Bolton, T. B., Lang, R. J. & Takewaki, T. (1985b) The mechanism of action of Ba^{2+} and TEA on single Ca^{2+}-activated K^+-channels in arterial and intestinal smooth muscle cell membranes. *Pflügers Archiv* **403**, 120–127.

Benham, C. D., Bolton, T. B., Lang, R. J. & Takewaki, T. (1986) Calcium-activated potassium channels in single smooth muscle cells of rabbit jejunum and guinea-pig mesenteric artery. *Journal of Physiology* **371**, 45–67.

Berger, W., Grygorcyk, R. & Schwarz, W. (1984) Single K^+ channels in membrane evaginations of smooth muscle cells. *Pflügers Archiv* **402**, 18–23.

Bielefeld, D. R., Hume, J. R. & Krier, J. (1990) Action potentials and membrane currents of isolated single smooth muscle cells of cat and rabbit colon. *Pflügers Archiv* **415**, 678–687.

Bilbaut, A., Hernandez-Nicaise, M-L., Leech, C. A. & Meech, R. W. (1988) Membrane currents that govern smooth muscle contraction in a ctenophore. *Nature* **331**, 533–535.

Bkaily, G., Peyrow, M., Sculptoreanu, A., Jacques, D., Chahine, M., Regoli, D. & Sperelakis, N. (1988) Angiotensin II increases I_{si} and blocks I_K in single aortic cells of rabbit. *Pflügers Archiv* **412**, 448–450.

Blatz, A. L. & Magleby, K. L. (1986) Single apamin-blocked Ca-activated K$^+$ channels of small conductance in cultured rat skeletal muscle. *Nature* **323**, 718–720.

Bolotina, V., Omelyanenko, V., Heyes, B., Ryan, V. & Bregestovski, P. (1989) Variations in membrane cholesterol after the kinetics of Ca^{2+} dependent K$^+$ channels and membrane fluidity in vascular smooth muscle cells. *Pflügers Archiv* **415**, 262–268.

Bolton, T. B. (1972) The depolarizing action of acetylcholine or carbachol in intestinal smooth muscle. *Journal of Physiology* **220**, 647–671.

Bolton, T. B. & Lim, S. P. (1989) Properties of calcium stores and transient outward currents in single smooth muscle cells of rabbit intestine. *Journal of Physiology* **409**, 385–401.

Bolton, T. B., Lang, R. J., Takewaki, T. & Benham, C. D. (1985) Patch and whole-cell voltage clamp of single mammalian visceral and vascular smooth muscle cells. *Experientia* **41**, 887–894.

Boyle, M. B., Azhderian, E. M., Maclusky, N. J., Naftolin, F. & Kaczmarek, L. K. (1987a) *Xenopus* oocytes injected with rat uterine RNA express very slowly activating potassium currents. *Science* **235**, 1221–1224.

Boyle, M. B., Maclusky, N. J., Naftolin, F. & Kaczmarek, L. K. (1987b) Hormonal regulation of K$^+$-channel messenger RNA in rat myometrium during oestrus cycle and in pregnancy. *Nature* **330**, 373–375.

Bregestovski, P. D., Bolotina, V. M. & Serebryakov, V. N. (1989) Fatty acid modifies Ca^{2+}-dependent potassium channel activity in smooth muscle cells from the human aorta. *Proceedings of the Royal Society London Series B* **237**, 259–266.

Bregestovski, P. D., Printseva, O. Yu., Serebryakov, J., Turmin, A. & Zamoyski, V. (1988) Comparison of Ca^{2+}-dependent K$^+$ channels in the membrane of smooth muscle cells isolated from adult and foetal human aorta. *Pflügers Archiv* **413**, 8–13.

Bregestovksi, P. D., Zamoyski, V. L. & Serebryakov, V. N. (1986) Action of quinine on Ca^{2+}-activated K$^+$ channels in smooth muscle cell membrane of human aorta. *Biological Membranes* **3**, 601–608.

Bregestovski, P. D., Zamoyski, V. L., Serebryakov, V. N., Topygin, A. Yu. & Antonov, A. C. (1985) Calcium-activated potassium channel with high conductance in cultured smooth muscle cell membranes of human aorta. *Biological Membranes* **2**, 487–498.

Brown, D. A. & Adams, P. R. (1980) Muscarinic suppression of a novel voltage-sensitive K$^+$ current in a vertebrate neurone. *Nature* **283**, 673–676.

Bülbring, E. (1955) Correlation between membrane potential, spike discharge and tension in smooth muscle. *Journal of Physiology* **128**, 200–221.

Bülbring, E. & Kuriyama, H. (1963) Effects of changes in external sodium and calcium concentrations on spontaneous electrical activity in smooth muscle of the guinea-pig taenia caeci. *Journal of Physiology* **166**, 29–58.

Buryi, V. A., Shuba, M. F. & Zholos, A. V. (1987) Potassium currents in the isolated smooth muscle cell membrane. In Ovchinnikov, Y. A. & Hucho, F. (eds), *Receptors and Ion Channels*. Walter de Gruyter & Co., Berlin, pp. 179–185.

Capiod, T. & Ogden, D. C. (1989) The properties of calcium-activated potassium ion channels in guinea-pig isolated hepatocytes. *Journal of Physiology* **409**, 285–295.

Carl, A. & Sanders, K. M. (1989) Ca^{2+}-activated K channels of canine colonic myocytes. *American Journal of Physiology* **257** (Cell Physiology 26), C470–C480.

Cecchi, X., Alvarez, O. & Wolff, D. (1986) Characterization of a calcium-activated potassium channel from rabbit intestinal smooth muscle incorporated into planar bilayers. *Journal of Membrane Biology* **91**, 11–18.

Cecchi, X., Wolff, D., Alvarez, O. & Latorre, R. (1987) Mechanisms of Cs$^+$ blockade in a Ca^{2+}-activated K$^+$ channel from smooth muscle. *Biophysical Journal* **52**, 707–716.

Cole, W. C. & Sanders, K. M. (1989) Characterization of macroscopic outward currents of canine colonic myocytes. *American Journal of Physiology* **257** (Cell Physiology **26**), C461–C469.

Cole, W. C., Carl, A. & Sanders, K. M. (1989) Muscarinic suppression of Ca^{2+}-dependent K current in colonic smooth muscle. *American Journal of Physiology* **257** (Cell Physiology **26**), C481–C487.

Coleman, H. A. & Parkington, H. C. (1987) Single channel Cl^- and K^+ currents from cells of uterus not treated with enzymes. *Pflügers Archiv* **410**, 560–562.

Connor, J. A. & Stevens, C. F. (1971a) Voltage-clamp studies of a transient outward membrane current in gastropod neural somata. *Journal of Physiology* **213**, 21–30.

Connor, J. A. & Stevens, C. F. (1971b) Prediction of repetitive firing behaviour from voltage-clamp data on an isolated neurone soma. *Journal of Physiology* **213**, 31–53.

Cook, D. L. & Hales, C. (1984) Intracellular ATP directly blocks K^+ channels in pancreatic β-cells. *Nature* **311**, 271–273.

Creed, K. E. & Kuriyama, H. (1971) Electrophysiological properties of the smooth muscle cells of the biliary system of the guinea-pig. *Japanese Journal of Physiology* **21**, 333–348.

Dean, P. M. & Matthews, E. K. (1970) Glucose-induced electrical activity in pancreatic islet cells. *Journal of Physiology* **210**, 255–264.

De Mey, J. G. & Vanhoutte, P. M. (1982) Heterogeneous behaviour of the canine arterial and venous wall. *Circulation Research* **51**, 439–447.

Den Hertog, A. (1981) Calcium and the α-action of catecholamines on guinea-pig taenia caeci. *Journal of Physiology* **316**, 109–125.

Den Hertog, A. (1982) Calcium and the action of adrenaline, adenosine triphosphate and carbachol on guinea-pig taenia caeci. *Journal of Physiology* **325**, 423–439.

Désilets, M., Driska, S. & Baumgarten, C-M. (1989) Current fluctuations and oscillations in smooth muscle cells from hog carotid artery. *Circulation Research* **65**, 708–722.

Dubois, J. M. (1981) Evidence for the existence of three types of potassium channels in the frog Ranvier node membrane. *Journal of Physiology* **318**, 297–316.

Edwards, F. R. & Hirst, G. D. S. (1988) Inward rectification in submucosal arterioles of guinea-pig ileum. *Journal of Physiology* **404**, 437–454.

Fedan, J. S., Hogaboom, G. K. & O'Donnell, J. P. (1984) Comparison of the effects of apamin, a Ca^{2+}-dependent K^+ channel blocker, and arylazido aminopropionyl ATP (ANAPP3), a P2-purinergic receptor antagonist, in the guinea-pig vas deferens. *European Journal of Pharmacology* **104**, 327–334.

Folander, K., Smith, J. S., Antanavage, J., Bennet, C., Stein, R. B. & Swanson, R. (1990) Cloning and expression of the delayed rectifier I_{sK} channel from neonatal rat heart and diethylstilbestrol-primed rat uterus. *Proceedings of the National Academy of Sciences USA* **87**, 2975–2979.

Fujii, K., Foster, C. D., Brading, A. F. & Parekh, A. B. (1990) Potassium channel blockers and the effects of cromakalim on the smooth muscle of the guinea-pig bladder. *British Journal of Pharmacology* **99**, 779–785.

Fujiwara, S. & Kuriyama, H. (1983) Effects of agents that modulate potassium permeability on smooth muscle cells of the guinea-pig basilar artery. *British Journal of Pharmacology* **79**, 23–35.

Garrino, M. G., Plant, T. D. & Henquin, J. C. (1989) Effects of putative activators of K^+ channels in mouse pancreatic β-cells. *British Journal of Pharmacology* **98**, 957–965.

Gater, P. R., Haylett, D. G. & Jenkinson, D. H. (1985) Neuromuscular blocking agents inhibit receptor-mediated increases in the potassium permeability of intestinal smooth muscle. *British Journal of Pharmacology* **86**, 861–868.

Gelband, C. H., Silberberg, S. D., Groschner, K. & van Breemen, C. (1990) ATP inhibits smooth muscle Ca^{2+}-activated K^+ channels. *Proceedings of the Royal Society of London, Series B* **242**, 23–28.

Gelband, C. H. & van Breemen, C. (1989) Reconstituted aortic Ca^{2+}-activated K^+ channels: Selectivity and pharmacological modulation by cromakalim (BRL 34915) and pinacidil. *Biophysical Journal* **55**, 545a.

Groschner, K., Silberberg, S. D., Gelband, C. H. & van Breemen, C. (1991) Ca^{2+}-activated K^+ channels in airway smooth muscle are inhibited by cytoplasmic ATP. *Pflügers Archiv* **417**, 517–522.

Hagiwara, S. & Takahashi, K. (1974) The anomalous rectification and cation selectivity of the membrane of a starfish egg cell. *Journal of Membrane Biology* **18**, 61–80.

Hagiwara, S., Kusano, K. & Saito, N. (1961) Membrane changes of *Onchidium* nerve cells in potassium rich media. *Journal of Physiology* **155**, 470–489.

Hamilton, T. C., Weir, S. W. & Weston, A. H. (1986) Comparison of the effects of BRL 34915 and verapamil on electrical and mechanical activity in rat portal vein. *British Journal of Pharmacology* **88**, 103–111.

Hara, Y., Kitamura, K. & Kuriyama, H. (1980) Actions of 4-aminopyridine on vascular smooth muscle tissues on the guinea-pig. *British Journal of Pharmacology* **68**, 99–106.

Hille, B. (1984) *Ionic Channels of Excitable Membranes.* Sinauer, Sunderland, MA.

Hisada, T., Kurachi, Y. & Sugimoto, T. (1990) Properties of membrane currents in isolated smooth muscle cells from guinea-pig trachea. *Pflügers Archiv* **416**, 151–161.

Hodgkin, A. L. & Huxley, A. F. (1952) A quantitative description of membrane current and its application to conduction and excitation in nerve. *Journal of Physiology* **117**, 500–544.

Horie, M., Irisawa, H. & Noma, A. (1987) Voltage-dependent magnesium block of adenosine-triphosphate-sensitive potassium channel in guinea-pig ventricular cells. *Journal of Physiology* **387**, 251–272.

Hoshi, T. & Aldrich, R. W. (1988) Voltage-dependent K^+ currents and underlying single K^+ channels in pheochromocytoma cells. *Journal of General Physiology* **91**, 73–106.

Hotta, K. & Yamamoto, Y. (1983) Ionic mechanisms involved in the strontium-induced spike and plateau in the smooth muscle of rat portal vein. *Journal of Physiology* **336**, 199–210.

Hu, S., King, H. S., Okolie, P. & Weiss, G. B. (1990) Alterations by glyburide of effects of BRL 34915 and P1060 on contraction, ^{86}Rb efflux and the maxi-K^+ channels in rat portal vein. *Journal of Pharmacology and Experimental Therapeutics* **253**, 771–777.

Hu, S. L., Yamamoto, Y. & Kao, C. Y. (1989a) The Ca^{2+}-activated K^+ channel and its functional roles in smooth muscle cells of guinea-pig taenia coli. *Journal of General Physiology* **94**, 833–847.

Hu, S. L., Yamamoto, Y. & Kao, C. Y. (1989b). Permeation, selectivity and blockade of the Ca^{2+}-activated potassium channel of the guinea-pig taenia coli myocyte. *Journal of General Physiology* **94**, 849–862.

Hughes, A. D., Hering, S. & Bolton, T. B. (1990) The action of caffeine on inward barium current through voltage-dependent calcium channels in single rabbit ear artery cells. *Pflügers Archiv* **416**, 462–466.

Hume, J. R. & Leblanc, N. (1989) Macroscopic K^+ currents in single smooth muscle cells of the rabbit portal vein. *Journal of Physiology* **413**, 49–73.

Imaizumi, Y., Muraki, K. & Watanabe, M. (1989) Ionic currents in single smooth muscle cells from the ureter of the guinea-pig. *Journal of Physiology* **411**, 131–159.

Imaizumi, Y., Muraki, K. & Watanabe, M. (1990) Characteristics of transient outward currents in single smooth muscle cells from the ureter of the guinea-pig. *Journal of Physiology* **427**, 301–324.

Inoue, I., Nakaya, Y., Nakaya, S. & Mori, H. (1989) Extracellular Ca^{2+}-activated K channel in coronary artery smooth muscle cells and its role in vasodilation. *FEBS Letters* **255**, 281–284.

Inoue, R., Kitamura, K. & Kuriyama, H. (1985) Two Ca-dependent K-channels classified by the application of tetraethylammonium distributes to smooth muscle membranes of the rabbit portal vein. *Pflügers Archiv* **405**, 173–179.

Inoue, R., Okabe, K., Kitamura, K. & Kuriyama, H. (1986) A newly identified Ca^{2+} dependent K^+ channel in the smooth muscle membrane of single cells dispersed from the rabbit portal vein. *Pflügers Archiv* **405**, 173–179.

Isacoff, E. Y., Jan, Y. N. & Jan, L. Y. (1990) Evidence for the formation of heteromultimeric potassium channels in *Xenopus* oocytes. *Nature* **345**, 530–534.

Ishikawa, Y., Takahashi, T. & Yamamura, T. (1983) Effect of apamin and theophylline on adenosine-5′-triphosphate-induced response of the guinea-pig gallbladder. *Digestion* **27**, 234–238.

Ito, Y. & Kuriyama, H. (1971) Membrane properties of the smooth muscle fibres of the guinea-pig portal vein. *Journal of Physiology* **214**, 427–441.

Ito, Y., Kuriyama, H. & Sakamoto, Y. (1970) Effects of tetraethylammonium chloride on the membrane activity of guinea-pig stomach smooth muscle. *Journal of Physiology* **211**, 445–460.

Josephson, I. R., Sanchez-Chapula, J. & Brown, A. M. (1984) Early outward current in rat single ventricular cells. *Circulation Research* **54**, 157–162.

Kajioka, S., Oike, M. & Kitamura, K. (1990) Nicorandil opens a calcium-dependent potassium-channel in smooth muscle cells of the rat portal vein. *Journal of Pharmacology and Experimental Therapeutics* **254**, 905–913.

Karashima, T. & Takata, Y. (1979) The effects of ATP related compounds on the electrical activity of the rat portal vein. *General Pharmacology* **10**, 477–487.

Kihira, M., Matsuzawa, K., Tokuno, H. & Tomita, T. (1990) Effects of calmodulin antagonists on calcium-activated potassium channels in pregnant rat myometrium. *British Journal of Pharmacology* **100**, 353–359.

Klöckner, U. & Isenberg, G. (1985a) Calcium currents of cesium loaded isolated smooth muscle cells (urinary bladder of the guinea-pig). *Pflügers Archiv* **405**, 340–348.

Klöckner, U. & Isenberg, G. (1985b) Action potentials and net membrane currents of isolated smooth muscle cells (urinary bladder of the guinea-pig). *Pflügers Archiv* **405**, 329–339.

Komori, S. & Bolton, T. B. (1990) Calcium release induced by inositol 1,4,5-triphosphate in single rabbit intestinal smooth muscle cells. *Journal of Physiology* **433**, 495–517.

Kume, H., Takagi, K., Satake, T., Tokuno, H. & Tomita, T. (1990) Effects of intracellular pH on calcium-activated potassium channels in rabbit tracheal smooth muscle. *Journal of Physiology* **424**, 445–457.

Kume, H., Takai, A., Tokuno, H. & Tomita, T. (1989) Regulation of Ca^{2+}-dependent K^+-channel activity in tracheal myocytes by phosphorylation. *Nature* **341**, 152–154.

Kuriyama, H., Ohshima, K. & Sakamoto, Y. (1971) The membrane properties of the smooth muscle of the guinea-pig portal vein in isotonic and hypertonic solutions. *Journal of Physiology* **217**, 179–199.

Lang, R. J. (1989) Identification of the major membrane currents in freshly dispersed single smooth muscle cells of the guinea-pig ureter. *Journal of Physiology* **412**, 375–395.

activated potassium channels in mammalian arterial myocytes by tetraethylammonium ions. *American Journal of Physiology* **260**, H927–H934.

McCann, J. D. & Welsh, M. J. (1986) Calcium-activated potassium channels in canine airway smooth muscle. *Journal of Physiology* **372**, 113–127.

McCann, J. D. & Welsh, M. J. (1987) Neuroleptics antagonize a calcium-activated potassium channel in airway smooth muscle. *Journal of General Physiology* **89**, 339–352.

Maas, A. J. J., Den Hertog, A. & van der Akker, J. (1980) The action of apamin on guinea-pig taenia caeci. *European Journal of Pharmacology* **67**, 265–274.

Martin, A. R. & Dryer, S. E. (1989) Potassium channels activated by sodium. *Quarterly Journal of Experimental Physiology* **74**, 1033–1041.

Marty, A. (1981) Ca-dependent K channels with large unitary conductance in chromaffin cell membranes. *Nature* **291**, 497–500.

Matsuda, H., Saigusa, A. & Irisawa, H. (1987) Ohmic conductance through the inwardly rectifying K channel and blocking by internal Mg^{2+}. *Nature* **325**, 156–159.

Mayer, M. L. & Sugiyama, K. (1988) A modulatory action of divalent cations on transient outward current in cultured sensory neurones. *Journal of Physiology* **396**, 417–433.

Meech, R. W. & Standen, N. B. (1975) Potassium activation in *Helix aspersa* neurones under voltage clamp: A component mediated by calcium influx. *Journal of Physiology* **249**, 211–239.

Miller, R. J. (1990) Glucose-regulated potassium channels are sweet news for neurobiologists. *Trends in Neuroscience* **13**, 197–199.

Mironneau, J. & Savineau, J-P. (1980) Effects of calcium ions on outward membrane currents in rat uterine smooth muscle. *Journal of Physiology* **302**, 411–425.

Mitra, R. & Morad, M. (1985) Ca^{2+} and Ca^{2+}-activated K^+ currents in mammalian gastric smooth muscle cells. *Science* **229**, 269–272.

Muraki, K., Imaizumi, Y., Kojima, T., Kawai, T. & Watanabe, M. (1990) Effects of tetraethylammonium and 4-aminopyridine on outward currents and excitability in canine tracheal smooth muscle cells. *British Journal of Pharmacology* **100**, 507–515.

Nakao, K. & Bolton, T. B. (1991) Cromakalim-induced potassium currents in single dispersed smooth muscle cells of rabbit artery and vein. *British Journal of Pharmacology* **102**, 155P.

Nakao, K., Inoue, R., Yamanaka, K. & Kitamura, K. (1986) Actions of quinidine and apamin on after-hyperpolarization of the spike in circular smooth muscle cells of the guinea-pig ileum. *Naunyn-Schmiedeberg's Archives of Pharmacology* **334**, 508–513.

Nakazawa, K., Matsuki, N., Shigenobu, K. & Kasuya, Y. (1987) Contractile response and electrophysiological properties in enzymatically dispersed smooth muscle cells of the rat vas deferens. *Pflügers Archiv* **408**, 112–119.

Nanjo, T. (1984) Effects of noradrenaline and acetylcholine on electro-mechanical properties of the guinea-pig portal vein. *British Journal of Pharmacology* **81**, 427–440.

Nelson, M. T., Huang, Y., Brayden, J. E., Hescheler, J. & Standen, N. B. (1990) Arterial dilations in response to calcitonin gene-related peptide involve activation of K^+ channels. *Nature* **344**, 770–773.

Noack, Th., Deitmer, P. & Golenhofen, K. (1990) Features of a calcium independent, caffeine sensitive outward current in single smooth muscle cells from guinea-pig portal vein. *Pflügers Archiv* **416**, 467–469.

Noack, Th., Edwards, G., Deitmer, P., Greengrass, P., Monita, T., Andersson, P.-O., Criddle, D., Wyllie, M. G. & Weston, A. H. (1992) The involvement of potassium channels in the action of ciclazindol in rat portal vein. *British Journal of Pharmacology* **106**, 17–24.

Noma, A. (1983) ATP-regulated K^+ channels in cardiac muscle. *Nature* **305**, 147–148.

Ohya, Y., Kitamura, K. & Kuriyama, H. (1987a) Cellular calcium regulates outward currents in rabbit intestinal smooth muscle cell. *American Journal of Physiology* **251** (Cell Physiology **21**), C401–C410.

Ohya, Y., Kitamura, K. & Kuriyama, H. (1987b) Modulation of ionic currents in smooth muscle balls of the rabbit intestine by intracellularly perfused ATP and cyclic AMP. *Pflügers Archiv* **408**, 465–473.

Ohya, Y., Terada, K., Kitamura, K. & Kuriyama, H. (1986) Membrane currents recorded from a fragment of rabbit intestinal smooth muscle cell. *American Journal of Physiology* **251** (Cell Physiology **20**), C335–C346.

Okabe, K., Kitamura, K. & Kuriyama, H. (1987) Features of 4-aminopyridine sensitive outward current observed in single smooth muscle cells from the rabbit pulmonary artery. *Pflügers Archiv* **409**, 561–568.

Ordway, R. W., Singer, J. J. & Walsh, J. V. (1991) Direct regulation of ion channels by fatty acids. *Trends in Neuroscience* **14**, 96–100.

Ordway, R. W., Walsh, J. V. & Singer, J. J. (1989) Arachidonic acid and other fatty acids directly activate potassium channels in smooth muscle cells. *Science* **244**, 1176–1179.

Osa, T. (1974) Effects of tetraethylammonium on the electrical activity of pregnant mouse myometrium and the interaction with manganese and cadmium. *Japanese Journal of Physiology* **24**, 119–133.

Papazian, D. M., Timpe, L. C., Jan, Y. N. & Jan, L. Y. (1991) Alteration of voltage-dependence of *Shaker* potassium channel by mutations in the S4 sequence. *Nature* **349**, 305–310.

Rimon, G., Hanski, E., Braun, S. & Levitzki, A. (1978) Mode of coupling between hormone receptors and adenylate cyclase elucidated by modulation of membrane fluidity. *Nature* **276**, 394–396.

Rogawski, M. A. (1985) The A-current: How ubiquitous a feature of excitable cells is it? *Trends in Neuroscience* **8**, 214–219.

Rudy, B. (1988) Diversity and ubiquity of K-channels. *Neuroscience* **25**, 729–749.

Ruppersberg, J. P., Schröter, K. H., Sakmanu, B. Stocker, M., Sewing, S. & Pongs, O. (1990) Heteromultimeric channels formed by rat brain potassium-channel proteins. *Nature* **345**, 535–537.

Sadoshima, J-I., Akaike, N., Kanaide, H. & Nakamura, M. (1988b) Cyclic AMP modulates Ca-activated K channel in cultured smooth muscle cells of rat aortas. *American Journal of Physiology* **255** (Heart Circulation Physiology **24**), H754–H759.

Sadoshima, J-I., Akaike, N., Tomoike, H., Kanaide, H. & Nakamura, M. (1988a) Ca-activated K channel in cultured smooth muscle cells of rat aortic media. *American Journal of Physiology* **255** (Heart Circulation Physiology **24**), H410–H418.

Schwarz, T. L., Tempel, B. L., Papazian, D. M., Jan, Y. N. & Jan, L. Y. (1988) Multiple potassium-channel components are produced by alternative splicing at the *Shaker* locus in *Drosophila*. *Nature* **331**, 137–142.

Silberberg, S. D. & van Breemen, C. (1990) An ATP, calcium and voltage sensitive potassium channel in porcine coronary artery smooth muscle cells. *Biochemical Biophysical Research Communications* **172**, 517–522.

Sims, S. M., Singer, J. J. & Walsh, J. V. (1985) Cholinergic agonists suppress a potassium current in freshly dissociated smooth muscle cells of the toad. *Journal of Physiology* **367**, 503–529.

Sims, S. M., Singer, J. J. & Walsh, J. V. (1988) Antagonist adrenergic–muscarinic regulation of M current in smooth muscle cells. *Science* **239**, 190–193.

Sims, S. M., Walsh, J. V. & Singer, J. J. (1986) Substance P and acetylcholine both suppress the same K$^+$ current in dissociated smooth muscle cells. *American Journal of Physiology* **251** (Cell Physiology **20**), C580–C587.

Singer, J. J. & Walsh, J. V. (1984) Large conductance of Ca^{++}-activated K^+ channels in smooth muscle cell membrane. *Biophysical Journal* **45**, 68–70.

Singer, J. J. & Walsh, J. V. (1987) Characterization of calcium-activated potassium channels in single smooth muscle cells using the patch-clamp technique. *Pflügers Archiv* **408**, 98–111.

Small, R. C. (1982) Electrical slow waves and tone of guinea-pig isolated trachealis muscle: Effects of drugs and temperature changes. *British Journal of Pharmacology* **77**, 45–54.

Somlyo, A. V., Vinall, P. & Somlyo, A. P. (1969) Excitation-contraction coupling and electrical events in two types of vascular smooth muscle. *Microvascular Research* **1**, 354–373.

Standen, N. B., Quayle, J. M., Davies, N. W., Brayden, J. E., Huang, Y. & Nelson, M. T. (1989) Hyperpolarizing vasodilators activate ATP-sensitive K^+ channels in arterial smooth muscle. *Science* **245**, 177–180.

Stanfield, P. R. (1983) Tetraethylammonium ions and the potassium permeability of excitable cells. *Reviews in Physiology, Biochemistry and Pharmacology* **97**, 1–67.

Strong, P. N., Weir, S. W., Beech, D. J., Hiestand, P. & Kocker, H. P. (1989) Effects of potassium channel toxins from *Leiurus quinquestriatus hebraeus* venom on responses to cromakalim in rabbit blood vessels. *British Journal of Pharmacology* **98**, 817–826.

Stuenkel, E. L. (1989) Single potassium channels recorded from vascular smooth muscle cells. *American Journal of Physiology* **257** (Heart Circulation Physiology **26**), H760–H769.

Suzuki, N. & Kasuya, Y. (1986) Effects of cocaine and tetraethylammonium on the spike potentials and contractions induced by trans-mural stimulation in the rat vas deferens. *Journal of Pharmacobio-Dyamics* **9**, 600–606.

Suzuki, T., Nishiyama, A. & Inomata, H. (1963) Effect of tetraethylammonium ion on the electrical activity of smooth muscle cell. *Nature* **197**, 908–909.

Szurszewski, J. H. (1978) A study of the canine gastric action potential in the presence of tetraethylammonium chloride. *Journal of Physiology* **277**, 91–102.

Takata, Y. (1980) Regional differences in electrical and mechanical properties of guinea-pig mesenteric vessels. *Japanese Journal of Physiology* **30**, 709–728.

Terada, K., Kitamura, K. & Kuriyama, H. (1987) Different inhibitions of the voltage-dependent K^+ current by Ca^{2+} antagonists in the smooth muscle cell membrane of rabbit small intestine. *Pflügers Archiv* **408**, 558–564.

Toro, L. & Stafini, E. (1987) Ca^{2+} and K^+ current in cultured vascular smooth muscle cells from rat aorta. *Pflügers Archiv* **408**, 417–419.

Toro, L., Amador, M. & Stefani, E. (1990a) ANG II inhibits calcium-activated potassium channels from coronary smooth muscle in lipid bilayers. *American Journal of Physiology* (Heart Circulation Physiology 27), H912–H915.

Toro, L., Ramos-Franco, J. & Stefani, E. (1990b) GTP-dependent regulation of myometrial KCa channel incorporated into lipid bilayers. *Journal of General Physiology* **96**, 373–394.

Toro, L., Stefani, E. & Erulkar, S. (1990c) Hormonal regulation of potassium currents in single myometrial cells. *Proceedings of the National Academy of Sciences USA* **87**, 2892–2895.

Trieschmann, U. & Isenberg, G. (1989) Ca^{2+}-activated K^+ channels contribute to the resting potential of vascular myocytes. Ca^{2+}-sensitivity is increased by intracellular Mg^{2+}-ions. *Pflügers Archiv* **414** (Suppl. 1), S183–S184.

Vassort, G. (1975) Voltage-clamp analysis of the transmembrane ionic currents in guinea-pig myometrium: Evidence for an initial potassium activation triggered by calcium influx. *Journal of Physiology* **252**, 713–734.

Vladimirova, I. A. & Shuba, M. F. (1978) The effect of strychnine, hydrastin and apamin on synaptic transmission in smooth muscle cells. *Neirofiziologiya* **10**, 295–299.

Vogalis, F. & Sanders, K. M. (1990) Cholinergic stimulation activates a non-selective cation current in canine pyloric circular muscle cells. *Journal of Physiology* **429**, 223–236.

Walsh, J. V. & Singer, J. J. (1981) Voltage-clamp of single freshly dissociated smooth muscle cells: Current–voltage relationships for three currents. *Pflügers Archiv* **390**, 207–210.

Walsh, J. V. & Singer, J. J. (1987) Identification and characterization of major ionic currents in isolated smooth muscle cells using the voltage-clamp technique. *Pflügers Archiv* **408**, 83–97.

Weigel, R. J., Connor, J. A. & Prosser, C. L. (1979) Two roles of calcium during the spike in circular muscle of small intestine in cat. *American Journal of Physiology* **237**, C247–C256.

Wilde, D. W. & Lee, K. S. (1989) Outward potassium currents in freshly isolated smooth muscle cell of dog coronary artery. *Circulation Research* **65**, 1718–1734.

Williams, D. L., Katz, G. M., Roy-Contancin, L. & Reuben, J. P. (1988) Guanosine 5'-monophosphate modulates gating of high-conductance Ca^{2+}-activated K^+ channels in vascular smooth muscle cells. *Proceedings of the National Academy of Sciences USA* **85**, 9360–9364.

Yamamoto, Y., Hu, S. L. & Kao, C. Y. (1989a) Inward current in single smooth muscle cells of the guinea-pig taenia coli. *Journal of General Physiology* **93**, 521–550.

Yamamoto, Y., Hu, S. L. & Kao, C. Y. (1989b) Outward current in single smooth muscle cells of the guinea-pig taenia coli. *Journal of General Physiology* **93**, 551–564.

Yamanaka, K., Furukawa, K. & Kitamura, K. (1985) The different mechanisms of action of nicorandil and adenosine triphosphate on potassium channels of circular smooth muscle of the guinea-pig small intestine. *Naunyn-Schmiedeberg's Archives of Pharmacology* **331**, 96–103.

Yanagisawa, A. & Lefer, A. M. (1987) Vasoactive effects of eicosapentanoic acid on isolated vascular smooth muscle. *Basic Research in Cardiology* **82**, 186–196.

Yool, A. J. & Schwarz, T. L. (1991) Alteration of ionic selectivity of a K^+ channel by mutation of the H5 region. *Nature* **349**, 700–704.

Zacour, M. E., Collier, B. & Martin, J. G. (1987) Apamin and nonadrenergic inhibition of guinea-pig trachealis. *Agents and Actions* **22**, 75–81.

Chapter 8
Potassium channels in the heart: physiological function and neurohormonal regulation

L. C. Freeman, W. M. Kwok, J. M. B. Anumonwo
and R. S. Kass

Introduction

In heart cells, as in other excitable tissue, K-channel currents are important in maintaining the normal cell resting potential and controlling the duration of the action potential. In the heart, these channels have particularly important roles because of the complex pattern of electrical activity that exists in different cell types ranging from the sinoatrial (SA) node in the right atrium to the Purkinje fibre in the ventricle. Resting potentials range from moderately depolarized nodal cells to fully polarized myocardial muscle and Purkinje fibre cells. Alterations in resting potential can directly influence conduction velocity by changing the number of available Na- or Ca-channels. In addition, the regular pattern of impulse conduction and muscle activation must be maintained over a wide range of stimulation frequencies because heart rate is under direct sympathetic and parasympathetic control.

It is thus not surprising that cardiac K-channels consist of a diverse group of membrane proteins that have many different forms of functional expression. These channels include the delayed rectifier (Noble & Tsien, 1969; Bennett et al., 1985; Sanguinetti & Jurkiewicz, 1990); the inward rectifier (Hall et al., 1963); the adenosine triphosphate (ATP)-sensitive K-channel (Noma, 1983; Trube & Hescheler, 1984; Noma & Shibasaki, 1985); a transient outward K-channel (Siegelbaum & Tsien, 1980; Giles & Van Ginneken, 1985; Kenyon & Sutko, 1987; Tseng & Hoffman, 1989) and the acetylcholine-regulated K-channel (Sakmann et al., 1983). Other K-channels reported include a time-independent plateau channel (Yue &

Marban, 1988) and a K-channel activated by a high concentration of intracellular sodium ($[Na^+]_i$) (Kameyama *et al.*, 1984).

This chapter will focus on the voltage dependence and regulatory properties of inward rectifier channels (K_{IR}); delayed rectifier channels (K_{dr})*; ATP-inhibited K-channels (K_{ATP}); and transient outward current channels (K_{to}). The basic properties of the channels including their voltage dependence as well as their regulation by neurohormones and some drugs will be discussed. Further details of cardiac K-channel pharmacology can be found in Chapter 12.

Physiological role of K-channels: regulation of the cardiac action potential

A key characteristic of electrical activity in all regions of the heart is the very slow time-course of the action potential. The duration of action potentials in nerve and skeletal muscle is typically on the order of 2–10 ms, and is relatively independent of stimulation frequency. In contrast, in the mammalian heart, the duration of the action potential ranges from 200 to 500 ms and is very sensitive to stimulation frequency and small perturbations in the cellular environment.

Underlying the prolonged electrical response of cardiac cells is the period of depolarization known as the action potential plateau. During this period, in which there are very slow time-dependent changes in membrane potential, cellular input resistance is high (Weidmann, 1951). As a result, small changes in membrane current can cause large changes in action potential configuration. The membrane current that generates the action potential plateau is small in magnitude and results from the energetically efficient sum of small inward and outward currents (Noble, 1978). Time- and voltage-dependent changes in either the inward or outward currents will thus have pronounced effects both on the start and time-course of repolarization of the action potential. The outward currents that regulate cardiac repolarization are K-currents. Clearly, an understanding of the voltage and time dependence of these currents is essential in the design of therapeutic agents that are intended to modify the time-course of cardiac action potentials.

Inwardly rectifying K-channels (K_{IR})

As discussed above, it has been known since the work of Weidmann (1951) that the plateau phase of the cardiac action potential is characterized by high cellular input resistance. One of the principal mechanisms underlying

*In other excitable cells, the delayed rectifier channel is abbreviated to K_V. As this chapter unfolds, it will be clear that the cardiac delayed rectifier channel is somewhat different from K_V and the designation K_{dr} has been adopted.

the low conductance action potential plateau is the unique non-linear voltage dependence of a background K-current that has been referred to as I_{K1}* or the inward rectifier (Noble, 1978). A conductance that rectifies passes current preferentially in one direction. An inwardly rectifying channel allows current to flow in the inward direction, but provides high resistance to flow in the outward direction. Thus the inwardly rectifying K-channel of heart cells has a high conductance when membrane potential is made negative to the Nernst or equilibrium potential for K^+ (E_K), but conducts relatively poorly when membrane potential is depolarized and the driving force for outward current flow is increased.

McAllister and Noble (1966) first measured the voltage-dependent properties of I_{IR} in calf Purkinje fibres. They used a two microelectrode voltage-clamp procedure and reduced overlapping membrane currents by recording currents in the absence of extracellular sodium ($[Na^+]_o$) and calcium ($[Ca^{2+}]_o$). They found that currents near the beginning of their voltage-clamp steps were measurable negative to E_K, but as the membrane potential was made more positive than E_K, currents reached a peak and then subsided. A characteristic current–voltage ($I–V$) relationship for I_{K1} and its block by tertiary clofilium are shown in Fig. 8.1. In the figure, obtained using whole-cell patch-clamp procedures in an isolated ventricular myocyte, it is clear that there is a small window of voltages positive to E_K over which outward current flows through this channel. At voltages near the action potential plateau (-10 to $+20$ mV), there is no outward current through this type of channel in normal physiological solutions.

Consequently, the physiological role of this channel is in the maintenance of the cellular resting potential and in the contribution of outward current to the final phases of repolarization. Computations have shown that block of I_{K1} can alter the resting potential and prolong the action potential due to these dual roles of the channel (Kass *et al.*, 1990).

The K_{IR} is a K-selective channel. As a result, the equilibrium potential of the channel is closely related to E_K (Noble, 1978). Thus, in elevated extracellular potassium concentration ($[K^+]_o$) the equilibrium potential of the channel, and in turn the cell resting potential becomes less negative. In addition to the influence of $[K^+]_o$ on the channel equilibrium potential there is a marker effect of $[K^+]_o$ on the magnitude of outward current that can flow in the limited voltage range positive to E_K; increasing $[K^+]_o$ enhances $I_{K(IR)}$.

The dual effects of $[K^+]_o$ cause the $I–V$ relationships of K_{IR} determined in different concentrations of $[K^+]_o$ to 'cross over'. The K-dependent cross-over of the inward rectifier $I–V$ relationship accounts for the anomalous shortening of the cardiac action potential in elevated $[K^+]_o$

---

*I_{K1} is typical terminology for the cardiac inward rectifier current. In the rest of this book, the term $I_{K(IR)}$ is used to describe similar current types in other excitable cells.

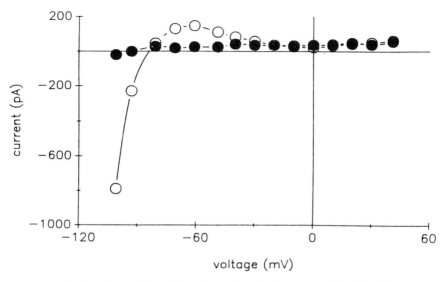

Fig. 8.1. Whole-cell recording of inward rectifier (I_{K1}) current and its block by tertiary clofilium (100 μM). Currents, measured at the end of 40 ms pulses applied to the voltages indicated along the abscissa from a -40 mV holding potential are plotted against test pulse voltage. Calcium-channel current was blocked by nisoldipine (500 nM). Open symbols indicate current in control. Filled symbols were recorded after steady-state had been obtained in the presence of 100 μM tertiary clofilium. (Unpublished data.)

(Weidmann, 1956) which is an effect opposite to that predicted by a linear background K-conductance.

Sakmann and Trube (1984) showed that these properties of I_{K1} exist at the single channel level. They found that single channel recordings could be made for K_{IR} when the holding potential was more negative than E_K. They also showed that the single channel conductance varied with the square root of $[K^+]_o$ and demonstrated cross-over of the single channel $I-V$ relationships in different $[K^+]_o$. The rectification of outward current through the channel was shown to develop within 1.5 ms of a step change in membrane potential. Thus, compared with the very slow time-course of the cardiac action potential, it was appropriate to refer to current through this channel as time-independent.

The K-dependent cross-over of the K_{IR} $I-V$ relationship provided evidence that the conductance of the channel was sensitive to the 'driving force' for K^+. The driving force is the difference between cell membrane potential and the equilibrium potential for the permeant ion. In the case of this channel, the channel conductance becomes very small as the driving force for outward current flow is increased. Conductance is large and constant when the driving force favours inward current flow, or when membrane potential is more negative than E_K. This type of driving force-dependent rectification had been demonstrated in K-channels of squid axons when quaternary ammonium ions were injected intracellularly suggesting that, perhaps, rectification of heart background currents might be due to an indigenous internal blocking particle (Armstrong, 1969).

Evidence for a blocking particle model of inward rectification was provided by the patch-clamp experiments of Vandenberg (1987) who showed that inward rectification could be abolished from excised inside-out membrane patches containing K_{IR} if Mg^{2+} was removed from the cytoplasmic side of the membrane. At intermediate concentrations of Mg^{2+}, intermediate degrees of rectification could be obtained. Matsuda et al. (1987) found a similar Mg^{2+}-dependent contribution to inward rectification, but also reported a voltage-dependent component to channel gating that causes these channels to close upon depolarization. Thus, Mg^{2+} is the physiological intracellular blocking particle that contributes to the marked inward rectification of K_{IR}.

In summary, because of the strong rectifying properties of these channels, the associated background K-conductance in the heart stabilizes resting potentials near E_K and provides a window of outward current that speeds the final phase of repolarization. This is responsible for the high input impedance of the plateau phase of the action potential as well as for the anomalous effects of $[K^+]_o$ on heart action potential duration.

Transient outward channel (K_{to})*

The current carried by the transient outward K-channel $I_{K(to1)}$ was originally investigated using two microelectrode voltage-clamp techniques in shortened Purkinje fibre strands (Dudel et al., 1967; Fozzard & Hiraoka, 1973). The name of the channel reflects the activating and inactivating components of its conductance. The channel was initially suggested to be selective for Cl^- (Fozzard & Hiraoka, 1973). However, evidence based largely on channel pharmacology was later provided to suggest strongly that $I_{K(to)}$ is carried by a K-selective channel (Kenyon & Gibbons, 1979).

Siegelbaum et al. (1977) and Siegelbaum and Tsien (1980) provided evidence that $I_{K(to)}$ was, at least in part, a $[Ca^{2+}]$-activated current. Their evidence was based on simultaneous measurements of membrane current and contractile activity in microelectrode-clamped shortened Purkinje fibres. The $I_{K(to)}$ was well correlated with activation of contraction, and in addition, removal of $[Ca^{2+}]_o$, replacement of $[Ca^{2+}]_o$ by other permeant divalent ions, and buffering $[Ca^{2+}]_i$ by injection of EGTA all inhibited $I_{K(to)}$.

Investigations from several groups have provided evidence that there are two components to $I_{K(to)}$: one that is voltage-dependent, $I_{K(to1)}$, and

*The channels responsible for carrying $I_{K(to)}$ are poorly characterized. The current seems to comprise two components, one of which, $I_{K(to1)}$ is voltage-dependent. The other, $I_{K(to2)}$, is Ca-dependent. We have not assigned a designation to the channels involved.

one, $I_{K(to2)}$, that is controlled by $[Ca^{2+}]_i$ (Giles & van Ginneken, 1985; Kenyon & Sutko, 1987; Tseng & Hoffman, 1989). The evidence which has accumulated is derived from both kinetic and pharmacological data. As shown by Kenyon and Sutko (1987), $I_{K(to1)}$ is sensitive to external application of aminopyridines and can be analysed within the framework of a voltage-gated (activation and inactivation gates) ion channel. $I_{K(to2)}$ is inhibited by ryanodine, which also inhibits the release of Ca^{2+} from the sarcoplasmic reticulum. Thus, these experiments strongly suggest that this $[Ca^{2+}]_i$-sensitive component is activated by release of Ca^{2+} from internal stores.

Figure 8.2 illustrates typical $I_{K(to)}$ records. Activation and inactivation occurs over a voltage range that is comparable with that of the L-type Ca-channel in cardiac preparations (Siegelbaum & Tsien, 1980). Because the channel is inactivated at positive potentials, it does not contribute strongly to the electrical activity of nodal cells, but is more prominent in cells that have resting or diastolic potentials near E_K.

The functional significance of $I_{K(to)}$ has, until recently, been limited to the characteristic early phase (2) of repolarization that is seen most clearly in Purkinje fibre preparations. Its activation and subsequent inactivation clearly cause the notch in the Purkinje fibre action potential. However, more recently, the possible contribution of a maintained component of $I_{K(to)}$ in the regulation of action potential duration has been explored.

Dukes & Morad (1989) have shown that tedisamil blocks $I_{K(to)}$ and shortens action potential duration in rat ventricular myocytes. Furthermore, Litovsky and Antzelevitch (1988, 1990) have reported regional differences in the density of channels which carry $I_{K(to)}$ in the canine heart. They found $I_{K(to)}$ prominent in the ventricular epicardium but not in the endocardium. As a result, one would predict that if there were a maintained component of $I_{K(to)}$ in epicardial cells, differences between epicardial and endocardial action potential durations would, in part, be caused by the relative contrast in channel density. If this were shown to be the case in other species, particularly in the human heart, then regional differences in channel density underlying $I_{K(to)}$ could be the mechanism responsible for the well-known phenomenon of T-wave inversion on the electrocardiogram.

Delayed rectifier channel*

Time-dependent changes in total membrane current underlie the time-course of the cardiac action potential plateau. Inactivation of L-type Ca-channels contributes to a net decrease in inward current during this

*The characteristics of the cardiac delayed rectifier currents $I_{K(dr)}$ designated individually in the literature as $I_{K(r)}$ and $I_{K(s)}$ have not been well-investigated. Many of their properties are quite different from those of more typical delayed rectifier currents $I_{K(V)}$ in other cells.

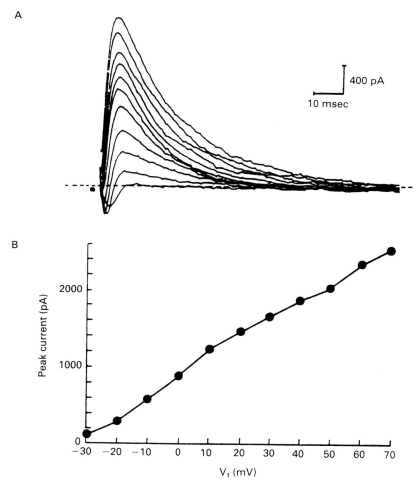

Fig. 8.2. Voltage-dependent component of I_{to}: activation and inactivation. A, Superimposed 4-aminopyride-sensitive currents measured from a -60 mV holding potential in response to voltage pulses (V_t) applied from -30 to $+70$ mV. Note rapid activation and subsequent inactivation of 4-aminopyridine-sensitive current. B, Peak 4-aminopyridine-sensitive current plotted against test potential from the data shown above. Whole-cell recording obtained from canine ventricular myocyte. (With permission from Tseng & Hoffman, 1989.)

time, and this combined with the slow activation of an outward current determines the start and speed of repolarization. In most cardiac preparations, the major time-dependent outward current that underlies repolarization of the action potential is the delayed rectifier current ($I_{K(dr)}$), so called because of its delay in activation.

Noble and Tsien (1969) provided the first quantitative description of time-dependent outward currents that contribute to repolarization in the

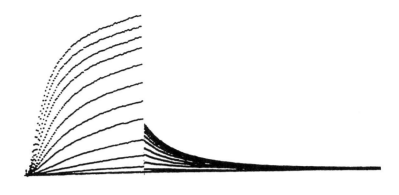

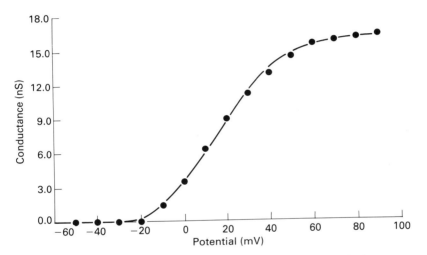

Fig. 8.3. Activation of total delayed rectification in guinea-pig ventricular myocyte. Traces show baseline-subtracted records of time-dependent outward current ($I_{K(dr)}$) recorded in response to a series of 2 s voltage pulses applied from a -30 mV holding potential. The I_{Ca} was blocked by the addition of 200 μM cadmium. The plot shows conductance determined from deactivating tail amplitude and driving force, plotted against conditioning pulse voltage. (Kass, R. S., unpublished data.)

heart. They used a two-microelectrode voltage-clamp procedure to study currents in isolated Purkinje fibres and found that two components of time-dependent outward current ($I_{K(dr)}$) could be distinguished by their kinetics and ion selectivity. One component was moderately selective for K^+, but a second, slower component, was found to be quite non-selective for K^+. Because of the multicellular nature of the Purkinje fibre preparation, subsequent studies indicated that this second, very slow component was most likely caused by accumulation and depletion of K^+ in intracellular spaces (Attwell & Cohen, 1977).

Recent pharmacological data (Sanguinetti & Jurkiewicz, 1990) have provided evidence for the existence of multiple types of delayed rectifier channels in ventricular cells of the guinea-pig. They found a very rapidly activating component that was marked by strong *inward* rectification of the maximally activated I–V relation. This current component, blocked by the benzenesulphonamide antiarrhythmic drug E-4031 and by lanthanum, has been labelled $I_{K(r)}$ because of its rectifying properties. A second, approximately 10-fold larger current component which is lanthanum and E-4031-insensitive and shows little rectification, was labelled $I_{K(s)}$ because of its slow kinetics; it is the dominant component of K-currents recorded during test pulses positive to $+20\,mV$, and is the current component most often referred to as delayed rectification in ventricular cells. Thus, as originally proposed by Noble and Tsien (1969), it now appears that multiple types of delayed rectifier channels exist in heart cells and it will be of increasing interest to determine the pharmacology and regulatory properties of these channels in different regions of the heart (*see below*).

The data discussed below describe properties of total delayed rectifier current without dissection by either lanthanum or E-4031. An example of total $I_{K(dr)}(I_{K(r)} + I_{K(s)})$ is shown in Fig. 8.3.

Modulation of cardiac delayed rectification

Physiological significance

Neuroendocrine control of cardiac function involves extensive regulation of K-currents in different anatomical regions of the heart. As heart rate changes, action potential duration must also be adjusted in order to ensure a proper temporal relationship between diastolic filling and systolic ejection. Because delayed rectifier channels are such major determinants of action potential duration, their neurohormonal regulation is the key to cardiac function. Understanding the modulation of cardiac delayed rectifier K-currents in different regions of the heart is critical to understanding how cardiac output is maintained when heart rate changes.

cAMP-dependent protein kinase

β-adrenergic agonists, cAMP (cyclic adenosine monophosphate) and its analogues, and phosphodiesterase inhibitors were first shown to increase $I_{K(dr)}$ in calf Purkinje fibres (Tsien et al., 1972; Kass & Weigers, 1982; Bennett et al., 1986) and other multicellular preparations (Brown & Noble, 1974; Pappano & Carmeliet, 1979; Umeno, 1984; Carmeliet & Mubagwa, 1986). Further support for the hypothesis that $I_{K(dr)}$ is regulated by a cytoplasmic, cAMP-dependent signalling pathway has been obtained from experiments performed using isolated cardiac myocytes (Bennett &

Begenisich, 1987; Duchatelle-Gourdon *et al.*, 1989; Harvey & Hume, 1989; Walsh *et al.*, 1989; Yazawa & Kameyama, 1990). The $I_{K(dr)}$ in guinea-pig ventricular cells is increased in response to elevation of intracellular cAMP via extracellular application of β-adrenoceptor agonists (Bennett & Begenisich, 1987; Duchatelle-Gourdon *et al.*, 1989; Harvey & Hume, 1989; Yazawa & Kameyama, 1990), forskolin (Harvey & Hume, 1989; Walsh *et al.*, 1989; Yazawa & Kameyama, 1990) or membrane permeable analogues of cAMP (Walsh & Kass, 1988; Walsh *et al.*, 1989). Intracellular application of cAMP (Duchatelle-Gourdon *et al.*, 1989; Yazawa & Kameyama, 1990) or the catalytic subunit of cAMP-dependent protein kinase (Walsh *et al.*, 1989; Yazawa & Kameyama, 1990) stimulates $I_{K(dr)}$ in the absence of agonist, while dialysis with either the regulatory subunit or a specific inhibitor of the enzyme prevents agonist-induced enhancement of $I_{K(dr)}$ (Kameyama *et al.*, 1986). β-adrenergic enhancement of $I_{K(dr)}$ is potentiated by concurrent exposure to okadaic acid and prevented by exposure to protein phosphatases (Kameyama *et al.*, 1986; Hescheler *et al.*, 1987). Together, these findings suggest that β-adrenergic enhancement of $I_{K(dr)}$ is associated with phosphorylation of an intracellular protein by protein kinase A. The response of guinea-pig ventricular $I_{K(dr)}$ to agents that promote cAMP-dependent phosphorylation is steeply temperature-dependent and appreciable at physiological temperatures but not room temperature (Walsh & Kass, 1988; Walsh *et al.*, 1989). The extreme temperature sensitivity of the delayed rectifier from rat brain encoded by *drk1* gene has been associated with cAMP-dependent phosphorylation of the channel protein (Fedulova *et al.*, 1991). This may also be true for the cardiac delayed rectifier (Walsh *et al.*, 1989). Phosphorylation-independent regulation of ventriculae $I_{K(dr)}$ by guanine nucleotides and β-adrenoceptor agonists has also been demonstrated (Freeman *et al.*, 1992).

Although muscarinic stimulation in the absence of protein kinase A activation has no effect on ventricular $I_{K(dr)}$, muscarinic receptor activation has been shown to antagonize the stimulatory effects of isoprenaline and forskolin on $I_{K(dr)}$ in guinea-pig ventricular cells (Harvey & Hume, 1989; Yazawa & Kameyama, 1990). Cholinergic stimulation has no effect on cAMP-stimulated $I_{K(dr)}$; this suggests that the antagonism occurs at a step in the signalling pathway that is proximal to stimulation of protein kinase A (PKA) by cAMP (Yazawa & Kameyama, 1990).

Protein kinase C (PKC)

Activation of PKC increases $I_{K(dr)}$ in isolated guinea-pig ventricular cells. The $I_{K(dr)}$ increases following either extracellular application of phorbol esters that activate PKC, such as 12-*O*-tetradecanoylphorbol-13-acetate (TPA), 1-oleolyl-2-acetylglycerol (OAG), and phorbol 12,13-dibutyrate (PDB) or cell dialysis with PKC in the presence of TPA (Tohse *et al.*, 1987;

Walsh & Kass, 1988; Tohse, 1990; Tohse *et al.*, 1990; Yazawa & Kameyama, 1990). Enhancement of $I_{K(dr)}$ by phorbol esters is seen at low concentrations in the absence of any change in I_{Ca} (Walsh & Kass, 1988; Tohse *et al.*, 1990), suggesting a specific effect of PKC on delayed rectifier K-channels.

Phorbol esters (TPA, PDB) can increase $I_{K(dr)}$, even after maximal stimulation of PKA by forskolin or a membrane permeable cAMP analogue (Walsh & Kass, 1988; Yazawa & Kameyama, 1990). The additive effects of PKA and PKC activation, in combination with the kinetic- and voltage-dependent differences in their effects on $I_{K(dr)}$ suggest that the phosphorylation sites for the two protein kinases may be distinct (Walsh & Kass, 1991). Interestingly, the stimulatory effects of PKC, as well as PKA, are temperature-dependent for $I_{K(dr)}$, but not for Ca-channel currents recorded in the same cells (Walsh & Kass, 1988). Muscarinic stimulation has no inhibitory effects on $I_{K(dr)}$ stimulated by PKC (Yazawa & Kameyama, 1990).

Regulation by divalent cations

Calcium

Intracellular Ca^{2+} concentration ($[Ca^{2+}]_i$) is important for a variety of cellular functions. Modulation of $I_{K(dr)}$ by $[Ca^{2+}]_i$ would be important physiologically, because $[Ca^{2+}]_i$ increases during each heartbeat. For these reasons, the $[Ca^{2+}]_i$ sensitivity of $I_{K(dr)}$ has been extensively investigated in multicellular preparations (Kass & Tsien, 1975, 1976; Goto *et al.*, 1983; Kass, 1984) and isolated cardiac cells (Tohse *et al.*, 1987; Tohse, 1990). Experimental evidence suggests that $I_{K(dr)}$ is sensitive to $[Ca^{2+}]_i$; it is unchanged by increasing $[Ca^{2+}]_i$ from 10 pM to 1 nM, but is increased progressively as $[Ca^{2+}]_i$ is raised from 10 nM to 1 μM (Tohse, 1990). Ensemble noise analysis suggests that elevation of $[Ca^{2+}]_i$ increases the number and open probability of functional $I_{K(dr)}$-channels (Tohse, 1990).

Despite its $[Ca^{2+}]_i$ sensitivity, $I_{K(dr)}$ should not be considered as a Ca-activated K-current. Its activation does not require Ca-influx or release of intracellular stores; $I_{K(dr)}$ is not suppressed when Ca-current and contractile activity of Purkinje fibres are blocked by nisoldipine (Kass, 1984). Furthermore, elevation of $[Ca^{2+}]_i$ has no effect on the voltage dependence of $I_{K(dr)}$ activation (Tohse, 1990).

Modulation of $I_{K(dr)}$ by β-adrenergic agonists is independent of changes in $[Ca^{2+}]_i$ that result from β-adrenergic enhancement of inward calcium current (I_{Ca}). β-adrenoceptor stimulation and activation of cAMP-dependent protein kinase can stimulate $I_{K(dr)}$ in the presence of Ca-channel blockers (Walsh & Kass, 1988; Duchatelle-Gourdon *et al.*, 1989; Yazawa & Kameyama, 1990). Furthermore, modulation of $I_{K(dr)}$ and I_{Ca} in mammalian cells differs in terms of temperature sensitivity (Walsh *et al.*, 1989), response to selective β_1-adrenoceptor stimulation (Iijima *et al.*, 1990), cAMP concentration dependence, and kinetics (Nerbonne *et al.*, 1984).

Modulation of $I_{K(dr)}$ by $[Ca^{2+}]_i$ cannot be completely attributed to an indirect action of PKC, although the $[Ca^{2+}]_i$ sensitivity of $I_{K(dr)}$ is modulated by PKC activation. The $I_{K(dr)}$ remains sensitive to $[Ca^{2+}]_i$, in the presence of PKC inhibition by H-7 (Tohse *et al.*, 1987). Activation of PKC by phorbol esters shifts the $I_{K(dr)}$ concentration–response curve in the direction of lower $[Ca^{2+}]_i$ (Tohse *et al.*, 1990), but the molecular basis of this modulation by $[Ca^{2+}]_i$ has not been elucidated. A direct interaction between Ca^{2+} and the $I_{K(dr)}$-channel has been.hypothesized (Tohse, 1990) but indirect Ca effects on intracellular proteins that regulate the channel have not been ruled out.

Magnesium

The delayed rectifier K-current $I_{K(dr)}$ in frog atrial myocytes is extremely sensitive to intracellular Mg concentration ($[Mg^{2+}]_i$); however, the underlying mechanisms are poorly understood. When $I_{K(dr)}$ is measured in frog heart cells using the whole-cell configuration of patch-clamp, $I_{K(dr)}$ amplitude increases progressively (run-up) if $[Mg^{2+}]_i < 1$ mM, but decreases progressively (run-down) if $[Mg^{2+}]_i$ is > 1 mM (Duchatelle-Gourdon *et al.*, 1989, 1991; Tarr *et al.*, 1989). Suppression of $I_{K(dr)}$ by millimolar $[Mg^{2+}]_i$ is independent of membrane potential or direction of current flow; thus, in the delayed rectifier K-channel, in contrast to the background inward rectifier channel, which carries the current I_{K1}, Mg^{2+} does not act simply as a blocking particle in the permeation pathway (Duchatelle-Gourdon *et al.*, 1989, 1991; Tarr *et al.*, 1989). Varying $[Mg^{2+}]_i$ does not shift the $I_{K(dr)}$ activation curve (Tarr *et al.*, 1989; Duchatelle-Gourdon *et al.*, 1991). This absence of a shift in the activation curve is inconsistent with screening of intracellular negative surface charges by Mg^{2+}.

Suppression of $I_{K(dr)}$ by $[Mg^{2+}]_i > 1$ mM is unrelated to the intracellular concentration of cAMP (Tarr *et al.*, 1989). Enhancement of $I_{K(dr)}$ by isoproterenol is independent of $[Mg^{2+}]_i$ between 0.1 and 2 mM $[Mg^{2+}]_i$, and the stimulatory effects of isoproterenol and $[Mg^{2+}]_i$ are additive at 0.1 mM $[Mg^{2+}]_i$ (Duchatelle-Gourdon *et al.*, 1991). Yet, the reversibility of isoproterenol stimulation of $I_{K(dr)}$ is dependent on $[Mg^{2+}]_i$. At $[Mg^{2+}]_i < 1$ mM, enhancement of $I_{K(dr)}$ by β-adrenergic agonist or cAMP becomes irreversible; the persistent response does not depend on continual activation of PKA (Duchatelle-Gourdon *et al.*, 1991). Together, these findings have been used to hypothesize that $[Mg^{2+}]_i$ modulates the dephosphorylation of delayed rectifier K-channels in frog atrial myocytes, by either allosteric interactions which affect channel susceptibility to dephosphorylation, or modulation of intracellular phosphatases required for channel dephosphorylation (Duchatelle-Gourdon *et al.*, 1991).

The nodal delayed rectifier

In mammalian sino-atrial and atrioventricular nodes, the repolarization phase of the action potential depends on a rectifying outward current that is mostly carried by K^+ (Noma & Irisawa, 1976; DiFrancesco *et al.*, 1979; Kokubun *et al.*, 1982). The decline in conductance of this channel, in the face of a background inward current (I_{K1}), has been implicated as one of the main mechanisms by which pacemaking nodal cells generate diastolic depolarizations (Irisawa, 1978; Brown, 1982).

Compared to ventricular cells, the $I_{K(dr)}$ current in nodal cells is less well characterized. Early studies using multicellular nodal preparations (Noma & Irisawa, 1976; DiFrancesco *et al.*, 1979; Kokubun *et al.*, 1982) reported the properties of the current as similar to those of the $I_{K(dr)}$ current described in other mammalian cardiac preparations (Noble & Tsien, 1968; Bennett *et al.*, 1985; Matsuura *et al.*, 1987). For example, Noma and Irisawa (1976) and DiFrancesco *et al.* (1979) showed that the kinetics of this current in the nodal preparations could be described as a first-order process using the Hodgkin–Huxley (1952) type of analysis. The onset of current activation was sigmoidal, and the activation variable changed from 0 at -50 mV, to 1 at about $+20$ mV. Outward current tails declined with a single (Noma & Irisawa, 1976) or a double-exponential time-course (DiFrancesco *et al.*, 1979). Subsequently, more quantitative studies have confirmed these properties of the current in isolated pacemaker cells. Shibata and Giles (1985) investigated the kinetics and ion selectivity of the channel in pacemaker cells of the bullfrog. Both current activation and decline were best described as single exponential processes, and K^+ acted as the primary charge carriers. Similar results have been obtained from mammalian pacemaker cells (Nakayama *et al.*, 1984; Shibasaki, 1987).

The first reported study of $I_{K(dr)}$ in isolated nodal cells was carried out by Nakayama *et al.* (1984) in experiments that determined electrophysiological properties of isolated sino-atrial and atrioventricular nodal cells. In this study, the time-course of the outward tail current could be separated into two components, one fast and the other slow, with time constants of 152 and 942 ms respectively. The fully activated *I–V* relationship crossed the voltage axis at -70 to -80 mV, and showed an inward-going rectification with a slightly negative slope at potentials positive to $+20$ mV.

A more extensive analysis of the nodal cell $I_{K(dr)}$ current was carried out by Shibasaki (1987) who used whole-cell and cell-attached patch-clamp techniques to determine the kinetics of both macroscopic and as single channel currents. Using high (50–300 mM) external K-concentrations to enable the observation of single channel activity, the issues of the different degrees of rectification (as reported by different investigators) and the mechanism of rectification were addressed.

Shibasaki (1987) showed that the kinetics of activation of the macroscopic current were dependent on membrane potential and were not affected by $[K^+]_o$. The I–V plot was shifted by approximately 60 mV when $[K^+]_o$ was increased 10-fold, indicating a high selectivity for K^+. The single channel conductance varied in relation to the square root of $[K^+]_o$ and was estimated as 1.6 pS in normal Tyrode ($[K^+]_o = 5.4$ mM) solution. Single channel open and closed times could be fitted, respectively, with single and biexponentials. Furthermore, it was estimated that there were approximately 0.7 channels/μm^2 on the nodal cells. Two important observations in the experiments were that: (i) shorter open times and longer closed times, i.e. decreased probability of channel opening, occurred with progressive depolarizations of the membrane—a rather unexpected observation for a current that increases in magnitude with increasing depolarizations; (ii) channel inactivation was observed during prolonged depolarizing voltage pulses. Inactivation is rapidly removed with repolarization. Removal of inactivation is seen as a 'hook' preceding the time-dependent decline of outward tail current. The inactivation process was suggested to be responsible for the inward-going rectification in the 'fully activated' channel. These properties resemble those reported by Sanguinetti and Jurkiewicz (1990) for the rectifying small component of ventricular delayed rectification ($I_{K(r)}$). Further studies are needed to determine whether nodal and ventricular $I_{K(r)}$ reflect populations of the same, or different, ion channels. A recent report suggests that some nodal $I_{K(dr)}$ currents may more closely resemble $I_{K(s)}$ (Anumowo et al., (1992)).

Neurotransmitter modulation of nodal $I_{K(dr)}$

There is very limited data on transmitter modulation of the nodal delayed rectifier. Evidence that adrenaline modulates an outward K-current comes from the observation that the maximum diastolic potential and the repolarization rates were enhanced in the nodal preparations (Brown et al., 1979a,b). Noma et al. (1980) determined the effect of epinephrine on $I_{K(dr)}$ recorded from small sinus nodal tissue strips, using the two-electrode voltage-clamp technique. They reported that there was a 10% increase in the current and that there was no shift in the steady-state activation curve in the presence of epinephrine. Further analysis also showed that the time constant of deactivation was not affected by epinephrine. Thus, it was concluded that epinephrine increased the current without affecting its kinetics.

Given the role of $I_{K(dr)}$ in pacemaker activity, it is important that the mechanisms underlying the neurotransmitter regulation of the current in the node be fully understood. Therefore, much data are needed, especially from whole-cell and single channel experiments, on the role of second messengers and other intracellular agents in the modulation of nodal $I_{K(dr)}$.

ATP-sensitive K-channels

The first reports of K_{ATP}-channels were from experiments carried out in heart cells and cell-free membrane patches (Noma, 1983; Trube & Hescheler, 1984). Subsequently, the channel has been reported to exist in a wide range of cell types including pancreatic β-cells (Cook & Hales, 1984), skeletal muscle cells (Spruce et al., 1985) and more recently, arterial smooth muscle cells (Standen et al., 1989). This channel is particularly interesting because it seems to be regulated by the metabolic state of the cell: channel activity is inhibited by the intracellular ATP concentration ([ATP]$_i$).

Dual effects of ATP on $I_{K(ATP)}$

In the heart as in other cell types, the K_{ATP}-channel is regulated by ATP in a complex manner. Channel activity is inhibited by [ATP]$_i$ in sub-millimolar concentrations, yet the channel requires ATP-dependent phosphorylation to maintain activity (Ashcroft, 1988). Studies involving patch-clamping of excised, inside-out membrane patches have shown that channel activity decreases with time (run-down) (Trube & Hescheler, 1984; Kakei et al., 1985). However, channel activity is sustained longer in the open-cell configuration, where the cell is structurally intact but permeabilized with detergent (Kakei et al., 1985). The run-down in channel activity in excised, inside-out membrane patches can be reversed by exposure to Mg–ATP (Findlay & Dunne, 1986; Findlay, 1987; Ohno-Shosaku et al., 1987; Takano et al., 1990). AMP–PNP, ATPγS, and Mg-free ATP are unable to mimic the reactivating effect of Mg–ATP, suggesting the involvement of a Mg-dependent channel phosphorylation in the maintenance of channel activity.

Although $I_{K(ATP)}$ may require ATP-dependent phosphorylation to maintain channel activity, the inhibitory effect of ATP does not involve a phosphorylation step since AMP–PNP, a non-hydrolysable ATP analogue, can also inhibit channel activity (Lederer & Nichols, 1989). Thus, the inhibitory effect of ATP involves the direct binding of ATP to the channel. Apparent Hill coefficients of 2 or 3 for channel inhibition as a function of [ATP]$_i$ have been obtained, suggesting multiple binding sites for ATP (Kakei et al., 1985; Lederer & Nichols, 1989; Nichols & Lederer, 1990). Other nucleotides have also been shown to inhibit $I_{K(ATP)}$, although not as effectively as ATP. In the absence of ATP or Mg^{2+}, adenosine diphosphate (ADP), cytidine triphosphate (CTP) and guanosine diphos-

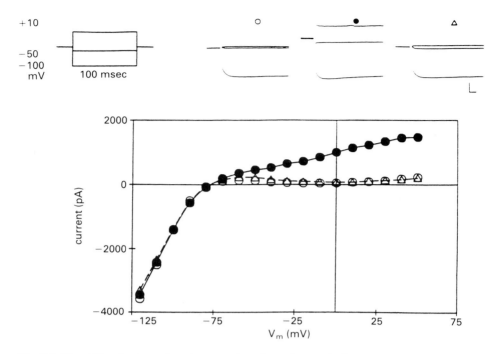

Fig. 8.4. Pinacidil activates outward current in guinea-pig ventricular myocyte. Whole-cell recordings of membrane current measured in response to 100 ms pulses applied to the voltages indicated along the abscissa from a $-40\,mV$ holding potential. Currents (inset) were measured in the absence and presence of $100\,\mu M$ pinacidil and following washout of the drug. The plot shows current plotted against test voltage for each condition. Filled symbols indicate currents in the presence of drug. (With permission from Arena & Kass, 1989a.)

phate (GDP) each showed inhibitory effects on the channel (Lederer & Nichols, 1989). More recently, nucleotide diphosphates such as uridine diphosphate, inosine diphosphate and cytidine diphosphate were found to activate dramatically K_{ATP} after the channel had run-down in the absence of ATP (Tung & Kurachi, 1991). The activation by nucleotide diphosphates, which was Mg-dependent and involved a dephosphorylated channel, potentially suggests the presence of a nucleotide diphosphate binding site on the K_{ATP}-channel protein. These results add further to the complexities of the modulatory mechanism of K_{ATP} by nucleotides.

Physiological role of K_{ATP}

Since this channel is regulated by the metabolic state of the cell, it may have important physiological roles. Under normal physiological conditions the $[ATP]_i$ range in cardiac cells is approximately $3-4\,mM$ and this is sufficient to inhibit K_{ATP}. Several investigators have suggested that

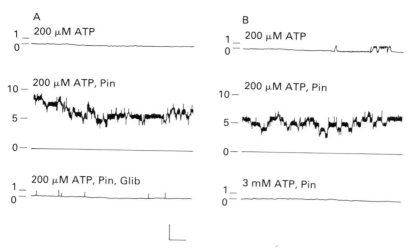

Fig. 8.5. Pinacidil (Pin)-activation of K_{ATP} is inhibited by glibenclamide (Glib) and ATP in cell-free membrane patches of guinea-pig ventricular cells. A, In the presence of 200 μM ATP, 200 μM pinacidil induces K_{ATP} channel activity. Subsequent exposure to glibenclamide (100 nM) inhibits this activity. B, In the presence of 200 μM ATP, exposure to 200 μM pinacidil stimulates K_{ATP} activity which can then be suppressed by raising the ATP concentration to 3 mM. (From Arena & Kass, 1989a.)

activity of this channel may become more pronounced under ischaemic and hypoxic conditions (Noma & Shibasaki, 1985; Wilde *et al.*, 1990; Lederer *et al.*, 1989), and may be largely responsible for the shortening of the action potential duration observed under these conditions. These suggestions are based largely on ischaemic models using metabolic blockade. In cardiac myocytes metabolically poisoned by 2,4-dinitrophenol (DNP), glibenclamide, an inhibitor of $I_{K(ATP)}$, suppressed the effects of DNP (Wilde *et al.*, 1990). Furthermore, in ventricular cells, outward current induced by metabolic inhibition of the cell by cyanide was depressed by injection of ATP (Taniguchi *et al.*, 1983). However, during ischaemic episodes, $[ATP]_i$ levels are not known to fall sufficiently to inhibit $I_{K(ATP)}$ (Elliott *et al.*, 1989). On the other hand, the relatively large conductance of the channel (approximately 80 pS in equimolar 150 mM K^+) and its high density in cardiac myocytes may require that only a small number of open channels are needed to shorten cardiac action potential during pathophysiological conditions (Noma & Shibasaki, 1985; Nichols & Lederer, 1990). Lederer and Nichols (1989) have demonstrated that low levels of ADP in the presence of ATP can stimulate $I_{K(ATP)}$. Since intracellular ADP rises during metabolic blockade (Allen *et al.*, 1985), it may be involved in the regulation of $I_{K(ATP)}$ under pathophysiological conditions. Thus, the physiological role of $I_{K(ATP)}$ remains unclear but factors other than $[ATP]_i$ may also be involved in the regulation of K_{ATP}.

The pharmacology of the cardiac $I_{K(ATP)}$ is discussed in more detail in Chapter 12, but is summarized briefly here. As in other cells, K_{ATP} can be activated by the novel class of drugs referred to as the K-channel openers. Pinacidil, diazoxide, nicorandil, cromakalim, and RP 49356 have all been reported to activate K_{ATP} in cardiac preparations, although generally at higher concentrations than those needed to relax smooth muscle preparations (Sanguinetti, *et al.*, 1988; Arena & Kass, 1989a,b; Escande *et al.*, 1989; Hiraoka & Fan, 1989; Tseng & Hoffman, 1990; Ripoll *et al.*, 1990). Furthermore, as is the case for pancreatic β-cells, the sulphonylureas, agents widely used in the treatment of diabetes mellitus, inhibit K_{ATP} in the heart at concentrations that do not block $I_{K(dr)}$, or I_{K1} (Arena & Kass, 1990a,b). Examples of the activation of K_{ATP} by pinacidil and its inhibition by glibenclamide are given in Figs 8.4 and 8.5. ·

Conclusions

Potassium channels are important to normal cardiac function because they are key factors in determining cell resting potential and action potential duration. The wide range of K-channel types in the heart as well as the diverse cellular mechanisms that regulate them contribute to the modulation of cardiac electrical and mechanical activity under normal physiological conditions. In the case of cardiac dysfunction, the variety of K-channels offers great potential as therapeutic targets for specific rhythm disturbances. The potential use of K-channel modulators as antiarrhythmic agents is the topic of Chapter 12.

References

Allen, D. G., Morris, P. G., Orchard, C. H. & Pirolo, J. S. (1985) A nuclear magnetic resonance study of metabolism in the ferret heart during hypoxia and inhibition of glycolysis. *Journal of Physiology* **361**, 185–204.

Anumonwo, J. M. B., Freeman, L. C., Kwok, W.-M. & Kass, R. S. (1992) Delayed rectification in single cells isolated from guinea pig sinoatrial node. *American Journal Physiology* **262**, H921–H925.

Arena, J. P. & Kass, R. S. (1989a) Enhancement of potassium–sensitive current in heart cells by pinacidil: evidence for modulation of the ATP-sensitive potassium channel. *Circulation Research* **65**, 436–445.

Arena, J. P. & Kass, R. S. (1989b) Activation of ATP-sensitive K channels in heart cells by pinacidil: dependence on ATP. *American Journal of Physiology* **257**, H2092–H2096.

Armstrong, C. M. (1969) Inactivation of the potassium conductance and related phenomena caused by quaternary ammonium ion injection in squid axons. *Journal of General Physiology* **54**, 553–575.

Ashcroft, F. M. (1988) Adenosine 5′-triphosphate-sensitive potassium channels. *Annual Review of Neuroscience* **11**, 97–118.

Attwell, D. & Cohen, I. (1977) The voltage clamp of multicellular preparations. *Progress in Biophysics* **31**, 201–245.

Bennett, P. B. & Begenisich, T. (1987) Catecholamines modulate the delayed rectifying potassium current (I_K) in guinea pig ventricular myocytes. *Pflügers Archiv* **410**, 217–219.

Bennett, P. B., McKinney, L., Begenisich, T. & Kass, R. S. (1986) Adrenergic modulation of the delayed rectifier potassium channel in calf cardiac Purkinje fibres. *Biophysical Journal* **49**, 839–848.

Bennett, P. B., McKinney, L. C., Kass, R. S. & Begenisich, T. (1985) Delayed rectification in the calf cardiac Purkinje fibre. *Biophysical Journal* **48**, 553–567.

Brown, H. F. (1982) Electrophysiology of the sinoatrial node. *Physiological Reviews* **62**, 505–530.

Brown, H. F. & Noble, S. J. (1974) Effects of adrenaline on membrane currents underlying pacemaker activity in frog atrial muscle. *Journal of Physiology* **238**, 51–52.

Brown, H. F., DiFrancesco, D. & Noble, S. J. (1979a) Cardiac pacemaker oscillation and its modulation by autonomic transmitters. *Journal of Experimental Biology* **81**, 175–204.

Brown, H. F., DiFrancesco, D. & Noble, S. J. (1979b) How does adrenaline accelerate the heart? *Nature* **280**, 235–236.

Carmeliet, E. & Mubagwa, K. (1986) Changes by acetylcholine of membrane currents in rabbit cardiac Purkinje fibres. *Journal of Physiology* **371**, 201–217.

Cook, D. L. & Hales, C. N. (1984) Intracellular ATP directly blocks K^+ channels in pancreatic β-cells. *Nature* **311**, 271–273.

DiFrancesco, D., Noma, A. & Trautwein, W. (1979) Kinetics and magnitude of the time-dependent potassium current in the rabbit sinoatrial node. *Pflügers Archiv* **381**, 271–279.

Duchatelle-Gourdon, I., Hartzell, H. C. & Lagrutta, A. A. (1989) Modulation of the delayed rectifier potassium current in frog cardiomyocytes by β-adrenergic agonists and magnesium. *Journal of Physiology* **415**, 251–274.

Duchatelle-Gourdon, I., Lagrutta, A. A. & Hartzell, H. C. (1991) Effects of Mg^{2+} on basal and β-adrenergic-stimulated delayed rectifier potassium current in frog atrial myocytes. *Journal of Physiology* **435**, 333–347.

Dudel, J., Peper, K., Rudel, R. & Trautwein, W. (1967) The dynamic chloride component of membrane current in Purkinje fibres. *Pflügers Archiv* **295**, 197–212.

Dukes, I. D. & Morad, M. (1989) Tedisamil inactivates transient outward K^+ current in rat ventricular myocytes. *American Journal of Physiology* **257**, H1746–H1749.

Elliott, A. C., Smith, G. L. & Allen, D. G. (1989) Simultaneous measurements of action potential duration and intracellular ATP in isolated ferret hearts exposed to cyanide. *Circulation Research* **64**, 583–591.

Escande, D., Thuringer, D., Le Guern, S., Courteix, J., Laville, M. & Cavero, I. (1989) Potassium channel openers act through an activation of ATP-sensitive K^+ channels in guinea-pig cardiac myocytes. *Pflügers Archiv* **414**, 669–675.

Fedulova, S. A., Drewe, J. A., Joho, R. H., Brown, A. M. & VanDongen, A. M. J. (1991) Structure–function analysis of the delayed rectifier K^+ channel *drk1:* temperature sensitivity. *Biophysical Journal* **59**, 453a.

Findlay, I. (1987) ATP-sensitive K^+ channels in rat ventricular myocytes are blocked and inactivated by internal divalent cations. *Pflügers Archiv* **410**, 313–320.

Findlay, I. & Dunne, M. J. (1986) ATP maintains ATP-inhibited K^+ channels in an operational state. *Pflügers Archiv* **407**, 238–240.

Fozzard, H. A. & Hiraoka, M. (1973) The positive dynamic current and its inactivation properties in cardiac Purkinje fibres. *Journal of Physiology* **234**, 569–586.

Freeman, L. C., Kwok, W.-M., & Kass, R. C. (1992) Phosphorylation-independent regulation of cardiac I_K by guanine nucleotides and isoproterenol. *American Journal of Physiology* **262**, H1298–H1302.

Giles, W. R. & van Ginneken, A. C. G. (1985) A transient outward current in isolated cells from the crista terminals of rabbit heart. *Journal of Physiology* **368**, 243–264.

Goto, M., Hyodo, T. & Ikeda, K. (1983) Ca-dependent outward currents in bullfrog myocardium. *Japanese Journal of Physiology* **33**, 837–854.

Hall, A. E., Hutter, O. F. & Noble, D. (1963) Current–voltage relations of Purkinje fibres in sodium deficient solutions. *Journal of Physiology* **166**, 225–240.

Harvey, R. D. & Hume, J. R. (1989) Autonomic regulation of delayed rectifier K^+ current in mammalian heart involves G proteins. *American Journal of Physiology* **257**, H818–H823.

Hescheler, J., Kameyama, M., Trautwein, W., Mieskes, G. & Soling, H. D. (1987) Regulation of the cardiac calcium channel by protein phosphatases. *European Journal of Biochemistry* **165**, 261–266.

Hiraoka, M. & Fan, Z. (1989) Activation of ATP-sensitive outward K^+ current by nicorandil (2-nicotinamidoethyl nitrate) in isolated ventricular myocytes. *Journal of Pharmacology and Experimental Therapeutics* **250**, 278–285.

Hodgkin, A. L. & Huxley, A. F. (1952) A quantitative description of membrane current and its application to conduction and excitation in nerve. *Journal of Physiology* **117**, 500–544.

Iijima, T., Imagawa, J. I. & Taira, N. (1990) Differential modulation by beta adrenoceptors of inward calcium and delayed rectifier potassium current in single ventricular cells of guinea pig heart. *Journal of Pharmacology and Experimental Therapeutics* **254**, 142–146.

Irisawa, H. (1978) Comparative physiology of the cardiac pacemaker mechanism. *Physiological Reviews* **58**, 461–498.

Kakei, M., Noma, A. & Shibasaki, T. (1985) Properties of adenosine-triphosphate-regulated potassium channels in guinea-pig ventricular cells. *Journal of Physiology* **363**, 441–462.

Kameyama, M., Hescheler, J., Mieskes, G. & Trautwein, W. (1986) The protein-specific phosphatase 1 antagonizes the β-adrenergic increase of the cardiac Ca current. *Pflügers Archiv* **407**, 461–463.

Kameyama, M., Kakei, M., Sato, R., Shibasaki, T., Matsuda, H. & Irisawa, H. (1984) Intracellular Na^+ activates a K^+ channel in mammalian cardiac cells. *Nature* **309**, 354–356.

Kass, R. S. (1984) Delayed rectification in the cardiac Purkinje fibre is not activated by intracellular calcium. *Biophysical Journal* **45**, 837–839.

Kass, R. S. & Tsien, R. W. (1975) Multiple effects of calcium antagonists on plateau currents in cardiac Purkinje fibres. *Journal of General Physiology* **66**, 169–192.

Kass, R. S. & Tsien, R. W. (1976) Control of action potential duration by calcium ions in cardiac Purkinje fibres. *Journal of General Physiology* **67**, 599–617.

Kass, R. S. & Weigers, S. E. (1982) The ionic basis of concentration-related effects of noradrenaline on the action potential of calf cardiac Purkinje fibres. *Journal of Physiology* **322**, 541–558.

Kass, R. S., Arena, J. P. & Walsh, K. B. (1990) Measurement and block of potassium channel currents in the heart: Importance of channel type. *Drug Development Research* **19**, 115–127.

Kenyon, J. L. & Gibbons, W. R. (1979) Influence of chloride, potassium, and tetraethyl-ammonium on the early outward current of sheep cardiac Purkinje fibers. *Journal of General Physiology* **73**, 117–138.

Kenyon, J. L. & Sutko, J. L. (1987) Calcium and voltage-activated plateau currents of cardiac Purkinje fibres. *Journal of General Physiology* **89**, 921–958.

Kokubun, S., Nishimura, M., Noma, A. & Irisawa, H. (1982) Membrane currents in the rabbit atrioventricular node cell. *Pflügers Archiv* **393**, 15–22.

Lederer, W. J. & Nichols, C. G. (1989) Nucleotide modulation of the activity of rat heart ATP-sensitive K⁺ channels in isolated membrane patches. *Journal of Physiology* **419**, 193–211.

Lederer, W. J., Nichols, C. G. & Smith, G. L. (1989) The mechanism of early contractile failure of isolated rat ventricular myocytes subjected to complete metabolic inhibition. *Journal of Physiology* **413**, 329–349.

Litovsky, S. H. & Antzelevitch, C. (1988) Transient outward current prominent in canine ventricular epicardium but not endocardium. *Circulation Research* **62**, 116–126.

Litovsky, S. H. & Antzelevitch, C. (1990) Differences in the electrophysiological response of canine ventricular subendocardium and subepicardium to acetylcholine and isoproterenol. A direct effect of acetylcholine in ventricular myocardium. *Circulation Research* **67**, 615–627.

McAllister, R. E. & Noble, D. (1966) The time and voltage dependence of the slow outward current in cardiac Purkinje fibres. *Journal of Physiology* **186**, 632–662.

Matsuda, H., Saigusa, A. & Irisawa, H. (1987) Ohmic conductance through the inwardly rectifying K channel and blocking by internal Mg^{2+}. *Nature* **325**, 156–158.

Matsuura, H., Ehara, T. & Imoto, Y. (1987) An analysis of the delayed outward current in single ventricular cells of the guinea pig. *Pflügers Archiv* **410**, 596–603.

Nakayama, T., Kurachi, Y., Noma, A. & Irisawa, H. (1984) Action potential and membrane currents of single pacemaker cells of the rabbit heart. *Pflügers Archiv* **402**, 248–257.

Nerbonne, J. M., Richard, S., Nargeot, J. & Lester, H. A. (1984) New photoactivatable cyclic nucleotides produce intracellular jumps in cyclic AMP and cyclic GMP concentrations. *Nature* **310**, 74–76.

Nichols, C. G. & Lederer, W. J. (1990) The regulation of ATP-sensitive K⁺ channel activity in intact and permeabilized rat ventricular myocytes. *Journal of Physiology* **423**, 91–110.

Noble, D. (1978) *The Initiation of the Heartbeat*, 2nd edn. Clarendon Press, Oxford.

Noble, D. & Tsien, R. (1968) The kinetics and rectifier properties of the slow potassium current in cardiac Purkinje fibres. *Journal of Physiology* **195**, 185–214.

Noble, D. & Tsien, R. W. (1969) Outward membrane currents activated in the plateau range of potentials in cardiac Purkinje fibres. *Journal of Physiology* **200**, 205–231.

Noma, A. (1983) ATP-regulated K⁺ channels in cardiac muscle. *Nature* **305**, 147–148.

Noma, A. & Irisawa, H. (1976) A time and voltage-dependent potassium current in the rabbit sinoatrial node cell. *Pflügers Archiv* **366**, 251–258.

Noma, A. & Shibasaki, T. (1985) Membrane current through adenosine-triphosphate-regulated potassium channels in guinea-pig ventricular cells. *Journal of Physiology* **363**, 463–480.

Noma, A., Kotake, H. & Irisawa, H. (1980) Slow inward current and its role in mediating the chronotropic effect of epinephrine in rabbit sino-atrial node. *Pflügers Archiv* **388**, 1–9.

Ohno-Shosaku, T., Zunkler, B. J. & Trube, G. (1987) Dual effects of ATP in K⁺ currents of mouse pancreatic B-cells. *Pflügers Archiv* **408**, 133–138.

Pappano, A. J. & Carmeliet, E. (1979) Epinephrine and the pace-making mechanism at plateau potentials in sheep cardiac Purkinje fibres. *Pflügers Archiv* **382**, 17–26.

Ripoll, C., Lederer, W. J. & Nichols, C. G. (1990) Modulation of ATP-sensitive K⁺ channel activity and contractile behavior in mammalian ventricle by the potassium channel openers cromakalim and RP 49356. *Journal of Pharmacology and Experimental Theraputics* **255**, 429–435.

Sakmann, B. & Trube, G. (1984) Conductance properties of single inwardly rectifying potassium channels in ventricular cells from guinea-pig heart. *Journal of Physiology* **347**, 641–657.

Sakmann, B., Noma, A. & Trautwein, W. (1983) Acetylcholine activation of single muscarinic K$^+$ channels in isolated pacemaker cells of the mammalian heart. *Nature* **303**, 250–253.

Sanguinetti, M. C. & Jurkiewicz, N. K. (1990) Two components of cardiac delayed rectifier K$^+$ current. *Journal of General Physiology* **96**, 195–215.

Sanguinetti, M. C., Scott, A. L., Zingaro, G. J. & Siegl, P. K. S. (1988) BRL 34915 (cromakalim) activates ATP-sensitive K$^+$ current in cardiac muscle. *Proceedings of the National Academy of Sciences USA* **85**, 8360–8364.

Shibasaki, T. (1987) Conductance and kinetics of delayed rectifier potassium channels in nodal cells of the rabbit heart. *Journal of Physiology* **387**, 227–250.

Shibata, E. & Giles, W. (1985) Ionic currents which generate spontaneous diastolic depolarization in individual cardiac pacemaker cells. *Proceedings of the National Academy of Sciences USA* **82**, 7796–7800.

Siegelbaum, S. A. & Tsien, R. W. (1980) Calcium-activated transient outward current in calf Purkinje fibres. *Journal of Physiology* **299**, 485–506.

Siegelbaum, S. A., Tsien, R. W. & Kass, R. S. (1977) Role of intracellular calcium in the transient outward current of calf Purkinje fibres. *Nature* **269**, 611–613.

Spruce, A. E., Standen, N. B. & Stanfield, P. R. (1985) Voltage-dependent ATP-sensitive potassium channels of skeletal muscle membrane. *Nature* **316**, 736–738.

Standen, N. B., Quayle, J. M., Davies, N. W., Brayden, J. E., Huang, Y. & Nelson, M. T. (1989) Hyperpolarizing vasodilators activate ATP-sensitive K$^+$ channels in arterial smooth muscle. *Science* **245**, 177–180.

Takano, M., Qin, D. & Noma, A. (1990) ATP-dependent decay and recovery of K$^+$ channels in guinea pig cardiac myocytes. *American Journal of Physiology* **258**, H45–H50.

Taniguchi, J., Noma, A. & Irisawa, H. (1983) Modification of the cardiac action potential by intracellular injection of adenosine triphosphate and related substances in guinea pig single ventricular cells. *Circulation Research* **53**, 131–139.

Tarr, M., Trank, J. W. & Goertz, K. K. (1989) Intracellular magnesium affects I_K in single frog atrial cells. *American Journal of Physiology* **257**, H1663–H1669.

Tohse, N. (1990) Calcium-sensitive delayed rectifier potassium current in guinea pig ventricular cells. *American Journal of Physiology* **258**, H1200–H1207.

Tohse, N., Kameyama, M. & Irisawa, H. (1987) Intracellular Ca^{2+} and protein kinase C modulate K$^+$ current in guinea pig heart cells. *American Journal of Physiology* **253**, H1321–H1324.

Tohse, N., Kameyama, M., Sekiguchi, K., Shearman, M. S., Kanno, M., Nishizuka, Y. & Irisawa, H. (1990) Protein kinase C activation enhances the delayed rectifier potassium current in guinea pig heart cells. *Journal of Molecular and Cellular Cardiology* **22**, 725–734.

Trube, G. & Hescheler, J. (1984) Inward-rectifying channels in isolated patches of the heart cell membrane: ATP-dependence and comparison with cell-attached patches. *Pflügers Archiv* **401**, 178–184.

Tseng, G. & Hoffman, B. F. (1989) Two components of transient outward current in canine ventricular myocytes. *Circulation Research* **64**, 633–647.

Tseng, G. N. & Hoffman, B. F. (1990) Actions of pinacidil on membrane currents in canine ventricular myocytes and their modulation by intracellular ATP and cAMP. *Pflügers Archiv* **415**, 414–424.

Tsien, R. W., Giles, W. & Greengard, P. (1972) Cyclic AMP mediates the effects of adrenaline on cardiac Purkinje fibers. *Nature* **240**, 181–183.

Tung, R. T. & Kurachi, Y. (1991) On the mechanism of nucleotide diphosphate-induced openings of the ATP-sensitive potassium channel in ventricular cells of the guinea-pig—a functional transducer unit hypothesis. *Biophysical Journal* **59**, 94a.

Umeno, T. (1984) β-actions of catecholamines on the K-related currents of the bullfrog atrial muscle. *Japanese Journal of Physiology* **34**, 513–528.

Vandenberg, C. A. (1987) Inward rectification of a potassium channel in cardiac ventricular cells depends on internal magnesium ions. *Proceedings of the National Academy of Sciences USA* **84**, 2560–2564.

Walsh, K. B. & Kass, R. S. (1991) Distinct voltage-dependent regulation of a heart-delayed I_k by protein kinase A and C. *American Journal of Physiology* **261**, C1081–C1090.

Walsh, K. B. & Kass, R. S. (1988) Regulation of a heart potassium channel by PKA and C. *Science* **242**, 67–69.

Walsh, K. B., Begenisich, T. B. & Kass, R. S. (1989) β-adrenergic modulation of cardiac ion channels: differential temperature-sensitivity of potassium and calcium currents. *Journal of General Physiology* **257**, 841–854.

Weidmann, S. (1951) Effect of current flow on the membrane potential of cardiac muscle. *Journal of Physiology* **115**, 227–236.

Weidmann, S. (1956) *Elektrophysiologie der Herzmuskelfase* Huber, Bern.

Wilde, A. A. M., Escande, D., Schumacher, C. A., Thuringer, D., Mestre, M., Fiolet, J. W. T. & Janse, M. J. (1990) Potassium accumulation in the globally ischemic mammalian heart. A role for the ATP-sensitive potassium channel. *Circulation Research* **67**, 835–843.

Yazawa, K. & Kameyama, M. (1990) Mechanism of receptor-mediated modulation of the delayed outward potassium current in guinea-pig ventricular myocytes. *Journal of Physiology* **421**, 135–150.

Yue, D. T. & Marban, E. (1988) A novel cardiac potassium channel that is active and conductive at depolarized potentials. *Pflügers Archiv* **413**, 127–133.

Chapter 9
Potassium channels in mammalian neurones: their properties and prospects for pharmacological manipulation
M. Galvan

Introduction

The primary function of nerve cells and their numerous processes is the rapid transmission of sensory and motor information from one part of the organism to another. In order to perform this function effectively and with a minimum of energy consumption, an elaborate combination of electrical and chemical transmission has evolved. Rapid events are signalled via electrical impulses (action potentials), which propagate from neurone to neurone via classical chemical neurotransmission. A superficial view of the functioning nervous system reveals that the electrical signals are in part 'binary' in nature, an action potential being an 'all-or-none' event. Thus information is encoded primarily in the frequency of action potentials and not in their amplitude. The control of neuronal action potential discharge is therefore central to the function of the nervous system and it is with part of the control system that this chapter deals.

In principle, two processes govern the excitability of mammalian neurones (Fig. 9.1): depolarization (changes of membrane potential towards zero) and hyperpolarization (changes of membrane potential towards more negative values). Both changes can be brought about in two ways: (i) synaptically, via the action of a neurotransmitter or circulating hormone on a chemical receptor at the cell surface; (ii) non-synaptically via changes in the activity of membrane channels, whose open and closed state is governed by membrane potential (voltage-dependent channels) or intracellular messengers such as Ca^{2+}, cyclic adenosine monophosphate (cAMP) or inositol triphosphate (IP_3). Some channels are coupled to membrane surface receptors, exhibit voltage dependence and are influ-

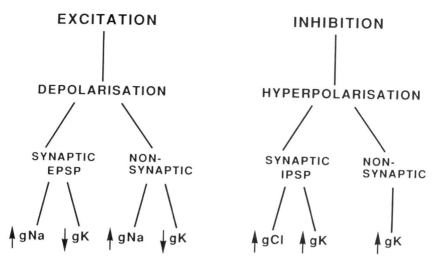

Fig. 9.1. The role of membrane ionic channels in the control of neuronal excitability. Synaptic events arise from neurotransmitter release and non-synaptic events result from the influence of voltage-dependent currents. In this simple scheme, K-currents participate in all forms of excitation and inhibition.

enced by changes in intracellular messenger concentration. Calcium-dependent K-channels are a good example of a channel with multiple control systems.

Synaptically induced membrane excitations (depolarizations) are termed excitatory postsynaptic potentials (EPSPs) and usually result from increases in membrane permeability to Na^+ and K^+. A simple example would be the action of acetylcholine on sympathetic ganglion cells. Non-synaptically induced depolarizations mainly result from changes in membrane permeability to Na^+ and/or Ca^{2+}. However, depolarization can also occur when hyperpolarizing influences are reduced: a reduction in outward K-current also leads to depolarization and excitation of the cell, as will be explained in more detail later in this chapter.

Synaptically induced inhibitions (hyperpolarizations) are termed inhibitory postsynaptic potentials (IPSPs) and usually result from increases in permeability to Cl^- or K^+. The non-synaptically induced hyperpolarizations result almost exclusively from increases in K-channel opening. A large variety of K-channels perform discrete tasks in the ongoing function of regulating neuronal activity. It is this multitude of channels which is the subject of this chapter and which will be discussed in detail.

A large number of excellent review articles describing the physiological and pharmacological properties of K-channels have been recently published (Adams & Galvan, 1986; Brown, 1988, 1990; Cook, 1988; Llinas, 1988; Nicoll, 1988; Rudy, 1988; Cook & Quast, 1990; Dreyer, 1990;

Halliwell, 1990). Therefore, a short summary of the physiology and pharmacology of the various channel types will suffice here and the reader is referred to this extensive library of review material for further details.

The primary object of this chapter is to summarize current views of the role of such channels in pathophysiological processes and to provide some information on past, present and possible future clinical uses of drugs modulating neuronal K-channel activity. In addition, the physiology and pharmacology of adenosine triphosphate (ATP)-coupled K-channels (K_{ATP}) is described in detail, since our knowledge of these channels has rapidly expanded in the last few years and this literature has not been extensively reviewed to date (Ashcroft & Ashcroft, 1990; Miller, 1990).

Background

The first formal description of the function of a K-current in a neuronal structure (the squid giant axon) was published by Hodgkin and Huxley in 1952. Their conclusion that the opening of so-called 'delayed rectifier' type K-channels contributed to the repolarizing phase of the axonal action potential is the foundation stone of our present knowledge. Research into neuronal K-channels continued using a variety of invertebrate (marine and terrestrial) animals possessing giant neurones or axons necessary for detailed voltage-clamp studies. Pioneer work on cat spinal motoneurones also contributed much information on the functional role of such channels in living mammals (Barrett et al., 1980).

The discovery of a second type of K-current in an invertebrate neurone, the 'transient outward current or A-current' $I_{K(A)}$ was reported by Neher (1971) and Connor and Stevens (1971a; see also Hagiwara et al., 1961). Connor and Stevens (1971b) also showed that $I_{K(A)}$ was involved in regulating interspike intervals and thus neuronal discharge frequency, a quite different role from that demonstrated for the 'delayed rectifier' ($I_{K(V)}$) by Hodgkin and Huxley (1952). In 1975, Meech and Standen published a detailed description of a third type of K-current elicited by increases in intracellular Ca concentration ($[Ca^{2+}]_i$), the 'Ca-dependent K-current' ($I_{K(Ca)}$). This epoch of research closed with the elegant demonstration by Thompson (1977) that all three of these K-currents were present in one type of neurone. Furthermore, Thompson showed that they could be distinguished not only on physiological grounds but also by using pharmacological tools.

By this time, microelectrode and voltage-clamp techniques had undergone enormous technical advances. The single electrode voltage-clamp technique (Brennecke & Lindeman, 1974; Wilson & Goldner, 1975) had been introduced enabling the study of membrane currents in small mammalian neurones previously inaccessible to the classical two-electrode voltage-clamp technique. In addition, the emphasis turned in general to vertebrate neurones, which were to provide electrophysiologists with a rich area of research for almost a decade. Brown and Adams (1980) described the muscarinic, (M) current as a novel K-current (inward) ($I_{K(M)}$) in bullfrog neurones. Anomalous rectifier currents ($I_{K(IR)}$), previously observed in invertebrates (Kandel & Tauc, 1966) and vertebrates (Nelson & Frank, 1967) were characterized in detail (Halliwell & Adams, 1982; Constanti & Galvan, 1983) and $I_{K(Ca)}$ currents were subdivided on the basis of their physiology and pharmacology (Brown & Griffith, 1983; Lancaster & Adams, 1986; Schwindt et al., 1988b). The characterization of neurotransmitter-dependent K-currents (Nicoll, 1988), a slowly-inactivating K-current (Storm, 1988) and finally an ATP-dependent K-current (Ashford et al., 1988) completes the story to date.

Functions of K-channels in neurones

The K-equilibrium potential (E_K) is normally negative to the resting membrane potential in nerve cells. Thus an increase in K-channel opening and, therefore, an increase in K-conductance leads to a membrane hyperpolarization. This is intrinsically inhibitory in nature, since the membrane potential is moved away from the threshold potential for action potential generation. Additionally, the increased membrane conductance *per se* (even without a change in membrane potential) reduces membrane excitability by short-circuiting any other excitatory electrical influences on the cell. Conversely, block of K-channels can lead to depolarization if the channels are open at resting potential as is the case for K_M-channels in many cell types (Constanti & Brown, 1981; Adams et al., 1982a,b). Even if block of K-channels does not directly influence membrane potential, membrane resistance is increased thus amplifying the effect of other currents on the membrane potential. Should these influences be excitatory in nature, overexcitation can be observed (Galvan & Behrends, 1985; Kawai & Watanabe, 1986; Stansfeld et al., 1986).

In order to understand the functional significance of K-channels and also to appreciate fully the possible modes of external (drug-induced) modulation of their function, the reader must be aware that a neurone is not at all similar to a smooth or a cardiac muscle cell. These latter structures are, as far as we know, homogeneous with regard to the distribution of K-channels over their cell surfaces. Organ differences are possible, but within-cell variations are, as yet, unknown. The situation with neurones is different. Most neurones are composed of four distinct parts: (i) the dendritic tree, which acts as a sort of antenna collecting information from incoming synaptic sources; (ii) the soma, a kind of central processing unit, whose function it is to integrate this information and to formulate an appropriate output signal; (iii) the axon, which has a cable function and is designed to transmit information over long distances from the soma to (iv) the nerve terminals. This latter structure, which on receipt of an action potential releases a chemical neurotransmitter is already well known to pharmacologists as a site where drug interventions can have significant and useful pharmacological effects.

Purely for reasons of size and accessibility to microelectrodes, most of our present knowledge about the distribution and properties of 'neuronal' K-channels is restricted to somata and axons. The fine dendrites and nerve terminals (sometimes only a few microns in diameter) have only been partially studied and thus a great deal of basic research is still needed in these areas. Nevertheless, enough is known about some dendrites and nerve terminals to state that the types of K-channel found in these structures resemble those in the soma in both their physiology and pharmacology. However, since only a few sites have been studied our knowledge is rudimentary and history has shown that somatic K-channels differ in character between neurones in adjacent regions in the brain. It is therefore reasonable to assume that their counterparts in dendrites, axons and nerve terminals could also differ from site to site.

In the following account emphasis has been placed on presenting the function of K-channels and the possible consequences of increases or decreases in function rather than a formal description of properties. For this more fundamental information, the reader is referred to the many review articles which have appeared and the original articles which are quoted therein (*see* references quoted in the Introduction).

It must also be considered that, contrary to the impression arising from the increasing amount of pharmacological literature containing references to blockers of various types of K-channel, selectivity is usually poor. Only a few of the commonly used blockers are highly specific, i.e. more than 100-fold more potent on one type of channel than on all others. The use of non-selective blockers to define function and further classification has, in the past, led to difficulties in the field of receptor pharmacology. The pharmacology of neuronal K-channels is still in its infancy and caution should therefore be exercised in the delicate task of assigning the word 'selective' to an existing or new blocker.

Types of K-channel

Delayed rectifier channels (K_V)

The delayed rectifier channel (K_V) carries a large current ($I_{K(V)}$) which is activated during the upstroke of the action potential and which contributes to the action potential repolarization (Hodgkin & Huxley, 1952; Hille, 1967; Thompson, 1977; Hagiwara *et al.*, 1981; Adams *et al.*, 1982a). Reduction of this current by tetraethylammonium (TEA) ions leads to a prolongation of the action potential. The consequences of this depend on the cell studied. In an axon where this current is the major or exclusive repolarizing current, action potential repolarization is slowed and after-hyperpolarization is reduced. On the other hand, in a neurone exhibiting both K_V- and K_{Ca}-channels, a reduction of $I_{K(V)}$ has a paradoxical effect. The reduced rate of repolarization prolongs the action potential and as a consequence, inward movement of Ca^{2+} is enhanced and therefore $I_{K(Ca)}$ is increased. The overall result is that after-hyperpolarization is increased in duration and/or amplitude (M. Galvan, unpublished observations; Schwartzkroin & Prince, 1980).

The K_V-channels open at potentials positive to about -20 mV, exhibit slow (1–100 ms) activation kinetics and little or no inactivation at depolarized potentials. They are not blocked by Ca- or Na-channel blockers but are sensitive to TEA in millimolar concentrations and to aminopyridines (Hille, 1967; Thompson, 1977; Kirsch & Narahashi, 1978; Hermann & Gorman, 1981; Adams *et al.*, 1982a; Galvan & Sedlmeir, 1984; Belluzzi *et al.*, 1985b; Numann *et al.*, 1987).

'A'-type transient outward channels (K_A)

The transient outward or A-channels (K_A) constitute a family of rapidly activating K-channels with fast (<10 ms) or medium (10–1000 ms) inactivation rates (Rogawski, 1985). This type of current exhibits almost complete steady state inactivation at potentials positive to about -50 mV and thus can only be activated by depolarizing stimuli from more hyperpolarized potentials. The original observation that $I_{K(A)}$ influences action potential discharge frequency (Connor & Stevens, 1971b) has been repeatedly confirmed. Thus 'non-selective' block of this current with aminopyridines [3,4-diaminopyridine is more potent than 4-aminopyridine (4-AP); Kirsch & Narahashi, 1978] leads to uncontrolled repetitive discharges (Fig. 9.2A, B). In central neurones with intact circuitry this can manifest as epileptic-like discharges (Baranyi & Fehér, 1979; Szente & Pongrácz, 1981).

In addition to a role in the regulation of action potential discharge frequency, $I_{K(A)}$ can also contribute to the repolarization of the action potential and to the latency to the first spike following a strong depolarizing stimulus (Galvan, 1982; Gustafsson *et al.*, 1982; MacDermott & Weight, 1982; Segal *et al.*, 1984; Belluzzi *et al.*, 1985a). Therefore, this current can retard or even prevent the initiation of action potential discharge.

Dendrotoxin is a very potent blocker of $I_{K(A)}$ in mammalian central neurones (Halliwell *et al.*, 1986; Dreyer, 1990). However, 4-AP which is more commonly used is far less potent (Gustafsson *et al.*, 1982; Segal *et al.*, 1984; Numann *et al.*, 1987). Unfortunately, neither of these compounds is particularly selective. Lastly, $I_{K(A)}$ can be modulated by activation of certain neurotransmitter receptors (Aghajanian, 1985).

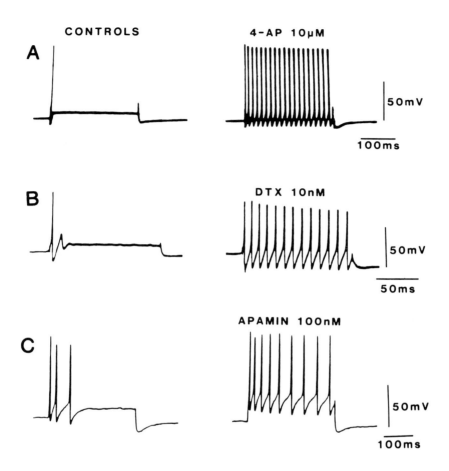

Fig. 9.2. Actions of three different K-channel blockers (A, 4-aminopyridine (4-AP);
B, dendrotoxin (DTX); and C, apamin) on the rate of action potential discharge in
rat visceral sensory ganglion cells (4-AP and DTX) and sympathetic ganglion cells
(apamin) *in vitro.* Cells were excited by injection of depolarizing current pulses (not
illustrated) in control solution *(left panels)* and after bath application of the
channel blocker *(right panels).* All three drugs, which are convulsant agents in
intact animals, blocked inhibitory outward K-currents resulting in trains of action
potentials during stimulation with depolarizing current. (A and B, from Stansfeld
et al. (1986) with permission; C, from J. Behrends & M. Galvan, unpublished.)

The slowly inactivating current (I_D) described by Storm (1988) in
hippocampal neurones is another form of transient outward current
involved in the control of latency to first spike following weak, near-
threshold depolarizations. This current is blocked by low concentrations
of 4-AP, (30–40 μM: Storm, 1988; Crépel *et al.*, 1992) and by glibenclamide
(10 μM: Crépel *et al.*, 1992).

Muscarinic channels (K_M)

Muscarinic channels (K_M), which are inhibited by acetylcholine acting via muscarinic receptors, serve a large variety of functions in mammalian central and peripheral neurones (reviewed by Brown, 1988). They are characterized by slow (several hundreds of milliseconds) activation and *de*activation kinetics and the current, $I_{K(M)}$, can be discriminated from almost all other K-currents in mammalian neurones by the fact that it does not exhibit steady-state inactivation. Thus at potentials positive to about $-60\,mV$ (the activation threshold), K_M-channels open and remain open as long as the membrane potential does not hyperpolarize. The lack of inactivation allows the M-current to contribute to the resting membrane potential of the cell.

The $I_{K(M)}$ also serves to limit the movement of the membrane potential towards or away from the action potential threshold (Adams *et al.*, 1982a). Thus this population of channels can dramatically reduce the frequency of cell firing, as is evident after pharmacological blockade with muscarine (Adams *et al.*, 1982b). It has also been suggested that $I_{K(M)}$ can modulate the change in membrane potential produced by released neurotransmitters (Brown, 1988).

The large number of neurotransmitter receptors coupled to K_M-channels (muscarinic, luteinizing hormone-releasing hormone, angiotensin, somatostatin and 5-hydroxytryptamine (5-HT)) lends great importance to the role of this system in regulating cell excitability (Constanti & Brown, 1981; Adams *et al.*, 1982b; Colino & Halliwell, 1987; Brown, 1988; Moore *et al.*, 1988). All of these substances except somatostatin lead to closure of the channels and an increase in cell excitability. Somatostatin has been reported to increase available $I_{K(M)}$ (Moore *et al.*, 1988). Lastly, it has been demonstrated that closure of K_M by synaptically released acetylcholine underlies the generation of some forms of slow EPSPs (Brown & Selyanko, 1985; Gähwiler & Brown, 1985; Madison *et al.*, 1987).

Calcium-dependent K-channels (K_{Ca})

The K_{Ca}-channels conduct a family of currents closely involved in the control of repetitive discharge and action potential repolarization (Blatz & Magelby, 1987; Lattore *et al.*, 1989; Marty, 1989). Although these channels are primarily opened via an increase in free $[Ca^{2+}]_i$, they are also voltage-dependent and often coupled to cell-surface receptors for endogenous neurotransmitters (Grafe *et al.*, 1980; Colino & Halliwell, 1987; Nicoll, 1988). The activator Ca^{2+} can enter the cell through voltage-dependent Ca-channels or be released from intracellular storage sites via the action of neurotransmitters on receptors coupled to second messenger systems.

There are at least two types of neuronal K_{Ca}-channel, the so-called large, high conductance (BK_{Ca}) channels and the small, low conductance (SK_{Ca}) channels (Marty, 1983; Romey & Lazdunski, 1984). These channels were originally discriminated by their pharmacology, BK_{Ca} being blocked by low millimolar concentrations of TEA and SK_{Ca} channels being blocked by nanomolar concentrations of apamin (Adams *et al.*, 1982c; Romey & Lazdunski, 1984; Galvan & Behrends, 1985; Pennefather *et al.*, 1985; Kawai & Watanabe, 1986; Numann *et al.*, 1987). The BK_{Ca}-channels appear to contribute to the repolarization of the action potential as demonstrated by the action of charybdotoxin, TEA or Cd^{2+} (Adams *et al.*, 1982c; Storm, 1987). As described below, BK_{Ca} are subject to control via the activation of a variety of neurotransmitter receptors.

Small, low conductance Ca-activated K-channels are involved in the generation of a long-lasting, apamin-sensitive spike after-hyperpolarization (Romey & Lazdunski, 1984; Pennefather *et al.*, 1985), and blockade of SK_{Ca} substantially reduces intrinsic cell inhibition resulting in repetitive action potentials following excitatory stimuli (Fig. 9.2C).

Inward rectifier K-channels (K_{IR})

In many types of neurones, a hyperpolarization to a potential negative to the E_K (about $-85\,mV$), opens a population of K-channels (K_{IR}) allowing *inward* current to flow. As a result of the inward flow of K-current, the membrane depolarizes slightly and this tends to counteract the hyperpolarizing drive on the cell membrane. Such a system can account for the depolarizing shifts in electrotonic potentials observed during strong hyperpolarizing current pulses (Kandel & Tauc, 1966; Nelson & Frank, 1967; Barrett *et al.*, 1980; Halliwell & Adams, 1982; Constanti & Galvan, 1983). It should be noted that these currents are not always pure K-currents (Halliwell & Adams, 1982; Halliwell, 1990) and are characterized by a lack of inactivation. They can be blocked by Cs^+ and/or Ba^{2+} ions.

The exact functions of K_{IR}-channels are not yet completely elucidated. An involvement in the pacemaker activity of neurones, as has been proposed for cardiac muscle, is one possibility (Noble, 1984). Second by the current could serve to limit hyperpolarization following periods of intense neuronal activity (Schwindt *et al.*, 1988a).

Receptor-coupled K-channels

The modulation of neuronal K-channels by neurotransmitter substances and synthetic ligands has been intensively studied over the last decade (see reviews by Nicoll, 1988; North, 1989; Nicoll *et al.*, 1990). It has been demonstrated (particularly clearly in rat hippocampal neurones *in vitro*) that K-channels can be opened or closed by the action of neurotransmit-

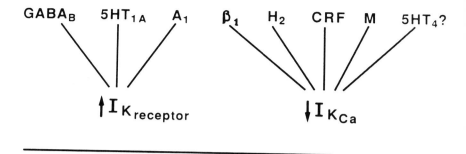

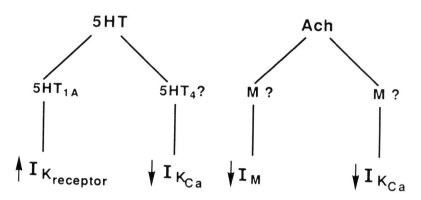

Fig. 9.3. The upper diagram illustrates the convergence that can occur in a single neurone between neurotransmitter receptors and the ion channel that is modulated. The lower diagram illustrates the divergence that can be observed in a single neurone. Question marks indicate uncertainty regarding receptor subtypes. (Redrawn with modifications from Nicoll (1988) with permission; copyright 1988 by the AAAS.)

ters (Nicoll, 1988). Figure 9.3 presents schematically the concept that the activation of several different receptor types can lead to the opening or closing of a single channel type. This phenomenon has been termed convergence since the final common pathway converges onto a single channel type. Activation of 5-HT$_{1A}$, γ-aminobutyric acid (GABA)$_B$ or adenosine A$_1$ receptors leads to the opening of K-channels, which accounts for the membrane hyperpolarization induced by agents acting as agonists at these receptors. In contrast, activation of adrenergic β$_1$, histamine H$_2$, corticotrophin releasing factor, muscarinic, or perhaps 5-HT$_4$ receptors leads to the closure of a population of K$_{Ca}$-channels and thus a reduction in action potential after-hyperpolarization (Nicoll, 1988).

In this scheme, 5-HT has an interesting position in that it simultaneously increases current through the ligand-gated channels while decreasing current flow through K$_{Ca}$-channels (Fig. 9.4; Colino & Halliwell, 1987). The opposite pathway in which one transmitter influences

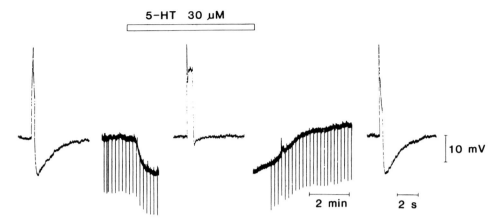

5-HT   30 μM

10 mV

2 min   2 s

Fig. 9.4. Modulation of two K-channels in a rat hippocampal CA1 neurone *in vitro* by 5-HT. Intracellular recording from a slice preparation showing that 5-HT hyperpolarized the membrane potential (via an increase in K-conductance) and also decreased action potential after hyperpolarization (via a decrease in Ca-dependent K-current). Downward deflections recorded at slow speed resulted from injection of brief current pulses to monitor membrane resistance. (P. Van Den Hooff & M. Galvan, unpublished.)

several K-channel types (Fig. 9.3), has been termed divergence (Nicoll, 1988).

ATP-sensitive K-channels (K_{ATP})

Neuronal-binding sites

Potassium channels regulated by intracellular levels of ATP (K_{ATP}) were first described in cardiac muscle by Noma (1983). These channels are open under conditions of low intracellular ATP and close as the concentration of this purine nucleotide rises. A physiological role for K_{ATP}-channels has been demonstrated in the insulin-secreting, pancreatic β-cells, where uptake of glucose leads to enhanced formation of ATP and closure of the ATP-sensitive channels (Petersen & Findlay, 1987; Ashcroft, 1988). The resulting depolarization elicits action potentials and initiates insulin secretion. A major discovery in this field was that many hypoglycaemic drugs, typified by the sulphonylureas, block these channels from the extracellular space (Sturgess *et al.*, 1985, Ashcroft, 1988; de-Weille *et al.*, 1989).

In recent years K_{ATP}-channels have been characterized in a number of other tissues, primarily in cardiac muscle (Noma, 1983; Sanguinetti *et al.*, 1988). By employing sulphonylurea binding to define potential ATP-coupled channels a substantial amount of evidence has also accumulated that such channels are present in neurones, particularly in the central nervous system. Kaubisch *et al.* (1982) described the presence of specific receptors for sulphonylureas in the brain by employing [^{3}H]-gliquidone as a radioligand. Saturable, specific binding was observed with a K_D of about 0.1 nM. In addition, these binding experiments demonstrated a rough correlation between the K_D of several sulphonylureas (glibenclamide, tolbutamide and chlorpropramide) and their clinical dosage. Although no physiological role of these binding sites (receptors) was postulated, the authors correctly pointed out that compounds yet to be shown to have a function in the brain can exhibit high affinity for neuronal membranes (Kaubisch *et al.*, 1982). A brief review of some possible physiological and pathological roles of neuronal K_{ATP}-channels has been published by Miller (1990).

An extensive study of the structure–activity relationship of the sulphonylurea binding sites in brain membranes was reported by Geisen *et al.* (1985). These authors introduced [^{3}H]-glibenclamide as a radioligand, which has continued to be widely used in such studies. An excellent correlation between the inhibition of [^{3}H]-glibenclamide binding to membranes from rat cerebral cortex and hypoglycaemic activity in rabbits was reported (Geisen *et al.*, 1985). Lupo and Bataille (1987) also published quantitative structure–activity data obtained using [^{3}H]-glipizide as the ligand. In addition, they further characterized the binding sites as being susceptible to proteolytic and lipolytic enzymes, suggesting a lipoprotein nature of the acceptor site. Competition binding experiments demonstrated that diazepam, nitrazepam, verapamil, nifedipine and quinine only reduced [^{3}H]-glipizide binding to brain membranes at high concentrations ($IC_{50} \geqslant 100\,\mu M$; Lupo & Bataille, 1987). Finally, they reported that glipizide did not modify adenylate cyclase activity; however the sulphonylureas gliquidone, glibenclamide and glipizide had an inhibitory effect on a crude fraction of cAMP-dependent phosphodiesterase. IC_{50} values were in the range 10–100 μM, and this effect should not be forgotten when interpreting experiments in which high (μM) concentrations of sulphonylureas are used to block certain pharmacological or physiological effects (see below).

Bernardi *et al.* (1988) reported a method for the purification of the [^{3}H]-glibenclamide-binding protein extracted from pig brain microsomes. After solubilization with digitonin, a four-step purification resulted in a 2500-fold concentration of the binding protein. Polyacrylamide gel electrophoresis or direct photoaffinity labelling of the receptor with [^{3}H]-glibenclamide showed that the sulphonylurea binding entity was composed of a single polypeptide chain with a molecular weight of about 150 000 (Bernardi *et al.*, 1988). An endogenous peptide ligand for the central sulphonylurea receptor has also been proposed to exist (Virsolvy-Vergine *et al.*, 1988); however, this report awaits confirmation.

Finally, Mourre *et al.* (1989, 1990) have mapped the distribution of sulphonylurea binding sites in the rat brain using autoradiographic techniques. [^{3}H]-glibenclamide binding sites were shown to be located throughout the brain, however, the pyramidal and extrapyramidal motor systems contained particularly high concentrations. The five structures with the highest density of binding were the substantia nigra, the globus and ventral pallidus, the motor neocortex and the molecular layer of the cerebellar cortex. Other motor regions and most sensory areas exhibited intermediate binding, the hypothalamic nuclei, the reticular formation and the medulla oblongata showed few binding sites. In contrast, the limbic system was rich in sites, particularly, the septohippocampal nucleus and the CA3 region of the hippocampus. Specific binding was reported to be undetectable in nerve fibres and cultured astrocytes. A reduction in glibenclamide receptor binding in rat brain (particularly in the hippocampus) was observed following transient forebrain ischaemia (Mourre *et al.*, 1990).

Iodinated glibenclamide was used by Gehlert *et al.* (1990) to detect sulphonylurea receptors autoradiographically in slices of rat brain. Since the iodine emissions are not quenched by white matter, a slightly different distribution to that reported by Mourre *et al.* (1989) was found. The highest levels of binding were in the globus pallidus followed by the substantia nigra and the molecular layer of the cerebellum. Several other brain regions were noted to exhibit a high density of binding sites, including the caudate–putamen, nucleus accumbens, interpenduncular nucleus, olfactory tubercle and cerebral cortex. Significant levels of binding were seen in the white fibres of the corpus callosum and the cerebellum (Gehlert *et al.*, 1990). Thus sulphonylurea sites appear to be located in soma and axonal regions of neurones.

Involvement in seizure-related phenomena

Alzheimer and ten Bruggencate (1988) first described the finding that cromakalim could decrease neuronal excitability in hippocampal brain slices and reduce epileptiform discharges. Intra- and extracellular recordings (Fig. 9.5A, B) revealed a reduction in synaptic potentials and a reduction in pacemaker activity of CA3 pyramidal neurones. However, the concentrations of cromakalim employed in this study (30–300 μM) are an order of magnitude higher than those required to produce effects in smooth muscle (Hamilton *et al.*, 1986; Standen *et al.*, 1989). More detailed voltage-clamp experiments indicated that these high concentrations produced a small (about 4 mV) hyperpolarization of the resting membrane potential, possibly via the activation of K_{IR} (Alzheimer *et al.*, 1989a). This action was shown to resemble that of adenosine (Alzheimer *et al.*, 1989b), which also activates K_{IR} (albeit via specific receptors). The conclusion from these studies was that cromakalim has weak effects on K-channels in hippocampal

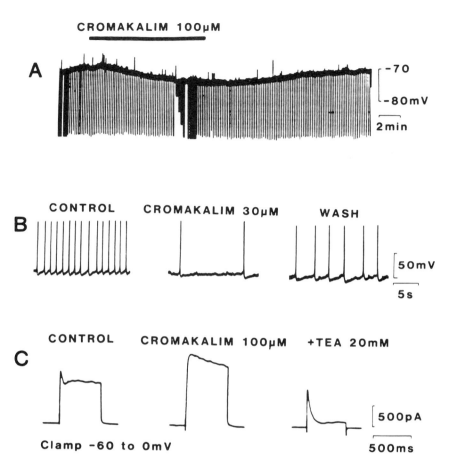

Fig. 9.5. Some actions of cromakalim on rat hippocampal neurones in slice preparations *in vitro* (A and B) and in culture (C). A, Chart record of the membrane potential of a CA3 neurone in the absence and presence of 100 μM cromakalim
(application period indicated by the bar). Action potentials were blocked by the
addition of 0.6 μmol/l TTX to the bathing solution. The downward deflections
represent voltage deviations produced by hyperpolarizing current pulses (300 ms,
0.2 nA) injected at a frequency of 0.1 Hz in order to monitor membrane resistance.
In this neurone, cromakalim hyperpolarized the membrane potential by 4 mV and
decreased membrane resistance by 10 MΩ. B, Effects of cromakalim upon spontaneous discharges recorded in a CA3 neurone before, during and after addition of
30 μM cromakalim to the bath solution. C, Tetraethylammonium blocks the outward
current increased by cromakalim (100 μM). Traces show current records obtained
with 500 ms voltage steps from −60 to 0 mV. TEA (20 mM) substantially reduces
the total sustained outward current during the continuous superfusion of cromakalim while the transient outward current is spared. (A, from Alzheimer *et al.*
(1989a); B, from Alzheimer & ten Bruggencate (1988); C, from Politi *et al.* (1989);
all with permission.)

Table 9.1. Anti-seizure effects of K-channel openers.

| Treatment (i.c.v.) | Frequency of seizures/min | | |
	MCD (0.15)	(nmol, i.c.v.) DTX (0.08)	4-AP (100)
Control	0.5	0.4	0.5
Vehicle	0.3	0.2	0.6
BRL 38227 100 nmol	0	0.3	0.2
RP 49356 10 nmol	0	0.4	0.9
RP 61419 10 nmol	0	0.4	0.9

Anti-seizure effects of novel K-channel opening drugs. The mean frequency of induced-crisis occurrence during 10 min after the first generalized seizures are given per min. A value of 1 indicates continuous seizures; absence of seizures is indicated by 0. Control rats were i.c.v.-injected with K-channel blocker alone. Vehicle-treated rats received vehicle injection prior to K-channel blocker administration. For each given dose, there was no significant difference in seizure frequencies between control, vehicle rats and cases when K-channel openers failed to prevent induced seizures. Mast cell degranulating peptide (MCD) seizures were prevented by BRL 38227 at a dose of 10 nmol given i.c.v. 15–20 min prior to MCD injection. Complete or almost complete prevention of MCD-induced (but not dendrotoxin, DTX, and 4-AP-induced) seizures were also seen with RP 49356 and RP 61419. Five control rats were investigated and six rats per group were treated with vehicle or drug. (Reproduced after modifications from Gandolfo *et al.* (1989b) with kind permission of the authors and the publishers.)

neurones resulting in an inhibition of cell firing. It remains to be excluded that cromakalim (at high concentrations) has an agonist action at adenosine A_1, $GABA_B$ or even $5-HT_{1A}$ receptors, all of which are coupled to a K_{IR}-channel (Nicoll, 1988).

Politi *et al.* (1989) investigated the effects of cromakalim on cultured hippocampal neurones. The results of their experiments confirm that the compound increases K-current under voltage-clamp conditions. However, in contrast to Alzheimer *et al.* (1989a,b), they found that cromakalim increased a sustained outward current activated by depolarization (Fig. 9.5C). This may be a delayed rectifier current, since it was blocked by TEA. The $I_{K(A)}$ was not affected by cromakalim (see Fig. 4B in Politi *et al.*, 1989). Once again these effects were observed during perfusion with high concentrations (10–500 μM) of the compound; the EC_{50} was given as 40 μM; (Politi *et al.*, 1989).

Evidence for anti-epileptic effects of K-channel openers stems from the experiments of Gandolfo *et al.* (1989a–c). Seizures resulting from the central administration of mast cell degranulating peptide (MCD) were inhibited by prior central administration of BRL 38227, RP 49356 or RP 61419 (Table 9.1). The action of the racemate cromakalim was stereo-specific: the (+)-enantiomer (BRL 38227) being inactive at doses at which the (−)-enantiomer (BRL 38227) was effective (Gandolfo *et al.*, 1989a).

Interestingly, these authors subsequently reported that the anti-epileptic effect of these three compounds was restricted to seizures induced by MCD. Apparently similar seizures elicited by 4-AP or dendrotoxin were unaffected by the three above-mentioned channel openers (see Table 9.1; Gandolfo et al., 1989b). Finally, spontaneously occurring seizures in genetically epileptic rats were also reduced by administration of BRL 38227 into the lateral ventricle (Gandolfo et al., 1989c).

Involvement in cerebral hypoxia and neuronal death

Evidence has accumulated within the last few years that K_{ATP}-channels may be involved in neurotoxic processes following cerebral hypoxia. It is, as yet, unclear whether this involvement is direct or whether it is simply that pharmacological interventions at K_{ATP} can influence the events taking place during and after the hypoxic insult. This situation is perhaps similar to that in smooth muscle, where Ca-antagonists are effective antihypertensive drugs, although there is little compelling evidence that a defect in Ca-channel function is the cause of hypertension. Nevertheless, there are at present two sets of evidence that K_{ATP} can modulate events taking place during or following hypoxic insult to brain tissue.

Abele and Miller (1990), working with cultured hippocampal neurones, demonstrated that neuronal death was increased 24 h after a 15 min exposure to a solution deficient in Mg^{2+} and supplemented with 0.1 μM glycine (Fig. 9.6). This procedure, which is thought to increase the synaptic activation of the N-methyl-D-aspartate (NMDA)-type glutamate receptors, resulted in large fluctuations in $[Ca^{2+}]_i$. Interestingly, both the increases in $[Ca^{2+}]_i$ and in cell death were inhibited by cromakalim (100 μM) or diazoxide (500 μM). These positive actions of the K-channel opening drugs were antagonized by glibenclamide (2 μM; Abele & Miller, 1990).

In a series of electrophysiological investigations, Ben Ari and associates have investigated the effects of anoxia (induced by superfusion with Krebs' solution gassed with 95% N_2/5% CO_2) on the properties of neurones in hippocampal slices (Ben Ari, 1989a,b, 1990; Ben Ari & Krnjević, 1989; Ben Ari & Lazdunski, 1989; Krnjević & Ben Ari, 1989; Ben Ari et al., 1990; see also Grigg & Anderson, 1989; Mourre et al., 1989). In summary, it was shown that brief (several minutes) periods of anoxia induced a depolarization of hippocampal CA3 neurones, which was followed by a postanoxic hyperpolarization. The hyperpolarization was probably due to activation of a Na^+/K^+ pump. The depolarization was often accompanied by increases in spontaneous synaptic activity leading to action potentials (Ben Ari, 1989b, 1990; Ben Ari & Lazdunski, 1989). In tetrodotoxin (TTX) containing solution, a postsynaptic hyperpolarization replaces the initial depolarization (Ben Ari, 1990).

Other experiments indicated that the anoxia-induced depolarization

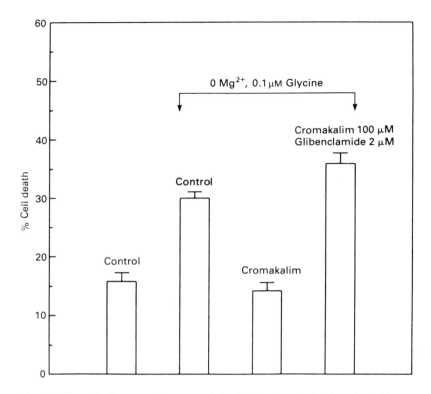

Fig. 9.6. Cromakalim prevents neuronal death. Treatment of cultured rat hippocampal pyramidal neurones with Mg^{2+}-free/glycine supplemented conditions ($-Mg/$ +Glycine) increased the number of dead cells compared with control conditions with Mg^{2+} present and without added glycine control. The effects of $-Mg/$ +Glycine were reversed by treatment with cromakalim (100 μM) and the effect of cromakalim was blocked by glibenclamide. Data represent the mean and SEM for between three and 12 separate experiments. Each separate experiment was performed in triplicate. (Reproduced from Abele & Miller (1990) with permission.)

was prevented by prior application of K_{ATP}-channel openers, such as galanin (1–5 μM; Fig. 9.7A, B; Ben Ari, 1989a), diazoxide (0.87 mM; Ben Ari & Krnjević, 1989) or somatostatin (1 μM; Ben Ari *et al.*, 1990). In contrast, the depolarization and associated increase in action potential activity was seemingly increased by glibenclamide (1–5 μM; Fig. 9.7C, D; Ben Ari, 1989a,b, 1990; Ben Ari & Lazdunski, 1989). The depolarization was blocked in the presence of the non-specific glutamate receptor antagonist kynurenate (Fig. 9.7E; Ben Ari, 1989a,b, 1990; Ben Ari & Lazdunski, 1989). The nature of the hypoxia-induced hyperpolarization (better seen in the presence of TTX) and its modulation by K_{ATP}-channel openers and blockers is, as yet, unclear.

Figure 9.8 presents a hypothetical scheme of events, which could

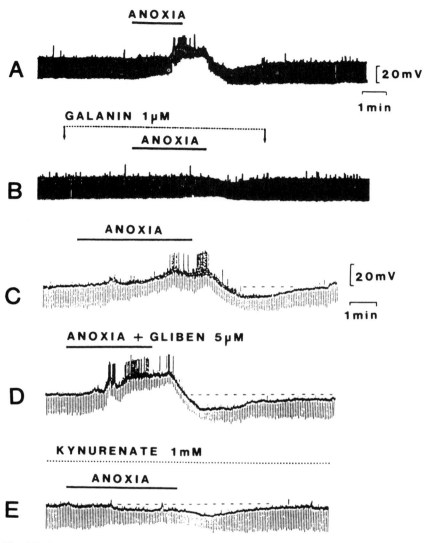

Fig. 9.7. A, Galanin blocks the effects of anoxia. Anoxia produced depolarization
and postanoxic hyperpolarization of a rat CA3 hippocampal neurone in a slice
preparation. B, Galanin (1 μM), which had no effect in oxygenated artificial cerebro-
spinal fluid (ACSF), fully blocked the anoxic response in oxygen deficient ACSF.
C–E, Kynurenate blocks glibenclamide-induced increase in the anoxic
depolarization. In control ACSF, anoxia (4 min, C) induced a depolarization;
reoxygenation was accompanied by a hyperpolarization. Bath-application of glibenclamide (GLIBEN, 5 μM, D) in the oxygen-deprived ACSF, augmented the anoxic
depolarization. Bath-application of kynurenate (1 mM, E) blocked the anoxic
depolarization indicating that this was mediated by glutamate. In the presence of
kynurenate, anoxia induced a hyperpolarization which was masked in control
ACSF by the anoxic depolarization. (A and B, from Ben Ari & Lazdunski (1989)
with permission. C–E, from Ben Ari (1990) with permission.)

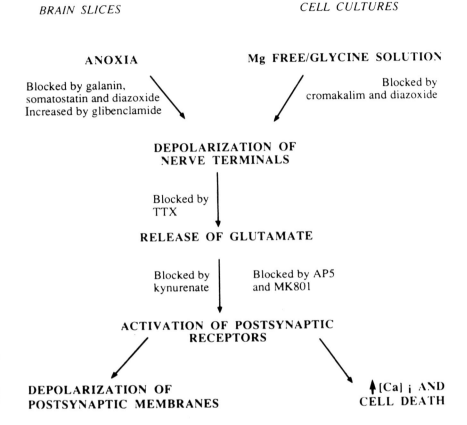

Fig. 9.8. Possible relationship between ATP-coupled channels, neurotoxic insult and cell death based on the data of Ben-Ari and co-workers (1989, 1990) and Abele and Miller (1990). Anoxia (elicited in CA3 neurones in rat hippocampal slices *in vitro*) or Mg-free/glycine-supplemented solution (in cultures of rat hippocampal pyramidal cells) may lead to depolarization of nerve terminals resulting in the release of glutamate. Activation of postsynaptic glutamate receptors leads to depolarization of postsynaptic membranes, an increase in $[Ca^{2+}]_i$ and perhaps thus to cell death. The postulated site of agonist and antagonist action is indicated by the position of the relevant compound name next to the arrows.

account for the results of both Ben Ari and coworkers and those of Abele and Miller (1990). Hypoxia or Mg^{2+}-free, glycine supplemented solution leads to action potential discharges in presynaptic nerve terminals. The resulting release of glutamate depolarizes postsynaptic membranes, increases intracellular Ca^{2+} and accelerates cell death. The initial (unknown) process in the nerve terminals is facilitated by sulphonylureas and blocked by K_{ATP}-channel openers. Action potential-dependent release of glutamate is blocked by TTX and finally, the postsynaptic action of glutamate is blocked by kynurenate, MK801 (dizocilpine) or 2-amino-5-phos-phonopentanoic acid (AP5). It remains to be seen if this sequence of events can be proven to be of physiological or pathological significance. However, it does appear that there may be a chance to pharmacologically influence the consequences of brain hypoxia and perhaps also of stroke, via K_{ATP}-channels.

Involvement in the substantia nigra

Following the demonstration by Mourre *et al.* (1989) that the substantia nigra contained the highest level of sulphonylurea-binding sites (K_{ATP}-channels?) in the rat central nervous system, Lazdunski and his colleagues (Amoroso *et al.*, 1990; Schmid-Antomarchi *et al.*, 1990) have systematic-ally explored the possible physiological and pathological roles of these channels. In an elegant series of publications they have presented several explanations for pathological phenomena, which may have a large impact on future therapeutic strategies.

Amoroso *et al.* (1990) and Schmid-Antomarchi *et al.* (1990) described the role of K_{ATP} in neurosecretion in the substantia nigra. [^{3}H]-GABA could be released by stimuli which led to closure of neuronal K_{ATP}-channels, such as increasing glucose or addition of sulphonylureas. On the other hand, stimuli which open K_{ATP} increased the efflux of $^{86}Rb^+$. Such stimuli included the K-channel openers cromakalim, pinacidil and nicorandil as well as oligomycin, 2-deoxyglucose and temporary anoxia. These latter effects were blocked by 100 nM gliquidone (Fig. 9.9). In their discussion, these authors propose that there is an intimate link between plasma glucose, GABA-mediated neurotransmission, cerebral ischaemia and the development of seizures (Amoroso *et al.*, 1990). One conclusion is that seizures in hypoglycaemic diabetic patients may result from a decrease in GABA release from substantia nigra nerve terminals due to the opening of K_{ATP}. Interestingly, it appears that the K_{ATP}-channels in the substantia nigra differ from those potassium channels interacting with K-channel openers in smooth muscle, since the K-channel openers showed a different order of potency in the nigra than in smooth muscle (Table 9.2). These drugs were also active at far lower concentrations than those required to open vascular K channels (Schmid-Antomarchi *et al.*, 1990).

Electrophysiological experiments on acutely-dissociated neurones from guinea-pig substantia nigra confirm the important role of K_{ATP}-channels in sculpting neuronal responses (Roeper *et al.*, 1990a). These authors showed that the membrane hyperpolarizations induced by activation of $GABA_B$ receptors (Fig. 9.10A) or dopamine-2 (D_2) receptors (Fig. 9.10B) are reversed by 100 μM tolbutamide, a blocker of K_{ATP}-channels. Thus these experiments demonstrate that ligand-gated K-channels can be

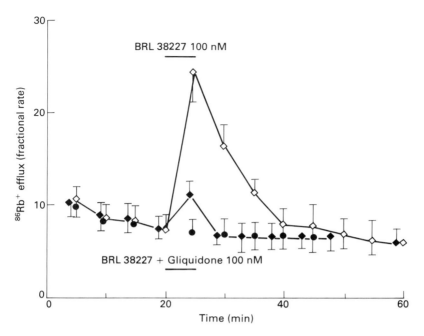

Fig. 9.9. Kinetics of $^{86}Rb^+$-efflux evoked by BRL 38227 in substantia nigra slices. Kinetics of $^{86}Rb^+$-efflux without ($\bullet$) or with ($\diamondsuit$, $\blacklozenge$) 100 nM ($-$)-cromakalim and in the absence ($\diamondsuit$) or presence ($\blacklozenge$) of 100 nM gliquidone. Horizontal bars represent the period of application of the effectors ($n = 5$). In experiments in which both BRL 38227 and gliquidone are used, the two drugs are added at the same time. (From Schmid-Antomarchi *et al.* (1990) with permission.)

Table 9.2. Effects of K-channel openers on $^{86}Rb^+$-efflux rates.

Compound	Substantia nigra $EC_{50\%}$ (nM)	Portal vein $EC_{15\%}$ (nM)
BRL 38227	10	500
Nicorandil	100	100 000
Pinacidil	400	5000

Approximate potencies of BRL 38227, nicorandil and pinacidil for the stimulation of $^{86}Rb^+$-efflux from rat substantia nigra slices or rat portal vein segments. The values for substantia nigra were obtained from full concentration–response curves; $EC_{50\%}$ is the concentration required to produce half-maximal stimulation. The data for portal vein were obtained from partial concentration–response curves; $EC_{15\%}$ is the concentration required to increase efflux rate by 15%. (Data from Schmid-Antomarchi *et al.*, 1990 and Cook & Quast, 1990.)

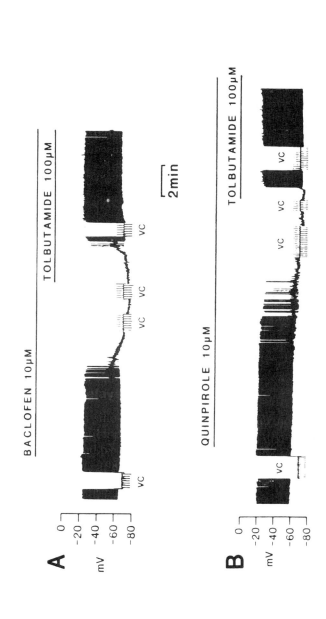

Fig. 9.10. Membrane potential of two guinea-pig isolated substantia nigra neurones recorded with the perforated patch technique. The cells were held under current-clamp control, except during the intervals marked VC when they were voltage-clamped to a potential of −70 and ±10 mV, 200 ms pulses were applied every 2 s. 10 μM baclofen, 10 μM quinpirole and 100 μM tolbutamide were added to the bath as indicated. Series resistance: A, 20 MΩ, and B, 16 MΩ; capacitance: A, 14 pF, and B, 18 pF. (From Roeper *et al.* (1990a) with permission.)

blocked by hypoglycaemic drugs. It is therefore likely that $GABA_B$- and D_2-receptors are linked to K_{ATP}-channels in this brain area. Furthermore, removal of glucose from the superfusate hyperpolarized substantia nigra neurones and decreased input resistance; these effects were abolished by tolbutamide (Roeper et al., 1990b). Patch-clamp experiments confirmed the presence of K_{ATP} in these cells (Roeper et al., 1990c).

In conclusion, there is an expanding body of experimental data supporting a role of K_{ATP}-channels in the functioning of substantia nigra neurones. Correct pharmacological manipulation of neurotransmission in this brain area could lead to significant advances in the understanding and treatment of Parkinson's disease, extrapyramidal motor disorders and some forms of seizure discharges.

Involvement in the hypothalamus

The central regulation of food intake involves hypothalamic neurones (Morley, 1980) and electrophysiological studies have shown that some of the neurones in this brain area are excited by increases in the extracellular glucose concentration (Ono et al., 1982; Minami et al., 1986). Several types of glucose-responsive neurones have been characterized (Minami et al., 1986): the so-called glucose-sensitive neurones exhibit decreases in action potential activity when glucose is applied (Oomura et al., 1974). The glucoreceptor neurones increase in activity during glucose application (Oomura et al., 1969). A similar pattern of changes has been observed in neurones in the rat nucleus tractus solitarius (Mizuno & Oomura, 1984).

More recent experiments indicate that K_{ATP}-channels are present in rat hypothalamic neurones and that they are involved in glucose-induced cell excitation (Ashford et al., 1989, 1990a–c; Boden et al., 1989). Interestingly, the pharmacology of these channels does not appear to be identical to that of the channels in pancreatic β-cells. Tolbutamide depolarized hypothalamic neurones and increased membrane resistance whereas glibenclamide (10–500 nM) had no effect on membrane properties. Prior application of glibenclamide blocked the effects of tolbutamide (Boden et al., 1989; Ashford et al., 1990a,c). Furthermore, patch-clamp experiments indicate that sulphonylureas may not directly block hypothalamic K_{ATP}-channels since the activity of single channels in inside-out patches was not affected by tolbutamide or glibenclamide (Ashford et al., 1990a,c). Similar observations were made on membrane patches excised from rat cultured cerebral cortex neurones (Ashford et al., 1990c).

Other central actions

Two types of ATP-sensitive K-channel were detected in single channel recordings from rat cultured cortical neurones (Ashford et al., 1988). One type was conventional in nature and blocked by cytoplasmic ATP, whereas the other showed an increase in open-state probability during application of ATP. A third type of ATP-sensitive channel was also observed. Preliminary experiments suggested that channels are also present in cerebellar neurones (Ashford et al., 1988).

Further evidence supporting a role of ATP-coupled K-channels in neuronal function is the finding that cromakalim can attenuate a behavioural response in mice elicited by administration of pilocarpine. Pilocarpine induces so-called 'purposeless chewing' by stimulating muscarinic receptors in the brain; this was reduced by i.p. or i.c.v. cromakalim indicating an interaction with muscarinic systems (Tricklebank et al., 1988).

A recent report (Ocana et al., 1990) presents experimental evidence that glibenclamide (10–40 μg, i.c.v.) antagonized morphine analgesia in mice; TEA or quinine, in similar doses, were without effect. It has previously been reported that glucose and insulin can modulate the analgesic effects of morphine (Singh et al., 1983).

Clinical uses of K-channel blockers

Finally, the question remains as to exactly which diseases are implicated in K-channel dysfunction and which diseases are not in themselves caused by channel dysfunction but may respond to therapeutic modification of K-channel activity. The largest body of evidence for K-channel dysfunction in a human disease is in epilepsy. Since this word embodies a whole range of diseases characterized by seizures and/or transient psychomotor disturbances, the discussion should, at first, be cautiously restricted to grand mal seizures, as this is the type most often studied in animal experiments.

4-Aminopyridine is a potent seizure-inducing agent, which has a well-documented blocking action on various K-channels (Hermann & Gorman, 1981; Galvan, 1982; Gustafsson et al., 1982; Thompson, 1982; Segal et al., 1984). Accidental poisoning of humans with this compound as well as its use in the treatment of humans suffering from botulinum toxin poisoning has been reported to induce grand mal-type seizures (Ball et al., 1979; Spyker et al., 1980). A variety of other potent K-channel blockers, such as apamin, MCD and dendrotoxin also provoke seizures in vivo and in vitro (Dreyer, 1990 for review). 4-Aminopyridine-induced seizures are characterized electrophysiologically by high frequency neuronal discharging, bursts of action potentials and prolongations of somatic and axonal action potentials (Baranyi & Fehér, 1979; Szente & Pongrácz, 1981; Galvan et al., 1982; Galvan et al., 1984). Voltage-clamp experiments demonstrated direct block of one or more types of K-channels (Thompson, 1977, 1982; Galvan, 1982; Gustafson et al., 1982).

In addition to the large body of evidence implicating inhibition of K-channels in the action of convulsant drugs, there are also some reports that anti-epileptic drugs can increase K-currents (e.g. Van Erp *et al.*, 1990; Zona *et al.*, 1990). Often such studies employed high concentrations and thus a question mark hangs over their significance. It should, however, be remembered that the mechanism of action of the 'classical' anti-epileptics is far from clear (Macdonald & McLean. 1986).

Based on this close link between K-channel dysfunction and seizure discharges, it is reasonably logical to propose that increasing the opening of certain types of K-channel could have anti-epileptic effects. This is, in terms of the number of patients affected, by far the most interesting area for development.

Interestingly, 4-AP has also been used postoperatively in Bulgaria to reverse the actions of curare (Paskov *et al.*, 1973; *see also* Booij *et al.*, 1978; Miller *et al.*, 1979). Although this compound is not significantly better than the usual anticholinesterase therapy, 4-AP potentiates the effects of the anticholinesterases. Therefore a combination of drugs, using lower doses of anticholinesterase than would otherwise be necessary, can be successfully employed.

Defects in neurotransmitter release, particularly at the neuromuscular junction could also respond to treatment with K-channel blockers. Several clinical trials of 4-AP have been reported on patients with such diseases with limited success (Elmquist & Lambert, 1968; Lundh *et al.*, 1979; Kim *et al.*, 1980). It is obvious to all parties involved that 4-AP is a poor first choice to test such a theory. 4-Aminopyridine and guanidine have been employed in humans suffering from the Eaton–Lambert syndrome. While guanidine has a rather toxic profile, 4-AP was an effective treatment, at least in the short-term trials published (Lundh *et al.*, 1977; Agoston *et al.*, 1978; Murray & Newsom-Davies, 1981).

As mentioned above, 4-AP was administered to patients suffering from botulinum toxin poisoning during the 'Birmingham outbreak' (Ball *et al.*, 1979). Despite severe side-effects and even convulsions, the authors came to the conclusion that, at that time, therapy with 4-AP was superior to other available substances in this fortunately rare, but life-threatening situation.

Demyelinating disease is associated with membrane channel defects and 4-AP improves axonal action potential conduction in demyelinated nerve fibres (Sherratt *et al.*, 1980). 4-Aminopyridine has also been tested in Huntingdon's chorea with disappointing results (Wesseling & Lakke, 1980; Uges, 1982). Lastly, 4-AP can dramatically reduce the recovery time following ketamine–diazepam anaesthesia (Martinez-Aguirre & Crul, 1979; Agoston *et al.*, 1980, 1982).

Regardless of the results of these various clinical trials, the reader is recommended to this literature as it forms the best account of the side effects and acute human toxicology of K-channel blockers. Clearly, safer compounds must be found to reappraise these potential therapeutic goals.

Conclusions

The pharmacological manipulation of neuronal K-channels as part of a rational therapy of human neurological disorders remains a target for the future. The basic sciences of physiology and pharmacology have success-fully disclosed the properties and functions of the various channel types. It is now up to medicinal chemists and clinical pharmacologists to charac-terize and develop novel K-channel modulating drugs for the treatment of, at present, therapy-resistant central and peripheral nervous system disorders.

Acknowledgements

I wish to thank the Deutsche Forschungs Gemeinschaft (Germany), the National Institute of Health (USA) and the Medical Research Council (UK) for generously supporting much of the research in which I was involved during the past years. In addition I would like to express my gratitude to Professors Paul Adams and David Brown and to Dr Andy Constanti for introducing me to voltage-clamp techniques and patiently discussing many of the problems and concepts described here. Finally, my thanks go to Dr Robert Miller for his helpful criticism of the manuscript.

References

Abele, A. E. & Miller, R. J. (1990) Potassium channel activators abolish excitotoxicity in cultured hippocampal pyramidal neurons. *Neuroscience Letters* **115**, 195–200.
Adams, P. R. & Galvan, M. (1986) Voltage-dependent currents of vertebrate neurons and their role in membrane excitability. In Delgado-Escueta, A. V., Ward, A. A. Jr, Woodbury, D. M. & Porter, R. J. (eds) *Advances in Neurology*, Vol. 44. Raven Press, New York, pp. 137–170.
Adams, P. R., Brown, D. A. & Constanti, A. (1982a) M-currents and other potassium currents in bullfrog sympathetic neurones. *Journal of Physiology* **330**, 537–572.
Adams, P. R., Brown, D. A. & Constanti, A. (1982b) Pharmacological inhibition of the M-current. *Journal of Physiology* **332**, 223–262.
Adams, P. R., Constanti, A., Brown, D. A. & Clark, R. B. (1982c) Intracellular Ca^{2+} activates a fast voltage-sensitive K^+ current in vertebrate sympathetic neurones. *Nature* **246**, 746–749.
Aghajanian, G. K. (1985) Modulation of transient outward current in serotonergic neurons by alpha$_1$-adrenoceptors. *Nature* **315**, 501–503.
Agoston, S., Salt, P. J., Erdmann, T., Hilkemeijer, T., Bencini, A. & Langrehr, D. (1980) Antagonism of ketamine–diazepam anaesthesia by 4-aminopyridine in human volunteers. *British Journal of Anaesthesia* **32**, 367–370.
Agoston, S., Uges, D. R. A. & Sia, R. L. (1982) Therapeutic applications of 4-amino-pyridine in anaesthesia. In: Lechat, P., Thesleff, S. & Bowman, W. C. (eds) *Amino-pyridines and Similarly Acting Drugs: Effects on Nerves, Muscles and Synapses*. Pergamon Press, Oxford, pp. 303–311.

Agoston, S., van Weerden, T., Westra, P. & Broekert, A. (1978) Effects of 4-amino-pyridine in Eaton–Lambert syndrome. *British Journal of Anaesthesia* **50**, 383–385.

Alzheimer, C. & ten Bruggencate, G. (1988) Actions of BRL 34915 (cromakalim) upon convulsive discharges in guinea pig hippocampal slices. *Naunyn-Schmiedeberg's Archives of Pharmacology* **337**, 429–434.

Alzheimer, C., Sutor, B. & ten Bruggencate, G. (1989a) Effects of cromakalim (BRL 34915) on potassium conductances in CA3 neurones of the guinea-pig hippocampus *in vitro*. *Naunyn-Schmiedeberg's Archives of Pharmacology* **340**, 465–471.

Alzheimer, C., Sutor, B. & ten Bruggencate, G. (1989b) Cromakalim (BRL 34915) acts on an inwardly-rectifying neuronal K^+ conductance, which is similar to that activated by adenosine. *Pflügers Archiv* **414** (Suppl. 1), S121–S122.

Amoroso, S., Schmid-Antomarchi, H., Fosset, M. & Lazdunski, M. (1990) Glucose, sulfonylureas, and neurotransmitter release: role of ATP-sensitive K^+ channels. *Science* **247**, 852–854.

Ashcroft, F. M. (1988) Adenosine, 5'-triphosphate-sensitive potassium channels. *Annual Review of Neuroscience* **11**, 97–118.

Ashcroft, S. J. & Ashcroft, F. M. (1990) Properties and functions of ATP-sensitive K-channels. *Cellular Signalling* **2**, 197–214.

Ashford, M. L. J., Boden, P. R. & Treherne, J. M. (1989) Glucose-induced excitation of rat hypothalamic neurones *in vitro* is mediated by ATP-sensitive K^+ channels. *Journal of Physiology* **415**, 31P.

Ashford, M. L. J., Boden, P. R. & Treherne, J. M. (1990a) Sulphonylurea excitation of dissociated glucose-responsive hypothalamic neurones in the rat. *Journal of Physiology* **420**, 93P.

Ashford, M. L. J., Boden, P. R. & Treherne, J. M. (1990b) Glucose-induced excitation of hypothalamic neurones is mediated by ATP-sensitive K^+ channels. *Pflügers Archiv* **415**, 479–483.

Ashford, M. L. J., Boden, P. R. & Treherne, J. M. (1990c) Tolbutamide excites rat glucoreceptive ventromedial hypothalamic neurones by indirect inhibition of ATP–K^+ channels. *British Journal of Pharmacology* **101**, 531–540.

Ashford, M. L. J., Sturgess, N. C., Trout, N. J., Gardner, N. J. & Hales, C. N. (1988) Adenosine-5'-triphosphate-sensitive ion channels in neonatal rat cultured central neurones. *Pflügers Archiv* **412**, 297–304.

Ball, A. P., Hopkinson, R. B., Farrell, I. D., Hutchinson, J. P. G., Paul, R., Watson, R. D. S., Page, A. J. F., Parker, R. G. F., Edwards, C. W., Snow, M., Scott, D. K., Leone-Ganado, A., Hastings, A., Ghosh, A. C. & Gilbert, R. J. (1979) Human botulism caused by botulinum type E: the Birmingham outbreak. *Quarterly Journal of Medicine* **191**, 473–491.

Baranyi, A. & Fehér, O. (1979) Convulsive effects of 3-aminopyridine on cortical neurones. *Electroencephalography and Clinical Neurophysiology* **47**, 745–751.

Barrett, E. F., Barrett, J. N. & Crill, W. E. (1980) Voltage-sensitive outward currents in cat motoneurones. *Journal of Physiology* **304**, 251–276.

Belluzzi, O., Sacchi, O. & Wanke, E. (1985a) A fast transient outward current in the rat sympathetic neurone studied under voltage clamp conditions. *Journal of Physiology* **358**, 91–108.

Belluzzi, O., Sacchi, O. & Wanke, E. (1985b) Identification of delayed potassium and calcium currents in the rat sympathetic neurone under voltage clamp. *Journal of Physiology* **358**, 109–129.

Ben Ari, Y. (1989a) Effects of galanin and glibenclamide on the anoxic response of rat hippocampal neurones *in vitro*. *Journal of Physiology* **415**, 78P.

Ben Ari, Y. (1989b) Effects of glibenclamide, a selective blocker of an ATP–K^+

channel, on the anoxic response of hippocampal neurones. *Pflügers Archiv* **414** (Suppl. 1), S111–S114.

Ben Ari, Y. (1990) Galanin and glibenclamide modulate the anoxic release of glutamate in rat CA3 hippocampal neurons. *European Journal of Neuroscience* **2**, 62–68.

Ben Ari, Y. & Krnjević, K. (1989) The ATP-sensitive K$^+$ channel opener diazoxide reduces anoxic depolarization in rat CA3 hippocampal neurones in isolated slices. *Journal of Physiology* **418**, 192P.

Ben Ari, Y. & Lazdunski, M. (1989) Galanin protects hippocampal neurons from the functional effects of anoxia. *European Journal of Pharmacology* **165**, 331–332.

Ben Ari, Y., Krnjević, K. & Crepel, V. (1990) Activators of ATP-sensitive K$^+$ channels reduce anoxic depolarization in CA3 hippocampal neurons. *Neuroscience* **37**, 55–60.

Bernardi, H., Fosset, M. & Lazdunski, M. (1988) Characterisation, purification, and affinity labelling of the brain [^{3}H] glibenclamide-binding protein, a putative neuronal ATP-regulated K$^+$ channel. *Proceedings of the National Academy of Sciences USA* **85**, 9816–9820.

Blatz, A. L. & Magelby, K. L. (1987) Calcium-activated potassium channels. *Trends in Neurosciences* **10**, 463–467.

Boden, P., Ashford, L. J. & Treherne, J. M. (1989) Actions of sulphonylureas on neurones of rat ventromedial hypothalamus *in vitro*. *British Journal of Pharmacology* **98**, 830P.

Booij, L. H. D. J., Miller, R. D. & Crul, J. F. (1978) Neostigmine and 4-aminopyridine antagonism of lincomycin–pancuronium neuromuscular blockade in man. *Anesthesia and Analgesia* **57**, 316–321.

Brennecke, R. & Lindeman, B. (1974) Design of a fast voltage clamp for biological membranes using discontinuous feedback. *Reviews of Scientific Instrumentation* **45**, 656–661.

Brown, D. A. (1988) M currents. In Narahashi, T. (ed.) *Ion Channels*, vol. 1. Plenum Publishing, New York, pp. 55–94.

Brown, D. A. (1990) G-proteins and potassium currents in neurons. *Annual Review of Physiology* **52**, 215–242.

Brown, D. A. & Adams, P. R. (1980) Muscarinic suppression of a novel voltage-sensitive K$^+$ current in a vertebrate neurone. *Nature* **283**, 673–676.

Brown, D. A. & Griffith, W. H. (1983) Calcium-activated outward current in voltage-clamped hippocampal neurones of the guinea-pig. *Journal of Physiology* **337**, 287–301.

Brown, D. A. & Selyanko, A. A. (1985) Membrane currents underlying the cholinergic slow excitatory post-synaptic potential in the rat sympathetic ganglion. *Journal of Physiology* **365**, 365–387.

Colino, A. & Halliwell, J. V. (1987) Differential modulation of three separate K-conductances in hippocampal CA1 neurons by serotonin. *Nature* **328**, 73–77.

Connor, J. A. & Stevens, C. F. (1971a) Voltage clamp studies of transient outward membrane current in a gastropod neural somata. *Journal of Physiology* **213**, 21–30.

Connor, J. A. & Stevens, C. F. (1971b) Prediction of repetitive firing behaviour from voltage clamp data on an isolated neurone soma. *Journal of Physiology* **213**, 31–53.

Constanti, A. & Brown, D. A. (1981) M-currents in voltage-clamped mammalian sympathetic neurones. *Neuroscience Letters* **24**, 289–294.

Constanti, A. & Galvan, M. (1983) Fast inward-rectifying current accounts for anomalous rectification in olfactory cortex neurones. *Journal of Physiology* **385**, 153–178.

Cook, N. S. (1988) The pharmacology of potassium channels and their therapeutic potential. *Trends in Pharmacological Sciences* **9**, 21–28.

Cook, N. S. & Quast, U. (1990) Potassium channel pharmacology. In Cook, N. S. (ed.) *Potassium Channels*. Ellis Horwood Ltd, Chichester, pp. 181–255.

Crépel, V., Krnjevic, K. & Ben-Ari, Y. (1992) Glibenclamide depresses the slowly inactivating outward current (I_D) in hippocampal neurons. *Canadian Journal of Physiology and Pharmacology* **70**, 306–307.

De Weille, J. R., Fosset, M., Mourre, C., Schmid-Antomarchi, H., Bernardi, H. & Lazdunski, M. (1989) Pharmacology and regulation of ATP-sensitive K$^+$ channels. *Pflügers Archiv* **414** (Suppl. 1), S80–S87.

Dreyer, F. (1990) Peptide toxins and potassium channels. *Reviews of Physiology, Biochemistry and Pharmacology* **115**, 93–136.

Elmquist, D. & Lambert, E. H. (1968) Detailed analysis of neuromuscular transmission in a patient with the myasthenic syndrome sometimes associated with bronchogenic carcinoma. *Mayo Clinic Proceedings* **43**, 689–713.

Gähwiler, B. H. & Brown, D. A. (1985) Functional innervation of cultured hippocampal neurones by cholinergic afferents from co-cultured septal explants. *Nature* **313**, 577–579.

Galvan, M. (1982) A transient outward current in rat sympathetic neurones. *Neuroscience Letters* **31**, 295–300.

Galvan, M. & Behrends, J. (1985) Apamin blocks calcium-dependent spike after-hyperpolarization in rat sympathetic neurones. *Pflügers Archiv* (Suppl. 403), R50.

Galvan, M. & Sedlmeir, C. (1984) Outward currents in voltage-clamped rat sympathetic neurones. *Journal of Physiology* **356**, 115–133.

Galvan, M., Grafe, P. & ten Bruggencate, G. (1982) Convulsant actions of 4-aminopyridine on the guinea-pig olfactory cortex slice. *Brain Research* **241**, 75–86.

Galvan, M., Franz, P. & Vogel-Wiens, C. (1984) Actions of potassium channel blockers on guinea-pig lateral olfactory tract axons. *Naunyn-Schmiedeberg's Archives of Pharmacology* **325**, 8–11.

Gandolfo, G., Gottesmann, C., Bidard, J-N. & Lazdunski, M. (1989a) K$^+$ channel openers prevent epilepsy induced by the bee venom peptide MCD. *European Journal of Pharmacology* **159**, 329–330.

Gandolfo, G., Gottesmann, C., Bidard, J-N. & Lazdunski, M. (1989b) Subtypes of K$^+$ channels differentiated by the effects of the K$^+$ channel openers upon K$^+$ channel blocker-induced seizures. *Brain Research* **495**, 189–192.

Gandolfo, G., Romettino, S., Gottesmann, C., van Luijtelaar, G., Coenen, A., Bidard, J-N. & Lazdunski, M. (1989c) K$^+$ channel openers decrease seizures in genetically epileptic rats. *European Journal of Pharmacology* **167**, 181–183.

Gehlert, D. R., Mais, D. E., Gackenheimer, S. L. Krushinski, J. H. & Robertson, D. W. (1990) Location of ATP sensitive potassium channels in the rat brain using a novel radioligand, [^{125}I]iodoglibenclamide. *European Journal of Pharmacology* **186**, 373–375.

Geisen, K., Hitzel, V., Okomonopoulos, R., Punter, J., Weyer, R. & Summ, H-D. (1985) Inhibition of ^{3}H-glibenclamide binding to sulphonylurea receptors by oral antidiabetics. *Arzneimittel-Forschung (Drug Research)* **35**, 707–712.

Grafe, P., Mayer, C. J. & Wood, J. (1980) Synaptic modulation of calcium-dependent potassium conductance in myenteric neurones in the guinea-pig. *Journal of Physiology* **305**, 235–248.

Grigg, J. J. & Anderson, E. G. (1989) Glucose and sulphonylureas modify different phases of the membrane potential change during hypoxia in rat hippocampal slices. *Brain Research* **489**, 302–310.

Gustafsson, B., Galvan, M., Grafe, P. & Wigstrom, H. (1982) A transient outward current in a mammalian central neurone blocked by 4-aminopyridine. *Nature* **299**, 252–254.

Hagiwara, S., Kusano, K. & Saito, N. (1961) Membrane changes of Onchidium nerve cells in potassium-rich media. *Journal of Physiology* **155**, 470–489.

Hagiwara, S., Yoshida, S. & Yoshii, M. (1981) Transient and delayed potassium currents in the egg cell membrane of the coelenterate, *Renilla koellikeri. Journal of Physiology* **318**, 123–141.

Halliwell, J. V. (1990) K$^+$ channels in the central nervous system. In Cook, N. S. (ed.), *Potassium Channels*. Ellis Horwood Ltd., Chichester, pp. 348–381.

Halliwell, J. V. & Adams, P. R. (1982) Voltage-clamp analysis of muscarinic excitation in hippocampal neurones. *Brain Research* **250**, 71–92.

Halliwell, J. V., Othman, I. B., Pelchan-Mathews, A. & Dolly, J. O. (1986) Central action of dendrotoxin: selective reduction of a transient K conductance in hippocampus and binding to localised receptors. *Proceedings of the National Academy of Sciences USA* **83**, 493–497.

Hamilton, T. C., Weir, S. W. & Weston, A. H. (1986) Comparison of the effects of BRL 34915 and verapamil on electrical and mechanical activity in rat portal vein. *British Journal of Pharmacology* **88**, 103–111.

Hermann, A. & Gorman, A. L. F. (1981) Effects of 4-aminopyridine on potassium currents in a molluscan neuron. *Journal of General Physiology* **78**, 63–86.

Hille, B. (1967) The selective inhibition of delayed potassium currents in nerve by tetraethylammonium ion. *Journal of General Physiology* **50**, 1287–1302.

Hodgkin, A. L. & Huxley, A. F. (1952) Currents carried by sodium and potassium through the membrane of the giant axon of *Loligo*. *Journal of Physiology* **116**, 449–472.

Kandel, E. R. & Tauc, L. (1966) Anomalous rectification in the metacerebral giant cells and its consequences for synaptic transmission. *Journal of Physiology* **183**, 287–304.

Kaubisch, N., Hammer, R., Wollheim, C., Renold, A. E. & Offord, R. E. (1982) Specific receptors for sulphonylureas in brain and in a β-cell tumor of the rat. *Biochemical Pharmacology* **31**, 1171–1174.

Kawai, T. & Watanabe, M. (1986) Blockade of Ca-activated K conductance by apamin in rat sympathetic neurones. *British Journal of Pharmacology* **87**, 225–232.

Kim, Y. I., Goldner, M. M. & Sanders, D. B. (1980) Facilitatory effects of 4-aminopyridine on neuromuscular transmission in disease states. *Muscle and Nerve* **3**, 112–119.

Kirsch, G. E. & Narahashi, T. (1978) 3,4-diaminopyridine. A potent new potassium channel blocker. *Biophysical Journal* **22**, 507–512.

Krnjević, K. & Ben Ari, Y. (1989) Anoxic changes in dentate granule cells. *Neuroscience Letters* **107**, 89–93.

Lancaster, B. & Adams, P. R. (1986) Calcium-dependent current generating the afterhyperpolarization of hippocampal neurons. *Journal of Neurophysiology* **55**, 1268–1282.

Latorre, R., Oberhauser, A., Labarca, P. & Alvarez, O. (1989) Varieties of calcium-activated potassium channels. *Annual Review of Physiology* **51**, 385–399.

Llinas, R. R. (1988) The intrinsic electrophysiological properties of mammalian neurons: insights into central nervous system function. *Science* **242**, 1654–1664.

Lundh, H., Nilsson, O. & Rosen, I. (1977) 4-aminopyridine—A new drug tested in the treatment of Eaton–Lambert syndrome. *Journal of Neurology, Neurosurgery and Psychiatry* **40**, 1109–1112.

Lundh, H., Nilsson, O. & Rosen, I. (1979) Effects of 4-aminopyridine in myasthenia gravis. *Journal of Neurology, Neurosurgery and Psychiatry* **42**, 171–175.

Lupo, B. & Bataille, D. (1987) A binding site for [^{3}H]glipizide in the rat cerebral cortex. *European Journal of Pharmacology* **140**, 157–169.

MacDermott, A. B. & Weight, F. F. (1982) Action potential repolarization may involve a transient Ca^{2+}-sensitive outward current in a vertebrate neurone. *Nature* **300**, 185–188.

Macdonald, R. L. & McLean, M. J. (1986) Anticonvulsant drugs: mechanisms of action. In Delgado-Escueta, A. V., Ward Jr, A. A., Woodbury, D. M. & Porter, R. J. (eds), *Advances in Neurology*, vol. 44. Raven Press, New York, pp. 713–736.

Madison, D. V., Lancaster, B. & Nicoll, R. A. (1987) Voltage-clamp analysis of cholinergic action in the hippocampus. *Journal of Neuroscience* **7**, 733–741.

Martinez-Aguirre, E. & Crul, J. F. (1979) Effect of tetrahydroaminoacridine and

4-aminopyridine on recovery from ketamine–diazepam anesthesia in the macacus rhesus monkey. *Acta Anaesthesiologica Belgica* **30**, 231–238.

Marty, A. (1983) Ca^{2+}-dependent K channels with large unitary conductance. *Trends in Neurosciences* **6**, 262–265.

Marty, A. (1989) The physiological role of calcium-dependent channels. *Trends in Neurosciences* **12**, 420–424.

Meech, R. W. & Standen, N. B. (1975) Potassium activation in *Helix aspersa* neurones under voltage clamp: a component mediated by calcium influx. *Journal of Physiology* **249**, 211–239.

Miller, R. D., Booij, L. H. D. J., Agoston, S. & Crul, J. F. (1979) 4-aminopyridine potentiates neostigmine and pyridostigmine in man. *Anesthesiology* **50**, 416–420.

Miller, R. J. (1990) Glucose-regulated potassium channels are sweet news for neurobiologists. *Trends in Neurosciences* **13**, 197–199.

Minami, T., Oomura, Y. & Sugimori, M. (1986) Electrophysiological properties and glucose responsiveness of guinea-pig ventromedial hypothalamic neurones *in vitro*. *Journal of Physiology* **380**, 127–143.

Mizuno, Y. & Oomura, Y. (1984) Glucose responding neurones in the nucleus tractus solitarius of the rat: *in vitro* study. *Brain Research* **307**, 109–116.

Moore, S. D., Madamba, S. G., Joels, M. & Siggins, G. R. (1988) Somatostatin augments the M-current in hippocampal neurons. *Science* **239**, 278–280.

Morley, J. E. (1980) The neuroendocrine control of appetite: the role of the endogenous opiates, cholecystokinin, TRH, gamma-aminobutyric-acid and the diazepam receptor. *Life Sciences* **27**, 355–368.

Mourre, C., Ben Ari, Y., Bernardi, H., Fosset, M & Lazdunski, M. (1989) Antidiabetic sulphonylureas: localization of binding sites in the brain and effects on the hyperpolarization induced by anoxia in hippocampal slices. *Brain Research* **486**, 159–164.

Mourre, C., Smith, M-J., Siesjo, B. K. & Lazdunski, M. (1990) Brain ischemia alters the density of binding sites for glibenclamide, a specific blocker of ATP-sensitive K^+ channels. *Brain Research* **526**, 147–152.

Murray, N. M. F. & Newsom-Davis, J. (1981) Treatment with oral 4-aminopyridine in disorders of neuromuscular transmission. *Neurology* **31**, 265–271.

Neher, E. (1971) Two fast transient current components during voltage clamp on snail neurones. *Journal of General Physiology* **58**, 36–53.

Nelson, P. G. & Frank, K. (1967) Anomalous rectification in cat spinal motoneurons and effects of polarizing currents on excitatory postsynaptic potentials. *Journal of Neurophysiology* **30**, 1097–1113.

Nicoll, R. A. (1988) The coupling of neurotransmitter receptors to ion channels in the brain. *Science* **241**, 545–551.

Nicoll, R. A., Malenka, R. C. & Kauer, J. A. (1990) Functional comparison of neurotransmitter receptor subtypes in mammalian central nervous system. *Physiological Reviews* **70**, 513–565.

Noble, D. (1984) The surprising heart: a review of recent progress in cardiac electrophysiology. *Journal of Physiology* **353**, 1–50.

Noma, A. (1983) ATP-regulated K^+ channels in cardiac muscle. *Nature* **305**, 147–148.

North, R. A. (1989) Drug receptors and the inhibition of nerve cells. *British Journal of Pharmacology* **98**, 13–28.

Numann, R. E., Wadman, W. J. & Wong, R. K. S. (1987) Outward currents of single hippocampal cells obtained from the adult guinea-pig. *Journal of Physiology* **393**, 331–353.

Ocana, M., Del Ponzo, E., Barrios, M., Robles, L. I. & Baeyens, J. M. (1990) An ATP-dependent potassium channel blocker antagonizes morphine analgesia. *European Journal of Pharmacology* **186**, 377–378.

Ono, T., Nishino, H., Fukuda, M., Sasaki, K., Muramoto, K-I,. & Oomura, Y. (1982) Glucoresponsive neurons in rat ventromedial hypothalamic tissue slices *in vitro*. *Brain Research* **232**, 494–499.

Oomura, Y., Ono, T., Ooyama, H. & Wayner, M. J. (1969) Glucose and osmosensitive neurons of the rat hypothalamus. *Nature* **222**, 282–284.

Oomura, Y., Ooyama, H., Sugimori, M., Nakamura, T. & Yamada, Y. (1974) Glucose inhibition of the glucose-sensitive neurone in the rat lateral hypothalamus. *Nature* **247**, 284–286.

Paskov, D. S., Staenov, E. A. & Mirov, V. V. (1973) New anticurare and analeptic drug pimadin (4-aminopyridine hydrochloride) and its use in anaesthesia. *Exsperimentalnaja Chirurgija i Anesthesiologija* **18**, 48–52.

Pennefather, P., Lancaster, B., Adams, P. R. & Nicoll, R. A. (1985) Two distinct Ca-dependent K-currents in bullfrog sympathetic ganglion cells. *Proceedings of the National Academy of Sciences USA* **82**, 3040–3044.

Petersen, O. H. & Findlay, I. (1987) Electrophysiology of the pancreas. *Physiological Reviews* **67**, 1054–1116.

Politi, D. M. T., Suzuki, S. & Rogawski, M. A. (1989) BRL 34915 (cromakalim) enhances voltage-dependent K^+ current in cultured rat hippocampal neurons. *European Journal of Pharmacology* **168**, 7–14.

Roeper, J., Hainsworth, A. H. & Ashcroft, F. M. (1990a) Tolbutamide reverses membrane hyperpolarisation induced by activation of D_2 receptors and $GABA_B$ receptors in isolated substantia nigra neurones. *Pflügers Archiv* **416**, 473–475.

Roeper, J., Hainsworth, A. & Ashcroft, F. M. (1990b) Tolbutamide reverses hypoglycemia-induced hyperpolarisation in guinea-pig isolated substantia nigra neurones. *Journal of Physiology* **426**, 68P.

Roeper, J., Hainsworth, A. H. & Ashcroft, F. M. (1990c) ATP-sensitive K channels in guinea-pig isolated substantia nigra neurones are modulated by cellular metabolism. *Journal of Physiology* **430**, 130P.

Rogawski, M. A. (1985) The A-current: how ubiquitous a feature of excitable cells is it? *Trends in Neurosciences* **8**, 214–219.

Romey, G. & Lazdunski, M. (1984) The coexistence in rat muscle cells of two distinct classes of Ca^{2+}-dependent K^+ channels with different pharmacological properties and different physiological functions. *Biochemical and Biophysical Research Communications* **118**, 669–674.

Rudy, B. (1988) Diversity and ubiquity of K channels. *Neuroscience* **25**, 729–749.

Sanguinetti, M. C., Scott, A. I., Zingaro, G. J. & Siegl, P. K. S. (1988) BRL 34915 (cromakalim) activates ATP-sensitive K^+ current in cardiac muscle. *Proceedings of the National Academy of Sciences USA* **85**, 8360–8364.

Schmid-Antomarchi, H., Ambroso, S., Fosset, M. & Lazdunski, M. (1990) K^+ channel openers activate brain sulfonylurea-sensitive K^+ channels and block neurosecretion. *Proceedings of the National Academy of Sciences USA* **87**, 3489–3492.

Schwartzkroin, P. A. & Prince, D. A. (1980) Effects of TEA on hippocampal neurons. *Brain Research* **185**, 169–181.

Schwindt, P. C., Spain, W. J. & Crill, W. E. (1988a) Influence of anomalous rectifier activation on afterhyperpolarizations of neurons from cat sensorimotor cortex *in vitro*. *Journal of Neurophysiology* **59**, 468–481.

Schwindt, P. C., Spain, W. J., Foehring, R. C., Stafstrom, C. E., Chubb, M. C. & Crill, W. E. (1988b) Multiple potassium conductances and their functions in neurons from cat sensorimotor cortex *in vitro*. *Journal of Neurophysiology* **59**, 424–499.

Segal, M., Rogawski, M. A. & Barker, J. L. (1984) A transient potassium conductance regulates the excitability of cultured hippocampal and spinal neurons. *Journal of Neuroscience* **4**, 604–609.

Sherratt, R. M., Bostock, H. & Sears, T. A. (1980) Effects of 4-aminopyridine on normal and demyelinated mammalian nerve fibres. *Nature* **283**, 570–572.

Singh, I. S., Chatterjee, T. K. & Ghosh, J. J. (1983) Modification of morphine antinociceptive response by blood glucose status: possible involvement of cellular energetics. *European Journal of Pharmacology* **90**, 437–439.

Spyker, D. A., Lynch, C., Shabanowitz, J. & Sinn, J. A. (1980) Poisoning with 4-aminopyridine: report of three cases. *Clinical Toxicology* **16**, 487–497.

Standen, N. B., Quale, J. M., Davies, N. W., Brayden, J. E. Huang, Y. & Nelson, M. T. (1989) Hyperpolarizing vasodilators activate ATP-sensitive K$^+$ channels in arterial smooth muscle. *Science* **245**, 177–180.

Stansfeld, C. E., Marsh, S. J., Halliwell, J. V. & Brown, D. A. (1986) 4-aminopyridine and dendrodotoxin induce repetitive firing in rat visceral sensory neurones by blocking a slowly inactivating outward current. *Neuroscience Letters* **64**, 299–304.

Storm, J. (1987) Action potential repolarization and a fast after-hyperpolarization in rat hippocampal pyramidal cells. *Journal of Physiology* **385**, 733–759.

Storm, J. (1988) Temporal integration by a slowly inactivating K$^+$ current in hippocampal neurons. *Nature* **336**, 379–381.

Sturgess, N. C., Ashford, M. L. J., Cook, D. L. & Hales, C. N. (1985) The sulfonylurea receptor may be an ATP-sensitive potassium channel. *Lancet* **ii**, 474–475.

Szente, M. & Pongrácz, F. (1981) Comparative study of aminopyridine-induced seizure activities in primary and mirror foci of cat's cortex. *Electroencephalography and Clinical Neurophysiology* **52**, 353–367.

Thompson, S. H. (1977) Three pharmacologically distinct potassium channels in molluscan neurones. *Journal of Physiology* **265**, 465–488.

Thompson, S. H. (1982) Aminopyridine block of transient potassium current. *Journal of General Physiology* **80**, 1–18.

Tricklebank, M. D., Flockhart, G. & Freedman, S. B. (1988) The potassium channel activator, BRL 34915, antagonises a behavioural response to the muscarinic receptor agonist, pilocarpine. *European Journal of Pharmacology* **151**, 349–350.

Uges, D. R. A. (1982) 4-aminopyridine, clinical pharmaceutical, pharmacological and toxicological aspects. PhD Thesis, State University of Groningen, The Netherlands.

Van Erp, M. G., Van Dongen, M. J. & Van den Berg, R. J. (1990) Voltage-dependent action of valproate on potassium channels in frog node of Ranvier. *European Journal of Pharmacology* **184**, 151–161.

Virsolvy-Vergine, A., Brück, M., Dufour, M., Cauvin, A., Lupo, B. & Bataille, D. (1988) An endogenous ligand for the central sulfonylurea receptor. *FEBS Letters* **242**, 65–69.

Wesseling, H. & Lakke, J. P. W. F. (1980) Observations with 4-aminopyridine in Huntingdon's chorea. *IRCS Medical Science* **8**, 332–333.

Wilson, W. A. & Goldner, M. M. (1975) Voltage clamping with a single microelectrode. *Journal of Neurobiology* **6**, 411–422.

Zona, C., Tancredi, V., Palma, E., Pirrone, G. C. & Avoli, M. (1990) Potassium currents in rat cortical neurons in culture are enhanced by the antiepileptic drug carbamazepine. *Canadian Journal of Physiology and Pharmacology* **68**, 545–547.

Chapter 10
Skeletal muscle potassium channels and their relevance to muscle disease

A. C. Wareham

Introduction

This chapter aims to survey the types of K-channel found in skeletal muscle and to describe some of the human disease states of this tissue which are attributable to altered membrane permeability. Furthermore, attention will be focused on the relatively small amount of recent work on modulating K-channels in normal or pathological skeletal muscle.

Although diseased states of skeletal muscle are well documented, very little experimental electrophysiology on single fibres has been carried out. The advent of the techniques of membrane patch-clamping, where intact fibres are not needed, has permitted analyses of biopsy specimens in some cases. There is, nevertheless, a paucity of work upon human skeletal muscle. Fortunately, it does appear that the electrophysiology of human skeletal muscle differs little from that of other mammals and vertebrates. Before considering the pathophysiology of muscle diseases it may be helpful to review briefly the electrophysiological properties of human and mammalian skeletal muscle fibres and to survey the role of K-channels in muscle function.

The resting membrane potential

The surface membrane, the sarcolemma, of a single skeletal muscle fibre can easily be penetrated with a microelectrode to measure the resting membrane potential. This was first determined for human fibres by Johns in 1963 who obtained a value of $-77.8 \pm 2.4\,$mV. Several subsequent studies have yielded similar values, close to typical values from muscle of experimental animals. The resting membrane potential is a consequence of an uneven distribution of the major ions Na^+, K^+ and Cl^- between the intracellular and extracellular spaces and of the differing ionic permeabilities, P_{Na}, P_K, P_{Cl} of the sarcolemma. As is the case for skeletal muscle of vertebrates, the mathematical description of the resting potential which gives the closest approximation to measured values is given by the constant field equation (Hodgkin & Katz, 1949). Owing to the relatively low electrical resistance of the sarcolemma any electrogenic contribution to the membrane potential from the Na^+–K^+ pump is small. Intracellular sodium concentration $[Na^+]_i$ is low and Cl^- passively distribute across the sarcolemma according to the membrane potential. Hence the resting membrane potential can be described by a simplified constant field equation. Thus, *in vivo*, the resting membrane potential is:

$$-61.5 \, \log \frac{[K]_i}{[K]_o + P_{Na}/P_K[Na]_o} \, \text{mV}.$$

This is more correctly written in terms of ionic activities (*a*) rather than ionic concentrations, thus:

$$-61.5 \, \log \frac{a[K]_i}{a[K]_o + P_{Na}/P_K(a[Na]_o)} \, \text{mV}.$$

Substitution of measured values for $[K^+]$ and $[Na^+]$ (Rudel, 1986) gives a calculated value for the resting membrane potential close to measured values from human intercostal muscle fibres (Kwieciński *et al.*, 1984). Clearly, the value recorded depends primarily upon $[K^+]_i$ and $[K^+]_o$ and P_K. Hence application of agents which alter membrane K-permeability can have significant effects upon the magnitude of the membrane potential (*see later*).

Sarcolemmal resistance and conductance

Membrane resistance is the second most frequently-determined electrical parameter of diseased muscle fibres after the resting membrane potential. Elmqvist *et al.* (1960) reported the specific membrane resistance of human intercostal fibres to be $4070 \pm 259\,\Omega cm^2$. More recently, values of about $6000\,\Omega cm^2$ have been recorded (Kwieciński *et al.*, 1984). The reciprocal of membrane resistance, the membrane conductance (g_m), may be easily split into its components, thus:

$$g_m = g_K + g_{Na} + g_{Cl}, \text{ etc.}$$

Component conductances are determined *in vitro* by removing ions or blocking specific conductances. At the resting membrane potential in human intercostal fibres, g_{Cl} is three to four times greater than g_K (Lipicky & Bryant, 1973; Kwieciński et al., 1984). The slope of the relationship between membrane potential and g_m becomes steeper for both depolarization and hyperpolarization from the normal resting level. Alterations in the characteristic current–voltage (I–V) curves can be used diagnostically.

Anomalous rectification

The increase in g_m seen with hyperpolarization was named anomalous rectification by Katz (1949) because, according to the Goldman constant field equation, rectification would be expected in the opposite direction, on the assumption that g_m would be almost equal to g_K at hyperpolarizing potentials. Anomalous rectification is due to K-channels in the transverse (T) tubular system of muscle fibres (Adrian et al., 1970) restricting the outward movement of K^+. Impulse propagation down T-tubules involves a flux of Na^+ into the myoplasm from the tubule lumen and a flux of K^+ in the reverse direction. Loss of K^+ into the tubule lumen is minimized by the rectified K-channel in the T-tubule membrane and by the high g_{Cl} of the sarcolemma which allows Cl^- influx to dissipate part of the depolarization of the action potential (Rudel, 1986). Disturbance of g_{Cl} or of tubule K-channels can result in decreased excitability (*see later*).

Membrane capacitance

Specific membrane capacitance is much larger in skeletal muscle fibres than in nerve axons, about $5\,\mu F/cm^2$ compared with $1\,\mu F/cm^2$ in a motor axon, due to the contribution of T-tubule membranes.

The action potential

The action potential of human skeletal muscle fibres largely conforms to the textbook description of the action potential of the squid giant axon. Depolarization is caused by an increase in g_{Na}, which is inactivated within a millisecond leading to repolarization. After a short delay g_K increases (delayed rectification) also promoting repolarization. Unlike the neuronal action potential there is only a very slow inactivation of g_K (Adrian et al., 1970). The greatest difference between nerve and muscle action potentials is the prolonged after-depolarization of the sarcolemma following an action potential. The early part of this is due to the rate of spread of activation along T-tubules (Adrian & Peachey, 1973). The later part is due to the accumulation of K^+ in the tubular system (Freygang et al., 1964) during repetitive activity (Adrian & Peachey, 1973).

Thus, electrophysiological investigations of whole fibres implicate dif-

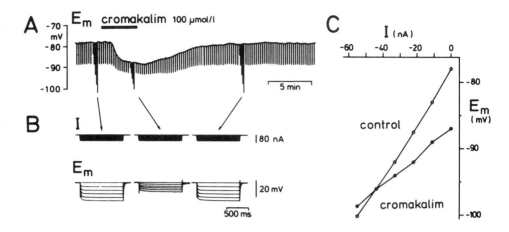

Fig. 10.1. Cromakalim enhances membrane conductance. A, Shows a continuous recording of membrane potential (E_m) and input resistance of a fibre from a skeletal muscle biopsy (not diseased). Input resistance was determined every 15 s by hyperpolarizing current pulses (40 nA, 1 s). B, Illustrates I–V relationships taken before, during and after the application of cromakalim. C, Current–voltage curves plotted before and during application of cromakalim. The reversal potential was −95 mV. (Reproduced with permission from Spuler *et al.*, 1989.)

ferent types of K-channel at two sites in skeletal muscle fibres: (i) in the sarcolemma involved with the generation of delayed rectifier currents; and (ii) in the T-tubule system responsible for inward or anomalous rectification. In addition, it is known that K-channels also are present in sarcoplasmic reticulum membranes (Young *et al.*, 1981; Williams & Tomlins, 1985), where they may be involved in the process of Ca release (Moutin & Dupont, 1988). Finally, a very large g_K of the sarcolemma which becomes apparent in conditions of metabolic exhaustion (Fink & Luttgau, 1976) may be due to activation of a family of adenosine triphosphate (ATP)-sensitive K-channels (Spruce *et al.*, 1985).

Alteration in the kinetics, density or distribution of any of the types of K-channel present could cause pathological changes in muscle excitability or in excitation–contraction coupling. In addition, manipulation of one type of K-channel by application of activators or blockers, e.g. the K-channel opener cromakalim enhances the membrane conductance of normal human skeletal muscle fibres (Fig. 10.1), could serve to correct pathological alterations in muscle electrophysiology caused by factors other than K-channels.

Early work investigating single K-channels in skeletal muscle has been carried out using patch-clamp techniques on cultured fibres, where the sarcolemma is clean enough to permit the establishment of high resistance seals with electrodes. However, it is likely that the types of channel, their concentrations and distributions in myoblasts and cultured fibres differ from those in mature fibres. For example, T-tubule systems do not differentiate fully until after the third postnatal week in rats. Hence, channels specifically associated with T-tubules may be absent, present in different concentrations or distributed in the sarcolemma, probably with different kinetics. In addition, it is of interest to apply patch-clamp techniques to the sarcolemma of mature diseased muscle. It was, therefore, important to develop suitable preparations from mature skeletal muscle fibres.

Preparation of membrane vesicles from mature muscle fibres

Standen *et al.* (1984) first described the enzymatic treatment of frog muscle with collagenase and protease. This resulted in the production of sarcolemmal vesicles of approximately $50\,\mu m$ diameter, which were clean, and which yielded gigaseal patch-clamp seals in the range of $10–100\,G\Omega$. Subsequently, this method has been adapted to produce vesicles suitable for patching from skeletal muscle from normal humans (Burton *et al.*, 1988) and rats (Wareham *et al.*, 1990). Standard patch-clamp techniques (Hamill *et al.*, 1981) can then be used to investigate the channels present in the vesicle membranes. Vesicles still attached to the fibres are the easiest to patch, probably because they are the cleanest. Some vesicles fall to the bottom of the recording chamber and can also be patched but the success rate for obtaining good seals is lower. In most cases, formation of a patch with a vesicle leads to a 'cell-free' or 'vesicle-free' configuration and an inside-out patch. It seems that, possibly due to the removal of the extracellular matrix by treatment with collagenase, vesicle membranes are relatively fragile and unable to maintain a 'vesicle attached' configuration with a patch electrode. Seals with resistances $10–30\,G\Omega$ are normal with rat and mouse muscle. Whilst this is lower than values reported for seals made with vesicles from frog skeletal muscles by Standen *et al.* (1984), such seals can be used to resolve single channels with conductances below $10\,pS$.

Recently, an alternative method has been described to produce membrane vesicles, which is attractive because no enzyme treatment is employed (Stein & Palade, 1989). In this method, frog semitendinosus muscle fibres are dissected free and pulled to five to eight times their resting length, causing them to stretch, break and then rapidly shorten. Over the next $5–15\,min$ surface spheres form and enlarge to $5–80\,\mu m$ diameter. These are reported to easily form high-resistance seals ($30–50\,G\Omega$) suitable for single channel recording. The authors claim that vesicles may also be prepared from similarly-treated giant barnacle muscle and from rabbit multifidus muscle. The method has the advantage over other methods of membrane production from skeletal muscle because vesicles can be made in minutes and no exogenous enzyme treatment is needed. Hence, from the

viewpoint of channel lability (Chad & Eckert, 1985) and possible alteration or loss of channel properties by proteolysis (Rousseau *et al.*, 1988),
this method promises the least disturbed view of native sarcolemmal
membrane channels.

To date, at least five types of K-channel with different properties and
proposed functions have been described in patch-clamped membrane
preparations from skeletal muscle. Not all of these are necessarily derived
from the sarcolemma alone.

Anomalous or inwardly rectifying K-channels (K_{IR})

Conductance through these channels increases with hyperpolarization,
allowing K^+ entry, and there is little outflow upon depolarization when
the driving force on internal cations is outwards. Rectification is around
E_K in cardiac muscle and is probably due to a block by intracellular Mg^{2+}
competing with K^+ for entry to the channel (Matsuda *et al.*, 1987; Vandenberg, 1987). In the T-tubule membrane, reduction of K^+ outflow upon
depolarization will help to maintain the depolarization of the action
potential and encourage propagation of the action potential into the
T-tubules (Lorkovic, 1976) where resistance is high. A K_{IR} has been
identified in vesicles prepared from human vastus lateralis and gluteus
medius (Burton *et al.*, 1988) and from mouse extensor digitorum longus
(EDL; Rowe *et al.*, 1990). Since the vesicles used for these studies do not
allow identification of the origin of the channels they could have been
derived from pure sarcolemmal membranes or from sarcolemmal membranes contaminated with T-tubule membranes. The K_{IR}-channel described
in human muscle preparations had a maximum conductance of about
20 pS at a membrane potential of -80 mV. Channel open probability never
rose above 0.5 even at very negative membrane potentials. It may be,
therefore, that activation of this channel in T-tubules is not as complete
at the resting potential as has been supposed (Leech & Stanfield, 1981) and
it might possess an intrinsic inactivating mechanism as does its counter-
part in cardiac muscle (Sakmann & Trube, 1984). In Mg^{2+}-free medium
the inward rectifier of skeletal muscle (Burton *et al.*, 1988) produced noisy
outward current events, suggesting, as for cardiac muscle (Matsuda *et al.*,
1987; Vandenberg, 1987) that Mg^{2+} is involved in this process.

In normal rat EDL the K_{IR}-channel in symmetrical 120 mM KCl
solution had a unitary conductance of 40 pS and the *I–V* relationship was
linear between -20 and -100 mV (Rowe *et al.*, 1990). Channel open
probability reached 0.8 at strongly negative potentials (Fig. 10.2). The
properties of K_{IR} were unchanged in preparations from dystrophic mouse
EDL. A higher single channel conductance of 90 pS in symmetrical
120 mM KCl solution has been found for this type of channel in neonate
rat muscle (Wareham *et al.*, 1990). Using voltage-clamp techniques it has

been calculated (Schwarz *et al.*, 1981) that in frog skeletal muscle, there are four inwardly rectifying channels per square micron of muscle surface.

Delayed rectifier K-channels (K_V)

This is another voltage-dependent channel. Conductance increases upon depolarization and only inactivates very slowly (Adrian *et al.*, 1970; Stanfield, 1970) during maintained depolarization. The K_V is a widely-distributed channel blocked by tetraethylammonium ions (TEA) and 4-aminopyridine (4-AP; Standen *et al.*, 1985). It has a single channel conductance of 15–20 pS and is characterized by bursting behaviour, depolarization increasing the frequency of bursts. In frog skeletal muscle K_V has a single channel conductance of 15 pS in physiological saline and about 30 pS in symmetrical 120 mM KCl solution (Standen *et al.*, 1985). These channels are highly K^+-selective and are primarily responsible for the efflux of K^+ during the action potential and thus contribute to membrane repolarization.

Calcium-activated K-channels (K_{Ca})

These are common to many preparations and are the most widely studied type of K-channel. They are activated by micromolar or lower concentrations of Ca^{2+} at the inner membrane surface and by depolarization. In cultured rat muscle (Barrett *et al.*, 1982) the presence of Ca^{2+} at the extracellular membrane surface was not sufficient to activate K-channels, while increasing $[Ca^{2+}]$ between 0.1 μM and 1 mM at the intracellular membrane surface or depolarization increased both the frequency and duration of the channel openings. Single channel conductance was independent of membrane potential between -50 and $+50$ mV but increased with temperature from 100 pS at 1°C to 300 pS at 37°C. This is comparable with the large conductance Ca^{2+}-activated K (BK_{Ca})-channel, one of the two main types of K_{Ca}-channel found in mature skeletal muscle. The other type is a small conductance channel (SK_{Ca}) with a conductance of 12 pS in symmetrical 140 mM KCl and which is blocked by apamin (Romey & Lazdunski, 1984; Blatz & Magleby, 1986). Such SK_{Ca}-channels found in membrane preparations of adult muscle probably originate from T-tubule membranes. Denervation and certain disease states result in their appearance in the sarcolemma. These smaller conductance channels have mainly been studied in cultured myotubes and muscle of newborn rats where T-tubules are absent or very immature.

The BK-channel described in cultured rat muscle by Barrett *et al.* (1982) is characteristic of the large conductance, 200–300 pS, BK_{Ca} channel described in muscle (Fig. 10.3) for mice (Rowe *et al.*, 1990), rats (Wareham *et al.*, 1990) and humans (Burton *et al.*, 1988), which is blocked

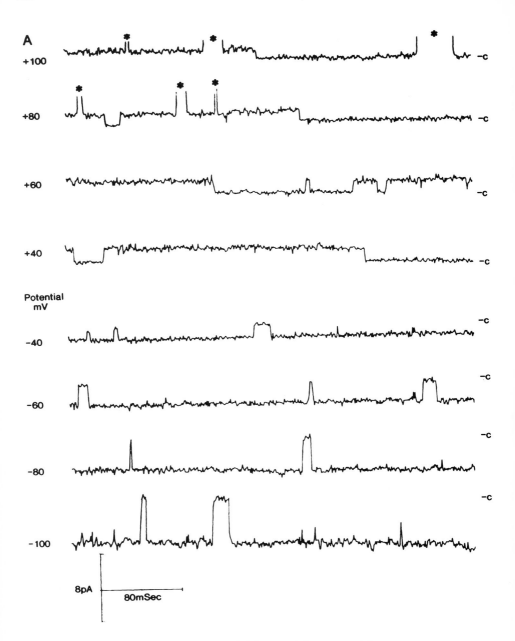

Fig. 10.2. Example of a K_{IR}-channel recorded from vesicles prepared from mouse EDL muscle. A, Single channel activity from an inside-out excised patch. The patch pipette contained 120 mM KCl, 10 mM NaCl, 0.1 mM $CaCl_2$, 5 mM Tris buffer, pH 7.2. The closed state is marked with a 'c' and the asterisks indicate activity of a BK_{Ca}-channel also present in this patch. (*Opposite*) B, Current–voltage relationship for K_{IR}. C, Open probability–voltage relationship of K_{IR}. (Reproduced with permission from Rowe *et al.*, 1990.)

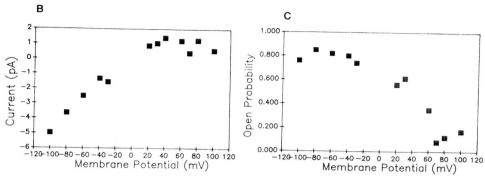

Fig. 10.2. Continued.

by external TEA or charybdotoxin (ChTX) (Blatz & Magleby, 1984; Romey & Lazdunski, 1984; Miller et al., 1985).

Studies of patches from cultured rat skeletal muscle (McManus & Magleby, 1988) reveal that the kinetics of BK_{Ca} are complex. Analysis of 10^6 open-and-shut intervals in patches containing a single such channel revealed four different kinetic modes: *normal* which included 96% of measured intervals: *intermediate* open mode with 3.2% of the intervals; *brief* open mode with 0.5% of the intervals and *buzz* mode with 0.1% of the intervals. The mean open-interval durations were 61% of normal during the intermediate open mode, 12% of normal during the brief open mode and 2.6% of normal during the buzz mode. The authors suggest that the data show that the BK-channel can enter three to four discrete open states and six to eight discrete shut states during normal activity.

There is evidence that Mg^{2+} may increase the apparent affinity of BK_{Ca} for Ca^{2+} (Golowasch et al., 1986). Channels were extracted from rat T-tubule membranes and inserted into planar phospholipid bilayers to study the activation by Ca^{2+}. On the cytoplasmic side of the channel, Ca^{2+} (10–100 μM) increased channel open probability in a sigmoid fashion, with an average Hill coefficient of about 2. Mg^{2+} (1–10 mM) increased the apparent affinity of the channel for Ca^{2+} and greatly enhanced the sigmoidal nature of the Ca^{2+}-activation curve. In the presence of 10 mM Mg^{2+}, the Hill coefficient for Ca^{2+}-activation increased to approximately 4.5. Magnesium was only effective on the cytoplasmic side of the channel.

Charybdotoxin (ChTX), a small basic protein from scorpion *(Leiurus quinquestriatus)* venom, strongly inhibits conduction of K^+ through BK_{Ca}. Interaction with ChTX has been studied isolating single channels from rat skeletal into uncharged planar phospholipid bilayers (Anderson et al., 1988). ChTX bound to the external side of the channel with an apparent dissociation constant of about 10 nM at physiological ionic strength. It blocked both open and closed channels but with an association rate seven times faster for the open channel. Depolarization enhanced the

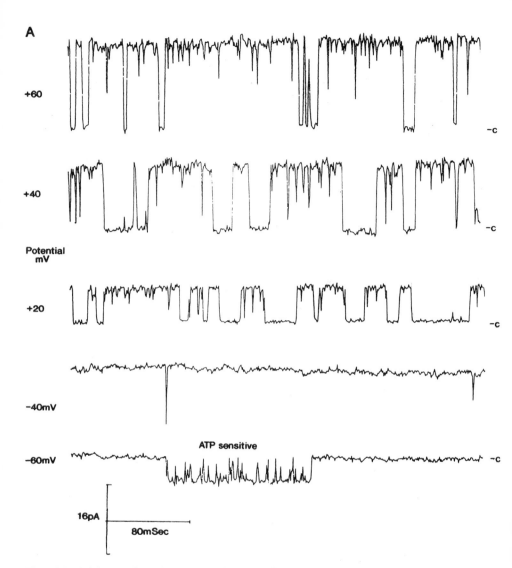

Fig. 10.3. Calcium-activated K-channel from vesicles prepared from normal adult mouse EDL muscle. A, Single channel activity recorded from an inside-out excised patch. The patch pipette contained 120 mM KCl, 10 mM NaCl, 0.1 mM CaCl$_2$, 5 mM Tris buffer, pH 7.2. The bathing solution had the same composition. Outward current is shown as an upward deflection and 'c' indicates the closed state. (*Opposite*) B, Mean *I–V* relationship for single channel activity in three excised patches taken from normal adult mouse EDL and in the same recording conditions as above. C, Mean open probability–voltage relationship for the same three channels. While K$_{Ca}$-channels were frequently encountered it was only rarely that patches were made with only one such channel and no other activity. Standard errors are shown in both B and C as vertical bars when the error exceeds the symbol size. (Reproduced with permission from Rowe *et al.*, 1990.)

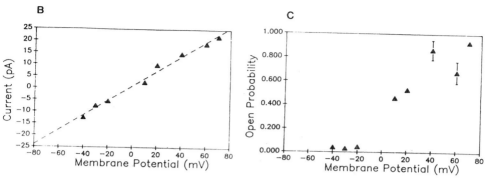

Fig. 10.3. Continued.

ChTX dissociation rate e-fold/28 mV. There was also evidence that the ChTX interaction sensed both voltage and the channels' conformational state. The authors concluded that a region of fixed negative charge exists near the ChTX-binding site. The BK_{Ca}-channel may have a number of functions in skeletal muscle, such as regulation of Ca^{2+} entry, action potential repolarization and duration of after-hyperpolarizations (Rudy, 1988).

The apamin-sensitive SK_{Ca}-channel has received far less attention, possibly because it has a far smaller conductance and is therefore more difficult to characterize. Cognard *et al.* (1984), using voltage-clamped single frog skeletal muscle fibres, showed that this polypeptide toxin from bee venon, at 50–100 nM, inhibited a slow outward K-current. Traore *et al.* (1986) showed that in frog skeletal muscle apamin partially blocked a slow outward K-current which was absent after detubulation. Hence it is likely, in the frog at least, that the SK_{Ca}-channel is located in the T-tubule membrane.

The SK_{Ca}-channels in patches of cultured rat skeletal muscle had slope conductances of about 12 pS in symmetrical 140 mM KCl solutions and exhibited little voltage sensitivity (Blatz & Magleby, 1986). In this preparation, SK_{Ca}-channels were more Ca^{2+}-sensitive than BK_{Ca}-channels at negative membrane potentials. They concluded that SK_{Ca} satisfied the criteria expected for channels underlying the prolonged after-hyperpolarization in cultured skeletal muscle fibres.

Apamin-sensitive K-channels could not be detected in adult rat muscle (Schmid-Antomarchi *et al.*, 1985). However, after denervation, in non-innervated rat myocytes in culture and *in vivo* during the embryonic period before the final innervation pattern was reached, apamin-sensitive channels were present. These channels have also been detected in diseased human muscle (see below).

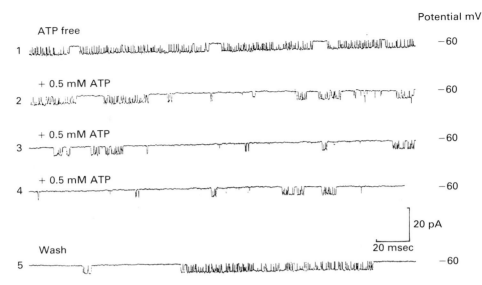

Fig. 10.4. K$_{ATP}$-channel activity recorded from an inside-out excised patch from a vesicle prepared from a normal adult mouse EDL muscle: 1, Single channel activity recorded with 120 mM KCl on both sides of the patch. 2, Single channel activity in the same patch 15 s after addition of 0.5 mM ATP to the inner membrane surface. 3, Single channel activity in the same patch 45 s after addition of 0.5 mM ATP to the inner membrane surface. 4, Single channel activity in the same patch 2 min after addition of 0.5 mM ATP. 5, Single channel activity in the same patch after washing ATP from the inner membrane surface. (Reproduced with permission from Rowe *et al.*, 1990.)

ATP-sensitive K-channels (K$_{ATP}$)

These have been described in several different tissues and also in skeletal muscle of frog (Spruce *et al.*, 1985; Quayle *et al.*, 1988), humans (Burton *et al.*, 1988), mice (Woll *et al.*, 1989; Rowe *et al.*, 1990) and neonate rats (Wareham *et al.*, 1990). The K$_{ATP}$-channels are identified by the fact that their open state probability is dramatically reduced by the presence of low concentrations of ATP (< 1 mM) at the cytoplasmic membrane surface (Fig. 10.4). External Cs$^+$ and Ba^{2+} block these channels in a voltage-dependent manner, the block increasing upon hyperpolarization (Quayle *et al.*, 1988). The single channel conductance for K$_{ATP}$ from frog skeletal muscle in symmetrical high K-solution was reported to be 42 pS (Spruce *et al.*, 1987). Similar values have been reported for these channels in mammalian skeletal muscle. In mouse EDL muscle we found values of 90 pS in both normal and dystrophic fibres (Rowe *et al.*, 1990). Burton *et al.* (1988), reported conductances of 60 pS in patches from human sarcolemma. In muscle from neonate rats, K$_{ATP}$-channels with much higher conductances have been found, in the region of 250–300 pS (Wareham *et al.*, 1990).

The K_{ATP}-channel of frog muscle has been characterized by Spruce *et al.* (1987). Opening of the channel, in the absence of ATP, was voltage-dependent and unitary conductance increased with increasing $[K]_0$. Rubidium substituted for K^+ almost equally and the channel was blocked by both internal and external TEA. Adenosine triphosphate hydrolysis was not necessary for channel closure. Reduction in channel open probability by ATP was consistent with $1:1$ binding with a dissociation constant of 0.13 mM ATP. Adenosine diphosphate (ADP) and adenosine monophosphate (AMP) were less effective than ATP although they retained some closing properties. Interestingly, myotubes cultured from thigh muscles of new-born rats lacked demonstrable K_{ATP}-channels (Spruce *et al.*, 1987), although the ATP-sensitivity of large conductance K-channels has been demonstrated in vesicles prepared from neonate rat muscle (Wareham *et al.*, 1990).

Single K_{ATP}-channels have also been studied in membrane patches from mouse toe muscles (Woll *et al.*, 1989). These had a conductance of 74 pS in symmetrical 160 mM KCl solution. Channel openings occurred in bursts and open probability increased upon depolarization. Three types of blocking agent were identified: (i) small internal cations (fast blockers at positive voltages); (ii) internal ATP (voltage-dependent decrease in open probability); (iii) tolbutamide (voltage-independent decrease in open probability). They concluded that K_{ATP} has an internal gate like that of other voltage-gated cation channels and that different blockers interfere with different transitions in channel gating.

Using the mouse toe muscle preparation, Weik and Neumcke (1990) studied the action of K-channel openers, such as cromakalim, pinacidil, RP 49356 and diazoxide, which are believed to target K_{ATP}-channels in smooth (Quast & Cook, 1989; Standen *et al.*, 1989) and cardiac (Escande *et al.*, 1988, 1989) muscle.* Cromakalim has been shown to produce an increase in the macroscopic K-conductance of human skeletal muscle (Spuler *et al.*, 1989). Using inside-out cell-free patches, Weik and Neumcke (1990) showed that cromakalim (0.2–0.8 mM) and pinacidil (0.4 mM) restored the open probability of channels blocked by 0.1 mM ATP to 50–90% of the value in ATP-free medium (Fig. 10.5). Diazoxide had little effect and none of the channel openers stimulated BK_{Ca}. This is in contrast to the situation in smooth muscle where Gelband *et al.* (1989) and Klöckner *et al.* (1989) have demonstrated activation of this channel type by diazoxide and by cromakalim.* RP 49356 differs in its action from cromakalim and pinacidil in that it is able to activate the K_{ATP}-channel of skeletal muscle in the absence of ATP. At concentrations of 0.4 and 0.8 mM, RP 49356 increased the channel open probability by a factor of

---

*For a full discussion of K_{ATP} as a site of action for the K-channel openers in smooth muscle, *see* Chapters 7 and 14.

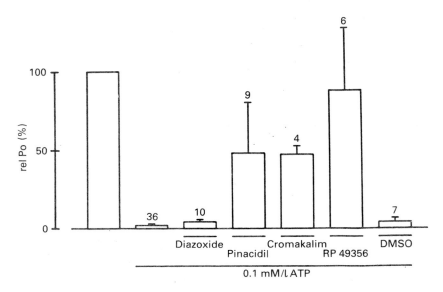

Fig. 10.5. Relative open probabilities (rel Po) of K_{ATP}-channels during treatment with several drugs dissolved in DMSO in the presence of internal ATP (0.1 mM). The probabilities are normalized with respect to measurements on the same patches in drug-free K^+-rich internal solution without ATP (first column on the left). The drugs used were diazoxide, pinacidil, RP 49356 (each 0.4 mM) and cromakalim (0.2 mM). Dimethylsulphoxide (DMSO) (1.6 μl/ml) without added drugs showed no effects. Bars and numbers above the columns indicate SEM values with corresponding number of measurements. Membrane potential – 50 mV. Temperatures 19–24°C (ATP without drug, diazoxide, pinacidil, RP 49356 and DMSO) and 30°C (cromakalim). (Reproduced with permission from Weik & Neumcke, 1990.)

2.7 and 17.4 respectively. Hence RP 49356 probably acts primarily not by displacing ATP from its binding site but by recruiting inactive channels (Thuringer & Escande, 1989). Similar activating effects have been described for the pulmonary artery (Eltze, 1989) and cardiac myocytes (Escande et al., 1989).

The actions of diazoxide in skeletal muscle are anomalous. Whilst this agent was hardly effective in skeletal muscle (Weik and Neumcke, 1990) and inhibited K_{ATP} in ventricular muscle cells (Faivre & Findlay, 1989), diazoxide showed remarkable activating effects at concentrations of 50–100 μM in smooth muscle (Quast & Cook, 1989; Standen et al., 1989). These diverse effects of diazoxide indicate that the K_{ATP}-channels in mouse sarcolemma may in some respects resemble those of cardiac cells more than those in smooth muscle. Nevertheless, 0.5 mM Mg^{2+} had little effect upon channel activity in frog skeletal muscle (Spruce et al., 1987; Davies, 1990) but did inhibit channel activity in cardiac cells (Findlay, 1987).

There has not been a very convincing proposal of a physiological role for K_{ATP}-channels which are present at a high density in the sarcolemma, a density as great as that found for the K_V-channels (Spruce et al., 1987). It seems reasonable, therefore, to expect them to have a significant physiological role to play in muscle function. It has been proposed (Spruce et al., 1987) that a fall in $[ATP]_i$ during metabolic exhaustion raises the open probability of the channels and that the resulting increase in K-conductance serves to stabilize the sarcolemma and protect the muscle fibre by decreasing its excitability. Certainly, metabolically-exhausted muscle fibres do develop a high g_K (Fink & Luttgau, 1976; Fink et al., 1983). Alternatively, it has been suggested (Spruce et al., 1987) that the K^+-efflux occurring through these channels in conditions of low $[ATP]_i$ could contribute significantly to vasodilation of skeletal arterioles and thus increase blood flow to exhausted fibres. However, the $[ATP]_i$ in muscle is buffered by creatine phosphate to about 5 mM and changes little, even during sustained activity (Carlson & Siger, 1960). Since the $[ATP]_i$ required to attain a 50% block of K_{ATP} in frog skeletal muscle is only 0.14 mM (Spruce et al., 1987), it seems unlikely that the open probability of these channels would ever be very significant. It is possible that an ATP concentration gradient exists within the cell due to ATP-consuming centres stationed just beneath the cell membrane (Weik & Neumcke, 1990). Alternatively a different regulating factor for these channels may be involved under (patho)physiological conditions.

Davies (1990) has presented evidence that a decrease of intracellular pH_i, which can fall by as much as 1 unit during sustained muscle activity (Renaud, 1989), markedly reduces the inhibitory effect of ATP on K_{ATP}-channels in excised patches from frog skeletal muscle. Davies proposes that under physiological conditions the activity of these channels is primarily regulated by protons. In the absence of ATP, a decrease of pH resulted in an increase in mean channel open time. Channel open probability was little changed so this effect arose via a reduction in duration of closings. There was a large decrease in the inhibitory effect of 0.5 mM ATP as pH_i was decreased. The activity of K_{ATP} was highly sensitive to changes in pH in the presence of Mg^{2+} and ATP, the greatest sensitivity lying between pH 7.2 and 6.0, which is within the physiological range for skeletal muscle (Renaud, 1989). Interestingly, all other major types of K-current in skeletal muscle are reduced by a fall in pH_i (Davies, 1990). Such an interaction between ATP and pH_i, or between ATP and another cellular factor sensitive to pH_i, provides an attractive basis for an explanation of the physiological control of K_{ATP} in skeletal muscle.

Potassium channels in sarcoplasmic reticulum membranes (K_{SR})

A K-selective channel (K_{SR}) has been identified in reconstituted membrane vesicles formed after solubilization of rabbit SR membranes (Young et al., 1981; Williams & Tomlins, 1985). Two open states have been described for this channel, a fully open one with a single channel conductance of 180 pS and a substate with a conductance of 125 pS (Williams & Tomlins, 1985). The channel was blocked in a voltage-dependent manner by gallamine with a greater degree of block at increasingly negative holding potentials (Gray *et al.*, 1988). Based on evidence that the rate of release of Ca^{2+} from isolated SR vesicles was influenced by the K-gradient across the SR membrane, it has been suggested that there is an influx of K^+ through K_{SR}-channels during Ca^{2+} release, allowing reconsideration of a possible influence of the SR membrane potential on Ca^{2+} release (Moutin & Dupont, 1988). Neither the gating properties nor conductance properties of single K_{SR}-channels from SR membranes was affected by ryanodine, suggesting that the site of action of ryanodine is limited only to Ca-channels in SR membranes (Campos de Carvalho & Cukierman, 1987).

Electrophysiological changes in skeletal muscle disease

Several pathological conditions of skeletal muscle are known to involve changes in membrane K-conductance or other ion conductances, which might be susceptible to treatment by drugs targeted at specific types of K-channel. An understanding of the role of different types of K-channel may also permit the treatment of other muscle pathologies, in which there is not necessarily an electrophysiological disturbance. For example, 4-AP, which blocks K_V, is known to augment the force of both indirectly and directly elicited muscle twitches of rat hemidiaphragm preparations (Harvey & Marshall, 1977). Two recent reviews have surveyed the potential clinical usefulness of a variety of peptide toxins acting on K-channels (Moczydlowski *et al.*, 1988; Castle *et al.*, 1989).

A limited number of skeletal muscle conditions will be considered, each with a pathology involving an altered sarcolemmal ionic conductance. Such changes result in membrane depolarization and often muscle weakness, and for these the development of therapeutic applications for K-channel modulators may be considered. The conditions are denervation, muscular dystrophy, myotonia and hypokalaemic and hyperkalaemic periodic paralyses.

Denervated skeletal muscle

The influence of innervation upon single K-channels has not been studied in any detail but it may repress the expression of apamin-sensitive SK_{Ca}-channels. Fibres from the fast-twitch EDL muscle of the rat have action potentials which are not followed by a long-lasting hyperpolarization. In contrast, cultured rat myotubes (non-innervated) exhibit action potentials with long-lasting after-hyperpolarizations which are apamin-sensitive. Embryonic fibres are similar but 1 week after birth, apamin sensitivity disappears (Schmid-Antomarchi *et al.*, 1985) at a time when intense rearrangement of muscle innervation is at a peak (Redfern, 1970). Two to four days after denervation of mature skeletal muscle, previously undetectable apamin-binding sites can be revealed with ^{125}I-labelled apamin, strongly suggesting an all-or-none effect of innervation on the expression of apamin-sensitive SK_{Ca}-channels (Schmid-Antomarchi *et al.*, 1985).

Denervation of mammalian skeletal muscle is known to result in a significant membrane depolarization and this has been postulated to be due to an increase in sarcolemmal P_{Na} (Robbins, 1977; Wareham, 1978). To date, no attempt has been made to characterize the K-channels in denervated muscle. In view of the intriguing relationship between the innervating motor nerve and muscle properties (Pette and Vrbova, 1985) such a study could be very rewarding. Duval and Leoty (1985) have shown that denervation of slow-twitch fibres leads to the appearance of a new population of Na-channels contributing 32% of total membrane Na-conductance and showing resistance to blockage by tetrodotoxin. Denervated fast-twitch fibres developed a slow component of the delayed outward current which was typical of normal slow fibres. This change was associated with a modification of channel sensitivity for TEA and 4-AP. The delayed outward K^+ current ($I_{K(V)}$) became resistant to 4-AP after denervation, whereas TEA became more effective in blocking the fast and less effective in blocking the slow component of this current. Such changes may be the result of loss of innervation *per se* or of the loss of muscle activity, a factor known to exert many controlling influences on the morphology and physiology of skeletal muscle (Pette & Vrbova, 1985).

Muscular dystrophy

The most serious, though not the most common form of this disease in humans, is the X-chromosome-linked Duchenne muscular dystrophy (DMD). It occurs in from 13 to 33 per 100 000 live male births. It has a sex-linked recessive mode of inheritance so that only boys are affected but girls act as carriers. Although plasma creatine levels may be very high there are few physical signs of the disease at birth, but by 3–4 years of age a delay in reaching the usual motor milestones becomes apparent. Thereafter, the sufferer has increasing difficulties with standing and walking and by the age of 20 years, the patient is usually confined to a wheelchair. Later, weakness of the respiratory muscles becomes a problem and death usually results before the age of 30. The pathophysiology displayed by muscles from the autosomal murine models of muscular dystrophy, strains 129/ReJ dy/dy and C57BL6J dy/dy, share a number of major similarities with that of DMD and the less severe form, Becker dystrophy. All show severe and progressive muscle weakness, progressive fibre degeneration, elevated serum creatinine kinase and a shortened life expectancy (Rowland, 1985). In a more recent animal model, the X-chromosome-linked defect of the *mdx* mouse results in a dystrophy which, although it is of similar genetic origin to the human Duchenne condition (Hoffman *et al.*, 1987), shows few clinical symptoms and does not shorten life expectancy (Brown & Hoffman, 1988).

The chromosomal location of the DMD gene is the Xp21 region of the short arm of the X-chromosome. The 427 kDa protein encoded by this locus, dystrophin, forms 0.002% of striated muscle protein and is expressed in apparently equal levels in all muscle cells and in the brain (Hoffman *et al.*, 1987; Chamberlain *et al.*, 1988).

Dystrophin, which is absent in DMD and at reduced levels in Becker dystrophy, has been shown by immunofluorescent staining to be associated with the plasma membrane (Bonilla *et al.*, 1988; Zubrzycka-Gaarn *et al.*, 1988). Electron microscope studies have localized dystrophin to the inner face of the sarcolemmal membrane where it may be arranged in a periodic network (Watkins *et al.*, 1988). The precise function of dystrophin is not known, but structural similarities with spectrin and α-actin and other characteristics (Brown & Hoffman, 1988) indicate that it is a cytoskeletal protein which stabilizes skeletal muscle membranes.

Few electrophysiological studies have been carried out on single muscle fibres from human dystrophics but such studies of muscle from dystrophic mice show a fibre depolarization which is associated with a greater than twofold increase in $[Na^+]_i$ (Ward & Wareham, 1984) and a 25% decrease in $[K^+]_i$ (Charlton *et al.*, 1981; Shalton & Wareham, 1981). Whether sarcolemmal K-conductance changes in dystrophy is not clear, since evidence in favour of a decrease (Sellin & Sperelakis, 1978) or an increase (Lipicky & Hess, 1974; Hertzberg *et al.*, 1975) has been obtained.

The $[Ca^{2+}]_i$ is significantly increased in dystrophic muscle. Resting levels of Ca^{2+} in intact single fibres from flexor digitorum brevis and EDL muscles of normal and dystrophic (129 ReJ dy/dy) mice have been determined with Fura-2 (Williams *et al.*, 1990). Fibres from phenotypically normal mice had an average free Ca-level of 106 nM, a value comparable with resting levels reported by other workers using a variety of techniques (Williams *et al.*, 1990). Two distinct types of fibre were identified in dystrophic muscles, both of which maintained $[Ca^{2+}]$ at levels elevated two to four times above normal. Those fibres with apparently normal morphology were found to have Ca^{2+} levels at rest that averaged 189 nM and were uniformly distributed. The second population of fibres had Ca^{2+} concentrations of 368 nM, often with a heterogeneous intrafibre distribution. Such elevated resting Ca^{2+} levels are near threshold for contraction of normal muscle (Head *et al.*, 1990) and are probably involved in promoting the fibre necrosis apparent in dystrophy via activation of proteases (Duncan, 1978).

The increased resting levels of Ca^{2+} may modify the state of K_{Ca} channels in these fibres. In a study of sarcolemmal vesicles from dystrophic muscle of mice (C57BL6J dy/dy), an apparent reduction of the Ca^{2+}-sensitivity of BK_{Ca} channels has been observed (Rowe et al., 1990). However, in other respects there was little detectable alteration in the characteristics of the K-channels studied (Fig. 10.6).

Myotonic syndromes

Myotonia is typified by the slow or delayed relaxation of a muscle after contraction. It differs from the delayed relaxation seen in fatigued muscle or in hypothyroidism in that the EMG shows continued electrical activity during relaxation. Myotonic stiffness affects limb muscles and a common complaint from sufferers is that they have difficulty in relaxing their grip. There are three major myotonic syndromes recognized, namely, myotonia congenita, myotonic dystrophy and paramyotonia congenita (Rudel, 1986).

Myotonia congenita

Two forms of myotonia congenita have been described. There is a less severe, dominantly-inherited, Thomsen type and a more severe, recessively-inherited, Becker type (Becker, 1977). Antiarrhythmic drugs have been used for the treatment of myotonia, although lignocaine derivatives, such as tocainine, are less effective in myotonia congenita than in paramyotonia (Rudel et al., 1980). The understanding of the basis to myotonia arose from electrophysiological studies of myotonic goats which were subsequently extended to human patients (Lipicky et al., 1971; Lipicky & Bryant, 1973). The major finding from these studies was a marked decrease in membrane g_{Cl} without any change in resting membrane potential. As a percentage of total membrane conductance g_{Cl} was only 20% in myotonia congenita compared with 80% in normal muscle. A reduced g_{Cl} could lead to electrical instability of the sarcolemma. Abnormal repetitive firing in response to a constant-current depolarizing pulse can be reproduced in computer simulations of the action potential, based on the Hodgkin–Huxley equations, by reducing the value for g_{Cl} (Bretag, 1973). From this, and from the work of Adrian and Bryant (1974), the repetitive discharges observed upon stimulation of myotonic congenita muscle can be explained (Rudel, 1986).

During repolarization K^+ leaves the muscle fibre and during repetitive activity this K^+ will accumulate in T-tubules, thereby lowering E_K. The tendency for the membrane potential to follow E_K is reduced in normal fibres because the large g_{Cl} tends to 'clamp' the membrane potential near to the Cl^- equilibrium potential of $-80mV$. In the absence of a high g_{Cl},

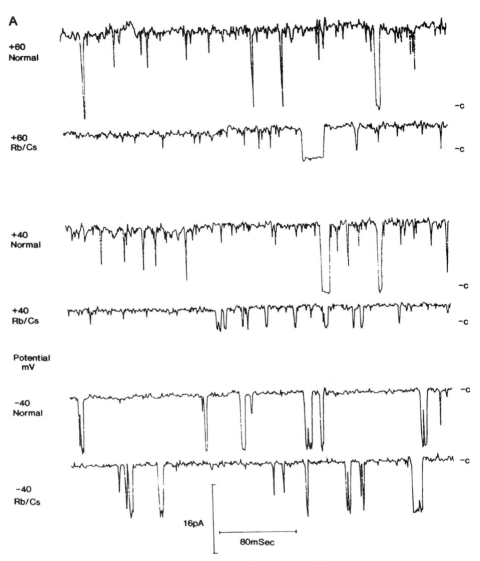

Fig. 10.6. Calcium-activated K-channel activity from dystrophic mouse muscle. A,
Single channel activity recorded from an inside-out excised patch from a vesicle
prepared from an adult dystrophic mouse (C57BL6J dy/dy) EDL muscle. The ionic
conditions were as in Fig. 10.3. The activity at + 60 mV was due to the presence of
an K$_{ATP}$-channel. (*Opposite*) B, Mean *I–V* relationship for single channel activity
in three patches from dystrophic adult mouse EDL recorded under the same
conditions. C, Mean open probability–voltage relationship for the same three
patches. Vertical bars represent standard errors. Note the shift to the right in the
open probability–voltage relationship for these channels from dystrophic muscle
compared to that for channels with the same conductance and *I–V* relationship
found in membrane patches from normal adult mouse muscle and shown in Fig.
10.3. (Reproduced with permission from Rowe *et al.*, 1990.)

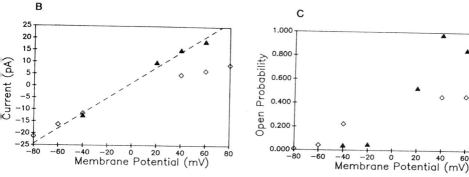

Fig. 10.6. Continued.

as in myotonic fibres, the cumulative late after-depolarization can become large enough to initiate self-maintaining activity. Potassium accumulation in the tubules may be reduced by increased activity of the Na^+–K^+ pump and might be the reason why muscle stiffness and weakness in myotonia can be worked off by a warm-up period of muscle activity (Birnberger et al., 1975).

A reduced g_{Cl} may not be the only reason for instability of myotonic muscle fibres (Adrian & Bryant, 1974). McComas (1977) has suggested that transient stretching of muscle fibres increases P_{Na} and leads to repetitive firing. Certainly, in myotonic goat muscle, the slope of the Na^+-current inactivation curve is reduced resulting in an increase in the steady state Na^+-current and a decrease in the rate of inactivation in the threshold region, leading to hyperexcitability. The goat studies have also shown that hereditary myotonia is not caused by blockade of Cl-channels but by a decrease in the number of channels.

Even though the primary cause of myotonic activity in myotonia congenita is not an alteration of K-channels it is possible that the decreased membrane conductance due to a reduction in g_{Cl} could be counteracted by inducing an increase in g_K. There has recently been a report on the effects of K-channel openers on the contractions of isolated bundles of fibres taken from four patients suffering from myotonia congenita (Quasthoff et al., 1990). One end of a fibre bundle was fixed in a perspex chamber and the other end fastened to a strain gauge and stimuli applied directly via two silver plates. In myotonic preparations an initial muscle twitch of approximately normal force and duration was followed by after-contractions lasting several seconds. Two potent K-channel openers, cromakalim and EMD 52692 (DePeyer et al., 1989), at concentrations of 1–10 and 10–100 μM respectively, completely suppressed the after-contractions, while only slightly increasing the force of the initial twitch (Fig. 10.7). In biopsy specimens, cromakalim effectively suppressed spontaneous myotonic activity. Removal of the channel openers led to a

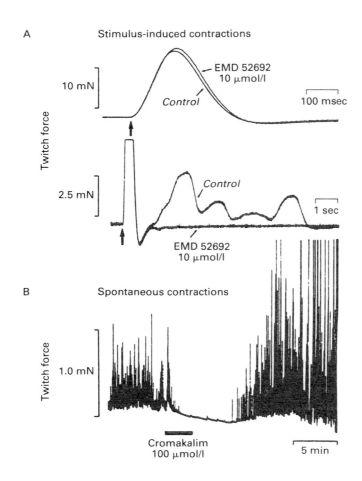

Fig. 10.7. Effects of K-channel openers on myotonic activity of a skeletal muscle fibre bundle from a patient with myotonia congenita. Cromakalim and EMD 52692 were applied via the bath solution. A, Examples of stimulus-induced muscle contractions (field stimulation with 2 ms duration and 100 V stimulus strength, indicated by arrows) obtained in normal bathing solution (control) and in the presence of EMD 52692 are superimposed. The upper panel shows the initial twitch, the lower one the after-contractions (note increase in twitch force amplification and slower time base). B, Continuous recording of spontaneous mechanical activity. (Reproduced with permission from Quasthoff *et al.*, 1990.)

prompt recovery of myotonic activity. In voltage-clamp experiments with non-myotonic human muscle, cromakalim (100 μM) increased membrane conductance four-fold without altering g_{Cl}. Hence K-channel openers may be of therapeutic use to treat electrophysiological defects of skeletal muscle even where the original lesion is not one of altered g_K.

Myotonic dystrophy

Although the myotonic aspects of this disease are not understood, there is no indication that a decrease in membrane g_{Cl} is responsible. The resting membrane potential is lower (Norris, 1962; Hofmann et al., 1966; McComas & Mrozek, 1968; Gruener et al., 1979) and $[Na^+]_i$ is increased (Horvath et al., 1955; Williams et al., 1957), factors consistent with an increased resting g_{Na} (Hofmann & DeNardo, 1968). Myotonia is a relatively minor complaint in this disease since spontaneous activity is less than in myotonia congenita (Gruener, 1977; Lipicky, 1977) and local anaesthetics, antiarrhythmic drugs and diphenylhydantoin are effective antimyotonic agents. Here again, there is a therapeutic potential for K-channel openers. In their study reported above, Quasthoff et al. (1990) also obtained skeletal muscle biopsies from four patients suffering from myotonic dystrophy. They found that the K-channel openers cromakalim and EMD 52692 totally suppressed the after-contractions which followed a single stimulus in untreated preparations.

An increased membrane g_{Na} is not the only change in membrane permeability. An apamin receptor has been found in muscle membrane of patients with myotonic dystrophy (Renaud et al., 1986) which may represent the reappearance of the SK_{Ca}-channel described in cultured myotubes (Blatz & Magleby, 1986) and in denervated skeletal muscle (Schmid-Antomarchi et al., 1985).

Paramyotonia congenita

This disease is characterized by myotonia and muscle weakness, both of which are provoked by cold, particularly during exercise (see Engel, 1986a), a phenomenon which led Eulenberg (1892) to name the disease paramyotonia. Again, there are associated myotonic discharges from affected muscles but at frequencies lower than in myotonia congenita.

Fibres have normal resting potentials of -80 mV at 37°C. On cooling, the fibres depolarize and spontaneous electrical activity sets in at a membrane potential of -60 mV (Lehmann-Horn et al., 1981). Further cooling reduces the membrane potential to -40 mV and fibres become inexcitable. An increased membrane g_{Na} is implicated in this cold-induced depolarization since it can be prevented by application of the Na-channel blocker tetrodotoxin. At 37°C, g_{Na}, g_K and g_{Cl} are normal but at 27°C, g_{Na} and g_{Cl} are abnormally high, while g_K remains normal. Hence the cold-induced weakness and paralysis are caused by a temperature-dependent increase in g_{Na} resulting in membrane depolarization and eventual paralysis. It may be that K-channel openers could be effective in opposing this depolarization, although a continued high g_{Na} might result in maintenance of an increased excitability. Currently, antiarrhythmic drugs such as tocainide and mexiletine are employed to block active Na-channels (*see* Rudel, 1986).

Primary periodic paralyses

These include a group of hereditary disorders characterized by transient attacks of muscle weakness without impairment of consciousness or sensation, usually related to transient changes of serum $[K^+]$. Hyperkalaemic, normokalaemic and hypokalaemic types of periodic paralyses are recognized, according to the direction of change of serum $[K^+]$. Classifications and descriptions of the various conditions are given by Engel (1986b). The altered membrane properties of two primary conditions will be considered.

Primary hyperkalaemia

Short duration episodes may occur frequently, several times a day, or attacks may be of longer duration and less frequent. The attacks often develop after exercise and can affect most muscles but spare cranial and respiratory muscles. In patients the administration of 1 meq K^+ per kilogram body weight provokes attacks by raising serum $[K^+]$ much more than it would in normal subjects (Lewis *et al.*, 1979). The occurrence of attacks can be lowered by administration of diuretics and acute attacks may be aborted by intravenous administration of Ca or by inhalation of salbutamol (Wang & Clausen, 1976; Dahl-Jorgensen & Michalsen, 1979).

Recordings of membrane potential *in vivo* show that the muscle resting potential is low between attacks and it is a further lowering which is the immediate reason for paralysis (Rudel, 1986; Ruff, 1989). It has also been reported that membrane excitability is also reduced (Brooks, 1969). *In vitro*, normal and affected muscle fibres in a physiological $[K^+]_o$ of 3.5 mM have normal resting potentials of -80 mV (Lehmann-Horn *et al.*, 1983). When $[K^+]_o$ was increased to 7 mM both normal fibres and affected depolarized to -65 mV. At this potential normal fibres remained excitable and could generate full force. In one variant of this disease, affected fibres further depolarize to -55 mV and become inexcitable. When $[K^+]_o$ is elevated, affected fibres respond with an activation of a non-inactivating Na^+-conductance (Lehmann-Horn *et al.*, 1983, 1987) and the membrane depolarizes more than would be predicted by the Nernst equation. Furthermore, the membrane remains depolarized even when $[K^+]_o$ is returned to normal. Tetrodotoxin has been shown to block this Na^+-conductance *in vitro* and to repolarize the membrane.

The hyperpolarizing effect of adrenaline on skeletal muscle has been shown to improve muscle strength in patients suffering from hyperkalaemic periodic paralysis (Wang & Clausen, 1976; Bendheim *et al.*, 1985). In addition, cromakalim has recently been shown to be effective *in vitro* in

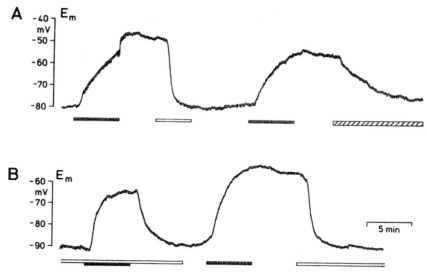

Fig. 10.8. Cromakalim repolarizes the membrane in two different fibres from a patient with hyperkalaemic periodic paralysis. A, Addition of 7 mM K$^+$ (▬▬▬) to the normal bathing solution resulted in a depolarization of the membrane; the membrane remained in this depolarized state even after [K$^+$]$_o$ was lowered to its normal resting level (3.5 mM). Cromakalim (100 μM, ▭) restored the normal resting potential. Such a repolarization was also induced by tetrodotoxin (TTX, 0.6 μM, ▨). B, When 7 mM K$^+$ were added in the presence of cromakalim no excessive membrane depolarization was seen. Later on, 7 mM K$^+$ were added to the normal bathing solution; this induced a membrane depolarization with the typical characteristics of a hyperkalaemic periodic paralysis muscle fibre. (Reproduced with permission from Spuler *et al.*, 1989.)

repolarizing fibres from two patients with hyperkalaemic paralysis (Spuler *et al.*, 1989). Initially, [K$^+$]$_o$ was elevated by 7 mM which resulted in a strong membrane depolarization. Repolarization did not occur upon lowering [K$^+$]$_o$ to the normal resting level of 3.5 mM. Adding 100 μM cromakalim to the bathing solution repolarized the membrane. Later, in the same fibre, tetrodotoxin was used to repolarize the fibre after depolarization (Fig. 10.8). In other experiments on human muscle fibres, the hyperpolarizing effect of cromakalim was blocked by tolbutamide, a specific antagonist of K$_{ATP}$-channels in β-cells of rat islets of Langerhans (Sturgess *et al.*, 1985). The authors concluded that the hyperpolarizing effect of cromakalim on human muscle fibres from patients with hyperkalaemic periodic paralysis was via an increase in membrane g_K caused by activation of a population of K$_{ATP}$-channels.

Hypokalaemic paralysis

In this disease there is a movement of K$^+$ from serum into muscle cells

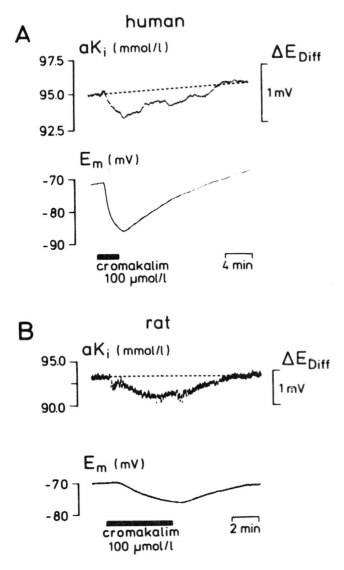

Fig. 10.9. Effects of cromakalim on intracellular K^+ activity (aK_i) and membrane potential (E_m) of a fibre in a normal human skeletal muscle segment, A, and in an isolated rat soleus muscle, B. ΔE_{Diff} is the difference between the voltage reading of the K^+-sensitive and the reference barrel of the double-barrelled ion-sensitive microelectrode. Cromakalim was applied via the bathing solution during the times indicated by the bars. (Reproduced with permission from Grafe *et al.*, 1990.)

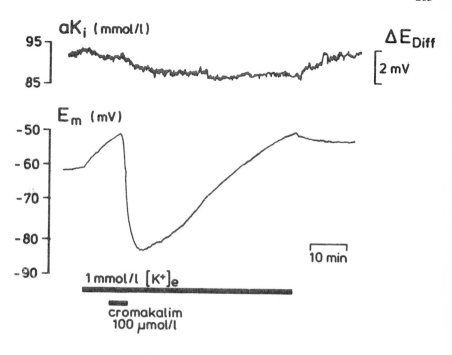

Fig. 10.10. Effects of cromakalim on intracellular K^+ activity (aK_i) and membrane potential (E_m) of a muscle fibre in a skeletal muscle segment obtained from a patient with hypokalaemic periodic paralysis. The $[K^+]_o$ at the beginning of the recording was 3.5 mmol/l. It was reduced to 1 mmol/l to imitate the clinical situation in which low levels of $[K^+]_o$ are observed. Other conditions are as in Fig. 10.9. (Reproduced with permission from Grafe *et al.*, 1990.)

during paralytic attacks. These attacks are less frequent than in hyperkalaemic paralysis but severe attacks can last for days and leave patients helpless and unable to move. Again, respiratory muscles are the least affected. Unlike the situation in normal skeletal muscle, lowering $[K^+]_o$ of affected fibres does not lead to a hyperpolarization but to a depolarization. At a normal $[K^+]_o$, the resting potential of muscle from affected patients was found to be 5–10 mV lower than normal and was unstable (Rudel *et al.*, 1984). Between attacks there is evidence that $[K^+]_i$ is reduced and that $[Na^+]_i$ may be increased to as much as 50 mM (Engel & Lambert, 1969).

The underlying cause for membrane depolarization and membrane inexcitability seems to be an abnormal ratio in the relative conductances to Na and K, probably due to a high Na-conductance (Rudel *et al.*, 1984). It might, therefore, be expected that inducing an increase in K-conductance would cause membrane repolarization and alleviate muscle weakness. There has been one recent report (Grafe *et al.*, 1990) of an investigation into the efficacy of the K-channel opener cromakalim on biopsied muscle from sufferers of hypokalaemic periodic paralysis. *In*

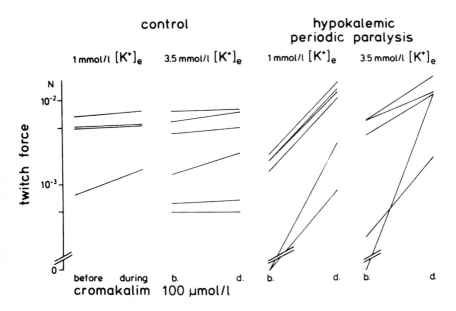

Fig. 10.11. Summary of the effects of cromakalim on the twitch force of 12 skeletal muscle bundles obtained from six control persons and from four patients with hyperkalaemic paralysis. The bundles were stimulated every 10 s. The values of the twitch force, which were taken before and 5–10 min after application of croma-kalim, are shown. Note the logarithmic scale. (Reproduced with permission from Grafe *et al.*, 1990.)

vitro, cromakalim, 100 μM, caused a hyperpolarization of normal human fibres of 10–15 mV and a very small decrease in intracellular K^+ activity (Fig. 10.9). Muscle specimens were obtained from four patients with hypokalaemic periodic paralysis. Even in solutions with normal, 3.5 mM $[K^+]$, these fibres were depolarized by 10 mV from normal. This is not due to a decrease in E_K since $[K^+]_i$ was normal at 93 mM. Reducing $[K^+]_o$ to 1 mM resulted in depolarization as typically found for hypokalaemic muscle fibres. Application of cromakalim induced a strong hyperpolariza-tion of over 30 mV at a concentration of 100 μM (Fig. 10.10). While the twitch force of normal muscle was unaffected by cromakalim, its applica-tion to fibres from patients with hypokalaemic paralysis increased twitch force several-fold (Grafe *et al.*, 1990; Fig. 10.11). This increased twitch force was only slowly reversed. After a 10 min exposure to cromakalim it took 30 min for the twitch force to recover to pretreatment levels. Gliben-clamide (1 μM) completely suppressed the membrane hyperpolarizing and force-facilitating effect of cromakalim. Since glibenclamide is a specific antagonist of K_{ATP}-channels (Fosset *et al.*, 1988) it seems likely that cromakalim exerts its beneficial effects upon muscle fibres from sufferers of hypokalaemic paralysis by an increase in membrane g_K via activation of K_{ATP}.

Therapeutic potential for K-channel modulators

Clearly, there are several pathological conditions in which there are therapeutic applications for membrane stabilizers and increasing g_m is one means by which this can be achieved. The presence of a high density of K_{ATP}-channels in the sarcolemma provides an attractive intervention site by which membrane conductance could be raised. There is a real lack of detailed electrophysiological measurements into many human muscle diseases which would be necessary before any clinical intervention of this sort could be undertaken. It should also be noted that the concentration of drugs such as cromakalim that have been used in *in vitro* experiments on skeletal muscle fibres has been in the high, micromolar range. *In vivo*, the greater sensitivity of vascular smooth muscle (nanomolar micromolar range) to these agents may prevent their therapeutic use on skeletal muscle unless a means of targeting skeletal muscle, or of protecting vascular muscle, can be developed.

References

Adrian, R. H. & Bryant, S. H. (1974) On the repetitive discharge in myotonic muscle fibres. *Journal of Physiology* **240**, 505–515.

Adrian, R. H. & Peachey, L. D. (1973) Reconstruction of the action potential of frog sartorius muscle. *Journal of Physiology* **234**, 103–131.

Adrian, R. H., Chandler, W. K. & Hodgkin, A. L. (1970) Voltage clamp experiments in striated muscle fibres. *Journal of Physiology* **208**, 607–644.

Anderson, C. S., MacKinnon, R., Smith, C. & Miller, C. (1988) Charybdotoxin block of single calcium-activated potassium channels. Effects of channel gating, voltage and ionic strength. *Journal of General Physiology* **91**, 317–333.

Barrett, J. N., Magleby, K. L. & Pallotta, B. S. (1982) Properties of single calcium-activated potassium channels in cultured rat muscle. *Journal of Physiology* **331**, 211–230.

Becker, P. E. (1977) Myotonia congenita and syndromes associated with myotonia: clinical–genetic studies of the nondystrophic myotonias. In Becker, P. E. (ed.) *Topics in Human Genetics*, vol. III. Thieme, Stuttgart.

Bendheim, P. E., Reale, E. O. & Berg, B. O. (1985) β-Adrenergic treatment of hyperkalaemic periodic paralysis. *Neurology* **35**, 746–749.

Birnberger, K. L., Rudel, R. & Struppler, A. (1975) Clinical and electrophysiological observations in patients with myotonic muscle disease and the therapeutic effect of N-propyl-ajmalin. *Journal of Neurology* **210**, 99–110.

Blatz, L. A. & Magleby, K. L. (1984) Ion conductance and selectivity of single calcium-activated potassium channels in cultured rat muscle. *Journal of General Physiology* **84**, 1–23.

Blatz, L. A. & Magleby, K. L. (1986) Single apamin-blocked Ca-activated K^+ channels of small conductance in cultured rat skeletal muscle. *Nature* **323**, 718–720.

Bonilla, E., Samitt, C. E., Miranda, A. F., Hays, A. P., Salviati, G., Dimauro, S., Kunkel, L. M., Hoffman, E. P. & Rowland, L. P. (1988) Duchenne muscular dystrophy: Deficiency of dystrophin at the muscle cell surface. *Cell* **54**, 447–452.

Bretag, A. H. (1973) Mathematical modelling of the myotonic action potential. In Desmedt, J. E. (ed.), *New Developments in Electromyography and Clinical Neurophysiology*, vol. 1. Karger, Basel, pp. 464–482.

Brooks, J. E. (1969) Hyperkalemic periodic paralysis. *Archives of Neurology* **20**, 13–18.

Brown, R. H. Jr & Hoffman, E. P. (1988) Molecular biology of Duchenne muscular dystrophy. *Trends in Neurosciences* **11**, 480–484.

Burton, F., Dorstelmann, U. & Hutter, O. F. (1988) Single-channel activity in sarcolemmal vesicles from human and other mammalian muscles. *Muscle and Nerve* **11**, 1029–1038.

Campos de Carvalho, A. C. & Cukierman, S. (1987) Ryanodine does not affect the potassium channel from the sarcoplasmic reticulum of skeletal muscle. *Biochemical and Biophysical Research Communications* **148**, 1137–1143.

Carlson, F. D. & Siger, A. (1960) The mechanochemistry of muscular contraction. 1. The isometric twitch. *Journal of General Physiology* **44**, 33–60.

Castle, N. A., Haylett, D. G. & Jenkinson, D. H. (1989) Toxins in the characterization of potassium channels. *Trends in Neurosciences* **12**, 59–66.

Chad, J. E. & Eckert, R. (1985) Inactivation of Ca^{2+} channels. *Progress in Biophysics and Molecular Biology* **44**, 215–245.

Chamberlain, J. S., Pearlman, J. A., Muzny, D. M., Gibbs, R. A., Ranier, J. E., Reeves, A. A. & Caskey, C. T. (1988) Expression of the murine Duchenne muscular dystrophy gene in muscle and brain. *Science* **239**, 1416–1418.

Charlton, M., Silverman, H. & Atwood, H. L. (1981) Intracellular potassium activities in muscles of normal and dystrophic mice: an *in vivo* electrometric study. *Experimental Neurology* **71**, 203–219.

Cognard, C., Traore, F., Potreau, D. & Raymond, G. (1984) Effects of apamin on the outward potassium current of isolated frog skeletal muscle fibers. *Pflügers Archiv* **402**, 222–224.

Dahl-Jorgensen, K. & Michalsen, H. (1979) Adynamia episodica hereditaria: Treatment with salbutamol. *Acta Paediatrica Scandinavica* **68**, 583–585.

Davies, N. W. (1990) Modulation of ATP-sensitive K^+ channels in skeletal muscle by intracellular protons. *Nature* **344**, 375–377.

DePeyer, J. E., Lues, I., Gericke, R. & Haeusler, G. (1989) Characterization of a novel K^+ channel activator, EMD 52962, in electrophysiological and pharmacological experiments. *Pflügers Archiv* **414**, S191.

Duncan, C. J. (1978) Role of intracellular calcium in promoting muscle damage: a strategy for controlling the dystrophic condition. *Experientia* **34**, 1532–1535.

Duval, A. & Leoty, C. (1985) Changes in the ionic current sensitivity to inhibitors in twitch rat skeletal muscles following denervation. *Pflügers Archiv* **403**, 407–414.

Elmqvist, D., Johns, T. R. & Thesleff, S. (1960) A study of some electrophysiological properties of human intercostal muscle. *Journal of Physiology* **154**, 602–607.

Eltze, M. (1989) Glibenclamide is a competitive antagonist of cromakalim, pinacidil and RP 49356 in guinea-pig pulmonary artery. *European Journal of Pharmacology* **165**, 231–239.

Engel, A. G. (1986a) The pathophysiologic basis of the mytonias and the periodic paralysis. In Engel, A. G. & Banker, B. Q. (eds) *Myology — Basic and Clinical*. McGraw-Hill, New York, pp. 1297–1311.

Engel, A. G. (1986b) Periodic paralysis. In Engel, A. G. & Banker, B. Q. (eds) *Myology — Basic and Clinical*. McGraw-Hill, New York, pp. 1843–1870.

Engel, A. G. & Lambert, E. H. (1969) Calcium activation of electrically inexcitable muscle fibres in primary hypokalaemic periodic paralysis. *Neurology* **19**, 851–858.

Escande, D., Thuringer, D., LeGuern, S. & Cavero, I. (1988) The potassium channel opener cromakalim (BRL 34915) activates ATP—dependent K^+ channels in isolated cardiac myocytes. *Biochemical and Biophysical Research Communications* **154**, 620–625.

Escande, D., Thuringer, D., LeGuern, S., Courtie, J., Laville, M. & Cavero, I. (1989)

Potassium channel openers act through an activation of ATP-sensitive K^+ channels in guinea-pig cardiac myocytes. *Pflügers Archiv* **414**, 669–675.

Eulenberg, A. (1892) Über eine familiäre, über 6 Generationen verfolgbare Form kongenitaler Paramyotonie. *Zentralblatt für Neurologie* **5**, 265–272.

Faivre, J-F., & Findlay, I. (1989) Effects of tolbutamide, glibenclamide and diazoxide upon action potentials recorded from rat ventricular muscle. *Biochimica et Biophysica Acta* **984**, 1–5.

Findlay, I. (1987) ATP-sensitive K^+ channels in rat ventricular myocytes are blocked and inactivated by internal divalent cations. *Pflügers Archiv* **410**, 313–320.

Fink, R. & Luttgau, H. C. (1976) An evaluation of the membrane constants and the potassium conductance in metabolically exhausted muscle fibres. *Journal of Physiology* **263**, 215–238.

Fink, R., Hase, S., Luttgau, H. C. & Wettwer, E. (1983) The effect of cellular energy reserves and internal calcium ions on the potassium conductance in skeletal muscle of the frog. *Journal of Physiology* **336**, 211–228.

Fosset, M., DeWeille, J. R., Green, R. D., Schmid-Antomarchi, H. & Lazdunski, M. (1988) Antidiabetic sulfonylureas control action potential properties in heart cells via high affinity receptors that are linked to ATP-dependent K^+ channels. *Journal of Biological Chemistry* **263**, 7933–7936.

Freygang, W. H. Jr., Goldstein, D. A. & Hellam, D. C. (1964) The after-potential that follows trains of impulses in frog muscle fibres. *Journal of General Physiology* **47**, 929–952.

Gelband, C. H., Lodge, N. J. & Van Breemen, C. (1989) A Ca^{2+}-activated K^+ channel from rabbit aorta: modulation by cromakalim. *European Journal of Pharmacology* **167**, 201–210.

Golowasch, J., Kirkwood, A. & Miller, C. (1986) Allosteric effects of magnesium on the gating of calcium-activated potassium channels from mammalian skeletal muscle. *Journal of Experimental Biology* **124**, 5–13.

Grafe, P., Quasthoff, S., Strupp, M. & Lehmann-Horn, F. (1990) Enhancement of K^+ conductance improves *in vitro* the contraction force of skeletal muscle in hypokalemic periodic paralysis. *Muscle and Nerve* **13**, 451–457.

Gray, M. A., Tomlins, B., Montgomery, R. A. P. & Williams, A. J. (1988) Structural aspects of the sarcoplasmic reticulum potassium channel revealed by gallium block. *Biophysical Journal* **54**, 233–239.

Gruener, R. (1977) *In vitro* membrane excitability of diseased human muscle. In Rowland, L. P. (ed.), *Proceedings of the 5th International Scientific Conference of the Muscular Dystrophy Association: Pathogenesis of Human Muscular dystrophies*. Excerpta Medica, New York, pp. 242–258.

Gruener, R., Stern, L. Z., Markovitz, D. & Gerdes, C. (1979) Electrophysiological properties of intercostal muscle fibres in human neuromuscular diseases. *Muscle and Nerve* **2**, 165–173.

Hamill, O. P., Marty, A., Neher, E., Sakmann, B. & Sigworth, F. J. (1981) Improved patch-clamp techniques for high resolution current recording from cells and cell-free membrane patches. *Pflügers Archiv* **391**, 85–110.

Harvey, A. L. & Marshall, I. G. (1977) A comparison of the effects of aminopyridines on isolated chicken and rat skeletal muscle preparations. *Comparative Biochemistry and Physiology C* **58**, 161–165.

Head, S. I., Stephenson, D. G. & Williams, D. A. (1990) Properties of enzymatically isolated skeletal fibres from mice with muscular dystrophy. *Journal of Physiology* **422**, 351–367.

Hertzberg, G. R., Challberg, M. D., Hess, B. C. & Howland, J. L. (1975) Elevated potassium efflux from dystrophic diaphragm: influence of diphenylhydantoin and lithium. *Biochemical and Biophysical Research Communications* **63**, 858–863.

Hodgkin, A. L. & Katz, B. (1949) The effect of sodium ions on the electrical activity of the giant axon of the squid. *Journal of Physiology* **108**, 37–77.

Hoffman, E. P., Brown, R. H. Jr & Kunkel, L. M. (1987) Dystrophin: The protein product of the Duchenne muscular dystrophy locus. *Cell* **51**, 919–928.

Hofmann, W. W. & DeNardo, G. L. (1968) Sodium flux in myotonic muscular dystrophy. *American Journal of Physiology* **214**, 330–336.

Hofmann, W. W., Alston, W. & Rowe, G. (1966) A study of individual neuromuscular junctions in myotonia. *Electroencephalography and Clinical Neurophysiology* **21**, 521–537.

Horvath, B., Berg, L., Cummings, D. J. & Shy, G. M. (1955) Muscular dystrophy cation concentrations in residual muscle. *Journal of Applied Physiology* **8**, 22–30.

Johns, R. J. (1963) The electrical and mechanical events of neuromuscular transmission. *American Journal of Medicine* **35**, 611–621.

Katz, B. (1949) Les constantes électriques de la membrane du muscle. *Archives Science et Physiologie* **3**, 285–300.

Klöckner, U., Trieschmann, U. & Isenberg, G. (1989) Pharmacological modulation of calcium and potassium channels in isolated vascular smooth muscle cells. *Arzneimittelforschung (Drug Research)* **39**, 120–126.

Kwieciński, H., Lehmann-Horn, F. & Rudel, R. (1984) The resting membrane parameters of human intercostal muscle at low, normal, and high extracellular potassium. *Muscle and Nerve* **7**, 60–65.

Leech, C. A. & Stanfield, P. R. (1981) Inward rectification in frog skeletal muscle fibres and its dependence on membrane potential and external potassium. *Journal of Physiology* **319**, 295–309.

Lehmann-Horn, F., Kuther, G., Ricker, K., Grafe, P., Ballanyi, K. & Rudel, R. (1987) Adynamia episodia hereditaria with myotonia: a non-inactivating sodium current and the effect of extracellular pH. *Muscle and Nerve* **10**, 363–374.

Lehmann-Horn, F., Rudel, R., Dengler, R., Lorkovic, H., Haass, A. & Ricker, K. (1981) Membrane defects in paramyotonia congenita with and without myotonia in a warm environment. *Muscle and Nerve* **4**, 396–406.

Lehmann-Horn, F., Rudel, R., Ricker, K., Lorkovic, H., Dengler, R. & Hopf, H. C. (1983) Two cases of adynamia episodica hereditaria: *In vitro* investigation of muscle cell membrane and contraction parameters. *Muscle and Nerve* **6**, 113–121.

Lewis, E. D., Griggs, R. C. & Moxley, R. T. (1979) Regulation of plasma potassium in hyperkalemic periodic paralysis. *Neurology* **29**, 1131–1137.

Lipicky, R. J. (1977) Studies in human myotonic dystrophy. In Rowland, L. P. (ed.), *Pathogenesis of Human Muscular Dystrophies*. Excerpta Medica, Amsterdam, pp. 729–738.

Lipicky, R. J. & Bryant, S. H. (1973) A biophysical study of the human myotonias. In Desmedt, J. E. (ed.) *New Developments in Electromyography and Clinical Neurophysiology*, vol. 1. Karger, Basel, pp. 451–463.

Lipicky, R. J. & Hess, J. (1974) Potassium permeability in isolated skeletal muscle from mice with muscular dystrophy. *American Journal of Physiology* **226**, 592–596.

Lipicky, R. J., Bryant, S. H. & Salmon, J. H. (1971) Cable parameters, sodium, potassium, chloride and water content, and potassium efflux in isolated external intercostal muscle of normal volunteers and patients with myotonia congenita. *Journal of Clinical Investigation* **50**, 2091–2103.

Lorkovic, H. (1976) Effect of sodium on voltage–current relationships in rat muscles. *Archives Internationales de Physiologie et de Biochemie* **84**, 839–854.

McComas, A. J. (1977) *Neuromuscular Function and Disorders*. Butterworth, London.

McComas, A. J. & Mrozek, K. (1968) The electrical properties of muscle fibre membranes in man. *Journal of Neurology, Neurosurgery and Psychiatry* **31**, 434–440.

McManus, O. B. & Magleby, K. L. (1988) Kinetic states and modes of single large-conductance calcium-activated potassium channels in cultured rat skeletal muscle. *Journal of Physiology* **402**, 79–120.

Matsuda, H., Saigusa, A. & Irisawa, H. (1987) Ohmic conductance through the inwardly rectifying K channel and blocking by internal Mg^{2+}, *Nature* **325**, 156–159.

Miller, C. Moczydlowski, E., Latorre, R. & Phillips, M. (1985) Charybdotoxin, a protein inhibitor of single Ca^{2+}-activated K^+ channels from mammalian skeletal muscle. *Nature* **313**, 316–318.

Moczydlowski, E., Lucchesi, K. & Ravindran, A. (1988) An emerging pharmacology of peptide toxins targeted against potassium channels. *Journal of Membrane Biology* **105**, 95–111.

Moutin, M. J. & Dupont, Y. (1988) Rapid filtration studies of calcium-induced calcium release from skeletal sarcoplasmic reticulum. Role of monovalent ions. *Journal of Biological Chemistry* **269**, 4228–4235.

Norris, F. H. (1962) Unstable membrane potential in human myotonic muscle. *Electroencephalography and Clinical Neurophysiology* **14**, 197–201.

Pette, D. & Vrbova, G. (1985) Invited review: Neural control of phenotypic expression in mammalian muscle fibres. *Muscle and Nerve* **8**, 676–689.

Quast, U. & Cook, N. S. (1989) *In vitro* and *in vivo* comparisons of two K^+ channel openers, diazoxide and cromakalim, and their inhibition by glibenclamide. *Journal of Pharmacology and Experimental Therapeutics* **250**, 261–271.

Quasthoff, S., Spuler, A., Spittelmeister, W., Lehmann-Horn, F. & Grafe, P. (1990) K^+ channel openers suppress myotonic activity of human skeletal muscle *in vitro*. *European Journal of Pharmacology* **186**, 125–128.

Quayle, J. M., Standen, N. B. & Stanfield, P. R. (1988) The voltage-dependent block of ATP-sensitive potassium channels of frog skeletal muscle by caesium and barium ions. *Journal of Physiology* **405**, 677–697.

Redfern, P. A. (1970) Neuromuscular transmission in newborn rats. *Journal of Physiology* **209**, 701–709.

Renaud, J-F., Desnuelle, C., Schmid-Antomarchi, H., Hughes, M., Serratrice, G. & Lazdunski, M. (1986) Expression of apamin receptor in muscles of patients with myotonic dystrophy. *Nature* **319**, 678–680.

Renaud, J. M. (1989) The effect of lactate on intracellular pH and force recovery of fatigued sartorius muscles of the frog *Rana pipiens*. *Journal of Physiology* **416**, 31–47.

Robbins, N. (1977) Cation movements in normal and short-term denervated rat fast twitch muscle. *Journal of Physiology* **271**, 605–624.

Romey, G. & Lazdunski, M. (1984) The coexistence in rat muscle cells of two distinct classes of Ca^{2+}-dependent K^+ channels with different physiological functions. *Biochemical and Biophysical Research Communications* **118**, 669–674.

Rousseau, E., Lai, F. A., Henderson, J. S. & Meissner, G. (1988) Activation and inactivation of the skeletal SR Ca^{2+} release channel by trypsin. *Biophysical Journal* **53**, 455a.

Rowe, I. C. M., Wareham, A. C. & Whittle, M. A. (1990) Potassium channel activity in sarcolemmal vesicles formed from skeletal muscle fibres of normal and dystrophic mice. *Journal of the Neurological Sciences* **98**, 51–61.

Rowland, L. P. (1985) Clinical perspective: phenotypic expression in muscular dystrophy. *Advances in Experimental and Medical Biology* **182**, 3–13.

Rudel, R. (1986) The pathophysiological basis of the myotonias and the periodic paralyses. In Engel, A. G. & Banker, B. Q. (eds) *Myology — Basic and Clinical*. McGraw-Hill, New York, pp. 1297–1311.

Rudel, R., Dengler, R., Ricker, K., Haass, K. & Emser, W. (1980) Improved therapy of myotonia with the lidocaine derivative tocainide. *Journal of Neurology* **222**, 275–278.

Rudel, R., Lehmann-Horn, F., Ricker, K. & Kuther, G. (1984) Hypokalemic periodic paralysis: *in vitro* investigation of muscle fiber membrane parameters. *Muscle and Nerve* **7**, 110–120.

Rudy, B. (1988) Diversity and ubiquity of K channels. *Neuroscience* **25**, 729–749.

Ruff, R. L. (1989) Periodic paralysis. In Seldin, D. W. & Giebisch, G. (eds), *The Regulation of Potassium Balance*. Raven Press, New York, pp. 303–323.

Sakmann, B. & Trube, G. (1984) Conductance properties of single inwardly rectifying potassium channels in ventricular cells from guinea-pig heart. *Journal of Physiology* **347**, 641–657.

Schmid-Antomarchi, H., Renaud, J. F., Romey, G., Hughes, M., Schmid, A. & Lazdunski, M. (1985) The all-or-none role of innervation in expression of apamin receptor and of apamin-sensitive calcium-activated potassium channel in mammalian skeletal muscle. *Proceedings of the National Academy of Sciences USA* **82**, 2188–2191.

Schwarz, W., Neumcke, B. & Palade, P. T. (1981) Potassium-current fluctuations in inward-rectifying channels of frog skeletal muscle. *Journal of Membrane Biology* **63**, 85–92.

Sellin, L. C. & Sperelakis, N. (1978) Decreased potassium permeability in dystrophic skeletal muscle. *Experimental Neurology* **62**, 605–617.

Shalton, P. M. & Wareham, A. C. (1981) Intracellular activity of potassium in normal and dystrophic skeletal muscle from C57BL/6J mice. *Experimental Neurology* **74**, 673–687.

Spruce, A. E., Standen, N. B. & Stanfield, P. R. (1985) Voltage dependent, ATP-sensitive potassium channels of skeletal muscle membrane. *Nature* **316**, 736–738.

Spruce, A. E., Standen, N. B. & Stanfield, P. R. (1987) Studies of the unitary properties of adenosine-5′-triphosphate-regulated potassium channels of frog skeletal muscle. *Journal of Physiology* **382**, 213–236.

Spuler, A., Lehmann-Horn, F. & Grafe, P. (1989) Cromakalim (BRL 34915) restores *in vitro* the membrane potential of depolarized human skeletal muscle fibres. *Naunyn-Schmiedeberg's Archives of Pharmacology* **339**, 327–331.

Standen, N. B., Quayle, J. M., Davies, N. W., Brayden, J. E., Huang, Y. & Nelson, M. T. (1989) Hyperpolarizing vasodilators activate ATP-sensitive K^+ channels in arterial smooth muscle. *Science* **245**, 177–180.

Standen, N. B., Stanfield, P. R. & Ward, T. A. (1985) Properties of single potassium channels in vesicles formed from the sarcolemma of frog skeletal muscle. *Journal of Physiology* **364**, 339–358.

Standen, N. B., Stanfield, P. R., Ward, T. A. & Wilson, S. W. (1984) A new preparation for recording of single-channel currents from skeletal muscle. *Proceedings of the Royal Society London Series B* **221**, 455–464.

Stanfield, P. R. (1970) The effect of the tetraethylammonium ion on the delayed currents of frog skeletal muscle. *Journal of Physiology* **209**, 209–229.

Stein, P. & Palade, P. (1989) Patch clamp of sarcolemmal spheres from stretched skeletal muscle fibres. *American Journal of Physiology* **256** (Cell Physiology **25**), C434–C440.

Sturgess, N. C., Ashford, M. L. J., Cook, D. L. & Hales, C. N. (1985) The sulphonylurea receptor may be an ATP-sensitive potassium channel. *Lancet ii*, 474–475.

Thuringer, D. & Escande, D. (1989) Apparent competition between ATP and the potassium channel opener RP 49356 on ATP-sensitive K^+ channels of cardiac myocytes. *Molecular Pharmacology* **36**, 897–902.

Traore, F., Cognard, C., Potreau, D. & Raymond, G. (1986) The apamin-sensitive potassium current in frog skeletal muscle: Its dependence on the extracellular calcium and sensitivity to calcium channel blockers. *Pflügers Archiv* **407**, 199–203.

Vandenberg, C. A. (1987) Inward rectification of a potassium channel in cardiac ventricular cells depends on internal magnesium ions. *Proceedings of the National Academy of Sciences USA* **84**, 2560–2564.

Wang, P. & Clausen, T. (1976) Treatment of attacks in hyperkalaemic familial periodic paralysis by inhalation of salbutamol. *Lancet i*, 221–227.

Ward, K. M. & Wareham, A. C. (1984) Intracellular activity of sodium in normal and dystrophic skeletal muscle from C57BL/6J mice. *Experimental Neurology* **83**, 629–633.

Wareham, A. C. (1978) Effect of denervation on the response of the resting membrane potential of rat skeletal muscle to potassium. *Pflügers Archiv* **373**, 225–228.

Wareham, A. C., Rowe, I. C. M. & Whittle, M. A. (1990) Sarcolemmal K⁺ channel activity in developing rat skeletal muscle membranes. *Journal of the Neurological Sciences* **96**, 321–331.

Watkins, S. C., Hoffman, E. P., Slayter, H. S. & Kunkel, L. M. (1988) Immunoelectron microscopic localization of dystrophin in muscle fibres. *Nature* **333**, 863–866.

Weik, R. & Neumcke, B. (1990) Effects of potassium channel openers on single potassium channels in mouse skeletal muscle. *Naunyn-Schmiedeberg's Archives of Pharmacology* **342**, 258–263.

Williams, A. J. & Tomlins, B. (1985) Solubilization and reconstitution of the potassium-selective channel of rabbit skeletal muscle sarcoplasmic reticulum. *Biochemical Society Transactions* **13**, 1247–1248.

Williams, D. A., Head, S. I., Bakker, A. J. & Stephenson, D. G. (1990) Resting calcium concentrations in isolated skeletal muscle fibres of dystrophic mice. *Journal of Physiology* **428**, 243–256.

Williams, J. D., Ansell, B. M., Reiffel, L., Stone, C. A. & Kark, R. M. (1957) Electrolyte levels in normal and dystrophic muscle determined by neutron activation. *Lancet ii*, 464–466.

Woll, K. H., Lonnendonker, U. & Neumcke, B. (1989) ATP-sensitive potassium channels in adult mouse skeletal muscle: Different modes of blockage by internal cations, ATP and tolbutamide. *Pflügers Archiv* **414**, 622–628.

Young, R. C., Allen, R. J. & Meissner, G. (1981) Permeability of reconstituted sarcoplasmic reticulum vesicles. Reconstitution of the potassium ion, sodium ion channel. *Biochimica et Biophysica Acta* **640**, 409–418.

Zubrzycka-Gaarn, E. E., Bulman, D. E., Karpati, G., Burghes, A. H. M., Belfall, B., Klamut, H. J., Talbot, J., Hodges, R. S., Ray, P. N. & Warton, R. G. (1988) The Duchenne muscular dystrophy gene is localized in sarcolemma of human skeletal muscle. *Nature* **333**, 466–469.

Chapter 11
Naturally-occurring
potassium channel blockers

B. S. Brewster and P. N. Strong

Introduction

Animal venom toxins are produced for either offensive or defensive purposes, the toxin's main role in the venom being the immobilization of the victim. The properties that a toxin must possess in order to achieve this end are potency and specificity. It is these characteristics that enable venom toxins to target specific sites with high affinity and it is this ability which makes them so useful to the biological scientist.

Venom toxins have proved to be extremely versatile tools in ion channel research. The ionic currents which are blocked by each toxin have been characterized by electrophysiological means. Binding assays using radiolabelled toxins enable ion channels to be characterized by their affinities and the binding site density to be determined. Autoradiographic studies reveal the distribution and density of binding sites in brain and other tissues. This information, coupled with behavioural studies involving the injection of toxin into a specific brain region, can identify the ion channels and brain regions responsible for particular behavioural patterns. Cross-linking of radiolabelled toxin to its receptor enables the molecular weight of the binding proteins to be determined. Finally, by using the toxin as an affinity ligand, K-channel proteins can be purified and further characterized.

The primary function of this article is to survey the more recent literature published during the past 18 months and to provide an update of a more comprehensive review published recently (Strong, 1990).

Features of animal venom toxins with activity at K-channels

β-Bungarotoxin

Structural features

β-Bungarotoxin, isolated from the venom of the Taiwan krait, *Bungarus multicinctus*, belongs to a group of presynaptically acting neurotoxins (other members include crotoxin, notexin and taipoxin) that possess Ca-dependent phospholipase activity (Howard & Gundersen, 1980; Strong, 1987). β-Bungarotoxin has two dissimilar chains, linked by a single disulphide bridge. The larger chain ($M_r = 13.5\,\text{kDa}$) shares considerable sequence homology with pancreatic phospholipase A_2 and other snake venom phospholipase enzymes. The smaller chain ($M_r = 7\,\text{kDa}$) has some sequence homology with Kunitz-type trypsin inhibitors, although the toxin has no protease inhibitor activity. Reduction of the interchain disulphide bonds leads to a complete loss of activity and it has not been possible to separate the two chains of β-bungarotoxin in their native state and demonstrate that either chain has any biological activity. Five isotoxins have been characterized and sequenced (Kondo *et al.*, 1978, 1982a,b) and they conveniently fall into two groups based on sequence analysis (three A-chain variants, and two B-chain variants). Recently, a fourth A-chain variant has been cloned from a cDNA library prepared from the venom gland of *B. multicinctus* (Danse *et al.*, 1990).

Crystallographic data of β_1-bungarotoxin at 2.3 Å (0.23 nm) resolution suggests that the two-chain, heterodimeric toxin is associated as two distinct tetramers, $(AB)_4$, each heterodimer having dihedral D_2 symmetry (Kwong *et al.*, 1989).

Phospholipase A_2 activity

The properties of β-bungarotoxin as a phospholipase A_2 enzyme are essentially indistinguishable from non-toxin pancreatic phospholipases. However, β-bungarotoxin, unlike the vast majority of phospholipase A_2 enzymes, selectively inhibits the release of acetylcholine at presynaptic motor endplates. Attempts to correlate phospholipid hydrolysis and loss of membrane integrity, following treatment of rat brain synaptosomes with either β-bungarotoxin or notexin (as compared with non-toxic phospholipases), have not been successful in explaining the presynaptic specificity (Yates *et al.*, 1990). The proposed correlation between phospholipid hydrolysis and the pharmacological properties of β-bungarotoxin and notexin, was examined by selective chemical modification of the two toxins. The results have proved equivocal, with some (but not all) pharmacological actions occurring independently of phospholipid hydrolysis

(Rosenberg et al., 1989). This trend, however, suggests that the N-terminal region of the phospholipase A_2 toxins is an important contributor to their β-type presynaptic neurotoxicity.

Effects on K-currents and channels

The facilitatory effects of β-bungarotoxin and crotoxin at the neuromuscular junction may be due to an inhibition of a subpopulation of K-currents at motor nerve endings. Using an extracellular microelectrode recording technique, part of the K-current contribution to the observed perineural waveform can be inhibited by these toxins. Inhibition can still be observed in zero Ca conditions, indicating that K-channel blockade is independent of phospholipase activity and that the toxins do not affect Ca-activated K-currents, $I_{K(Ca)}$ (Dreyer & Penner, 1987; Rowan & Harvey, 1988; Rowan et al., 1990). β-Bungarotoxin also blocks a subtype of the non-inactivating, slow outward K-current in guinea-pig dorsal root ganglion neurones (Petersen et al., 1986). This current is also blocked by dendrotoxin (see later).

β-Bungarotoxin is also active in the central nervous system and produces irreversible blockade of neurotransmission in nerve terminals of the cerebellum, olfactory cortex and hippocampus (Halliwell et al., 1982). Using autoradiographic techniques on brain sections, binding sites for the iodinated toxin have been found enriched in grey matter areas and synaptic regions, consistent with the pharmacological data (Pelchen-Matthews & Dolly, 1988). In contrast to the peripheral nervous system, β-bungarotoxin appears to inhibit the effects of a number of different neurotransmitters in the brain.

The toxin also perturbs many functions of brain synaptosomes, including the enhancement of neurotransmitter release (Wernicke et al., 1975), the inhibition of transport systems (Dowdall et al., 1977), the release of cytoplasmic markers (Rugolo et al., 1986) as well as the depolarization and eventual collapse of the synaptosomal membrane potential (Ng & Howard, 1978; Nicholls et al., 1985). Benishin (1990) has recently shown that β-bungarotoxin blocks K (^{86}Rb) efflux from mammalian synaptosomes ($EC_{50} = 1$ nM). The toxin selectively inhibits the slowly inactivating component of ^{86}Rb-efflux in the absence of Ca^{2+}. The reduced and carboxymethylated, isolated single B chain of the toxin is surprisingly even more effective ($EC_{50} = 0.1$ nM) at inhibiting the non-inactivating component of ^{86}Rb efflux. This is an intriguing result, since all previous attempts to separate the two chains of the toxin in their native state have not been successful; yet this result would suggest that the denatured, isolated B-chain retains biological activity. Thus, in accordance with electrophysiological data, it appears that β-bungarotoxin affects more than one type of voltage-activated K-channel. Identification is complicated by the fact that the kinetics of K-channel subtypes in the peripheral and central nervous systems may be different. Experiments with mammalian synaptosomes are further complicated by their diverse neurotransmitter populations. An interesting attempt to address this problem has recently been made by partitioning cerebrocortical synaptosomes in dextran-polyethylene glycol two-phase systems (Garcia-Garayo *et al.*, 1990). β-Bungarotoxin induces cholinergic synaptosomes to selectively and completely partition into the low density phase.

Triton X-100 successfully solubilizes the β-bungarotoxin binding protein from chick brain (Rehm & Betz, 1984; Black *et al.*, 1988). Gel filtration and sedimentation analysis indicated that the solubilized binding protein had a molecular mass of approximately 430 kDa. The affinity of the binding protein was only slightly decreased by solubilization and β-bungarotoxin binding to the solubilized protein was inhibited by dendrotoxin.

Binding sites

Original experiments cross-linking β-bungarotoxin to its high affinity binding site on chick brain membranes, with a photoactivatable cross-linking agent, resulted in the identification of a 115–120 kDa toxin-binding protein adduct (Rehm & Betz, 1983). In a more recent study from the same laboratory, two major binding proteins ($M_r = 75$ kDa, $M_r = 28$ kDa) have been identified, using different bivalent cross-linking agents (Schmidt & Betz, 1989). Formation of both adducts in the latter experiment was inhibited by both dendrotoxin and mast cell degranulating (MCD) peptide (*see later*). This result, coupled with the fact that the same toxin-binding polypeptides were identified under reducing and non-reducing conditions, suggest that they are two subunits of a hetero-oligomeric complex, representing the putative β-bungarotoxin sensitive neuronal K-channel. The previously identified larger adduct could not be observed and the authors suggest that this earlier result might be due to the formation of an oligomeric product of these two smaller peptides by the hydrophobic, membrane permeant cross-linking agent.

Dendrotoxins

Dendrotoxins are another group of snake toxins which act on K-channels in presynaptic nerve terminals. They have been isolated from African mambas (Harvey & Karlsson, 1980; Joubert & Taljaard, 1980; Harvey & Anderson, 1985) but unlike β-bungarotoxin, dendrotoxins enhance rather than block neuromuscular transmission.

Structural features and enzyme activity

Dendrotoxin, isolated from the venom of the green mamba *Dendroaspis angusticeps* (Harvey & Karlsson, 1980; Joubert & Taljaard, 1980) has been the most intensively studied member of this group; other members include toxins I and K from the venom of the black mamba *Dendroaspis polyepis* (Strydom, 1972). An exhaustive purification of all the peptides in this latter venom has identified as many as 14 different toxins, structurally and functionally related to dendrotoxin I (Schweitz *et al.*, 1990). Dendrotoxin and its homologues all have 57–61 amino acid residues including six half-cysteines. All of the dendrotoxins are highly homologous to Kunitz-type protease inhibitors, e.g. bovine pancreatic trypsin inhibitor (Dufton, 1985). More detailed structural analysis of both dendrotoxins I and K and bovine pancreatic trypsin inhibitor has been obtained using circular-dichroism spectroscopy (Hollecker & Larcher, 1989). Native forms of toxin K and more particularly toxin I, are less stable relative to their completely reduced forms than bovine pancreatic trypsin inhibitor. This might have functional significance, as toxin I, the less stable of the two toxins, is also the more potent. Lower stability probably reflects increased conformational freedom in the fully folded native molecule. Dendrotoxins are unable to inhibit the protease activity of either trypsin or chymotrypsin and these subtle differences in structural mobility may contribute to the functional differences between the toxins and protease inhibitors. Conversely, protease inhibitors do not possess dendrotoxin-line activity, nor do they inhibit radiolabelled dendrotoxin binding to brain membranes. In contrast to β-bungarotoxin, the dendrotoxins are not phospholipase A_2 enzymes. This makes the dendrotoxins more useful than β-bungarotoxin as specific tools for studying neurotransmitter release, since the enzymatic properties of β-bungarotoxin can mask toxin-acceptor interactions by hydrolysing phospholipids of the nerve terminal membrane (Strong *et al.*, 1977; Strong & Kelly, 1977; Kelly *et al.*, 1979; Rugolo *et al.*, 1986).

Effects on K-currents and channels

Dendrotoxin and its homologues increase acetylcholine released in response to motor nerve stimulation at the mammalian neuromuscular junction, without causing spontaneous contractions. There is both an increase in quantal content and the development of repetitive endplate potentials, in response to a single stimulus. These effects have a slow onset (minutes to hours) and are irreversible (Harvey & Karlsson, 1980; Anderson & Harvey, 1988). In a manner similar to β-bungarotoxin, dendrotoxins increase their potency several thousand-fold upon direct intracerebellar injection, causing severe convulsions and death (Mehraban *et al.*, 1985; Silveira *et al.*, 1988). There is a toxin-induced generalized increase in neuronal activity, affecting the release of both excitatory and inhibitory neurotransmitters (Halliwell *et al.*, 1986). Dendrotoxin causes a slight depolarization of mammalian synaptosomes, releasing both γ-aminobutyric acid (GABA) and glutamate in a Ca-dependent manner (Weller *et al.*, 1985; Nicholls *et al.*, 1985; Tibbs *et al.*, 1989a; Barbeito *et al.*, 1990). All these results are consistent with the notion that dendrotoxin blocks certain K-currents in both peripheral and central nerve endings.

Molecular genetic analyses of the *Shaker* gene in *Drosophila* have suggested the existence of multiple subtypes of closely related K-channel proteins. It appears that dendrotoxin does not simply affect one unique channel subtype, but rather a family of K-channels each with fast activation kinetics. For example, voltage-clamp studies on a variety of preparations have indicated that the sensitivity of K-channels to dendrotoxin in different excitable cells, does not necessarily reflect a similarity in channel function. Dendrotoxin suppresses a fast activating K-current at the frog node of Ranvier (Benoit & Dubois, 1986; Poulter *et al.*, 1989) and the non-inactivating or slowly inactivating K-currents in nodose ganglion neurones, dorsal root ganglion neurones (Penner *et al.*, 1986) and in visceral sensory neurones (Stansfeld *et al.*, 1986). Dendrotoxin also acts on the rapidly inactivating transient current in hippocampal neurones (Halliwell *et al.*, 1986), although a rapidly-inactivating variant of $I_{K(A)}$ in superior cervical ganglion neurones is reportedly not sensitive to dendrotoxin. The toxin also reduces A-type currents in both *Drosophila* larval muscle membrane and motor endplate preparations (Wu *et al.*, 1989). The dendrotoxin-sensitive K-current in dorsal root ganglia is carried by a K-channel with a maximum single channel conductance of 5–10 pS in a physiological K-gradient; the toxin appears to block this channel directly (Stansfeld & Feltz, 1988).

Dendrotoxin has recently been shown to block (albeit with lower affinity), large conductance Ca-activated K (BK_{Ca})-channels from rat skeletal muscle incorporated into planar bilayers (Lucchesi & Moczydlowski, 1990). This observation is complementary to other studies showing that charybdotoxin, a high affinity blocker of BK_{Ca}-channels (*see later*), also blocks some voltage-activated K-channels. Taken together, these results suggest that both dendrotoxin and charybdotoxin are recognizing similar structural motifs in both K_A- and BK_{Ca}-type channels. A most intriguing observation, however (Lucchesi & Moczydlowski, 1990), is that dendrotoxin appears to block BK_{Ca} internally. Although most characterized properties of dendrotoxin are more compatible with an external site of action, the effects of dendrotoxin at the neuromuscular junction (slow time of onset, irreversibility and temperature dependence) are consistent with such an intracellular action.

Binding sites

Iodinated dendrotoxin-binding sites are widely distributed in the brain, with high densities in synapse-rich areas of the hippocampus, the cerebellum and along nerve tracts (Pelchen-Matthews & Dolly, 1989). High affinity dendrotoxin-binding sites have been identified on both chick and rat brain membranes (Black & Dolly, 1986; Rehm & Lazdunski, 1988a). Using sequential toxin I and wheat germ lectin affinity columns, a several thousand-fold enrichment of the solubilized putative ion channel protein has been obtained (Rehm & Lazdunski, 1988b). The specific activity of these preparations (0.4–1.6 nmol toxin-binding sites/mg) is similar to the calculated value of 2.2 nmol/mg for the pure binding protein. The purified channel complex appears to be a multimeric protein and subunits of 76–80, 38 and 35 kDa have been identified (Rehm & Lazdunski, 1988b; Parcej & Dolly, 1989). The larger subunit, which binds dendrotoxin, can also be phosphorylated by a cyclic adenosine monophosphate (cAMP)-dependent protein kinase and by an endogenous protein kinase, which might be a K-channel specific kinase (Rehm et al., 1989b). After reconstitution into liposomes the purified protein induces a K-channel with a single channel conductance of 21 pS (150 mM symmetrical K^+) when it is incorporated into a lipid bilayer. Phosphorylation of the channel protein activates channel activity by increasing the proportion of time that the channel remains open (Rehm et al., 1989b). The toxin-binding subunit, but not the two smaller subunits, appears to be glycosylated (Rehm, 1989). Interestingly, the K_A-type channel cloned from *Drosophila* contains peptides of 70 and 35 kDa. Antibodies raised against synthetic peptides derived from the mouse brain homologue of the cloned *Drosophila* K-channel, recognize the toxin-binding subunit of the mammalian dendrotoxin-binding protein (Rehm et al., 1989a). This suggests that the isolated dendrotoxin-binding protein is related to the expression products of the mammalian homologue of the *Shaker* gene.

Homologues of α-dendrotoxin

Other dendrotoxin homologues (β- and γ-dendrotoxins) have been shown to block preferentially non-inactivating K-tracer fluxes in mammalian synaptosomes. In contrast to this, δ-dendrotoxin and the prototype α-dendrotoxin block inactivating K-tracer fluxes in this same preparation (Benishin et al., 1988). Using a rat brain synaptosomal preparation, the three new isotoxins all inhibit α-dendrotoxin binding and all elevate cytosolic-free Ca. These results suggest that the interaction of α- and δ-dendrotoxins with their acceptor protein, is tightly coupled to inhibition of K-currents, while the interactions of β- and γ-dendrotoxins are not (Muniz et al., 1990a). All isotoxins covalently label a 65 kDa membrane polypeptide in mammalian brain (Sorensen & Blaustein, 1989), whereas δ-dendrotoxin has additionally been shown to label an 82 kDa polypeptide

(Muniz *et al.*, 1990a). Such data suggest that K_A-type and non-inactivating voltage-gated K-channels in rat brain may have similar subunits.

Mast cell degranulating peptide

General properties

Mast-cell degranulating (MCD) peptide (peptide 401) is an extremely basic 2.6 kDa peptide isolated from the venom of the European honey bee, *Apis mellifera*. Mast cell degranulating peptide was originally found to trigger histamine release from mast cells (Habermann, 1972) and was initially thought to be an anti-inflammatory agent (Billingham *et al.*, 1973). Recent studies have shown that this is not strictly true; more precisely, the peptide degranulates mast cells *in vivo* (Banks *et al.*, 1990). Other MCD agents do not displace MCD peptide and the ability of MCD peptide to trigger histamine release is probably non-specific and is due to its polycationic structure. Subsequent to the discovery of its effects on mast cells, it was shown that much lower MCD concentrations caused convulsions upon direct intraventricular injection into the brain (Habermann, 1977). High-affinity binding sites for MCD peptide have been described, both in rat brain (Taylor *et al.*, 1984), and more specifically, on hippocampal membranes (Bidard *et al.*, 1987a). Mast cell degranulating peptide initially produces long-lasting hippocampal θ-rhythms associated with an increased level of wakefulness; this is followed by the induction of epileptic discharges, particularly at higher doses (Bidard *et al.*, 1987a). The epileptic discharges can in turn, be inhibited by K-channel openers such as cromakalim (Gandolfo *et al.*, 1989).

In rats injected with MCD peptide or dendrotoxin, similar symptoms of convulsions and hyperactivity are seen, suggesting that both toxins have similar cellular targets. Biochemical and electrophysiological experiments confirm this. Dendrotoxin is a non-competitive inhibitor of MCD peptide-binding sites on synaptosomal membranes (Bidard *et al.*, 1987b). An MCD peptide-binding protein from rat brain co-purifies with and is identical in size to, the dendrotoxin-binding protein discussed earlier (Rehm & Lazdunski, 1988a,b; Rehm *et al.*, 1988). High-affinity binding sites for both dendrotoxin and MCD peptide are located in synapse-rich areas, but are not identical in distribution. Autoradiographic studies on brain sections show a heterogeneous distribution of MCD peptide-binding sites in rat brain sections. High densities of binding sites occur in the pons, neocortex and parts of the hippocampus while low densities are found in white matter and the granular area of the brain (Mourre *et al.*, 1988). (*See earlier* for dendrotoxin-binding site distribution.) These subtle differences in the distribution of MCD and dendrotoxin-binding sites in brain have their counterparts in the origins of the epileptic seizures induced by the two toxins. The MCD peptide-induced seizures originate in the hippocampal region, while dendrotoxin-induced seizures have their origins in the cortex and the limbic system (Bidard *et al.*, 1989).

Effects on K-currents and channels

Electrophysiological experiments have shown that the dendrotoxin-sensitive, fast-activating A-type current in nodose ganglia is also blocked by MCD peptide at slightly higher concentrations (Stansfeld *et al.*, 1987). In contrast, both toxins were unable to block transient outward A-type currents in superior cervical ganglion cells. The MCD peptide also selectively blocks the same fast-inactivating component of K-current in *Xenopus* nerve fibres as does dendrotoxin (Brau *et al.*, 1990).

The most elegant proof that MCD peptide and dendrotoxin also block a non-inactivating, delayed rectifier K-channel comes from an experiment involving the expression of K-channel genes in *Xenopus* oocytes (Stühmer *et al.*, 1988). Using low stringency hybridization techniques with a *Drosophila Shaker* cDNA probe, an homologous cDNA was isolated from a rat cerebral cortex library. *In vitro* transcription of this isolated rat brain cDNA into mRNA and subsequent injection into *Xenopus* oocytes, resulted in the expression of a functional K-channel with delayed rectifier properties which was inhibited by both MCD peptide and dendrotoxin.

Binding sites

There is increasing evidence to suggest that there are mutual interactions between discrete binding sites for dendrotoxin, MCD peptide and β-bungarotoxin with several studies having demonstrated allosteric interactions between the three toxins (Rugolo *et al.*, 1986; Breeze & Dolly, 1989; Pelchen-Matthews & Dolly, 1989; Rehm & Lazdunski, 1988a; Schmidt *et al.*, 1988; Rehm *et al.*, 1988). Although it is extremely difficult to provide an accurate estimate, present data would suggest that the ratio of high affinity binding sites for dendrotoxin : MCD peptide : β-bungarotoxin is approximately 6 : 3 : 2. In some cases the physiological effects of one toxin can be antagonized by another, e.g. the effects of β-bungarotoxin on motor nerve terminals and brain synaptosomes can be partially inhibited by dendrotoxin (Harvey & Karlsson, 1982). It appears that MCD peptide, dendrotoxin and β-bungarotoxin probably all bind to the same ancestral voltage-sensitive K-channel (K_V). Biophysical differences in K_V subtypes will probably be reflected, both in the differences in affinity that these three toxins have evolved for an individual channel subtype and also in the subtle differences of their allosteric binding relationships. Although many attempts have been made, no plausible structural correlations between the three toxins have been put forward which would account for their similar physiological targets.

Apamin

Structural features

Apamin is a toxin found in the venom of the European honey bee, *Apis mellifera* (Habermann, 1984), consisting of 18 amino acids and having a molecular mass of 2 kDa. Although slightly smaller than the MCD peptide, it has a similar structure, possessing two intramolecular disulphide bridges and an amidated C-terminus (Gauldie *et al.*, 1976). It is very stable and is the smallest K-channel toxin characterized to date.

Apamin can be purified from bee venom (Banks *et al.*, 1981), or obtained by chemical synthesis (Cosland & Merrifield, 1977; Granier *et al.*, 1978); synthetic apamin possesses full biological activity. Three-dimensional structure predictions based on primary structure (Hider & Ragnarsson, 1980, 1981; Freeman *et al.*, 1986) and spectroscopic studies (Wemmer & Kallenbach, 1983; Pease and Wemmer, 1988) concur that apamin possesses an α-helical core which is attached by two disulphide bonds to a folded N-terminal region. Immunological studies indicate that those residues which contribute most to antigenic recognition are located in the α-helical core and second turn region (Komissarenko *et al.*, 1981; Defendini *et al.*, 1990a,b).

Within the α-helical core of apamin are a pair of arginine residues (Arg 13,14) which are essential for toxicity (Vincent *et al.*, 1975). While destroying toxicity, modifications of Arg 13 and Arg 14 do not alter the general conformation of apamin, as determined by circular-dichroism spectra (Defendini *et al.*, 1990b). Disulphide-bond reduction also destroys the biological activity.

Apamin was originally described as a centrally-acting neurotoxin which was able to cross the blood–brain barrier, producing motor hyperactivity and convulsions (Habermann, 1977). The molecular target for apamin is a small conductance, Ca-activated K-channel (SK_{Ca}), this fact only being determined some years after the initial demonstration of apamin's neurotoxicity (Banks *et al.*, 1979).*

Tissue localization

Autoradiographic studies of brain sections using radiolabelled apamin show that toxin binding sites have a wide but heterogeneous distribution. High receptor densities are found in the limbic and motor systems (Habermann, 1984; Mourre *et al.*, 1986) although no receptors have been found in regions that are rich in myelin (Mourre *et al.*, 1987). Microinjection of apamin into the A10 dopamine region of rat brain produces a dose-depen-

*In smooth muscle, the apamin-sensitive K-channel has been designated $SK_{Ca(Ap)}$. For further details, *see* Chapter 7.

dent increase in motor activity. This effect is blocked by pretreatment with the dopamine receptor antagonist, haloperidol. A role for dopaminergic transmission in this response is further supported by the fact that apamin microinjection increases the levels of dopamine metabolites in the nucleus accumbens and A10 region (Steketee & Kalivas, 1990). The mesolimbic dopamine system consists of cell bodies in the A10 dopamine region, that terminate in a number of limbic forebrain structures. Apamin block of SK_{Ca} (*see later evidence*) may lead to depolarization of dopamine neurones followed by an increase in dopaminergic transmission.

Effects on K-currents and channels

Apamin blocks receptor-mediated, Ca-activated K-permeabilities ($IC_{50} = 1$–7 nM) in intestinal smooth muscle (Maas *et al.*, 1980; Hugues *et al.*, 1982b; Weir & Weston, 1986) and hepatocytes (Burgess *et al.*, 1981; Cook & Haylett, 1985). It also blocks Ca-ionophore induced K-tracer efflux ($IC_{50} = 0.5$–2 nM) in primary neuronal cultures (Seagar *et al.*, 1984) and brown adipocytes (Nanberg *et al.*, 1985).

Action potentials in many cells are often followed by a slow after-hyperpolarization (AHP) which is a result of the activation of Ca-dependent K-conductances. Apamin (0.5–100 nM) has been shown to block AHPs in skeletal muscle (Hugues *et al.*, 1982d, Schmid-Antomarchi *et al.*, 1985; Traore *et al.*, 1986), smooth muscle (Fujii *et al.*, 1990), and a wide range of cells of neuronal origin (Kawai & Watanabe, 1986; Bourque & Brown, 1987; Goh & Pennefather, 1987; Zhang & Krnjevic, 1987; Brown & Higashida, 1988). Apamin increased the firing rate in 30% of spontaneously pacing cells of the GH_3 anterior pituitary cell line (Lang & Ritchie, 1990), and enhanced the frequency of spontaneous action potentials in smooth muscle of guinea-pig bladder (Fujii *et al.*, 1990). This suggests that the apamin-sensitive SK_{Ca}-channel may regulate the spontaneous action potential firing rate by hyperpolarizing the membrane following an action potential (Lang & Ritchie, 1990).

Apamin also blocks naturally occurring slow action potentials of cultured cell reaggregates from chick hearts and isoproterenol-induced slow action potentials in freshly isolated chick ventricular muscles (Bkaily *et al.*, 1985). These findings led to the conclusion that apamin is a highly specific blocker of Ca^{2+} entry into chick heart. In adult guinea-pig ventricular papillary muscles, apamin (1–100 nM) hyperpolarized the resting membrane potential and shortened the action potential duration of the fast response. The slow response action potential duration was also decreased without a significant decrease in the maximal rate of increase (V_{max}) of the action potential (Nakagawa *et al.*, 1989). These later findings therefore suggest that apamin increases K-conductance in the mammalian ventricular myocardium. Attempts to determine more precisely the effects of apamin on ionic currents were unsuccessful, as apamin could not be shown to affect the membrane currents of enzymatically isolated single ventricular cells (Nakagawa et al., 1989). Data obtained from heart tissue are therefore contradictory (perhaps due to the species difference), and are unsupported by results obtained with apamin in other tissues. Independent confirmation of these unique results in cardiac muscle is therefore awaited with interest.

The apamin-sensitive SK_{Ca}-channel has been characterized at the single channel level in cultured rat myotubes (Blatz & Magleby, 1986), guinea-pig hepatocytes (Capiod & Ogden, 1989) and a GH_3 anterior pituitary cell line (Lang & Ritchie, 1990). A single channel conductance (9–20 pS) was observed in symmetrical (140–150 mM) K^+ solution. This value decreased by one third when a physiological K-gradient (5 mM K^+ external/135 mM K^+ internal) was used (Capiod & Ogden, 1989) and suggests that potassium has a regulatory binding site on the channel's external face.

Binding sites

High affinity $[^{125}I]$monoiodoapamin-binding sites (K_d = 10–400 pM) have been identified on muscle cells (Hugues et al., 1982b,d; Schmid-Antomarchi et al., 1985; Marqueze et al., 1987), cells of neuronal origin (Hugues et al., 1982c; Seagar et al., 1984) and hepatocytes (Marqueze et al., 1987; Strong & Evans, 1987). Binding affinity is sensitive to cations and is optimal when $[K^+]$ = 5 mM (Hugues et al., 1982a; Seagar et al., 1984). It is thought that cations compete for an electrostatic binding site with the two arginine residues on apamin which are essential for toxicity.

Apamin-binding sites are of high affinity but extremely low density (B_{max} < 30 fmol/mg protein). Attempts to purify apamin-binding proteins have used rat brain (Schmid-Antomarchi et al., 1984; Seagar et al., 1987a). A molecular mass of approximately 700 kDa has been calculated for the purified detergent/protein complex by density gradient centrifugation, but up to half of this weight could be due to detergent. Radiation inactivation analysis studies using $[^{125}I]$monoiodoapamin binding to the solubilized protein have calculated relative masses of 250 kDa (Schmid-Antomarchi et al., 1984), or 84–115 kDa (Seagar et al., 1986), depending on the membrane preparations used.

Apamin-binding proteins of assorted molecular weights have been identified using chemical cross-linking or photoaffinity labelling. The most comprehensive study so far is that performed by Auguste et al. (1989) who used membrane preparations from both pheochromocytoma PC12 cells and rat brain with five different affinity labelling methods. The major component in both cases was a 30 kDa apamin-binding protein with other binding proteins of M_r = 86, 58, 45 and 28 kDa identified in brain membranes and $M_r = 86$, 58 and 28 kDa in PC12 cell membranes. Apamin-binding proteins have been affinity-labelled in other studies using membranes from cultured neurones (Seagar *et al.*, 1985), astrocytes (Seagar *et al.*, 1987b), heart, smooth muscle and liver (Marqueze *et al*, 1987). There is good evidence that different subtypes of the apamin-binding protein are expressed in different tissues (Marqueze *et al.*, 1987; Auguste *et al.*, 1989). Care must be taken in interpreting these results, as the apparent molecular weight of the apamin-binding protein is dependent both on the cross-linker and on whether gels are run under reducing or non-reducing conditions (Auguste *et al.*, 1989).

Expression of apamin-binding sites has been shown to be developmentally regulated in foetal and postnatal rat muscle. Expression of apamin-binding sites appears to be suppressed by a neuronal factor (Schmid-Antomarchi *et al.*, 1985). Expression could be regulated by recycling of apamin-binding proteins from the cell surface to the cell interior, a process which has been shown to occur in liver cells (Strong & Evans, 1987).

Using an apamin radioimmunoassay (Schweitz & Lazdunski, 1984) and other assays for apamin-like activity, an endogenous apamin-like molecule has been purified from pig brain. This peptide is present at minute levels and its role is unknown. An endogenous MCD-like peptide has also been purified from pig brain by a similar method (Cherubini *et al.*, 1987).

Apamin is one of the most specific K-channel toxins yet characterized. Although results from cardiac muscle (Bkaily *et al.*, 1985; Nakagawa *et al.*, 1989) and its apparently inhibitory effect on the electrogenic effect of the Na : K pump (Zemkova *et al.*, 1988), contradict this view, such data have yet to be independently confirmed.

Noxiustoxin

Noxiustoxin was the first K-channel modulator to be isolated from a scorpion venom. It is found in the venom of the Mexican scorpion, *Centruroides noxius* Hoffman (Possani *et al.*, 1981a, 1982) with venom from 1000 scorpions being required for the isolation of 0.1 mg of pure noxiustoxin (Gurrola *et al.*, 1989). A noxiustoxin homologue has been isolated from the venom of both *C. noxius* Hoffman venom and that of the Brazilian scorpion, *Tityus serrulatus* (Possani *et al.*, 1981b). Noxiustoxin is a 39-amino acid polypeptide ($M_r = 4.2$ kDa) containing six cysteine residues. As well as these six residues (which help to confer a common tertiary structure), noxiustoxin shares may sequence homologies with other scorpion venom K-channel toxins, namely, charybdotoxin, leiurotoxin and iberiotoxin.

Noxiustoxin has been shown to block the delayed rectifier channel

(K_V) of the squid giant axon (Carbone *et al.*, 1982, 1987). The toxin also blocks (but with lower affinity), BK_{Ca}-channels isolated from skeletal muscle T-tubules (Valdivia *et al.*, 1988). Nanomolar concentrations of noxiustoxin (and charybdotoxin, *see later*) block 'type n' voltage-gated K-channels on murine thymocytes (Sands *et al.*, 1989). In mouse brain synaptosomes, noxiustoxin stimulates [^{3}H]GABA release and inhibits ^{86}Rb-efflux ($K_i = 3$ nM) (Sitges *et al.*, 1986), both results consistent with K-channel blockade.

Studies with synthetic peptides suggest that the N-terminal region of noxiustoxin might be responsible for its interaction with mouse brain K-channels (Gurrola *et al.*, 1989). Neither synthetic noxiustoxin nor synthetic peptide fragments of the toxin, are as potent as native noxiustoxin.

Charybdotoxin

General features

Charybdotoxin is a K-channel toxin from the venom of the Old World scorpion *Leiurus quinquestriatus hebraeus* (LQH). Charybdotoxin consists of 37 amino acids, has a molecular weight of 4.3 kDa and shares many sequence homologies with the other scorpion venom K-channel toxins (Gimenez-Gallego *et al.*, 1988; Galvez *et al.*, 1990). A minor isoform of charybdotoxin has also been purified from LQH venom, which contains eight amino acid substitutions, four of which are conservative (Lucchesi *et al.*, 1989). The minor charybdotoxin isoform is a less potent blocker of BK_{Ca} in rat skeletal muscle than the major isoform.

Two-dimensional nuclear magnetic resonance (2D-NMR) spectroscopy studies indicate that charybdotoxin is built on a foundation of three antiparallel β-strands which are attached to other parts of the sequence by three disulphide bridges (Lambert *et al.*, 1990; Massefski *et al.*, 1990). Charybdotoxin is thought to be ellipsoidal in shape with axes of approximately 2.5 and 1.5 nm. All of charybdotoxin's 37 amino acid residues are exposed to solvent, with seven of its eight positively charged residues lying in a strip along one side of the molecule. Biologically-active charybdotoxin has been produced by both solid phase (Sugg *et al.*, 1990) and solution synthesis methods (Lambert *et al.*, 1990).

Effects on K-currents and channels

Charybdotoxin was initially isolated and characterized by its ability to block the tetraethylammonium (TEA)-sensitive, voltage-dependent, BK_{Ca}-channel (100–250 pS) of rat skeletal muscle, inserted into planar lipid bilayers (Miller *et al.*, 1985; Smith *et al.*, 1986). The BK_{Ca}-channels sensitive to blockade by low concentrations of charybdotoxin (2–50 nM) have subsequently been electrophysiologically characterized in a wide range of cells. These include cultured kidney epithelial cells (Guggino *et al.*, 1987), smooth muscle cells (Talvenheimo *et al.*, 1988; Strong *et al.*, 1989; Vázquez *et al.*, 1989), cultured human macrophages (Gallin & McKinney, 1988), PC12 pheochromocytoma cells (Hoshi & Aldrich, 1986), the GH_3 anterior pituitary cell line (Lang & Ritchie, 1990) and the C6 rat glioma cell line (Reiser *et al.*, 1990). Charbydotoxin also blocks Ca-activated K-currents ($I_{BK(Ca)}$), in rat hippocampal neurones (Lancaster & Nicoll, 1987), bullfrog sympathetic ganglia (Adams *et al.*, 1986; Goh & Pennefather, 1987), mouse and frog motor nerve terminals (Anderson *et al.*, 1987; Anderson *et al.*, 1988) and *Drosophila* longitudinal flight muscle (Elkins *et al.*, 1986).

BK_{Ca} subtypes exist which are insensitive to block by charybdotoxin. These include a slowly-activating BK_{Ca}-channel (236 pS) found in rat brain (Reinhart *et al.*, 1989).

Charybdotoxin is by no means solely a blocker of BK_{Ca}-channels, having been shown to block intermediate conductance (18–60 pS), Ca-activated K-channels ($I K_{Ca}$). In rat brain, for example, charybdotoxin blocks multiple types of K_{Ca}-channels (Farley & Rudy, 1988; Reinhart *et al.*, 1989), whilst an $I K_{Ca}$-channel (35 pS) is blocked by charybdotoxin in *Aplysia* ganglia (Hermann & Erxleben, 1987).

In human erythrocytes charybdotoxin blocks a 25 pS $I K_{Ca}$-channel (Beech *et al.*, 1987; Strong *et al.*, 1989) which may play a pathophysiological role in erythrocytes of patients with sickle-cell anaemia (Bookchin *et al.*, 1987). Charybdotoxin partially inhibits the formation of dense and irreversibly sickled cells in sickle-cell blood (Ohnishi *et al.*, 1989). The K_{Ca}-channel found in erythrocytes is a distinct subtype which unlike BK_{Ca}, is blocked equipotently by both homologues of charybdotoxin (Lucchesi *et al.*, 1989). There is no evidence to suggest the existence of a BK_{Ca}-channel in erythrocytes.

A *c*harybdotoxin-sensitive, *l*ow-conductance, *i*nwardly rectifying, *c*alcium-activated K-channel (K_{clic}), which is TEA-insensitive, has been identified in airway epithelial cells. This K_{clic}-channel may play a role, both in maintaining the driving force for transepithelial chloride secretion by the airways epithelium, as well as preventing cell swelling (McCann *et al.*, 1990).

An $I_{K(Ca)}$ sensitive to charybdotoxin has been identified in rat thymic lymphocytes (Grinstein & Smith, 1989, 1990). In human blood lymphocytes both Ca-activated, and Ca-independent K-conductances sensitive to charybdotoxin are thought to exist (Grinstein & Smith, 1990). These conductances were characterized using fluorescent probes and by measurement of ^{86}Rb flux. In human T-lymphocytes, a charybdotoxin-sensitive ($K_i = 0.3$ nM) K_V-type channel, has been identified by whole-cell patch-clamping (Price *et al.*, 1989; Sands *et al.*, 1989), but no evidence for a K_{Ca}-channel was found. Charybdotoxin inhibits the mitogen- and antigen-stimulated proliferation of human T-lymphocytes, possibly by blockade of K_V (Price et al., 1989). Cleavage of the two N-terminal residues from charybdotoxin results in the toxin having an unchanged affinity for the T-lymphocyte K-channel. In contrast, the cleaved toxin is rendered inactive against the BK_{Ca}-channel (Price et al., 1989), which supports the notion that the channel in T-lymphocytes is a distinct pharmacological subtype.

Charybdotoxin has also been shown to block a dendrotoxin-sensitive voltage-activated current on cultured rat dorsal root ganglia cells ($IC_{50} \approx 30 \, nM$). The toxin blocks the binding of both toxin I and MCD peptide to their receptors on rat brain synaptosomes (Schweitz et al., 1989b). A complementary study showed that charybdotoxin also blocked synaptosomal ^{86}Rb-efflux through K_A-type channels ($IC_{50} \approx 40 \, nM$) and K_{Ca}-type channels ($IC_{50} \approx 15 \, nM$) (Schneider et al., 1989).

Further studies have revealed that toxin I, charybdotoxin and MCD peptide all evoke [^{3}H]GABA release from preloaded synaptosomes (Schweitz et al., 1989a). In isolated central nerve terminals, nanomolar concentrations of charybdotoxin or dendrotoxin increased $[Ca^{2+}]_i$ (Tibbs et al., 1989b; Muniz et al., 1990b). These effects are consistent with the hypothesis that charybdotoxin, dendrotoxin and MCD peptide can block the same K_A-type channel. Additional evidence of this inter-relationship comes from binding studies. The relatively broad spectrum of K-channel blockade by charybdotoxin may be partially due to impurities (see Chapter 5).

Binding sites

Initial attempts to produce a ^{125}I-labelled charybdotoxin derivative suitable for use in binding studies, gave a radiolabelled product with a 1000-fold lower affinity for BK_{Ca}-channels than native charybdotoxin (Lucchesi et al., 1989). In a more successful study, a K_d value of 730 pM was reported for ^{125}I-charybdotoxin binding to rat brain synaptosomes (Schweitz et al., 1989a), with an apparent IC_{50} value of 142 pM for the inhibition of binding by native charybdotoxin. Binding and cross-linking experiments of this radiolabelled charybdotoxin to rat brain membranes, and the purified toxin I binding protein, showed that the α-subunit ($M_r = 76-78 \, kDa$) of the toxin I-sensitive K-channel contains a charybdotoxin binding site. The binding sites for toxin I, MCD peptide and charybdotoxin are in negative allosteric interaction with each other (Schweitz et al., 1989a,b).

A further binding study to rat brain synaptic membranes reported a K_d value for ^{125}I-charybdotoxin of 25–30 pM (Vázquez et al., 1990) with an IC_{50} value one order of magnitude lower than that discussed earlier

(Schweitz *et al.*, 1989). This is the most potent radiolabelled derivative of charybdotoxin reported to date, with an affinity two to three times lower than that of native charybdotoxin. Low concentrations of Na^+ and K^+ stimulated the binding of ^{125}I-charybdotoxin (by an allosteric interaction) while at high concentrations, binding was inhibited due to ionic strength effects. Tetraethylammonium ions did not inhibit charybdotoxin binding to rat brain membranes (indicating that the binding site is not the BK_{Ca}-channel) but tetrabutylammonium ions (a blocker of inactivating, voltage-dependent K-channels) did inhibit binding. Noxiustoxin and α-dendrotoxin non-competitively inhibited the binding of ^{125}I-charybdotoxin. These results suggest that charybdotoxin binds to inactivating, K_A-type channels on isolated brain membranes (Vázquez *et al.*, 1990).

^{125}I-charybdotoxin binds to bovine aortic smooth muscle membranes ($K_d = 100$ pM); binding is inhibited by Ba^{2+}, K^+, Ca^{2+} and TEA. ^{125}I-charybdotoxin also blocked a large BK_{Ca}-channel from the same membrane preparation, but with a 10-fold loss in affinity for these channels, compared with native charybdotoxin (Vázquez *et al.*, 1989).

^{125}I radiolabelling of charybdotoxin, with retention of biological activity, appears to be a difficult procedure (Harvey *et al.*, 1989; Lucchesi *et al.*, 1989). Two studies of binding to rat brain synaptosomes, using high-performance liquid chromatography-purified ^{125}I-charybdotoxin reported widely differing K_d and B_{max} values (Schweitz *et al.*, 1989a; Vázquez *et al.*, 1990). This could possibly be due to the use of different isoforms of the toxin (Lucchesi *et al.*, 1989). Clearly charybdotoxin blocks dendrotoxin-sensitive, K_A-type channels in the brain. The failure to detect ^{125}I-charybdotoxin binding to K_{Ca}-channels in brain is surprising in the light of other studies (Farley & Rudy, 1988; Reinhart *et al.*, 1989; Schneider *et al.*, 1989). This may be due either to a low channel density or to an anomalously low affinity of ^{125}I-charybdotoxin for the brain channel subtype of K_{Ca} (Vázquez *et al.*, 1990).

Charybdotoxin also blocks the K_A-channel encoded by the *Shaker* gene of *Drosophila melanogaster* (MacKinnon *et al.*, 1988). Charybdotoxin has been shown, by mechanistic studies and competition for binding by TEA, to block K^+ movement by binding in the external mouth of the pore (Anderson *et al.*, 1988; MacKinnon *et al.*, 1988). Site-directed mutagenesis of the *Shaker* gene indicated that toxin binding involves an electrostatic focusing onto the binding site by negatively charged residues of the ion-channel protein (MacKinnon & Miller, 1989). Such a mechanism is supported by the fact that charybdotoxin binding is sensitive to ionic strength (Vázquez *et al.*, 1989, 1990) and has a faster 'on' rate (k_1) than that calculated for a peptide of its size (Vázquez *et al.*, 1989). Residues involved in charybdotoxin binding must be located on the external face of the channel protein, close to the K-channel pore. Site-directed mutagenesis studies of K-channels and the concomitant effect on charybdotoxin binding can be used in modelling studies of the channel protein. The size of charybdotoxin itself has already indicated the minimum possible dimensions of the external mouth of the K-channel (Massefski *et al.*, 1990).

The blockade of both K_{Ca} and voltage-dependent K-channels (especially those of the K_A-type) by charybdotoxin indicates that the structures of different K-channel subtypes, particularly the ion-selective pore, may actually be quite similar.

Leiurotoxin

General properties

Charybdotoxin is not the only component of LQH venom which blocks K-channels. In guinea-pig hepatocytes, crude venom has been shown to block the Ca-activated K-permeabilities which are sensitive to apamin but not to pure charybdotoxin (Abia *et al.*, 1986; Castle & Strong, 1986; Strong *et al.*, 1989). The toxin which exhibits this blocking activity has been purified to homogeneity and sequenced (Chicchi *et al.*, 1988). This toxin, known as leiurotoxin (or scyllatoxin—Martins *et al.*, 1990), has 31 amino acids (M_r = 3.4 kDa) and shows some sequence homology with both noxiustoxin and charybdotoxin. The structure of leiurotoxin has been determined by 2D-NMR. It consists of an N-terminal α-helical region located by three disulphide bridges on one side of a C-terminal double-stranded antiparallel β-pleated sheet (Martins *et al.*, 1990).

There are at least two leiurotoxin isoforms. The most potent and abundant possesses an amidated C-terminus, and the other is apparently identical in all but this respect (Auguste *et al.*, 1990).

Biological activity

Leiurotoxin has been shown to block adrenaline-induced relaxation of guinea-pig taenia coli (Chicchi *et al.*, 1988; Auguste *et al.*, 1990) and the long-lasting AHP seen in cultured rat myotubes (Auguste *et al.*, 1990). Both of these effects are also sensitive to blockade by apamin (Maas *et al.*, 1980; Hugues *et al.*, 1982b,d).

Biologically-active leiurotoxin has been synthesized, as well as a leiurotoxin analogue ([Tyr^2]leiurotoxin) in which phenylalanine^2 is substituted by a tyrosine. This analogue can be monoiodinated with ^{125}I to yield biologically active ^{125}I-[Tyr^2]leiurotoxin (Auguste *et al.*, 1990). The iodinated toxin has been shown to bind specifically to sites on rat brain membranes (K_d = 80 pM), with a sensitivity to K^+ similar to that previously observed for ^{125}I-monoiodoapamin (Cook *et al.*, 1983; Hugues *et al.*, 1982a). Binding could be fully inhibited by apamin in a competitive fashion (Auguste et al., 1990). ^{125}I-monoiodoapamin binding to rat brain membranes is fully inhibited by native leiurotoxin, although there is disagreement over whether this inhibition is competitive (Auguste et al., 1990), or of a more complex nature (Chicchi et al., 1988).

Chemical cross-linking of ^{125}I-[Tyr^2]leiurotoxin to rat brain membranes revealed specific labelling of two polypeptides ($M_r = 27$, 57 kDa), the 27 kDa polypeptide being the most intensively labelled (see earlier for the labelling pattern with apamin). No chemical cross-linking was observed in the presence of an excess of [Tyr^2]leiurotoxin or apamin, again indicating that binding sites for ^{125}I-[Tyr^2]leiurotoxin and apamin are identical (Auguste et al., 1990).

Leiurotoxin and apamin would appear to bind to the same site in brain, smooth muscle, cultured rat myotubes (Chicchi et al., 1988; Auguste et al., 1990) and hepatocytes (Castle & Strong, 1986; Strong et al., 1989). Although there is no evident sequence homology between leiurotoxin and apamin, leiurotoxin does possess two arginine residues which may be in a structural arrangement similar to those possessed by apamin and which are essential for its toxicity (Vincent et al., 1975). An apparent difference in the site of action of the two toxins is that cromakalim-activated K-channels are blocked by leiurotoxin (Weir & Strong, 1988; Strong et al., 1989) but not by apamin (Weir & Weston, 1986; Quast & Cook, 1988; Fujii et al., 1990).

Iberiotoxin

Iberiotoxin is a 37-amino acid peptide ($M_r = 4.3$ kDa), purified from the venom of the scorpion, *Buthus tamulus*, by its ability to inhibit ^{125}I-charybdotoxin binding to bovine aortic sarcolemmal membranes. Iberiotoxin displays 68% sequence homology with charybdotoxin and like charybdotoxin it blocks the BK$_{Ca}$-channels of bovine aortic smooth muscle (IC$_{50} \approx 250$ pM). It is thought to act at a site on the BK$_{Ca}$ distinct from that for charybdotoxin. Iberiotoxin, unlike charybdotoxin, does not appear to block other types of voltage-dependent K-channel (Galvez et al., 1990).

Other toxins

The number of known K-channels and other naturally-occurring K-channel modulators is increasing steadily. This section contains evidence for the existence of new K-channel toxins that have yet to be fully characterized.

Crude venom of the African scorpion, *Pandinus imperator*, has been shown to block voltage-activated K-currents of the frog myelinated nerve and in GH$_3$ pituitary cells (Pappone & Cahalan, 1987; Pappone & Lucero, 1988). The venom also facilitates acetylcholine release at the neuromuscular junction by selectively blocking 3,4-diaminopyridine sensitive K-currents (Marshall & Harvey, 1989). Snake venoms from *Notechis scutatus, Vipera russelli russelli* and *Oxyuranus scutellatus* have all been shown to inhibit the Ca-dependent K transport of human erythrocytes.

The inhibitory effect of these venoms was additive to that of LQH venom (Alvarez & Garcia-Sancho, 1989). Another peptide, in addition to iberiotoxin, has been partially purified from the venom of the scorpion *B. tamulus*, which also inhibits charybdotoxin binding to aortic sarcolemmal vesicles (Galvez *et al.*, 1990) and brain membranes (Vázquez *et al.*, 1990). Crude venoms from the scorpions *Centruroides sculpturatus, Androctonus amourexi, Androctonus australis, Parabuthus raudus, Parabuthus transvaalicus, Buthus occitanus* var. *mardochei, Buthus occitanicus* var. *tunetanus* and *B. tamulus* all inhibit ^{125}I-charybdotoxin binding to aortic sarcolemmal vesicles (Galvez *et al.*, 1990). A fraction from LQH venom, other than charybdotoxin or leiurotoxin, blocks the cromakalim-mediated increase in [86]Rb$^+$ efflux from rabbit aorta (Strong *et al.*, 1989). This fraction may correspond to a toxin named 'leiurotoxin II', mentioned by Dunnwiddie, C. *et al.* as an unpublished observation (Vázquez *et al.*, 1989). Potassium-channel blockers also exist in organisms other than snakes, bees and scorpions. Crude venom from the marine snail, *Conus striatus*, blocks $I_{K(V)}$-type currents in *Aplysia* (Cheshunt *et al.*, 1987) while components of sea anemone (*Actinia equina*) venom are also active against voltage-gated K-channels (Suput, 1988). Plant toxins such as capsaicin (Petersen *et al.*, 1987) have also been shown to block K-currents. Naturally occurring modulators of potassium currents have also been isolated from non-venomous animals such as the endogenous apamin-like and MCD-like molecules found in pig brain (Fosset *et al.*, 1984; Cherubini *et al.*, 1987) and a cobalt-induced 70 kDa protein of the epileptogenic cortex of rat cerebrum (Onozuka *et al.*, 1990). The fact that so many K$^-$ and other ion channels specifically bind with high affinity such a wide range of peptide toxins indicates that these binding sites may primarily exist as sites for the interaction of endogenous modulatory peptides.

Conclusions

Potassium-channel toxins have contributed greatly to our present knowledge of K-channels. This contribution looks likely to increase still further as more and more different toxins are isolated.

Similarities in the primary structures of the scorpion toxins, noxiustoxin, charybdotoxin, leiurotoxin and iberiotoxin indicate that all evolved from a common ancestral toxin. That toxins with such similar structures can act on such a diverse range of K-channel subtypes, suggests that these must share common structural features. Proof of this, however, will have to await the cloning and sequencing of more K-channels.

Acknowledgements

We thank the Muscular Dystrophy Group of Great Britain and the Wellcome Trust for support of this research.

References

Abia, A., Lobaton, C. D., Moreno, A. & Garcia-Sancho, J. (1986) *Leiurus quinquestriatus* venom inhibits different kinds of Ca^{2+}-dependent K^+ channels. *Biochimica et Biophysica Acta* **856**, 403–407.

Adams, P. R., Jones, S. W., Pennefather, P., Brown, D. A., Koch, C. & Lancaster, B. (1986) Slow synaptic transmission in frog sympathetic ganglia. *Journal of Experimental Biology* **124**, 259–285.

Alvarez, J. & Garcia-Sancho, J. (1989) Inhibition of red-cell Ca^{2+}-dependent K^+ channels by snake-venoms. *Biochimica et Biophysica Acta* **980**, 134–138.

Anderson, A. J. & Harvey, A. L. (1988) Effects of the potassium channel blocking dendrotoxins on acetylcholine and motor nerve terminal activity. *British Journal of Pharmacology* **93**, 215–221.

Anderson, A. J., Harvey, A. L., Rowan, E. G. & Strong, P. N. (1988) Effects of charybdotoxin, a blocker of Ca^{2+}-activated K^+ channels, on motor nerve terminals. *British Journal of Pharmacology* **95**, 1329–1335.

Anderson, A. J., Harvey, A. L. & Strong, P. N. (1987) Characterization of calcium-activated potassium channels in motor nerve terminals of the mouse triangularis sterni muscle preparation. *Journal of Physiology* **392**, 117P.

Auguste, P., Hugues, M., Grave, B., Gesquiere, J. C., Maes, P., Tartar, A., Romey, G., Schweitz, H. & Lazdunski, M. (1990) Leiurotoxin-I (scyllatoxin), a peptide ligand for Ca^{2+}-activated K^+ channels—chemical synthesis, radiolabelling, and receptor characterization. *Journal of Biological Chemistry* **265**, 4753–4759.

Auguste, P., Hugues, M. & Lazdunski, M. (1989) Polypeptide constitution of receptors for apamin, a neurotoxin which blocks a class of Ca^{2+}-activated K^+ channels. *FEBS Letters* **248**, 150–154.

Banks, B. E. C., Burgess, G. M., Burnstock, C., Claret, M., Cocks, T. M. & Jenkinson, D. H. (1979) Apamin blocks certain neurotransmitter-induced increases in potassium permeability. *Nature* **282**, 415–417.

Banks, B. E. C., Dempsey, C. E., Pearce, F. L., Vernon, C. A. & Wholly, T. E. (1981) New methods of isolating bee venom peptides. *Analytical Biochemistry* **116**, 48–52.

Banks, B. E. C., Dempsey, C. E., Vernon, C. A., Warner, J. A. & Yamey, J. (1990) Anti-inflammatory activity of bee venom peptide-401 (mast-cell degranulating peptide) and compound 48/80 results from mast-cell degranulation *in vivo*. *British Journal of Pharmacology* **99**, 350–354.

Barbeito, L., Siciliano, J. & Dajas, F. (1990) Depletion of the Ca^{++}-dependent releasable pool of glutamate in striatal synaptosomes associated with dendrotoxin-induced potassium channel blockade. *Journal of Neural Transmission* **80**, 67–179.

Beech, D. J., Bolton, T. B., Castle, N. A. & Strong, P. N. (1987) Characterization of a toxin from scorpion (*Leiurus quinquestriatus*) venom that blocks *in vitro* both large (BK) K^+-channels in rabbit vascular smooth muscle and intermediate (IK) conductance Ca^{2+}-activated K^+ channels in human red cells. *Journal of Physiology* **387**, 32P.

Benishin, C. G. (1990) Potassium channel blockade by the B-subunit of β-bungarotoxin. *Molecular Pharmacology* **38**, 164–169.

Benishin, C. G., Sorensen, G., Brown, E., Bruce, K., Krueger & Blaustein, M. P. (1988) Four polypeptide components of green mamba venom selectively block certain potassium channels in rat brain synaptosomes. *Molecular Pharmacology* **34**, 152–159.

Benoit, E. & Dubois, J. M. (1986) Toxin I from the snake *Dendroaspis polylepis*: a highly specific blocker of one type of potassium channel in myelinated nerve fibre. *Brain Research* **377**, 374–377.

Bidard, J. N., Gandolfo, G., Mourre, C., Gottesmann, C. & Lazdunski, M. (1987a) The brain response to the bee venom peptide MCD. Activation and desensitisation of a hippocampal target. *Brain Research* **418**, 235–244.

Bidard, J. N., Mourre, C. & Lazdunski, M. (1987b) Two potent central convulsant peptides, a bee venom toxin, MCD peptide, and a snake venom toxin, dendrotoxin I, known to block K$^+$ channels, have interacting receptor sites. *Biochemical and Biophysical Research Communications* **143**, 383–389.

Bidard, J. N., Widmann, C., Mourre, C., Lazdunski, M., Gottesmann, C., Gandolfo, G. & Schweitz, H. (1989) Analogies and differences in the mode of action and properties of binding-sites (localization and mutual interactions) of 2 K$^+$ channel toxins, MCD peptide and dendrotoxin-I. *Brain Research* **495**, 45–57.

Billingham, M. E. J., Morley, J., Hanson, J. M., Shipolini, R. A. & Vernon, C. A. (1973) An anti-inflammatory peptide from bee venom. *Nature* **245**, 163–164.

Bkaily, G., Sperelakis, N., Renaud, J. F. & Payet, M. D. (1985) Apamin, a highly specific Ca^{2+} blocking agent in heart muscle. *American Journal of Physiology* **248**, H961–H965.

Black, A. R. & Dolly, J. O. (1986) Two acceptor sub-types for dendrotoxin in chick synaptic membranes distinguishable by beta-bungarotoxin. *European Journal of Biochemistry* **156**, 609–617.

Black, A. R., Donegan, C. M., Denny, B. J. & Dolly, J. O. (1988) Solubilization and physical characterization of acceptors for dendrotoxin and β-bungarotoxin from synaptic membranes of rat brain. *Biochemistry* **27**, 6814–6820.

Blatz, A. L. & Magleby, K. L. (1986) Single apamin-blocked Ca-activated K$^+$ channels of small conductance in cultured rat skeletal muscle. *Nature* **323**, 718–720.

Bookchin, R. M., Ortiz, O. E. & Lew, V. L. (1987) Activation of calcium-dependent potassium channels in deoxygenated sickled red cells. *Progress in Biological and Clinical Research* **240**, 193–200.

Bourque, C. W. & Brown, D. A. (1987) Apamin and D-tubocurarine block the after-hyperpolarization of rat supraoptic neurosecretory neurons. *Neuroscience Letters* **82**, 185–190.

Brau, M. E., Dreyer, F., Jonas, P., Repp, H. & Vogel, W. (1990) A K$^+$ channel in *Xenopus* nerve-fibers selectively blocked by bee and snake toxins. Binding and voltage-clamp experiments. *Journal of Physiology* **420**, 365–385.

Breeze, A. L. & Dolly J. O. (1989) Interactions between discrete neuronal membrane-binding sites for the putative K$^+$ channel ligands beta-bungarotoxin, dendrotoxin and mast-cell-degranulating peptide. *European Journal of Biochemistry* **178**, 771–778.

Brown, D. A. & Higashida, H. (1988) Voltage- and calcium-activated potassium currents in mouse neuroblastoma × rat glioma hybrid cells. *Journal of Physiology* **397**, 149–165.

Burgess, G. M., Claret, M. & Jenkinson, D. H. (1981) Effects of quinine and apamin on the calcium-dependent potassium permeability of mammalian hepatocytes and red cells. *Journal of Physiology* **317**, 67–90.

Capiod, T. & Ogden, D. C. (1989) The properties of calcium-activated potassium channels in guinea-pig isolated hepatocytes. *Journal of Physiology* **409**, 285–295.

Carbone, E., Prestipino, G., Spadavecchia, L., Franciolini, F. & Possani, L. D. (1987) Blocking of the squid axon K$^+$ channel by noxiustoxin: a toxin from the venom of the scorpion *Centruroides noxius*. *Pflügers Archiv* **408**, 423–431.

Carbone, E., Wanke, E., Prestipino, G., Possani, L. D. & Maelicke, A. (1982) Selective blockage of voltage-dependent K$^+$ channels by a novel scorpion toxin. *Nature* **296,** 90–91.

Castle, N. A. & Strong, P. N. (1986) Identification of two toxins from scorpion (*Leiurus quinquestriatus*) venom which blocks distinct classes of calcium-activated potassium channel. *FEBS Letters* **209,** 117–121.

Cherubini, E., Ben-Ari, Y., Goh, M., Bidard, J. N. & Lazdunski, M. (1987) Long term potentiation of synaptic transmission in the hippocampus induced by a bee venom peptide. *Nature* **328,** 70–73.

Cheshunt, T. J., Carpenter, D. O. & Strichartz, G. R. (1987) Effects of venom from *Conus striatus* on the delayed rectifier potassium current of molluscan neurones. *Toxicon* **25,** 267–278.

Chicchi, G. G., Gimenez-Gallego, G., Ber, E., Garcia, M. L., Winquist, R. & Cascieri, M. A. (1988) Purification and characterization of a unique, potent inhibitor of apamin binding from *Leiurus quinquestriatus hebraeus* venom. *Journal of Biological Chemistry* **263,** 10 192–10 197.

Cook, N. S. & Haylett, D. G. (1985) Effects of apamin, quinine and neuromuscular blockers on calcium-activated potassium channels in guinea-pig hepatocytes. *Journal of Physiology* **358,** 373–394.

Cook, N. S., Haylett, D. G. & Strong, P. N. (1983) High affinity binding of [^{125}I]-monoiodoapamin to isolated guinea-pig hepatocytes. *FEBS Letters* **152,** 265–269.

Cosland, W. L. & Merrifield, R. B. (1977) Concept of internal structural controls for evaluation of inactive synthetic peptide analogs: synthesis of [Orn 13,14] apamin and its guanidination to an apamin derivative with full neurotoxic activity. *Proceedings of the National Academy of Sciences USA* **74,** 2771–2775.

Danse, J. M., Toussaint, J. L. & Kempf, J. (1990) Nucleotide-sequence encoding β-bungarotoxin A2-chain from the venom glands of *Bungarus multicinctus. Nucleic Acids Research* **18,** 4609.

Defendini, M. L., Bahraoui, E. M., Labbe-Jullie, C., Regnier-Vigouroux, A., Elayeb, M., Van Reitschoten, J., Rochat, H. & Granier, C. (1990a) Identification of antigenic residues on apamin recognized by polyclonal antibodies. *Molecular Immunology* **27,** 37–44.

Defendini, M. L., Pierres, M., Regnier-Vigouroux, A., Rochat, H. & Granier, C. (1990b) Epitope mapping of apamin by means of monoclonal antibodies raised against free or carrier-coupled peptide. *Molecular Immunology* **27,** 551–558.

Dowdall, M. J., Fohlman, J. P. & Eaker, D. (1977) Inhibition of high affinity choline transport in peripheral cholinergic endings by presynaptic snake venom neurotoxins. *Nature* **269,** 700–702.

Dreyer, F. & Penner, R. (1987) The actions of presynaptic snake toxins on membrane currents of mouse motor nerve terminals. *Journal of Physiology* **386,** 445–463.

Dufton, M. J. (1985) Protease inhibitors and dendrotoxins. Sequence classification, structural prediction and structure/activity. *European Journal of Biochemistry* **153,** 647–654.

Elkins, T., Ganetzky, B. & Wu, C. (1986) A *Drosophila* mutation that eliminates a calcium-dependent potassium current. *Proceedings of the National Academy of Sciences USA* **83,** 8415–8419.

Farley, J. & Rudy, B. (1988) Multiple types of voltage-dependent Ca^{2+} activated K$^+$ channels of large conductance in rat brain synaptosomal membranes. *Biophysical Journal* **53,** 919–934.

Fosset, M., Schmid-Antomarchi, H., Hugues, M., Romey, G. & Lazdunski, M. (1984) The presence in pig brain of an endogenous equivalent of apamin the bee venom peptide that specifically blocks Ca^{2+}-dependent K$^+$-channels. *Proceedings of the National Academy of Sciences USA* **81,** 7228–7232.

Freeman, C. E., Catlow, C. R. A., Hemmings, A. M. & Hider, R. C. (1986) The conformation of apamin. *FEBS Letters* **197**, 289–296.

Fujii, K., Foster, C. D., Brading, A. F. & Parekh, A. B. (1990) Potassium channel blockers and the effects of cromakalim on the smooth muscle of the guinea-pig bladder. *British Journal of Pharmacology* **99**, 779–785.

Gallin, E. K. & McKinney, L. W. (1988) Patch-clamp studies in human macrophages: single-channel studies and whole-cell characterization of two K⁺ conductances. *Journal of Membrane Biology* **103**, 55–66.

Galvez, A., Gimenez-Gallego, G., Reuben, J. P., Roy-Contancin, L., Feigenbaum, P., Kaczorowski, G. J. & Garcia, M. L. (1990) Purification and characterization of a unique, potent, peptidyl probe for the high conductance calcium-activated potassium channel from venom of the scorpion *Buthus tamulus*. *Journal of Biological Chemistry* **265**, 1083–1090.

Gandolfo, G., Gottesmann, C., Bidard, J. N. & Lazdunski, M. (1989) K⁺ channel openers prevent epilepsy induced by the bee venom peptide MCD. *European Journal of Pharmacology* **159**, 329–330.

Garcia-Garayo, J. J., Cebrian, J. A., Muino, M. T. & Lopez-Perez, M. J. (1990) Phase partitioning of beta-bungarotoxin-treated cerebrocortical synaptosomes. Quantitation of the toxin-vulnerable population. *Research Communications in Chemical Pathology and Pharmacology* **68**, 55–63.

Gauldie, J., Hanson, J. M., Shipolini, R. A. & Vernon, C. A. (1976) The structures of some peptides from bee venom. *European Journal of Biochemistry* **83**, 405–410.

Gimenez-Gallego, G., Navia, M. A., Reuben, J. P., Katz, G. M., Kaczorowski, G. J. & Garcia, M. L. (1988) Purification, sequence, and model structure of charybdotoxin, a potent selective inhibitor of calcium-activated potassium channels. *Proceedings of the National Academy of Sciences USA* **85**, 3329–3333.

Goh, J. W. & Pennefather P. S. (1987) Pharmacological and physiological properties of the after-hyperpolarization current of bullfrog ganglion neurones. *Journal of Physiology* **394**, 315–330.

Granier, C., Muller, E. P. & Van Reitschoten, J. (1978) Use of synthetic analogs for a study on the structure–activity relationship of apamin. *European Journal of Biochemistry* **82**, 293–299.

Grinstein, S. & Smith, J. D. (1989) Ca²⁺ induces charybdotoxin-sensitive membrane-potential changes in rat lymphocytes. *American Journal of Physiology* **257**, C197–C206.

Grinstein, S. & Smith, J. D. (1990) Calcium-independent cell-volume regulation in human lymphocytes-inhibition by charybdotoxin. *Journal of General Physiology* **95**, 97–120.

Guggino, S. E., Guggino, W. B., Green, N. & Sacktor, B. (1987) Blocking agents of Ca²⁺-activated K⁺ channels in cultured medullary thick ascending limb cells. *American Journal of Physiology* **252**, C128–C137.

Gurrola, G. B., Bayon, A., Possani, L. D., Molinar-Rode, R. & Sitges, M. (1989) Synthetic peptides corresponding to the sequence of noxiustoxin indicate that the active-site of this K⁺ channel blocker is located in its amino-terminal portion. *Journal of Neural Transmission* **77**, 11–20.

Habermann, E. (1972) Bee and wasp venoms. *Science* **177**, 314–322.

Habermann, E. (1977) Neurotoxicity of apamin upon central application. *Naunyn-Schmiedeberg's Archives of Pharmacology* **300**, 189–191.

Habermann, E. (1984) Apamin. *Pharmacology and Therapeutics* **25**, 255–270.

Halliwell, J. V., Othman, I. B., Pelchen-Matthews, A. & Dolly, J. O. (1986) Central action of dendrotoxin: selective reduction of a transient K⁺ conductance in hippocampus and binding of localized acceptors. *Proceedings of the National Academy of Sciences USA* **83**, 493–497.

Halliwell, J. V., Tse, C. K., Spokes, J. W., Othman, I. B. & Dolly, J. O. (1982) Biochemical and electrophysiological demonstrations of the actions of β-bungarotoxin on synapses in brain. *Journal of Neurochemistry* **39**, 543–550.

Harvey, A. L. & Anderson, A. J. (1985) Dendrotoxins: snake toxins that block potassium channels and facilitate neurotransmitter release. *Pharmacology and Therapeutics* **31**, 33–55.

Harvey, A. L. & Karlsson, E. (1980) Dendrotoxin from the venom of the green mamba *Dendroaspis angusticeps*, a neurotoxin that enhances acetylcholine release at neuromuscular junctions. *Naunyn-Schmiedeberg's Archives of Pharmacology* **312**, 1–6.

Harvey, A. L. & Karlsson, E. (1982) Protease inhibitor homologues from mamba venoms: facilitation of acetylcholine release and interactions with prejunctional blocking toxins. *British Journal of Pharmacology* **77**, 153–161.

Harvey, A. L., Marshall, D. L., De-Allie, F. A. & Strong, P. N. (1989) Interactions between dendrotoxin, a blocker of voltage-dependent potassium channels, and charybdotoxin, a blocker of calcium-activated potassium channels, at binding-sites on neuronal membranes. *Biochemical and Biophysical Research Communications* **163**, 394–397.

Hermann, A. & Erxleben, C. (1987) Charybdotoxin selectively blocks small Ca-activated K^+ channels in *Aplysia* neurons. *Journal of General Physiology* **90**, 27–47.

Hider, R. C. & Ragnarsson, U. (1980) A proposal for the structure of apamin. *FEBS Letters* **111**, 189–193.

Hider, R. C. & Ragnarsson, U. (1981) A comparative structural study of apamin and related bee venom peptides. *Biochimica et Biophysica Acta* **667**, 197–208.

Hollecker, M. & Larcher, D. (1989) Conformational forces affecting the folding pathways of dendrotoxins-I and dendrotoxins-K from black mamba venom. *European Journal of Biochemistry* **179**, 87–94.

Hoshi, T. & Aldrich, R. W. (1986) Four distinct classes of voltage-dependent K^+ channels in PC12 cells. *Neuroscience Abstracts* **12**, 763.

Howard, B. D. & Gundersen, C. B. (1980) Effects and mechanisms of polypeptide neurotoxins that act presynaptically. *Annual Review of Pharmacology and Toxicology* **20**, 307–336.

Hugues, M., Duval, D., Kitabgi, P., Lazdunski, M. & Vincent, J-P. (1982a) Preparation of a pure monoiodoapamin derivative of the bee venom neurotoxin apamin and its binding properties to rat brain synaptosomes. *Journal of Biological Chemistry* **257**, 2762–2769.

Hugues, M., Duval, D., Schmid, H., Kitabgi, P., Lazdunski, M. & Vincent, J-P. (1982b) Specific and pharmacological interactions of apamin, the neurotoxin from bee venom, with guinea pig colon. *Life Sciences* **31**, 437–443.

Hugues, M., Romey, G., Duval, D., Vincent, J-P. & Lazdunski, M. (1982c) Apamin as a selective blocker of the calcium-dependent potassium channel in neuroblastoma cells: Voltage-clamp and biochemical characterization of the toxin receptor. *Proceedings of the National Academy of Sciences USA* **79**, 1308–1312.

Hugues, M., Schmid, H., Romey, G., Duval, D., Frelin, C. & Lazdunski, M. (1982d) The Ca^{2+}-dependent slow K^+ conductance in cultured rat muscle cells: characterization with apamin. *EMBO Journal* **1**, 1039–1042.

Joubert, F. J. & Taljaard, N. (1980) The amino acid sequence of two proteinase inhibitor homologues from *Dendroaspis angusticeps* venom. *Hoppe-Seylers Zeitschrift Physiological Chemistry* **361**, 661–674.

Kawai, T. & Watanabe, M. (1986) Blockade of Ca^{2+}-activated K^+ conductance by apamin in rat sympathetic neurones. *British Journal of Pharmacology* **87**, 225–232.

Kelly, R. B., von Wedel, R. J. & Strong, P. N. (1979) Phospholipase-dependent and phospholipase-independent inhibition of transmitter release by β-bungarotoxin. In Ceccarelli, B. & Clementi, F. (eds), *Advances in Cytopharmacology*, vol. 3. Raven Press, New York, pp. 77–85.

Komissarenko, S. V., Vasilenko, S. V., Elyakova, E. G., Surina, E. A. & Miróshnikov, A. I. (1981) Immunochemistry of apamin-bee venom neurotoxin-I. Radioimmunoassay with apamin and its derivatives. *Molecular Immunology* **18**, 533–536.

Kondo, K., Narita, K. & Lee, C.Y. (1978) Amino acid sequences of the two polypeptide chains in β_1-bungarotoxin from the venom *Bungarus multicinctus*. *Journal of Biochemistry* **83**, 101–115.

Kondo, K., Toda, H., Narita, K. & Lee, C.Y. (1982a) Amino acid sequence of β_2-bungarotoxin from *Bungarus multicinctus* venom. The amino acid substitution in the B chains. *Journal of Biochemistry* **91**, 1519–1530.

Kondo, K., Toda, H., Narita, K. & Lee, C.Y. (1982b) Amino acid sequences of three β-bungarotoxins (β_3, β_4 and β_5-bungarotoxin) from *Bungarus multicinctus* venom. Amino acid substitutions in the A chains. *Journal of Biochemistry* **91**, 1531–1548.

Kwong, P. D., Hendrickson, W. A. & Sigler, P. B. (1989) Beta-bungarotoxin—preparation and characterization of crystals suitable for structural-analysis. *Journal of Biological Chemistry* **264**, 9349–9353.

Lambert, P., Kuroda, H., Chino, N., Watanabe, T. X., Kimura, T. & Sakakibara, S. (1990) Solution synthesis of charybdotoxin (Chtx), a K$^+$ channel blocker. *Biochemical and Biophysical Research Communications* **170**, 684–690.

Lancaster, B. & Nicoll, R. A. (1987) Properties of two calcium-activated hyperpolarizations in rat hippocampal neurones. *Journal of Physiology* **389**, 187–203.

Lang, D .G. & Ritchie, A. K. (1990) Tetraethylammonium blockade of apamin-sensitive and insensitive Ca^{2+}-activated K$^+$ channels in a pituitary cell-line. *Journal of Physiology* **425**, 117–132.

Lucchesi, K. & Moczydlowski, E. (1990) Subconductance behavior in a maxi Ca^{2+}-activated K$^+$ channel induced by dendrotoxin-I. *Neuron* **4**, 141–148.

Lucchesi, K., Moczydlowski, E., Ravindran, A. & Young, H. (1989) Analysis of the blocking activity of charybdotoxin homologs and iodinated derivatives against Ca^{2+} activated K$^+$ channels. *Journal of Membrane Biology* **109**, 269–281.

Maas, A. J. J., Den Hertog, A., Ras, R. & Van den Akker, J. (1980) The action of apamin on guinea-pig taenia caeci. *European Journal of Pharmacology* **67**, 265–274.

McCann, J. D., Matsuda, J., Garcia, M., Kaczorowski, G. & Welsh, M. J. (1990) Basolateral K$^+$ channels in airway epithelia. 1. Regulation by Ca^{2+} and block by charybdotoxin. *American Journal of Physiology* **258**, 334–342.

MacKinnon, R. & Miller, C. (1989) Mutant potassium channels with altered binding of charybdotoxin, a pore-blocking peptide inhibitor. *Science* **245**, 1382–1385.

MacKinnon, R., Reinhart, P. H. & White, M. M. (1988) Charybdotoxin block of *Shaker* K$^+$ channels suggests that different types of K$^+$ channels share common structural features. *Neuron* **1**, 997–1001.

Marqueze, B., Seagar, M. & Couraud, C. (1987) Photoaffinity labeling of the K$^+$-channel-associated apamin-binding molecule in smooth muscle, liver and heart membranes. *European Journal of Biochemistry* **169**, 295–298.

Marshall, D. L. & Harvey, A. L. (1989) Block of potassium channels and facilitation of acetylcholine release at the neuromuscular-junction by the venom of the scorpion, *Pandinus imperator*. *Toxicon* **27**, 493–498.

Martins, J. C., Zhang, W. Tartar, A. Lazdunski, M. & Borremans, F. A. M. (1990) Solution confirmation of leiurotoxin I (scyllatoxin) by ^{1}H nuclear magnetic resonance. Resonance assignment and secondary structure. *FEBS Letters* **260**, 249–253.

Massefski, W., Redfield, A. G., Hare, D. R. & Miller, C. (1990) Molecular-structure of charybdotoxin, a pore-directed inhibitor of potassium-ion channels. *Science* **249**, 521–524.

Mehraban, F., Black, A., Breeze, L., Green, D. & Dolly, J. O. (1985) A functional membranous acceptor for dendrotoxin in rat brain: solubilization of the binding component. *Biochemical Society Transactions* **13**, 507–508.

Miller, C., Moczydlowski, E., Latorre, R. & Phillips, M. (1985) Charybdotoxin, a protein inhibitor of single Ca^{2+}-activated K^+ channels from mammalian skeletal muscle. *Nature* **313**, 316–318.

Mourre, C., Bidard, J. N. & Lazdunski, M. (1988) High affinity receptors for the bee venom MCD peptide. Quantitative autoradiographic localization at different stages of brain development and relationship with MCD neurotoxicity. *Brain Research* **446**, 106–112.

Mourre, C., Cervera, P. & Lazdunski, M. (1987) Autoradiographic analysis in rat brain of the postnatal ontogeny of voltage-dependent Na^+ channels, Ca^{2+}-dependent K^+ channels and slow Ca^{2+} channels identified as receptors for tetrodotoxin, apamin and (−)-desmethoxyverapamil. *Brain Research* **417**, 21–32.

Mourre, C., Hugues, M. & Lazdunski, M. (1986) Quantitative autoradiographic mapping rat brain of the receptor of apamin, a polypeptide toxin specific for one class of Ca^{2+}-dependent K^+ channel. *Brain Research* **382**, 239–249.

Muniz, Z. M., Diniz, C. R. & Dolly, J. O. (1990a) Characterization of binding-sites for sigma-dendrotoxin in guinea-pig synaptosomes. Relationship to acceptors for the K^+-channel probe alpha-dendrotoxin. *Journal of Neurochemistry* **54**, 343–346.

Muniz, Z. M., Tibbs, G. R., Maschot, P., Bougis, P., Nicholls, D. G. & Dolly, J. O. (1990b) Homologs of a K^+ channel blocker alpha-dendrotoxin. Characterization of synaptosomal binding-sites and their coupling to elevation of cytosolic free calcium-concentration. *Neurochemistry International* **16**, 105–112.

Nakagawa, A., Nakamura, S. & Arita, M. (1989) Possible increases in potassium conductance by apamin in mammalian ventricular papillary-muscles. A comparison with the effects on enzymatically isolated ventricular cells. *Journal of Cardiovascular Pharmacology* **14**, 38–45.

Nanberg, E., Connolly, E. & Nedergaard, J. (1985) Presence of a Ca^{2+}-dependent K^+ channel in brown adipocytes. Possible role in maintenance of α_1-adrenergic stimulation. *Biochimica et Biophysica Acta* **844**, 42–49.

Ng, R. H. & Howard, B. D. (1978) De-energization of nerve terminals by β-bungarotoxin. *Biochemistry* **17**, 4978–4986.

Nicholls, D., Snelling, R. & Dolly, O. J. (1985) Bioenergetic actions of β-bungarotoxin, dendrotoxin and bee-venom phospholipase A_2 on guinea-pig synaptosomes. *Biochemical Journal* **229**, 653–662.

Ohnishi, S. T., Katagi, H. & Katagi, C. (1989) Inhibition of the *in vitro* formation of dense cells and of irreversibly sickled cells by charybdotoxin, a specific inhibitor of calcium-activated potassium efflux. *Biochimica et Biophysica Acta* **1010**, 199–203.

Onozuka, M., Imai, S., Ozono, S. & Sugimura, Y. (1990) A specific 70 kDa protein-induced in the epileptogenic cortex of rats, elicits bursting activity and inactivation of potassium current in snail neurons. *Neuroscience Letters* **115**, 49–54.

Pappone, P. A. & Cahalan, M. D. (1987) *Pandinus imperator* scorpion venom blocks voltage-gated potassium channels in nerve fibres. *Journal of Neuroscience* **7**, 3300–3305.

Pappone, P. A. & Lucero, M. (1988) *Pandinus imperator* scorpion venom blocks voltage-gated potassium channels in GH$_3$ cells. *Journal of General Physiology* **91**, 817–833.

Parcej, D. N. & Dolly, J. O. (1989) Dendrotoxin acceptor from bovine synaptic plasma-membranes. Binding-properties, purification and subunit composition of a putative constituent of certain voltage-activated K$^+$ channels. *Biochemical Journal* **257**, 899–903.

Pease, J. H. B. & Wemmer, D. (1988) Solution structure of apamin determined by nuclear magnetic resonance and distance geometry. *Biochemistry* **27**, 8491–8498.

Pelchen-Matthews, A. & Dolly, J. O. (1988) Distribution of acceptors for β-bungarotoxin in the central nervous system of the rat. *Brain Research* **441**, 127–138.

Pelchen-Matthews, A. & Dolly, J. O. (1989) Distribution in the rat central nervous-system of acceptor sub-types for dendrotoxin, a K$^+$ channel probe. *Neuroscience* **29**, 347–361.

Penner, R., Petersen, M., Pierau, F. K. & Dreyer, F. (1986) Dendrotoxin: a selective blocker of a non-inactivating potassium current in guinea-pig dorsal root ganglion neurones. *Naunyn-Schmiedeberg's Archives of Pharmacology* **332**(Suppl.), R93.

Petersen, M., Pierau, F-K. & Weyrich, M. (1987) The influence of capsaicin on membrane currents in dorsal root ganglion neurones of guinea-pig and chicken. *Pflügers Archiv* **409**, 403–410.

Petersen, P., Penner, R., Pierau, K. F. & Dreyer, F. (1986) β-Bungarotoxin inhibits a non-inactivating potassium current in guinea pig dorsal root ganglion neurones. *Neuroscience Letters* **68**, 141–145.

Possani, L. D., Dent, M. A. R., Martin, B. M., Maelicke, A. & Svendsen, I. (1981a) The amino terminal sequence of several toxins from the venom of the Mexican scorpion *Centruroides noxius* Hoffman. *Carlsberg Research Communications* **46**, 207–214.

Possani, L. D., Dent, M. A. R., Martin, B. M., Maelicke, A. & Svendsen, I. (1981b) Purification and chemical characterization of the major toxins from the venom of the Brazilian scorpion *Tityus serrulatus* Lutz and Mello. *Carlsberg Research Communications* **46**, 195–205.

Possani, L. D., Martin, B. M. & Svendsen, I. (1982) The primary structure of noxius-toxin: A K$^+$ channel blocking peptide, purified from the venom of the scorpion *Centruroides noxius* Hoffman. *Carlsberg Research Communications* **47**, 285–289.

Poulter, M. O., Padjen, A. L. & Hashiguchi, T. (1989) Dendrotoxin blocks accommodation in frog myelinated axons. *Journal of Neurophysiology* **62**, 174–184.

Price, M., Lee, S. C. & Deutsch, C. (1989) Charybdotoxin inhibits proliferation and interleukin-2 production in human peripheral-blood lymphocytes. *Proceedings of the National Academy of Sciences USA* **86**, 171–175.

Quast, U. & Cook, N.S. (1988) *Leiurus quinquestriatus* venom inhibits BRL 34915-induced ^{86}Rb$^+$ efflux from the rat portal vein. *Life Sciences* **42**, 805–810.

Rehm, H. (1989) Enzymatic deglycosylation of the dendrotoxin-binding protein. *FEBS Letters* **247**, 28–30.

Rehm, H. & Betz, H. (1983) Identification by cross-linking β-bungarotoxin binding polypeptide in chick brain membranes. *EMBO Journal* **7**, 1119–1122.

Rehm, H. & Betz, H. (1984) Solubilization and characterization of the β-bungarotoxin-binding protein of chick brain membranes. *Journal of Biological Chemistry* **259**, 6865–6869.

Rehm, H. & Lazdunski, M. (1988a) Existence of different populations of the dendro-toxin I binding protein associated with neuronal K$^+$ channels. *Biochemical and Biophysical Research Communications* **153**, 231–240.

Rehm, H. & Lazdunski, M. (1988b) Purification and subunit structure of a putative K$^+$-channel protein identified by its binding properties for dendrotoxin I. *Proceedings of the National Academy of Sciences USA* **85**, 4919–4923.

Rehm, H., Bidard, J. N., Hugues, S. & Lazdunski, M. (1988) The receptor site for bee venom mast cell degranulating peptide. Affinity labelling and evidence for a common molecular target for mast cell degranulating peptide and dendrotoxin I, a snake toxin active on K$^+$ channels. *Biochemistry* **27**, 1827–1832.

Rehm, H., Cochet, C., Chambaz, E., Lazdunski, M., Pelzer, D., Pelzer, S., Trautwein, W. & Tempel, B. L. (1989b) Dendrotoxin-binding brain membrane protein displays a K$^+$ channel activity that is stimulated by both cAMP-dependent and endogenous phosphorylations. *Biochemistry* **28**, 6455–6460.

Rehm, H., Newitt, R. A. & Tempel, B. L. (1989a) Immunological evidence for a relationship between the dendrotoxin-binding protein and the mammalian homolog of the *Drosophila-Shaker* K$^+$ channel. *FEBS Letters* **249**, 224–228.

Reinhart, P. H., Chung, S. & Levitan, I. B. (1989) A family of calcium-dependent potassium channels from rat brain. *Neuron* **2**, 1031–1041.

Reiser, G., Binmoller, F. J., Strong, P. N. & Hamprecht, B. (1990) Activation of a K$^+$ conductance by bradykinin and by inositol 1,4,5-triphosphate in rat glioma cells: involvement of intracellular and extracellular Ca^{2+}. *Brain Research* **506**, 205–214.

Rosenberg, P., Ghassemi, A., Condrea, E., Dhillon, D. & Yang, C. C. (1989) Do chemical modifications dissociate between the enzymatic and pharmacological activities of beta-bungarotoxin and notexin? *Toxicon* **27**, 493–498.

Rowan, E. G. & Harvey, A. L. (1988) Potassium channel blocking actions of β-bungarotoxin and related toxins on mouse and frog motor nerve terminals. *British Journal of Pharmacology* **94**, 839–847.

Rowan, E. G., Pemberton, K. E. & Harvey, A. L. (1990) On the blockade of acetylcholine-release at mouse motor-nerve terminals by β-bungarotoxin and crotoxin. *British Journal of Pharmacology* **100**, 301–304.

Rugolo, M., Dolly, J. O. & Nicholls, D. G. (1986) The action of β-bungarotoxin at the presynaptic plasma membrane. *Biochemical Journal* **233**, 519–523.

Sands, S. B., Lewis, R. S. & Cahalan, M. D. (1989) Charybdotoxin blocks voltage-gated K$^+$ channels in human and murine T-lymphocytes. *Journal of General Physiology* **93**, 1061–1074.

Schmid-Antomarchi, H., Hugues, M., Norman, R., Ellory, C., Borsotto, M. & Lazdunski, M. (1984) Molecular properties of the apamin binding component of the Ca^{2+}-dependent K$^+$ channel. Radiation inactivation, affinity-labelling and solubilization. *European Journal of Biochemistry* **142**, 1–6.

Schmid-Antomarchi, H., Renaud, J-F., Romey, G., Hugues, M., Schmid, A. & Lazdunski, M. (1985) The all-or-none role of innervation in expression of apamin receptor and of apamin-sensitive Ca^{2+}-activated K$^+$ channel in mammalian skeletal muscle. *Proceedings of the National Academy of Sciences USA* **82**, 2188–2191.

Schmidt, R. R. & Betz, H. (1989) Cross-linking of beta-bungarotoxin to chick brain membranes identification of subunits of a putative voltage-gated K$^+$ channel. *Biochemistry* **28**, 8346–8350.

Schmidt, R. R., Betz, H. & Rehm, H. (1988) Inhibition of β-bungarotoxin binding to brain membranes by mast cell degranulating peptide, toxin I and ethylene glycol *bis*(β-aminoethylether)-*N,N,N,N*-tetraacetic acid. *Biochemistry* **27**, 963–967.

Schneider, M. J., Rogowski, R. S., Krueger, B. K. & Blaustein, M. P. (1989) Charybdotoxin blocks both Ca-activated K-channels and Ca-independent voltage gated potassium channels in rat brain synaptosomes. *FEBS Letters* **250**, 433–436.

Schweitz, H. & Lazdunski, M. (1984) A micro-radioimmunoassay for apamin. *Toxicon* **22**, 985–988.

Schweitz, H., Bidard, J. N. & Lazdunski, M. (1990) Purification and pharmacological characterization of peptide toxins from the black mamba (*Dendroaspis polylepis*) venom. *Toxicon* **28**, 847–856.

Schweitz, H., Bidard, J. N., Lazdunski, M. & Maes, P. (1989a) Charybdotoxin is a new member of the K$^+$ channel toxin family that includes dendrotoxin-I and mast-cell degranulating peptide. *Biochemistry* **28**, 9708–9714.

Schweitz, H., Stansfeld, C. E., Maes, P., Lazdunski, M., Fagni, L. & Bidard, J. (1989b)

Charybdotoxin blocks dendrotoxin-sensitive voltage-activated K$^+$ channels. *FEBS Letters* **250**, 519–522.

Seagar, M. J., Deprez, P., Martin-Moutot, N. & Couraud, F. (1987b) Detection and photoaffinity labeling of the Ca^{2+}-activated K$^+$ channel-associated apamin receptor in cultured astrocytes from rat brain. *Brain Research* **411**, 226–230.

Seagar, M. J., Granier, C. & Couraud, F. (1984) Interactions of the neurotoxin apamin with a Ca^{2+}-activated K$^+$ channel in primary neuronal cultures. *Journal of Biological Chemistry* **259**, 1491–1495.

Seagar, M. J., Labbe-Jullie, C., Granier, C., Goll, A., Glossman, H., Van Rietschoten, J. & Couraud, F. (1986) Molecular structure of rat brain apamin receptor: Differential photoaffinity labelling of putative K$^+$ channel subunits and target size analysis. *Biochemistry* **25**, 4051–4057.

Seagar, M. J., Labbe-Jullie, C., Granier, C., Van Reitschoten, J. & Couraud, F. (1985) Photoaffinity labelling of components of the apamin-sensitive K$^+$ channel in neuronal membranes. *Journal of Biological Chemistry* **260**, 3895–3898.

Seagar, M. J., Marqueze, B. & Couraud, F. (1987a) Solubilization of the apamin receptor associated with a calcium-activated potassium channel from rat brain. *Journal of Neuroscience* **7**, 565–570.

Silveira, R., Siciliano, J., Abo, V., Veira, L. & Dajas, F. (1988) Intrastriatal dendrotoxin injection; behavioural and neurochemical effects. *Toxicon* **26**, 1009–1015.

Sitges, M., Possani, L. D. & Bayon, A. (1986) Noxiustoxin, a short chain toxin from the Mexican scorpion *Centruroides noxius*, induces transmitter release by blocking K$^+$ permeability. *Journal of Neuroscience* **6**, 1570–1574.

Smith, C. D., Phillips, M. & Miller, C. (1986) Purification of charybdotoxin, a specific inhibitor of the high conductance Ca^{2+}-activated K$^+$ channel. *Journal of Biological Chemistry* **261**, 14607–14613.

Sorensen, R. G. & Blaustein, M. P. (1989) Rat-brain dendrotoxin receptors associated with voltage-gated potassium channels. Dendrotoxin binding and receptor solubilization. *Molecular Pharmacology* **36**, 689–698.

Stansfeld, C. E. & Feltz, A. (1988) Dendrotoxin-sensitive K$^+$ channels in dorsal root ganglion cells. *Neuroscience Letters* **93**, 49–55.

Stansfeld, C. E., Marsh, S. J., Halliwell, J. V. & Brown, D. A. (1986) 4-Aminopyridine and dendrotoxin induce repetitive firing in rat visceral sensory neurones by blocking a slowly inactivating outward current. *Neuroscience Letters* **64**, 299–304.

Stansfeld, C. E., Marsh, S. J., Parcej, D. N., Dolly, J. O. & Brown, D. A. (1987) Mast cell degranulating peptide and dendrotoxin selectively inhibit a fast-activating potassium current and bind to common neuronal proteins. *Neuroscience* **23**, 893–902.

Steketee, J. D. & Kalivas, P. W. (1990) Effect of microinjections of apamin into the A10-dopamine region of rats. A behavioral and neurochemical analysis. *Journal of Pharmacology and Experimental Therapeutics* **254**, 711–719.

Strong, P. N. (1987) Presynaptic phospholipase A$_2$ neurotoxins: Relationship between biochemical and electrophysiological approaches to the mechanism of toxin action. In Dowdall, M. J. & Hawthorne, J. N. (eds), *The Cellular and Molecular Basis of Cholinergic Function*. Ellis Horwood Ltd, Chichester, pp. 534–549.

Strong, P. N. (1990) Potassium channel toxins. *Pharmacology and Therapeutics* **46**, 137–162.

Strong, P. N. & Evans, W. H. (1987) Receptor-mediated endocytosis of apamin by liver cells. *European Journal of Biochemistry* **163**, 267–273.

Strong, P. N. & Kelly, R. B. (1977) Membranes undergoing phase transitions are preferentially hydrolysed by β-bungarotoxin. *Biochimica et Biophysica Acta* **469**, 231–235.

Strong, P. N., Heuser, J. E. & Kelly, R. B. (1977) Selective enzymatic hydrolysis of nerve terminal phospholipids by β-bungarotoxin: biochemical and morphological studies. In Hall, Z. W., Kelly, R. B. & Fox, F. (eds), *Cellular Neurobiology*. Alan Liss, New York, pp. 227–249.

Strong, P. N., Weir, S. W., Beech, D. J., Hiestand, P. & Kocher, H. P. (1989) Effects of potassium channel toxins from *Leiurus quinquestriatus hebraeus* venom on responses to cromakalim in rabbit-blood vessels. *British Journal of Pharmacology* **98**, 817–826.

Strydom, D. J. (1972) Snake venom toxins. The amino acid sequences of two toxins from *Dendroaspis polylepis* (black mamba). *Journal of Biological Chemistry* **247**, 4029–4042.

Stühmer, W., Stocker, M., Sakmann, B., Seeburg, P., Baumann, A., Grupe, A. & Pongs, O. (1988) Potassium channels expressed from rat brain cDNA have delayed rectifier properties. *FEBS Letters* **242**, 199–206.

Sugg, E. E., Garcia, M. L., Reuben, J. P., Patchett, A. A. & Kaczorowski, G. J. (1990) Synthesis and structural characterization of charybdotoxin, a potent peptidyl inhibitor of the high conductance Ca^{2+}-activated K^+ channel. *Journal of Biological Chemistry* **265**, 18 745–18 748.

Suput, D. (1988) Effects of equinatoxin on single myelinated nerve-fibres. *Toxicon* **26**, 40.

Talvenheimo, J. A., Lam, G. & Gelband, C. (1988) CTX inhibits the 250 pŚ Ca^{2+}-activated K^+-channel in aorta and contracts aorta smooth muscle. *Biophysical Journal* **53**, 258a.

Taylor, J. W., Bidard, J-N. & Lazdunski, M. (1984) The characterisation of high affinity binding sites in rat brain for the mast cell-degranulating peptide from bee venom using the purified monoiodinated peptide. *Journal of Biological Chemistry* **259**, 13 957–13 967.

Tibbs, G. R., Dolly, J. O. & Nicholls, D. G. (1989a) Dendrotoxin, 4-aminopyridine, and beta-bungarotoxin act at common loci but by 2 distinct mechanisms to induce Ca^{2+}-dependent release of glutamate from guinea-pig cerebrocortical synaptosomes. *Journal of Neurochemistry* **52**, 201–206.

Tibbs, G. R., Nicholls, D. G. & Dolly, J. O. (1989b) Dendrotoxin and charybdotoxin increase the cytosolic concentration of free Ca^{2+} in cerebrocortical synaptosomes —an effect not shared by apamin. *FEBS Letters* **255**, 159–162.

Traore, F., Cognard, C., Potreau, D. & Raymond, G. (1986) The apamin-sensitive potassium current in frog skeletal muscle: its dependence on the extracellular calcium and sensitivity to calcium channel blockers. *Pflügers Archiv* **407**, 199–203.

Valdivia, H. H., Smith, J. S., Martin, B., Coronado, R. & Possani, L. D. (1988) Charybdotoxin and noxiustoxin, two homologous peptide inhibitors of the K^+ (Ca^{2+}) channel. *FEBS Letters* **226**, 280–284.

Vázquez, J., Feigenbaum, P., King, V. F., Kaczorowski, G. J. & Garcia, M. L. (1990) Characterization of high-affinity binding-sites for charybdotoxin in synaptic plasma membranes from rat brain. Evidence for a direct association with an inactivating, voltage-dependent, potassium channel. *Journal of Biological Chemistry* **265**, 5564–5571.

Vázquez, J., Reuben, J. P., Roy-Contancin, L., Slaughter, R. S., Garcia, M. L., Feigenbaum, P., Kaczorowski, G. J., Katz, G. & King, V. F. (1989) Characterization of high-affinity binding-sites for charybdotoxin in sarcolemmal membranes from bovine aortic smooth-muscle. Evidence for a direct association with the high conductance calcium-activated potassium channel. *Journal of Biological Chemistry* **264**, 902–909.

Vincent, J-P., Schweitz, H. & Lazdunski, M. (1975) Structure–function relationships and the site of action of apamin, a neurotoxic polypeptide of bee venom with an action on the central nervous system. *Biochemistry* **14**, 2521–2525.

Weir, S. W. & Strong, P. N. (1988) Inhibition of BRL 34915-stimulated ^{86}Rb^{+} efflux in rabbit aorta by fractionated *Leiurus quinquestriatus hebraeus* scorpion venom. *British Journal of Pharmacology* **93**, 202P.

Weir S. W. & Weston, A. H. (1986) Effect of apamin on responses to BRL 34915, nicorandil and other relaxants in the guinea pig taenia caeci. *British Journal of Pharmacology* **88**, 113–120.

Weller, U., Bernhardt, U., Siemen, D., Dreyer, F., Vogel, W. & Habermann, E. (1985) Electrophysiological and biochemical evidence for the blockade of a potassium channel by dendrotoxin. *Naunyn-Schmiedeberg's Archives of Pharmacology* **330**, 77–83.

Wemmer, D. & Kallenbach, N. R. (1983) Structure of apamin in solution. A two-dimensional nuclear magnetic resonance study. *Biochemistry* **22**, 1901–1906.

Wernicke, J. F., Vanker, A. D. & Howard, B. D. (1975) The mechanism of action of β-bungarotoxin. *Journal of Neurochemistry* **25**, 483–496.

Wu, C. F., Zhong, Y., Lee, C. Y., Tsai, M. C., Singh, S. & Chen, M. L. (1989) Actions of dendrotoxin on K^{+} channels and neuromuscular transmission in *Drosophila melanogaster*, and its effects in synergy with K^{+} channel-specific drugs and mutations. *Journal of Experimental Biology* **147**, 21–41.

Yates, S. L., Burns, M., Condrea, E., Ghassemi, A., Shina, R. & Rosenberg, P. (1990) Phospholipid hydrolysis and loss of membrane integrity following treatment of rat-brain synaptosomes with β-bungarotoxin, notexin, and *Naja-naja-atra* and *Naja-nigricollis* phospholipase A$_2$. *Toxicon* **28**, 847–856.

Zemkova, H., Teisinger, J. & Vyskocil, F. (1988) Inhibition of the electrogenic Na, K pump and Na,K-ATPase activity by tetraethylammonium, tetrabutylammonium, and apamin. *Journal of Neuroscience Research* **19**, 497–503.

Zhang, L. & Krnjevic, K. (1987) Apamin depresses selectively the after-hyperpolarisation of cat spinal motor neurones. *Neuroscience Abstracts* **12**, 1199.

Chapter 12
Potassium channel blockers: synthetic agents and their antiarrhythmic potential

T. J. Colatsky

Introduction

Although the antiarrhythmic benefit of prolonging repolarization in the heart has been recognized for some time, only recently has there been a concerted effort to synthesize and develop agents that selectively produce this therapeutic effect. Initial speculation about the mechanism of action of quinidine, one of the first antiarrhythmic drugs introduced into clinical practice, centred on its ability to increase the time-course of ventricular repolarization as measured by the QT interval, while its effects on conduction and the QRS interval were viewed primarily as signs of potential toxicity (Lewis & Drury, 1926). With the advent of intracellular microelectrode recordings in cardiac tissue, emphasis was shifted to conduction slowing and Na-channel block as primary determinants of antiarrhythmic activity (Weidmann, 1955; Vaughan Williams, 1958), actions which later became the basis for classifying these drugs as class I antiarrhythmic agents (Vaughan Williams, 1970, 1984). Whilst clear differences are recognized among the class I agents in their effects on repolarization (Harrison, 1985), these have been generally considered to be of secondary importance in directing the course of antiarrhythmic therapy (Cobbe, 1987).

During the past 15 years, the focus on Na-channel block as an important antiarrhythmic mechanism has been sustained by an intensive experimental and theoretical effort directed toward characterizing the time- and voltage-dependent interactions between class I antiarrhythmic drugs and the cardiac Na-channel (Hille, 1977; Hondeghem & Katzung, 1977, 1984; Courtney, 1980, 1987; Starmer & Grant, 1985), and the development of a number of very potent channel blockers (e.g. flecainide, encainide, indecainide) that were found to be extremely effective in suppressing the frequent and repetitive runs of premature ventricular complexes (PVCs) typically recognized as independent markers of an increased risk of sudden cardiac death. However, the validity of the Na-channel approach has been recently brought into question by the troubling results of the Cardiac Arrhythmia Suppression Trial (CAST). In this National Institutes of Health sponsored multicentre study, which was designed to test the hypothesis that suppression of ventricular arrhythmias by antiarrhythmic drugs improves survival postinfarction, patients treated with the class I agents encainide and flecainide were found to have a 3.6-fold greater risk of arrhythmic death and/or cardiac arrest than their respective placebo control groups, even though PVCs were effectively controlled on therapy (CAST Investigators, 1989). Although the reason for the drug-related increases in mortality remains in doubt, proarrhythmia due to excessive conduction slowing has been suggested as a probable cause (Task Force of the Working Group on Arrhythmias of the European Society of Cardiology, 1990).

The CAST findings have led to a critical re-evaluation of the adequacy of existing antiarrhythmic therapy (Pratt et al., 1990), and renewed interest in alternate approaches, particularly those based on a selective prolongation of repolarization and refractoriness. The validity of this strategy has been supported by recent studies correlating antiarrhythmic efficacy with increases in refractory period rather than conduction slowing, for both ventricular (Kus et al., 1990; Sheldon et al., 1990) and atrial arrhythmias (Feld et al., 1986, 1988).

The present chapter attempts to provide an overview of the different organic and synthetic agents known to block K-channels in the heart, concentrating on their potential therapeutic utility in the treatment of cardiac arrhythmias. Since the ability to block K-channels appears to be a property that is widely shared by a number of compounds, including the majority of class I antiarrhythmics, special consideration is given to the chemical requirements for gaining K-channel specificity and selectivity, and to the molecular mechanisms underlying the drug–K-channel interaction. Where necessary, results obtained in non-cardiac preparations will be used to help characterize the mechanism of drug action. The final portion of the chapter will deal with the antiarrhythmic and cardioprotective effects of agents known to increase K-conductance in the heart and their antagonists. While the list of references cited in this chapter is extensive, reflecting the tremendous advances in this field over the last 2–3 years, it is by no means exhaustive, and the reader is referred to the following recent reviews on this topic for additional information (Arrowsmith & Cross, 1989; Cook & Quast, 1990; Robertson & Steinberg, 1990).

Potential targets for K-channel blockers in the heart

As reviewed in detail elsewhere in this book (*see* Chapter 8), the repolarization phase of the cardiac action potential is determined by the interaction of several overlapping inward and outward currents which flow through discrete ion channels. At last count, at least eight different K-currents, together with some of the associated K-channels have been identified in the heart and proposed to contribute to the repolarization process. These include both rapidly and slowly activating subtypes of the delayed rectifier $(I_{K(dr)})$* current $(I_{K(r)}, I_{K(s)}$; Noble & Tsien, 1969; Shibasaki, 1987; Sanguinetti & Jurkiewicz, 1990a), the background (inward rectifier) K-channel (K_{IR}; Sakmann & Trube, 1984), a voltage-dependent transient outward current ($I_{K(to1)}$; Giles & Van Ginneken, 1985; Kenyon & Sutko, 1987; Tseng & Hoffman, 1989), a Ca-activated transient outward current ($I_{K(to2)}$; Siegelbaum & Tsien, 1980; Tseng & Hoffman, 1989), a high conductance plateau channel (K_p; Yue & Marban, 1988), and K-channels regulated by adenosine triphosphate (ATP) (K_{ATP}; Noma & Shibasaki, 1985) and acetylcholine (K_{ACh}; Sakmann *et al.*, 1983). The K_{ACh}-channel is modulated by arachidonic acid metabolites released intracellularly by the activation of phospholipase A_2 (Kurachi *et al.*, 1987; Kim *et al.*, 1989), and novel K-channels activated by arachidonic acid and phosphatidylcholine have also been described and suggested to shorten action potential duration during myocardial ischaemia (Kim & Clapham, 1989). In addition, a K-channel activated by extremely high intracellular Na ion concentrations has been described (Kameyama *et al.*, 1984), but its physiological role remains uncertain.

A large number of organic and inorganic agents are known to block myocardial K-channels. A partial list of some of the more commonly used agents and their relative selectivity for the various myocardial K-channels is given in Table 12.1. It should be remarked, however, that agents used to isolate specific K-currents in nerve and skeletal muscle (e.g. tetraethylammonium (TEA) ions) have generally failed to discriminate adequately between different myocardial K-channels to be useful as pharmacologic probes of channel activity. As a result, considerable uncertainty still remains about the number and type of K-channels actually present in the myocardial membrane and the role each plays in the repolarization process. Fortunately, the synthesis of new molecules with improved selectivity for certain K-channel subtypes, like the class III agent E4031, which was found to be a potent and selective blocker of the rapidly activating component of the delayed rectifier current $I_{K(r)}$ (Sanguinetti & Jurkiewicz,

---

*The macro delayed rectifier current in the heart is often designated I_K. This literally means 'potassium current' and is a most uninformative abbreviation. In this chapter the cardiac delayed rectifier current will be designated $I_{K(dr)}$ and its slowly and rapidly activating subtypes as $I_{K(r)}$ and $I_{K(s)}$, respectively.

Table 12.1. Specificity of myocardial K-channel blockers.

Current	Cations	Class I	Class III	Other
I_{K1}	TEA_o† Cs^+, Ba^{2+}, 4-AP*	Quinidine Disopyramide	RP 58866 Sematilide	Bepridil Bupivacaine
$I_{K(dr)}$	TEA_i, Cs^+, Ba^{2+}	Cibenzoline Disopyramide Encainide Flecainide Pirmenol Procainamide Quinidine	Acecainide Bretylium Clofilium E-4031 Risotilide Sematilide Sotalol Tedisamil UK68,798	Bupivacaine D-600 Diltiazem Nisoldipine*
$I_{K(to1)}$	TEA_i, Cs^+, 4-AP	Disopyramide Quinidine	Tedisamil	Bepridil
$I_{K(to2)}$	TEA_i, Cs^+, Ba^{2+}, Si^{2+}, Mn^{2+}	—	—	Caffeine D-600 Ryanodine
$I_{K(p)}$	Ba^{2+}; not sensitive to TEA_i	—	—	—
$I_{K(ATP)}$	TEA_o Cs^+, Ba^{2+}, 4-AP	Quinidine	Amiodarone?‡ E4031?‡	Glibenclamide Phentolamine Tolbutamide

*High concentrations only.
†Also blocked by internal TEA.
‡Not confirmed in other studies.
i, Applied to inner surface; o, applied to outer surface.

1990a), has provided a means to begin addressing some of these basic questions.

Blockers of myocardial K-channels

Inorganic cations

Monovalents

As in nerve and skeletal muscle, K-channels in heart can be blocked by a variety of inorganic cations that resemble K^+ in their hydrated or free crystal radius, as well as by some relatively simple organic molecules, such as the quaternary tetraalkylammonium derivatives (e.g., TEA^+), which bear K^+-like cationic head groups attached to hydrocarbon chains of increasing length. The alkali cation Cs^+ is a non-specific blocker of cardiac K-channels, and has been reported to inhibit $I_{(K1)}$, $I_{K(to1)}$, $I_{K(to2)}$ and $I_{K(ATP)}$ when applied extracellularly at concentrations of 5–20 mM, or when introduced into the cell using iontophoresis or other loading techniques (Isenberg, 1976; Meier & Katzung, 1981; Marban & Tsien, 1982; Tourneur *et al.*, 1987; Arena & Kass, 1989). In addition, external Cs^+ also effectively inhibits the cationic pacemaker current, I_f, and in fact may show some selectivity for this current at lower (approximately 1 mM) concentrations (Isenberg, 1976). In squid axon, block by external Cs^+ is steeply voltage-dependent and favoured by hyperpolarization (French & Shoukimas, 1985). In cat ventricular myocytes, a similar type of voltage dependence is observed, together with a rapid 'inactivation' of I_{K1} that is most evident at low concentrations (e.g. 0.01 mM) and strong hyperpolarizations (Harvey & ten Eick, 1989).

Divalents

Like Cs^+, Ba^{2+} (0.5–5 mM) is relatively non-specific in blocking K-channels. Since Ba^{2+} is very close to K^+ in atomic radius, it can enter the K-channel and bind to a blocking site within the pore. Numerous studies in a variety of excitable cells have established that Ba^{2+} block depends on both time and voltage. In the heart, as in skeletal muscle, application of Ba^{2+} causes a gradual decay or 'inactivation' of the inward rectifier current (I_{K1}) that is enhanced by hyperpolarization and relieved by depolarization (Standen & Stanfield, 1978; DiFrancesco *et al.*, 1984; Hirano & Hiraoka, 1986; Tourneur *et al.*, 1987). Modelling of results from skeletal muscle suggests that Ba^{2+} competes with K^+ for a binding site within the channel which experiences about 70% of the total membrane electrical field (Standen & Stanfield, 1978).

Effects of Ba^{2+} on the cardiac delayed rectifier channel are less clearly defined, primarily because of the difficulty in studying $I_{K(dr)}$ in isolation from other components of membrane current in cardiac preparations. Evidence suggests that $I_{K(dr)}$ is suppressed in myocytes isolated from guinea pig ventricle (Hirano & Hiraoka, 1986) and rabbit sinoatrial node (Yanagihara & Irisawa, 1980; Osterreider *et al.*, 1982), but not frog atrium (Simmons *et al.*, 1986). In squid axon, where $I_{K(dr)}$ can be clearly separated from other ionic currents, block by external Ba^{2+} exhibits a different time- and voltage-dependence than is observed when Ba^{2+} is applied to the cytoplasmic side of the membrane (Armstrong *et al.*, 1982). For internal Ba^{2+}, block is enhanced by strong depolarizations and characterized by an apparent 'inactivation' of the current (Armstrong & Taylor, 1980). In contrast, block of $I_{K(dr)}$ by external Ba^{2+} increases as membrane potential is made more negative, and the time-course of $I_{K(dr)}$ is relatively unaltered. It has been postulated that Ba^{2+} can move within the delayed rectifier channel to reach two different blocking sites. One site is near the outer mouth of the channel and is preferentially accessed by internal Ba^{2+} during depolarizations when the activation gates are open; the other site is two-thirds of the way into the channel and is accessed by external Ba^{2+} when the activation gates are closed (Armstrong et al., 1982). Increasing the $[K^+]_0$ concentration reduces the degree of Ba^{2+} block for both $I_{K(dr)}$ and I_{K1}, consistent with a 'knock off' mechanism in which K^+ and Ba^{2+} compete for the same binding site (Standen & Stanfield, 1978; Armstrong & Taylor, 1980; Hirano & Hiraoka, 1986). In the heart, $I_{K(dr)}$ tail currents have been reported to increase in the presence of Ba^{2+}, and similar data have recently been obtained in cat ventricular myocytes exposed to $200\,\mu M\,Cd^+$ (Lodge et al., 1990). This increase in tail amplitude may reflect the ability of the divalent cations to modify membrane surface charge and shift the voltage dependence of channel gating to more positive potentials (Agus et al., 1989).

In contrast to the results above, block of Ca^{2+}-activated K-channels by Ba^{2+} and other divalent cations may be indirect and involve interference with steps in the K-channel activation mechanism, such as interference with the transmembrane entry of Ca^{2+} entry (e.g. Mn^{2+}), the modification of Ca^{2+}-release from the sarcoplasmic reticulum (e.g. Ba^{2+}, Sr^{2+}), or a failure to substitute for Ca^{2+} at the channel activation site. As noted above, some divalent cations (e.g. Cd^{2+}) may also modify membrane surface charge.

Magnesium must be considered separately as a blocker of K-channels, since it is normally present inside cells and has been proposed to impart to myocardial K-channels the property of inward rectification that is so important in helping to maintain the cardiac action potential plateau. In the absence of internal Mg^{2+}, the background current–voltage relationship of myocytes becomes linear (ohmic). Subsequent addition of physiological concentrations of Mg^{2+} ($K_d = 1.7\,mM$) to the internal side of the membrane reduces outward currents through the background K^+ channel without affecting inward currents, thereby restoring inward rectification (Matsuda, 1988). Internal Mg^{2+} has also been reported to decrease the maximum amplitude of the delayed rectifier current (Duchatelle-Gourdon et al., 1989), and to block the K_{ATP} (Horie et al., 1987).

Trivalents

The trivalent cation lanthanum (La^{3+}) has recently been reported to block the rapidly activating delayed rectifier current ($I_{K(r)}$) in guinea-pig without altering the slower component ($I_{K(s)}$) (Balser & Roden, 1988; Sanguinetti & Jurkiewicz, 1990b). In addition to a direct block of the channel, La^{3+}, like Cd^{2+}, can also screen negative membrane surface charge and shift the voltage dependence of channel activation to more positive potentials.

Small organic molecules

TEA and its analogues

The tetra-n-alkylammonium ions have been widely used by electrophysiologists as tools to separate out K-currents from currents generated by
other ions. Selectivity for K-channels is based on the similarity in size
between the molecular radius of TEA$^+$ and K$^+$ with a single hydration
shell. In general, these molecules are more effective K-channel blockers
when introduced into the cytoplasm, and block only weakly when applied
in the external bathing solution, suggesting that the blocking site is accessible only from the internal side of the membrane. Increasing the length of
the hydrocarbon side chain attached to the quaternary ammonium head-
group has been shown to increase the potency and efficacy of block (Kass
et al., 1982), an effect that has been attributed to the larger size and
consequently greater hydrophobicity of the substituted molecule (Armstrong, 1971; French & Shoukimas, 1981). Tetraethylammonium and its
derivatives, however, like Cs$^+$ and Ba^{2+}, tend to be rather non-specific in
their block of the various myocardial K-channels, although some selectivity
is apparent in the insensitivity of the high conductance plateau K-current,
$I_{K(p)}$, to internally-applied TEA$^+$ (Yue & Marban, 1988) and in the complete block of $I_{K(ATP)}$ produced by external TEA$^+$ at concentrations having
only modest effects on other K-channels (20 mM; Arena & Kass, 1989).

Block of the delayed rectifier current by TEA$^+$ and its analogues has
been particularly well-characterized in squid axon (for a comprehensive
review, see Armstrong, 1975), and the results obtained in that preparation
provide a useful basis for a more general understanding of the molecular
aspects of K-channel block. Summarized briefly, these studies established
that: (i) TEA$^+$ blocks most effectively when added to the cytoplasm, rather
than to the bathing medium; (ii) analogues with larger hydrophobic
substituent groups are more potent blockers than TEA$^+$ itself; (iii) block
is not instantaneous, but develops with time after the channels are opened,
producing an apparent 'inactivation' of the current; and (iv) block can be
relieved by increasing the external K$^+$-concentration, as if the inward
movement of K$^+$ displaces the blocking particles from their binding sites
by a 'knock-off' mechanism. These results are consistent with a blocking
site for the quaternary ammonium compounds located within the K-
channel pore, which is accessible only from the inside of the cell and only
when the channel is open. In addition, approximate dimensions can be
placed on the internal 'antechamber' of the K-channel based on the relative
abilities of TEA$^+$ derivatives with increasingly larger head groups to block
the channel. Tetraethylammonium block is voltage-dependent, and increased
by more positive membrane potentials, as though the membrane field were
driving the molecule into the channel. However, this effect is rather small

(tetrabutylammonium (TBA^+) appears to sense only about 15% of the total membrane field), suggesting that the blocking site is located close to the internal opening of the pore. It should be noted that, whereas external TEA^+ has no effect on $I_{K(dr)}$ in squid axon, it is an effective blocker of $I_{K(dr)}$ in frog node of Ranvier (Hille, 1967) and skeletal muscle (Stanfield, 1970). Mutations in the S5–S6 linker regions of the *Shaker* H4 K-channel suggest that differences in sensitivity to external TEA^+ may be determined by the composition of specific amino acid residues at sites near the outer mouth of the channel (MacKinnon & Yellen, 1990).

External TEA^+ is a weak blocker of most myocardial K-channels, but eliminates nearly all time-dependent outward currents when applied intracellularly (Kass *et al.*, 1982). These results suggest that the mechanism of block may be similar to that described above for squid axon. Surprisingly little has been done in cardiac preparations with TEA^+ derivatives larger than TBA^+, so that comparative estimates of internal pore size and the location of the blocking site within the K-channel cannot be determined for the heart. However, TBA^+ appears to be a more potent blocker than TEA^+, consistent with the data obtained in nerve, which indicate a nearly 10-fold increase in blocking potency with TBA^+ over TEA^+ (French & Shoukimas, 1981). Block of $I_{K(dr)}$ by TEA^+ and TBA^+ occurs in squid axon within less than 5 ms, which is sufficiently fast to be beyond the resolution of most voltage-clamp studies in heart. No evidence for voltage dependence of TEA^+ block has yet been demonstrated for any myocardial K-channel.

4-Aminopyridine

4-Aminopyridine (4-AP) is a small lipid soluble molecule that has been routinely used to block K-channels in cardiac muscle (Kenyon & Gibbons, 1979a; Van Bogaert & Snyders, 1982; Shibate *et al.*, 1989). In nerve, the effects of 4-AP differ from those of TEA^+ in that 4-AP is equally effective when applied from either inside or outside the membrane. Moreover, low (μM) concentrations of 4-AP delay the activation of $I_{K(dr)}$ and produce a block that can be relieved by strong and repetitive depolarizations (Yeh *et al.*, 1976; Meves & Pichon, 1977), and it has been proposed that the reduction in block represents a voltage-dependent dissociation of 4-AP from its blocking site. In skeletal muscle, however, block by 4-AP appears as an accelerated inactivation of $I_{K(dr)}$ which depends on the channels being in an open state, and is enhanced by depolarization, suggesting differences between these two types of tissue similar to those seen with TEA^+.

In heart, low concentrations (< 0.5 mM) of 4-AP block $I_{K(to1)}$ with fairly good selectivity; however, higher concentrations (5 mM) also exert effects on I_{K1} and the pacemaker current I_f (Van Bogaert & Snyders, 1982). Effects on $I_{K(dr)}$ appear negligible. Whilst the mechanisms of 4-AP block of cardiac

K-channel have not been fully elucidated, preliminary studies on $I_{K(tol)}$ in ferret ventricular myocytes indicate a complex time- and voltage-dependent block in which 4-AP associates with a closed state of the channel at negative potentials, and which is removed upon depolarization (Campbell *et al.*, 1991).

Class I antiarrhythmic agents

The class I agents have been separated into three subclasses based on their ability to prolong, shorten or have no effect on repolarization and refractoriness (Harrison, 1985). The class Ia agents, which include quinidine, disopyramide and procainamide, tend to increase action potential duration, although some variability in this response is seen. Quinidine is perhaps the most thoroughly studied of these agents, and its effects on various ion channels have been well characterized. The tendency for quinidine to prolong repolarization has been shown to result primarily from a potent block of the delayed rectifier current (Colatsky, 1982; Hiraoka *et al.*, 1986; Furukawa *et al.*, 1989). In rabbit Purkinje fibres and in nodal cells under voltage-clamp, nearly complete block of the outward tails associated with $I_{K(dr)}$ can be seen at concentrations of quinidine that produce only a relatively modest depression of action potential upstroke velocity (Mirro *et al.*, 1981). In guinea-pig ventricular myocytes, which exhibit both fast and slow components of $I_{K(dr)}$, quinidine appears to suppress $I_{K(r)}$ preferentially (Roden *et al.*, 1988). Other myocardial K-channels are affected by quinidine as well. The inward rectifier K-channel, K_{IR}, has been reported to be unaltered by quinidine (Colatsky, 1982) or decreased in a non-specific manner (Hiraoka *et al.*, 1986; Salata & Wasserstrom, 1988). Quinidine also blocks the voltage-dependent transient outward current (Imaizumi & Giles, 1987) and the acetylcholine activated K-channel in the heart (Kurachi *et al.*, 1987).

Recent studies have confirmed block of K-channels by other class Ia agents including cibenzoline (Kotake *et al.*, 1987), disopyramide (Coraboeuf *et al.*, 1988) and pirmenol (Reichardt *et al.*, 1990). Like quinidine, disopyramide is non-specific in its K-channel blocking actions, inhibiting $I_{K(dr)}$, the voltage-dependent transient outward current ($I_{K(tol)}$ and I_{K1}), whilst initial studies suggest that pirmenol is relatively selective for $I_{K(dr)}$ (Reichardt *et al.*, 1990). In contrast, the class Ib agent lidocaine appears to have little effect on K-currents until concentrations much higher than those used clinically are examined (Colatsky, 1982; Coraboeuf *et al.*, 1988).

The failure to obtain a consistent prolongation of repolarization with potent K-channel blockers such as quinidine is due to the concomitant effects of these agents on steady-state or slowly inactivating Na- and Ca-currents supporting the plateau phase of the cardiac action potential (Colatsky, 1982; Carmeliet & Saikawa, 1982; Salata & Wasserstrom,

1988). On the other hand, the consistent shortening of action potential duration by class Ib drugs like lidocaine is related to a relative absence of K-channel blocking activity, which allows their effects on the tetrodotoxin (TTX)-sensitive Na-channels to predominate and lead to an early termination of the plateau. The absence of an effect of the class Ic agents on repolarization suggests that these compounds may possess a major component of K-channel block that balances a potent effect on the plateau Na-current (Colatsky & Follmer, 1990). This postulate has been confirmed in voltage-clamp studies on cat ventricular myocytes showing that therapeutic concentrations (1–10 μM) of flecainide can selectively inhibit $I_{K(dr)}$ without affecting I_{K1} or $I_{K(to1)}$ (Follmer & Colatsky, 1990). Similar data have also been obtained for the class Ic agent encainide (Colatsky et al., 1990), and it is likely that the 3-methoxy-O-desmethyl metabolite of encainide exhibits even greater potency as a K-channel blocker since it consistently lengthens repolarization and the QT interval in animal (Davy et al., 1986) and in human (Barbey et al., 1988) studies.

The contribution of K-channel block to the activity of class I agents is most evident and perhaps clinically important during premature stimulation. Action potentials elicited early during diastole (< 50–100 ms) tend to show a significant drug-induced prolongation, even with agents such as mexiletine which are commonly accepted to shorten repolarization during repetitive pacing at fixed diastolic intervals (Varro et al., 1985a,b; Nakaya et al., 1989). It seems reasonable to suggest that the efficacy of these agents against re-entrant arrhythmias, albeit limited, may be related to changes in repolarization time-course rather than to conduction slowing, a relationship that has been clearly established for the class Ia agents (Feld et al., 1986; Kus et al., 1990; Sheldon et al., 1990). These considerations led to the proposal of a new classification scheme in which the class I agents are grouped according to the degree of K-channel block each possesses (Colatsky & Follmer, 1990). In theory, increasing the level of K-channel block would predict increasing antiarrhythmic efficacy, while increasing potency and persistence of Na-channel block would more generally be a measure of proarrhythmic potential (Courtney, 1987).

Class III antiarrhythmic agents

By definition, class III antiarrhythmic agents lengthen repolarization without slowing intracardiac conduction, and consequently represent a logical extension of the concepts discussed above. The earliest compounds in this class were developed for indications other than the treatment of cardiac arrhythmias, and their class III effects were discovered serendipitously during clinical use. As a result, these early agents tend to possess prominent ancillary pharmacologic activities that can either complement or diminish their utility as antiarrhythmic agents. For example, amiodarone, initially used as an antianginal agent, was the first drug generally recognized as exerting relatively selective effects on repolarization. It is now well known that amiodarone blocks Ca-channels and possesses some class I and anti-adrenergic properties (Singh & Vaughan Williams, 1970a) that may underlie its marked efficacy and help reduce its proarrhythmic potential (Lazzara, 1989). Bretylium, a quaternary benzylammonium compound bearing a close resemblance to TEA^+ and its alkyl derivatives, was originally introduced as an adrenergic neuronal blocking agent for the treatment of hypertension, but was subsequently found to lengthen refractoriness and to exert antifibrillatory and antiarrhythmic actions (Baccaner, 1966; Wit et al., 1970; Gibson et al., 1983). Likewise, the antiarrhythmic effects of D,L-sotalol, developed initially as a β-blocker for the treatment of hypertension, appear to derive primarily from its ability to prolong repolarization (Singh & Vaughan Williams, 1970b).

Initial explorations into the rational development of 'pure' class III agents used the quaternary ammonium K-channel blockers as a starting point. Several permanently charged compounds including clofilium (Steinberg et al., 1984) and a series of propranolol derivatives, including pranolium (UM272: Eller et al., 1983), UM301 (Gibson et al., 1986) and UM424 (Gibson et al., 1985) were synthesized and found to have significant antiarrhythmic and antifibrillatory activity in a number of experimental models and did not produce effects on catecholamine release or adrenergic blockade. However, the oral bioavailability of these quaternary compounds was not optimal and their clinical development was curtailed.

Further insight into the development of selective class III agents came from the observation that the N-acetylated metabolite of procainamide (N-acetylprocainamide, NAPA) possessed a completely different electrophysiologic profile than its parent compounds, in that it produced a uniform prolongation of action potential duration with only limited effects on intracardiac conduction (Dangman & Hoffman, 1981). The inversion of pharmacologic activity produced by N-acetylation was exploited in the design of the class III agent sematilide (Lumma et al., 1987), which incorporated the (methylsulphonyl)amino substituent group characteristic of sotalol and most other class III agents under clinical and preclinical investigation today.

General profile of the class III agents

The basic properties shared by the class III agents are summarized in Table 12.2. Available clinical evidence suggests that the class III antiarrhythmics should be more effective than conventional class I drugs against both supraventricular and life-threatening ventricular arrhythmias, but less effective against low grade ectopy (Anderson, 1990). In addition, they should be better tolerated in patients with ventricular dysfunction, since

Table 12.2. General properties of class III antiarrhythmic agents.

Pharmacology
Prolongs repolarization and refractoriness uniformly:
increases QT and QTc intervals
no effect on intracardiac conduction
Slight improvement or no change in ventricular function
Slows heart rate
Effects may be attenuated by increases in heart rate and ischaemia

Antiarrhythmic efficacy
Ineffective in models predicting class I activity:
24–48 h Harris dog
ouabain toxicity
Prevents induction of tachyarrhythmias using programmed electrical stimulation in atrium and ventricle
Increases survival in canine sudden death models
Elevates ventricular fibrillation threshold
Can produce spontaneous defibrillation
Lowers or does not change energy requirements for electrical defibrillation

Proarrhythmic potential
May produce excessive prolongation of repolarization at long cycle lengths
Proarrhythmia diagnosed as toursade de pointes:
predictable from QT changes
suppressed by rapid pacing, catecholamines
may involve early after-depolarizations as mechanism
Exacerbated by interventions that prolong repolarization, e.g. hypokalaemia induced by use of diuretics

they do not depress myocardial contractility but may in fact exert a modest positive inotropic effect through their ability to prolong the duration of the cardiac action plateau. From the standpoint of preclinical drug discovery, the class III agents are largely ineffective in experimental arrhythmias models previously central to the selection of class I anti-arrhythmics, such as the 24–48 h Harris dog and ouabain toxicity, whereas they are extremely effective in suppressing the re-entrant ventricular tachy-cardias induced by programmed electrical stimulation and in protecting against the onset of ventricular fibrillation in models of secondary infarc-tion, both of which bear greater relevance to the arrhythmias seen clinically.

At this time, there are insufficient data, apart from potency, to distin-guish between the various K-channel blockers as antiarrhythmic drugs. Most of the agents block the delayed rectifier channel, all exhibit signifi-cant activity in critical arrhythmia models based on a selective and uniform prolongation of refractoriness, and, apart from a tendency to slow heart rate, all have negligible haemodynamic effects. A major concern, however, remains the relative safety of these agents and the availability of a reliable means of assessing their proarrhythmic potential (Jackman *et al.*, 1988; Sasyniuk *et al.*, 1989; Hondeghem & Snyders, 1990).

Table 12.3. Status of investigational class III agents.

Agent	Company	Status
D-Sotalol	Bristol-Myers-Squibb	Phase II
Sematilide	Berlex	Phase III
E4031	Eisai	Phase II
UK68,798	Pfizer	Phase III
RP 58866	Rhône-Poulenc-Rorer	Phase I
MS551	Mitsui	Phase I
Ibutilide	Upjohn	Phase I
Tedisamil	Kali-Chemie	Phase I
MDL11,939	Marion-Merrell-Dow	Preclinical
H234/09	Hässle	Phase I

A strong correlation has been noted in α-chloralose anaesthetized rabbits, between the ability of class III agents to prolong the QT interval, and the production of a toursades-like ventricular tachycardia (Carlsson et al., 1990). The generation of proarrhythmia in this study was dependent on continuous administration of the α_1-adrenoceptor agonist methoxamine, and could be prevented by the α_1-adrenoceptor antagonist prazosin. Since both α-chloralose (Schwartz & Herre, 1989) and the α-adrenoceptor agonists (Shah et al., 1988; Tohse et al., 1990) have been reported to prolong repolarization, most likely mediated through an inhibition of K-conductance, it is possible that the interactions between anaesthetics, α_1-agonists and class III agents may have introduced sufficient non-specificity in the profile of K-channel block to favour the occurrence of pause-dependent proarrhythmia (Colatsky et al., 1990).

There are currently a number of 'pure' class III agents reported to be at various stages of clinical and preclinical development (Table 12.3). These include sematilide (CK-1752) (Lumma et al., 1987; Chi et al., 1990a; Poizot et al., 1990), MDL-11,939 (Koerner & Dage, 1990; Li et al., 1990), UK68,798 (Cross et al., 1990; Tande et al., 1990; Gwilt et al., 1991; Zuanetti & Corr, 1991), E-4031 (Adaniya & Hiraoka, 1990; Katoh et al., 1990; Lynch et al., 1990; Oinuma et al., 1990), RP 58866 (Mestre et al., 1990), U70226E (Cimini & Gibson, 1990; Buchanan et al., 1990; Lee et al., 1990), MS551 (Ishii et al., 1990; Kamiya et al., 1990), tedisamil (KC8857) (Dukes & Morad, 1989; Beatch et al., 1990; Dukes et al., 1990; Tsuchi-hashi & Curtis, 1990), and H234/09 (Duker & Almgren, 1990). In addition, several compounds have entered clinical trials and been with-drawn for reasons of clinical toxicity, e.g. UK66,914 (Gwilt et al., 1988) and risotilide (WY48,986) (Colatsky et al., 1989; Follmer et al., 1989; Rials et al., 1990) or limited bioavailability (e.g., clofilium). In the discussion below, emphasis will be placed on the newer agents currently advancing through clinical trial (UK68,798, sematilide, E4031), and on agents reputed to have novel mechanisms of action (ibutilide, tedisamil).

UK68,798

The most potent synthetic class III agent described to date is UK68,798, which prolongs cardiac action potential duration at concentrations below 5 nM (Gwilt et al., 1991). Studied in vitro, Purkinje fibres appear to be more sensitive to UK68,798 (EC_{50} = 5.3 nM) than ventricular muscle (EC_{50} = 30 nM). In anaesthetized dogs, lengthening of both atrial and ventricular refractory periods began at doses of 3 μg/kg, i.v., with increases of 63% and 30% in atrium and ventricle, respectively, noted at the maximal dose studied, 100 μg/kg, i.v. (Gwilt et al., 1989; Cross et al., 1990). Antiarrhythmic efficacy was initially determined using measurements of ventricular fibrillation threshold in anaesthetized dogs, in which UK68,798 produced a more or less linear dose-dependent increase after administration of 3 (+74%)–100 (+683%) μg/kg, i.v. (Gwilt et al., 1989). During the course of this study, an impressive spontaneous termination of fibrillation and return to sinus rhythm were frequently observed following treatment. In dogs with healed myocardial infarction subjected to programmed electrical stimulation, UK68,798 (30 μg/kg, i.v.) prevented arrhythmia induction in six of seven dogs with sustained ventricular tachycardia, but, somewhat surprisingly, did not suppress ventricular fibrillation in any of the four animals in which this was the only arrhythmia induced during control testing (Zuanetti & Corr, 1991). Mapping studies indicated that the ventricular fibrillation induced in these animals was the result of a rapid non-re-entrant or focal mechanism, and consequently would be expected to be relatively insensitive to the increase in refractory period produced by the drug. The bearing of these latter findings on the potential of UK68,798 to prevent sudden death in the clinical situation remains to be established.

Reports of early clinical studies with UK68,798 have been published. Oral bioavailability in humans is 100%, which is somewhat greater than the estimate of 72% obtained in dogs (Cross et al., 1990). Dose-dependent increases in QT interval of 36 ms (9%), 52 ms (13%) and 83 ms (22%) were observed in 18 patients following 1.5, 3.0 and 4.5 μg/kg UK68,798 given i.v., with no changes in QRS duration or other adverse effects noted (Sedgwick et al., 1990, 1991). These doses produced peak plasma levels ranging from 1.74 to 5.11 ng/ml, which decayed with a mean elimination half-life of 8.7 h, which is slightly greater than that observed in dogs (4–6 h; Cross et al., 1990). Dosing with UK68,798 (0.25 mg/kg, b.i.d.) for 5 days did not have any significant effect on the pharmacokinetics of digoxin or its effects on the electrocardiogram (Rasmussen et al., 1990). No information is yet available on the metabolism of UK68,798 after oral dosing, or on its safety and antiarrhythmic efficacy in humans.

Sematilide (CK1752)

Sematilide is the most senior of the rationally-designed class III agents currently in clinical trials. *In vitro*, sematilide is 17-fold less potent than clofilium and sixfold more potent than sotalol in its ability to prolong Purkinje fibre action potential duration (Lumma *et al.*, 1987; Lumma, 1989). Intravenous administration at doses of 0.3–3.0 mg/kg increased both atrial (15–50%) and ventricular (4–18%) refractory periods with only modest haemodynamic changes. Sematilide was effective in preventing induction of sustained ventricular tachycardia in eight out of eight conscious dogs with 3–8 day-old healed infarctions at a mean oral dose of 2.5 mg/kg. In addition, sematilide prevented the occurrence of ventricular fibrillation in dogs subjected to an acute ischaemic event superimposed on a prior myocardial infarction (Chi *et al.*, 1990a). Preliminary results suggest that, unlike sotalol, the ability of sematilide to prolong repolarization is preserved under conditions of simulated ischaemia *in vitro* (Poizot *et al.*, 1990). In humans, sematilide is rapidly cleared after a single i.v. bolus ($t_{1/2} = 4$ h) but shows prolonged clearance after repeated oral dosing (50–200 mg every 8 h), which is characterized by a predominant β-phase (5 h) and a γ-phase (13 h), giving rise to variable peak/trough concentration ratios ranging from 1 to 4 within each dosing interval (Wong *et al.*, 1990). Induction of sustained ventricular tachycardia was prevented by sematilide (225–450 mg/day) in six of 19 patients (31%) subjected to programmed stimulation (Nademanee *et al.*, 1990). These effects were associated with a significant prolongation of monophasic action potential duration (+ 48 ms), ventricular refractory period (+ 20 ms) and paced QT interval (58 ms) with no effect on any parameters of intracardiac conduction. In initial clinical studies in patients with chronic non-sustained ventricular arrhythmias, sematilide produced a 25% increase in QTc at 1.7 µg/ml after i.v. administration (Wong *et al.*, 1989). One patient given 1 mg/kg exhibited a marked prolongation of the corrected QT interval (> 100 ms) and developed an increase in arrhythmia frequency marked by 5 beat runs of polymorphic tachycardia.

E4031

The ability of E4031 to block $I_{K(dr)}$ selectively has been well characterized in ventricular myocytes from guinea-pig ($IC_{50} = 397$ nM: Sanguinetti & Jurkiewicz, 1990a) and cat (Follmer & Colatsky, 1990), and its specificity for $I_{K(r)}$ has become a basis for distinguishing the presence of two delayed rectifier subtypes in different cells (Colatsky *et al.*, 1990; Sanguinetti &

Jurkiewicz, 1991). E4031 prolongs cardiac action potential duration at concentrations as low as 100 nM. In animal studies, E4031 (30–300 µg/kg, i.v.) prevented the induction of sustained ventricular tachycardia in seven of 10 dogs subjected to programmed electrical stimulation, and suppressed ventricular fibrillation in a canine reinfarction model of sudden death (Lynch et al., 1990; Chi et al., 1991). Refractory periods were prolonged by E4031 in both normal and infarcted zones (Katoh et al., 1990; Lynch et al., 1990). Administration of E4031 at 0.03–3.0 mg/kg, i.v. neither suppressed nor aggravated spontaneous ecotopic activity studied 48 h after myocardial infarction (Lynch et al., 1990). In other studies, E4031 protected heart mitochondria from the effects of ischaemia and prevented the leakage of lysosomal enzymes, as did amiodarone and sotalol (Sano et al., 1990), suggesting a possible additional mechanism of action for the class III agents. In rabbit isolated atrial preparations, E4031 (0.1 and 1.0 µM) increased atrial and arteriovenous nodal refractory periods, and prevented induction of re-entrant tachyarrhythmias by premature stimulation (Adaniya & Hiraoka, 1990). It has been suggested that E4031 may exert part of its antiarrhythmic effects via block of the K_{ATP}-channel (Chi et al., 1990b); however, this has not been confirmed in patch-clamp studies in cat ventricular myocytes (I. Moubarak & W. Spinelli, personal communication). E4031 is orally active, with a bioavailability in dogs of 56–79% and a final elimination half-life of 1.3–2.9 h (Oinuma et al., 1990). Although this compound is reported to be in phase II trials in Japan and Europe, no clinical data have yet been published.

Ibutilide (U7022E)

Ibutilide is a recently-disclosed class III agent resembling sotalol in its chemical structure. In contrast to the other class III antiarrhythmics, ibutilide has been reputed to act by a completely novel mechanism that involves the activation of a slow inward Na-current at subnanomolar concentrations, and the activation of an outward K-current at concentrations 100-fold higher (Lee et al., 1990). As a consequence of this dual mechanism of action, action potential duration is prolonged at lower concentrations, but shortened at higher concentrations, producing a bell-shaped dose–response curve. Sodium-channel activation, brought about by the removal of the normal fast inactivation process, has also been described for the novel cardiotonic agent DPI201,106 (Kohlhardt et al., 1986) and underlies its class III effects on repolarization (Scholtysik et al., 1985). In isolated rabbit ventricular muscle, ibutilide increased the effective refractory period by 12% at 1 µM and 18% at 10 µM, with frequency-dependent increases in conduction time evident at 10 µM (15–31%) but not 1 µM, suggesting that ibutilide, like sotalol, may block excitatory Na-channels at higher concentrations (Cimini & Gibson, 1990). Ibutilide

(0.03–0.3 mg/kg, i.v.) increased ventricular refractory period and mono-phasic action potential duration, and prevented programmed stimulation-induced sustained ventricular tachycardia without effects on spontaneous ectopy in anaesthetized dogs studied 24 h after myocardial infarction (Buchanan *et al.*, 1990).

Tedisamil (KC8857)

Tedisamil is a heterocyclic compound related to sparteine that exerts class III effects by blocking and speeding the inactivation of the transient outward current (Dukes & Morad, 1989; Dukes *et al.*, 1990). Its anti-arrhythmic efficacy has primarily been demonstrated in the rat, in which it has been shown to protect against ischaemia and reperfusion-induced ventricular fibrillation (Walker & Beatch, 1988; Tsuchihashi & Curtis, 1990). In rat ventricular muscle, which lacks a delayed rectifier current, tedisamil (1–20 μM) prolonged action potential duration by blocking $I_{K(to1)}$ with an IC_{50} of about 6 μM (Dukes & Morad, 1989). The effects on $I_{K(to1)}$ were both voltage- and rate-independent. Tedisamil was slightly more potent at blocking $I_{K(dr)}$ in guinea-pig ventricular myocytes (IC_{50} = 2.5 μM), and at 10 μM completely inhibited the time-dependent outward currents flowing during depolarization, as well as the tail currents seen upon return to the holding potential (Dukes *et al.*, 1990). These results are intriguing, since they suggest that tedisamil, unlike E4031 and many other class III agents, does not discriminate very well between $I_{K(r)}$ and $I_{K(s)}$, the components of $I_{K(dr)}$. No effect on I_{K1} or Ca-current was noted up to 50 μM, although concentrations greater than 20 μM produced an inhibition of the excitatory Na-current (Dukes *et al.*, 1990).

The therapeutic advantages offered by blocking the voltage-dependent transient outward current as a mechanism of class III action can be argued. Characterization of this current in a variety of cardiac prepara-tions indicates that it possesses a very long time constant of recovery from reactivation (100–500 ms; Tseng & Hoffman, 1989), so that its contribu-tion to the action potential should be minimal at short cycle lengths, and increase as cycle length is prolonged. Thus, in the absence of a unique voltage dependence like that recently reported for 4-AP block (Campbell *et al.*, 1991), one might anticipate a greater liability for excessive prolonga-tion of repolarization and the generation of new pause-dependent arrhyth-mias for agents that work by this mechanism. However, several studies suggest that $I_{K(to1)}$ is the predominant outward repolarizing current in the atrium (Imaizumi & Giles, 1987), and consequently, selective inhibition of this current may provide some specificity for the treatment of supraven-tricular arrhythmias. Demonstration of the ultimate utility of any of these approaches will clearly need to await more extensive clinical evaluation.

Molecular mechanisms of K-channel block

While voltage-clamp data are not yet available for all of the compounds under investigation, it appears that most of the currently available class III agents show good selectivity for the delayed rectifier current $I_{K(dr)}$ (Colatsky et al., 1990), in particular the rapidly activating component $I_{K(r)}$ (Sanguinetti & Jurkiewicz, 1990a). A notable exception is tedisamil, which blocks the transient outward current in addition to its effects on $I_{K(dr)}$ (Dukes & Morad, 1989; Dukes et al., 1990). D,L-sotalol has been shown to block delayed rectifier current, $I_{K(dr)}$, at concentrations producing little or no effect on I_{K1} and the excitatory Na-channel, although these additional effects may become apparent at higher drug concentrations (Carmeliet, 1985). The effects of sotalol on both action potential duration and $I_{K(dr)}$ appear to reside equally in both D- and L-isomers, indicating that stereochemical factors are relatively unimportant in the interactions between sotalol and the K-channel. This is in direct contrast to the class I agents quinidine and disopyramide, both of which show stereoselective effects on repolarization in the heart (Mirro et al., 1981).

Some selectivity for the delayed rectifier channel has been found for clofilium, a quaternary compound. When applied externally for brief exposures ($< 15\,min$), clofilium markedly depresses $I_{K(dr)}$ but has little effect on I_{K1} (Arena & Kass, 1988). Interestingly, this apparent selectivity for $I_{K(dr)}$ over I_{K1} is lost when tertiary analogues of clofilium (LY-97241 and LY-97119) are examined, since both of these compounds appear to block $I_{K(dr)}$ and I_{K1} equally well. The ability of the tertiary analogues, but not clofilium, to inhibit I_{K1} suggests the possible importance of lipid phase drug-channel interactions in producing I_{K1} block. However, neither clofilium nor its analogues was effective when introduced inside the cell by dialysis, suggesting an external site of action for these compounds. Among the newer agents, specificity of $I_{K(dr)}$ block has been clearly established for E4031 (Follmer & Colatsky, 1990; Sanguinetti & Jurkiewicz, 1990a), risotilide (Follmer et al., 1989), and UK68,798 (Gwilt et al., 1991). Sematilide appears to block both $I_{K(dr)}$ and I_{K1} (Lumma, 1989), while RP 58866 is reported to be a specific blocker of I_{K1} (Escande et al., 1989).

Unlike the situation with local anaesthetic and class I antiarrhythmic block of the excitatory Na-channel, there is little direct information currently available about the site and mechanism by which the K-channel blockers exert their effects on the heart. The studies in nerve and skeletal muscle described above for TEA^+ and the inorganic cations indicate that multiple blocking sites can exist, and that their location and properties may vary from tissue to tissue. While the smaller inorganic K-channel blockers like Ba^{2+} and Cs^+ are equally effective when applied internally or externally, TEA^+ appears to require internal application to block most myocardial K-channels. Where block by external TEA^+ is observed, it tends to be weak and better achieved with internal application. No information exists about the voltage dependence of TEA$^+$ block, but by analogy with data obtained in squid axon, one would expect that block by internal TEA$^+$ would be enhanced by depolarization and removed by repolarization. Block of $I_{K(dr)}$ in squid axon occurs within 5 ms, which is sufficiently fast to be beyond the resolution of most voltage-clamp studies in heart. Preliminary data on 4-AP block of $I_{K(to1)}$ support an external site of action for this agent, and a voltage dependence opposite to that predicted for TEA$^+$, i.e. relief of block by depolarization (Campbell et al., 1991).

Quinidine block of $I_{K(dr)}$ in nodal cells has been shown to exhibit a voltage dependence similar to that proposed for the Na-channel blockers (Furukawa et al., 1989), in that: (i) block appears to require open channels, since voltage-clamp depolarizations to membrane potentials below the activation range of $I_{K(dr)}$ produce little or no block; (ii) both the level and rate of quinidine block are increased as membrane potential is made more positive; and (iii) repolarization leads to release of the drug from its binding site, leading to channel unblocking as evidenced by the slowing of the $I_{K(dr)}$ tail current time-course. Additionally, the $I_{K(dr)}$ activation curve is shifted toward more negative potentials with a steepening in slope, consistent with voltage-dependent drug binding to the delayed rectifier channel. These actions of quinidine are well-fitted by a simplified version of the modulated receptor model (Hondeghem & Katzung, 1977) that postulates steeply voltage-dependent time constants for block of open delayed rectifier channels ranging from 300 ms at -30 mV to 50 ms at 0 mV. This type of drug-channel interaction has been recently confirmed in cat ventricular myocytes using the class Ic agents flecainide and encainide (Colatsky et al., 1990). Discrepancies between these results and results obtained in guinea-pig ventricular myocytes, in which quinidine block exhibits a 'reverse use-dependence' (Roden et al., 1988; Hondeghem & Snyders, 1990) can be explained by recent studies using the class III agent E4031. These established that the delayed rectifier current $I_{K(dr)}$ consists of two components, $I_{K(r)}$ and $I_{K(s)}$, only one of which ($I_{K(r)}$) is blocked by drug (Sanguinetti & Jurkiewicz, 1990a).

Why do K-channel blockers slow the heart rate?

The bradycardic properties of the class III agents appear to derive directly from their ability to block K-channels, rather than from any ancillary β-adrenoceptor antagonism, as was initially believed for D,L-sotalol and amiodarone. The cellular basis for this effect has not yet been clearly defined, although several mechanisms have been proposed. The most simple explanation is that these agents prolong the duration of the sinus node action potential. Increasing sinus node action potential duration would, by itself, slow heart rate in the absence of any change in pacemaker potential, since it would increase sinus node cycle length. For example it has been shown in isolated guinea-pig sinus node preparations that increases in sinus node action potential duration can account for nearly all of the slowing of spontaneous rate produced by D,L- and D-sotalol (Campbell, 1987a), with changes in the pacemaker potential becoming prominent only at high drug concentrations. Similarly, the tendency for class I antiarrhythmic agents to slow spontaneous rate in the same species appears to correlate with the relative ability of these drugs to prolong sinus node action potential duration (Campbell, 1987b), although some compounds within the class IB subcategory also tend to inhibit the pacemaker potential as well. The ability of these agents to prolong the duration of the sinus node action potential closely parallels their ability to block myocardial K-channels.

An alternative mechanism that may also play a role in producing bradycardia is a modulation of the pacemaker potential itself. Although the hyperpolarization-activated inward current I_f* has been characterized as the principal current underlying phase 4 depolarization in pacemaker tissue (van Ginneken & Giles, 1991), deactivation of K-channels upon repolarization may also contribute to the pacemaker potential. As characterized in embryonic chick atrial cells, which are spontaneously active in culture, the decay of the delayed rectifier current $I_{K(dr)}$ can account for the initial phase of the pacemaker depolarization (Clay et al., 1988). A similar mechanism may also be relevant in the mammalian sinus node. Nishimura et al. (1990) found that the class III antiarrhythmic E-4031 suppressed automaticity in rabbit sinus nodal cells by blocking $I_{K(dr)}$ tails in a voltage-dependent fashion. Moreover, Furukawa et al. (1989) suggest that unblocking of the delayed rectifier channel by quinidine at diastolic potentials would further depress the pacemaker potential, by permitting the additional hyperpolarizing current to flow during diastole through recovered (i.e. unblocked) $I_{K(dr)}$-channels.

Some agents with K-channel blocking properties (e.g. tedisamil) are currently under development as 'specific bradycardic agents', with possible utility as antianginal agents. However, K-channel block does not appear to be an exclusive approach, since a number of other compounds with different mechanisms of action also produce similar therapeutic benefits. For example, zatabradine (UL-FS 49), which is chemically related to the Ca-channel blockers verapamil and AQ-A39, exerts its bradycardic effect through a potent voltage- and frequency-dependent block of the L-type Ca-current in nodal cells (Doerr & Trautwein, 1990).

---

*The current I_f is a mixed cation current carried by both Na^+ and K^+ through a so-called non-selective cation channel.

Structure–activity relations for K-channel blockade

Despite the growing sophistication in our understanding of the molecular basis for class III antiarrhythmic activity as manifested through specific block of myocardial K-channels, rarely is screening performed at the level of macroscopic currents in isolated cardiac cells. The objective of most new drug discoveries in this area is an increase in repolarization time with no change in conduction time. These endpoints are usually determined in an initial *in vitro* screen, using measurements of action potential duration or effective refractory period in isolated tissue, followed by *in vivo* tests using changes in the electrocardiogram (QT interval, QRS duration) or in atrial and ventricular refractory periods as indices of class III activity. Given this gross empirical starting point, the ability to synthesize compounds as potent and specific as UK68,798 in blocking the delayed rectifier K-channel seems an extraordinary feat (Cross *et al.*, 1990).

Figure 12.1 illustrates the basic pharmacophore required for class III activity mediated by selective block of $I_{K(dr)}$. The importance of the methanesulphonamide (CH_3SO_2NH-) group was recognized early on (Lumma *et al.*, 1987) and a clear advantage in potency and efficacy is seen when this substituent is placed in the para position on the aryl ring. Whilst some electron-withdrawing groups (e.g. NO_2) also impart class III activity when substituted at this position (Colatsky & Follmer, 1990; Kamiya *et al.*, 1990), substitution within the methanesulphonamide group itself at the C or N tends to abolish activity (Lumma *et al.*, 1987). The atom or group linking the aryl ring to the basic N appears to be less critical, and a variety of substituents have yielded active agents with good potency. Favourable connector groups include alcohol (sotalol, ibutilide), ether (UK68,798), sulphonamide (risotilide), carbamide (sematilide), and carbonyl (E4031), which may be separated from the basic nitrogen by 1, 2 or 3 methylene groups. While class III activity is present in both secondary and tertiary amine analogues, a variety of cyclic and heterocyclic modifications of the basic amine have also yielded active compounds. MDL11,939 contains an unsubstituted aryl ring, but otherwise resembles the other compounds in this series. In contrast, tedisamil, a sparteine derivative, and the benzopyran RP 58866 are chemically distinct from the above agents, and accordingly display different K^+-channel blocking effects. Tedisamil blocks both $I_{K(dr)}$ and $I_{K(to1)}$, whilst RP 58866 is reported to be a selective blocker of I_{K1}.

Activators and blockers of the myocardial K$_{ATP}$-channel

Cardioprotective effects of the K-channel openers

A number of compounds have been reported to open myocardial K-channels, including nicorandil (Kakei *et al.*, 1986; Habuchi, *et al.*, 1987;

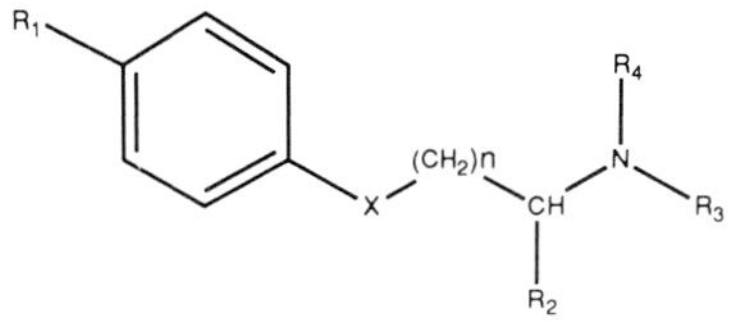

COMPOUND	R$_1$	X	n	R$_2$	R$_3$	R$_4$
Sotalol	CH$_3$SO$_2$NH-	OH $\mid$ -CH-	-	H	H	-CH(CH$_2$)$_3$
Sematilide	CH$_3$SO$_2$NH-	O $\parallel$ -CNH-	1	H	C$_2$H$_5$	-C$_2$H$_5$
Risotilide	CH$_3$SO$_2$NH-	O $\parallel$ -SNCH(CH$_3$)$_2$- $\parallel$ O	1	H	H	-CH(CH$_3$)$_2$
Ibutilide	CH$_3$SO$_2$NH-	OH $\mid$ -CH-	2	H	C$_2$H$_5$	C$_7$H$_{15}$
UK-68,798	CH$_3$SO$_2$NH-	- O -	1	H	CH$_3$	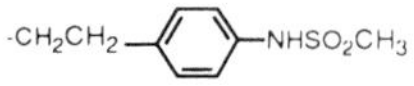 -CH$_2$CH$_2$— ⬡ —NHSO$_2$CH$_3$
E-4031	CH$_3$SO$_2$NH-	O $\parallel$ -C-	-	(4-piperidyl)		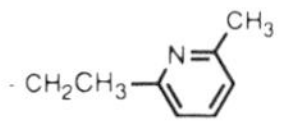 -CH$_2$CH$_3$— (pyridyl-CH$_3$)
MS-551	NO$_2$-	-	2	H	CH$_2$CH$_2$OH	-CH$_2$CH$_2$NH— (dimethyl-pyrimidinedione)
MDL-11,939	H	OH $\mid$ CH	-	(4-piperidyl)		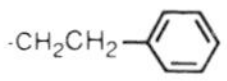 -CH$_2$CH$_2$— ⬡

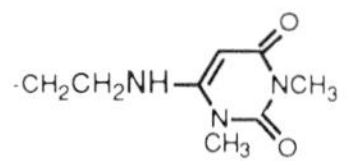

Fig. 12.1. Basic pharmacophore required for class III activity mediated by block of myocardial K-channels.

Hiraoka & Fan, 1989; Takano & Noma, 1990), pinacidil (Steinberg *et al.*, 1988, 1991; Arena & Kass, 1989; Fan *et al.*, 1990; Tseng & Hoffman, 1990), cromakalim (Escande *et al.*, 1988; Osterreider, 1988; Sanguinetti *et al.*, 1988; Bril & Man, 1990), and the newer agents RP 49356 (Thuringer & Escande, 1989; Ripoll *et al.*, 1990) and SR 44866 (Faivre & Findlay, 1990). The current activated by these agents can be blocked by low concentrations of the sulphonylurea compounds glyburide (= glibenclamide) and tolbutamide, suggesting that the channel opened is the ATP-sensitive channel (K$_{ATP}$). The effect of these drugs is to shorten the duration of the cardiac action potential without altering upstroke velocity.

Antiarrhythmic activity

Decreases in action potential duration are generally considered to be arrhythmogenic. However, a number of investigators have found that K-channel openers may in fact exert antiarrhythmic and cardioprotective effects in various experimental models, particularly when cells are abnormally depolarized or exhibit excessive prolongation as occurs in subendocardial Purkinje fibres surviving in regions of infarction (Friedman *et al.*, 1973; Bril & Man, 1990). Cromakalim was found to suppress spontaneous activity in isolated cardiac Purkinje fibres, and to antagonize positive chronotropic responses induced by norepinephrine, Ba^{2+} and strophanthidin (Liu *et al.*, 1988). In addition, oscillatory activity at both high (negative) and low (depolarized) membrane potentials was suppressed by this agent. Consistent with these data is the observation that pinacidil was able to suppress the arrhythmias present in 24 h Harris dogs (Kerr *et al.*, 1985). A clinical report of the effects of glibenclamide (10 mg in two divided doses) on ventricular arrhythmias in non-insulin-dependent diabetics indicates significant reductions in the frequency of ectopic beats and episodes of non-sustained ventricular tachycardia (Cacciapuoti *et al.*, 1991). These data suggest a possible beneficial role for K-channel openers in the treatment of certain cardiac arrhythmias.

Anti-ischaemic activity

In addition to their electrophysiological effects, the K-channel openers have also been shown to exert direct anti-ischaemic effects in the heart and to reduce infarct size. In anaesthetized open chest dogs, nicorandil reduced infarct size by 31% when administered 15 min after occlusion of the left anterior descending coronary artery (Endo *et al.*, 1988). However, this cardioprotective effect occurred in association with large falls in arterial blood pressure, total peripheral resistance and rate–pressure product, suggesting that the reduction in infarct size may have resulted, at least in part, from a decrease in myocardial oxygen demand. The incidence of ventricular fibrillation, however, was similar in both control and nicorandil-treated groups. Similar beneficial effects were obtained following ligation of the left circumflex artery in dogs treated with cromakalim (Grover *et al.*, 1990). In this study, cromakalim also reduced the incidence of fibrillation and the number of ectopic beats, with no effect on haemodynamic status. Both cromakalim and pinacidil reduced infarct size and improved the recovery of ventricular function following global ischaemia in isolated perfused rat heart preparations (Grover *et al.*, 1989, 1990). However, in contrast to the antiarrhythmic effects observed in the anaesthetized dog study, a profibrillatory effect was seen in the rat, as evidenced by a doubling of the incidence of fibrillation in the presence of cromakalim. Nicorandil was found to limit infarct size in the dog and to enhance the recovery of contractile function following reperfusion (Gross *et al.*, 1989). Of particular note in this study was the ability of nicorandil to inhibit superoxide production by neutrophils, which, along with favourable changes in haemodynamics and coronary blood flow, could contribute to the preservation of the ischaemic reperfused myocardium.

Proarrhythmic effects of the K-channel openers

There are additional data suggesting that K-channel openers may exert proarrhythmic effects under various conditions. *In vitro*, concentrations of pinacidil of 30 μM and greater cause spontaneous action potentials in 20% of the Purkinje fibre preparations studied (Steinberg *et al.*, 1988). The close coupling of these observed extra beats to the previously driven action potential, and the sensitivity of the arrhythmia to termination by an appropriately timed extrastimulus suggested that it was produced by a re-entrant mechanism. In isolated perfused rat hearts, both pinacidil and cromakalim increased the rate of ventricular tachycardia elicited by 30 min of low flow ischaemia and quickened the onset of fibrillation (Wolleben *et al.*, 1989; Grover *et al.*, 1990).

Proarrhythmic ventricular responses have also been reported in several studies in intact animals. Atrial arrhythmias (repetitive atrial responses or runs of atrial tachycardia) were occasionally seen in open-chest pentobarbital anaesthetized dogs following administration of cromakalim (three of five animals at 0.25–0.50 mg/kg, i.v.) or pinacidil (one of five animals at 1.0–2.0 mg/kg, i.v.), but only at doses producing a marked (40–50%) reduction in systemic blood pressure (Spinelli *et al.*, 1990). These arrhythmias were usually associated with rapid pacing (basic cycle length, 300 ms), but could also occur spontaneously. While no ventricular arrhythmias occurred in the above study, these have been induced in animals with prior myocardial infarction. It has been reported (Chi *et al.*, 1990c) that pinacidil (3 mg/kg, i.v.) significantly reduced ventricular refractory periods and increased mortality in a conscious dog model of sudden cardiac death. Changes in the electrocardiogram (T-wave inversion or flattening) consistent with effects on ventricular repolarization time-course have been observed in some patients treated with minoxidil (Hall *et al.*, 1980) and pinacidil (Goldberg, 1988). However, the relevance of these studies to the clinical situation must be carefully evaluated, since no clear cases of arrhythmia aggravation have been documented for any of the K-channel openers tested to date. Nevertheless, the potential proarrhythmic, as well as antiarrhythmic, activities of this new family of compounds appear to warrant further consideration.

Blockers of K_{ATP}

As indicated above, K_{ATP}, like other K-channels in excitable cells, can be blocked by Cs^+, Ba^{2+} and TEA^+ (Arena & Kass, 1989), although its sensitivity to external TEA^+ is greater than other K-channels. The channel is also blocked non-specifically by several antiarrhythmic drugs, including quinidine, verapamil and amiodarone (Haworth et al., 1989), as well as by the α-adrenoceptor antagonist phentolamine and several structurally-related compounds, including alinidine, tramazoline and naphazoline (McPherson & Angus, 1989). In the latter case, block is unrelated to α-adrenoceptor antagonism since clonidine, prazosin and phenoxybenzamine were inactive.

In contrast to the low potency and lack of specificity of the agents noted above, the effects of the K-channel openers on the cardiac action potential and cardiac membrane currents can be antagonized by low concentrations of glibenclamide and other sulphonylureas, which are considered to be highly specific inhibitors of K_{ATP}. These compounds bind with high affinity to sites in guinea-pig heart microsomes with the rank potency of glibenclamide ($K_d = 2.5\,nM$) > glisoxepide ($K_d = 40\,nM$) > glibornuride ($K_d = 2500\,nM$) > tolbutamide ($K_d = 15\,000\,nM$) (Fosset et al., 1988), which is similar to the order seen in insulin-secreting cells.

When ventricular muscle is exposed to hypoxic conditions or metabolic inhibition, there is a marked decrease in action potential duration that is accompanied by an increase in time-independent outward current and a linearization of the steady-state current–voltage relation (Vleugels et al., 1980; Conrad et al., 1983). In response to the increase in K-conductance, K^+ leave the myocardial cells and accumulate in the extracellular space, producing further abnormalities in conduction and repolarization that tend to destabilize the heart and promote serious arrhythmias. It had been suggested previously that the increase in outward current and consequent loss of K^+ from the cells was due to changes in the properties of the background K-current I_{K1}, but recent studies have implicated the activation of K_{ATP} in these effects.

Initial in vitro studies established that the shortening of action potential duration and effective refractory period induced by hypoxia could be effectively reversed by 0.03–10.0 μM glibenclamide (Sanguinetti et al., 1988). In isolated perfused rat hearts rendered globally ichaemic, glibenclamide (10 μM) exerted potent antifibrillatory effects and reduced the rate of K^+ loss from the tissue (Kantor et al., 1990). Similar results were obtained in hearts from rat, rabbit and guinea-pig in which extracellular K^+ accumulation during metabolic inhibition or hypoxia was measured directly using ion sensitive electrodes (Wilde et al., 1990). Glibenclamide also prevents the increased incidence of ventricular fibrillation produced by cromakalim, but worsened the recovery of contractile function post-ischaemia (Grover et al., 1989) and has been found to lack intrinsic anti-fibrillatory activity in another study (Adams et al., 1990).

Glibenclamide (0.15 mg/kg, i.v.) also reduced myocardial K^+ efflux in anaesthetized dogs subjected to brief (10 min) repeated occlusions of the left anterior descending coronary artery, and reduced the severity of the ischaemia-induced conduction delays (Bekheit *et al.*, 1990). The plasma levels of glibenclamide reached (500 ng/ml) caused a significant reduction in plasma glucose levels, from 110 to 72–76 mg/dl. In rabbits, glibenclamide (0.3–3.0 mg/kg, i.v.) did not alter the time-course of repolarization at baseline, but prevented the reductions in monophasic action potential duration induced by ischaemia (Smallwood *et al.*, 1990). Ventricular effective refractory period was increased by glibenclamide (0.5 mg/kg, i.v.) in anaesthetized dogs, although the magnitude of this change (5%) was not impressive. Glibenclamide reversed the increase in ventricular fibrillation threshold produced by ischaemia (Smallwood *et al.*, 1990). Overall, these data support the ability of glibenclamide to antagonize the effects of acute ischaemia on cardiac conduction and arrhythmias, although it may compromise a protective effect of K-channel activation and decreased action potential duration on contractility and its recovery following reperfusion.

Conclusions

The ability to modulate K-channel activity as a means of preventing cardiac arrhythmias and protecting the ischaemic myocardium represents an exciting new approach to a therapeutic area that has been plagued by agents with modest efficacy and patient tolerability. The incentive provided by CAST to explore new avenues of drug discovery, and a better understanding of arrhythmogenesis and drug action has led to an intense effort to develop rationally-designed antiarrhythmic agents directed at specific membrane targets. Clearly, research in this area remains at a relatively early stage and numerous questions concerning mechanism of action, safety and efficacy will need to be addressed in order to establish the ultimate viability of these approaches.

References

Adams, D., Crome, R., Lad, N. & Manning, A. S. (1990) Failure of the ATP-dependent K$^+$ channel inhibitor, glibenclamide, to reduce reperfusion-induced or ischaemic arrhythmias in rat hearts. *British Journal of Pharmacology* **100**, 438P.

Adaniya, A. & Hiraoka, M. (1990) Effects of a novel class III antiarrhythmic agent, E-4031, on reentrant tachycardias in rabbit right atrium. *Journal of Cardiovascular Pharmacology* **15**, 976–982.

Agus, Z. S., Dukes, I. D. & Morad, M. (1989) Divalent cations modulate transient outward current in isolated rat ventricular myocytes. *Journal of Physiology* **418**, 28P.

Anderson, J. L. (1990) Clinical implications of new studies in the treatment of benign, potentially malignant and malignant ventricular arrhythmias. *American Journal of Cardiology* **65**, 36B–42B.

Arena, J. P. & Kass, R. S. (1988) Block of heart potassium channels by clofilium and its tertiary analogs: relationship between drug structure and type of channel blocked. *Molecular Pharmacology* **34**, 60–66.

Arena, J. P. & Kass, R. S. (1989) Enhancement of potassium sensitive current in heart cells by pinacidil: evidence for modulation of the ATP-sensitive potassium channel. *Circulation Research* **65**, 436–445.

Armstrong, C. M. (1971) Interaction of tetraethylammonium ion derivatives with the potassium channels of giant axons. *Journal of General Physiology* **58**, 413–437.

Armstrong, C. M. (1975) Ionic pores, gates, and gating currents. *Quarterly Review of Biophysics* **7**, 179–210.

Armstrong, C. M., Swenson, R. P. Jr & Taylor, S. R. (1982) Block of squid axon K channels by internally and externally applied barium ions. *Journal of General Physiology* **80**, 663–682.

Armstrong, C. M. & Taylor, S. R. (1980) Interaction of barium with potassium channels in squid giant axons. *Biophysical Journal* **30**, 473–488.

Arrowsmith, J. E. & Cross, P. E. (1989) Antiarrhythmic agents. *Annual Reports in Medicinal Chemistry* **25**, 79–88.

Baccaner, M. B. (1966) Bretylium tosylate for the suppression of induced ventricular fibrillation. *American Journal of Cardiology* **17**, 528–534.

Balser, J. R. & Roden, D. M. (1988) Lanthanum-sensitive current contaminates I_K in guinea pig ventricular myocytes. *Biophysical Journal* **53**, 642a.

Barbey, J. T., Thompson, K. A., Echt, D. S., Woosley, R. L. & Roden, D. M. (1988) Antiarrhythmic activity, electrocardiographic effects and pharmacokinetics of the encainide metabolites O-desmethyl encainide and 3-methoxy-O-desmethyl encainide in man. *Circulation* **77**, 380–391.

Beatch, G. N., MacLeod, B. A., Abraham, S. & Walker, M. J. A. (1990) The *in vivo* electrophysiological actions of the new potassium channel blockers, tedisamil and UK 68,798. *Proceedings of the Western Pharmacology Society* **33**, 5–8.

Bekheit, S-S., Restivo, M., Boutjdir, M., Henkins, R., Gooyandeh, K., Assadi, M., Khatob, S., Gough, W. B. & El-Sherif, N. (1990) Effects of glyburide on ischemia-induced changes in extracellular potassium and local myocardial activation: a potential new approach to the management of ischemia-induced malignant ventricular arrhythmias. *American Heart Journal* **119**, 1025–1033.

Bril, A. & Man, R. Y. K. (1990) Effects of the potassium channel activator, BRL 34915, on the action potential characteristics of canine cardiac Purkinje fibers. *Journal of Pharmacology and Experimental Techniques* **253**, 1090–1096.

Buchanan, L. V., Turcotte, U. M., Gibson, J. K. & Kabell, G. G. (1990) Antiarrhythmic effects of ibutilide, a new class III agent, in 24 hour canine myocardial infarction. *Circulation* **82**, III-638.

Cacciapuoti, F., Spieza, R., Bianchi, U., Lama, D., D'Avino, M. & Varricchio, M. (1991) Effectiveness of glibenclamide on myocardial ischemic ventricular arrhythmias in non-insulin-dependent diabetes mellitus. *American Journal of Cardiology* **67**, 843–847.

Campbell, D. L., Qu, Y., Rasmusson, R. L. & Strauss, H. C. (1991) Interaction of 4-AP with I_{to} in ferret ventricular myocytes. *Biophysical Journal* **59**, 280a.

Campbell, T. J. (1987a) Differing electrophysiological effects of class IA, IB and IC antiarrhythymic drugs on guinea-pig sinoatrial node. *British Journal of Pharmacology* **91**, 395–401.

Campbell, T. J. (1987b) Cellular electrophysiological effects of D- and DL-sotalol in guinea-pig sinoatrial node, atrium and ventricle and human atrium: differential tissue sensitivity. *British Journal of Pharmacology* **90**, 593–599.

Cardiac Arrhythmia Suppression Trial (CAST) Investigators (1989) Preliminary report: effect of encainide and flecainide on mortality in a randomized trial of arrhythmia suppression after myocardial infarction. *New England Journal of Medicine* **321**, 406–412.

Carlsson, L., Almgren, O. & Duker, G. (1990) QTU-prolongation and toursades de pointes induced by putative class III antiarrhythmic agents in the rabbit: etiology and considerations. *Journal of Cardiovascular Pharmacology* **16**, 276–285.

Carmeliet, E. (1985) Electrophysiologic and voltage clamp analysis of the effects of sotalol on isolated cardiac muscle and Purkinje fibers. *Journal of Pharmacology and Experimental Therapeutics* **232**, 817–825.

Carmeliet, E. & Saikawa, T. (1982) Shortening of the action potential and reduction of pacemaker activity by lidocaine, quinidine and procainamide in sheep cardiac Purkinje fibers. An effect on Na or K currents? *Circulation Research* **50**, 257–272.

Chi, L., Mu, D-X., Driscoll, E. M. & Lucchesi, B. R. (1990a) Antiarrhythmic and electrophysiologic actions of CK-3579 and sematilide in a conscious canine model of sudden coronary death. *Journal of Cardiovascular Pharmacology* **16**, 312–324.

Chi, L., Mu, D-X, & Lucchesi, B. R. (1990b) Electrophysiologic and antiarrhythmic actions of E-4031 in the experimental animal model and isolated atrial tissue. *Circulation* **82**, III-638.

Chi, L., Mu, D-X. & Lucchesi, B. R. (1991) Electrophysiologic and antiarrhythmic actions of E-4031 in the experimental animal model of sudden coronary death. *Journal of Cardiovascular Pharmacology* **17**, 285–295.

Chi, L., Uprichard, A. C. G. & Lucchesi, B. R. (1990c) Profibrillatory actions of pinacidil in a conscious canine model of sudden death. *Journal of Cardiovascular Pharmacology* **15**, 452–464.

Cimini, M. G. & Gibson, J. K. (1990) The electrophysiologic effects of U-70226E on isolated rabbit myocardium. *Journal of Molecular and Cellular Cardiology* **22**, S17.

Clay, J. R., Hill, C. E., Roitman, D. & Shrier, A. (1988) Repolarization current in embryonic chick atrial heart cells. *Journal of Physiology* **403**, 525–537.

Cobbe, S. M. (1987) Clinical usefulness of the Vaughan Williams classification system. *European Heart Journal* **8**, 65–69.

Colatsky, T. J. (1982) Mechanisms of action of lidocaine and quinidine on action potential duration in rabbit cardiac Purkinje fibers: an effect on steady-state sodium currents? *Circulation Research* **50**, 17–27.

Colatsky, T. J. & Follmer, C. F. (1990) Potassium channels as targets for antiarrhythmic drug action. *Drug Development Research* **19**, 129–140.

Colatsky, T. J., Follmer, C. F. & Starmer, C. F. (1990) Channel specificity in antiarrhythmic drug action: mechanism of potassium channel block and its role in suppressing and aggravating cardiac arrhythmias. *Circulation* **82**, 2235–2342.

Colatsky, T. J., Jurkiewicz, N. K., Follmer, C. F. & Bird, L. B. (1989) Antiarrhythmic efficacy of Wy-48,986, a novel class III antiarrhythmic agent, on ventricular arrhythmias induced by coronary ligation in dogs and pigs: effects on acute, sub-acute and chronic phase post-ligation arrhythmias. *Journal of Molecular and Cellular Cardiology* **21**, S10.

Conrad, C. H., Mark, R. G. & Bing, O. H. L. (1983) Outward current and repolarization in hypoxic rat myocardium. *American Journal of Physiology* **244**, H341–H359.

Cook, N. S. & Quast, U. (1990) Potassium channel pharmacology. In Cook, N. S. (ed.), *Potassium Channels: Structure, Classification, Function and Therapeutic Potential.* Ellis Horwood Ltd., Chichester, pp. 181–255.

Coraboeuf, E., Deroubaix, E., Escande, D. & Coulombe, A. (1988) Comparative effects of three class I antiarrhythmic drugs on plateau and pacemaker currents of sheep cardiac Purkinje fibers. *Cardiovascular Research* **22**, 375–384.

Courtney, K. R. (1980) Interval-dependent effects of small antiarrhythmic drugs on excitability in guinea-pig myocardium. *Journal of Molecular and Cellular Cardiology* **12**, 1273–1286.

Courtney, K. R. (1987) Review: quantitative structure/activity relations based on use-dependent I_{Na} block and repriming kinetics in myocardium. *Journal of Molecular and Cellular Cardiology* **19**, 318–330.

Cross, P. E., Arrowsmith, J. E., Thomas, G. N., Gwilt, M., Burges, R. A. & Higgins, A. J. (1990) Selective class III antiarrhythmic agents. 1. Bis(arylaklyl)amines. *Journal of Medicinal Chemistry* **33**, 1151–1155.

Dangman, K. H. & Hoffman, B. F. (1981) *In vivo* and *in vitro* antiarrhythmic and arrhythmogenic effects of *N*-acetylprocainamide. *Journal of Pharmacology and Experimental Therapeutics* **217**, 851–862.

Davy, J-M., Dorian, P., Kantelip, J-P, Harrison, D. C. & Kates, R. E. (1986) Qualitative and quantitative comparison of the cardiac effects of encainide and its three major metabolites in the dog. *Journal of Pharmacology and Experimental Therapeutics* **237**, 907–911.

DiFrancesco, D., Ferroni, A. & Visentin, S. (1984) Barium-blockade of the inward rectifier in calf Purkinje fibers. *Pflügers Archiv* **402**, 446–453.

Doerr, T. & Trautwein, W. (1990) On the mechanism of the 'specific bradycardic action' of the verapamil derivative UL-FS 49. *Naunyn-Schmiedeberg's Archives of Pharmacology* **341**, 331–340.

Duchatelle-Gourdon, I., Hartzell, H. C. & Lagrutta, A. A. (1989) Modulation of the delayed rectifier potassium current in frog cardiomyocytes by β-adrenergic agonists and magnesium. *Journal of Physiology* **415**, 251–274.

Duker, G. D. & Almgren, O. S. (1990) H 234/09 — a new potent class III antiarrhythmic agent. *Journal of Molecular and Cellular Cardiology* **22**, S82.

Dukes, I. D. & Morad, M. (1989) Tedisamil inactivates transient outward K^+ current in rat ventricular myocytes. *American Journal of Physiology* **257**, H1746–H1749.

Dukes, I. D., Cleeman, L. & Morad, M. (1990) Tedisamil blocks the transient and delayed rectifier K^+ currents in mammalian cardiac and glial cells. *Journal of Pharmacology and Experimental Therapeutics* **254**, 560–569.

Eller, B. T., Patterson, E. & Lucchesi, B. R. (1983) Ventricular fibrillation in a conscious canine model — its prevention by UM-272. *European Journal of Pharmacology* **87**, 406–413.

Endo, T., Nejima, J., Kiuchi, K., Fujita, S., Kikuchi, K., Hayakawa, H. & Okumura, H. (1988) Reduction of size of myocardial infarction with nicorandil, a new antianginal drug, after coronary artery occlusion in dogs. *Journal of Cardiovascular Pharmacology* **12**, 587–592.

Escande, D., Mestre, M., Hardy, J-C. & Cavero, I. (1989) RP 58866, a pure class III antiarrhythmic agent, specifically blocks the inwardly rectifying K^+ current in heart cells. *Circulation* **80**, II-607.

Escande, D., Thuringer, D., Leguern, S. & Cavero, I. (1988) The potassium channel opener cromakalim (BRL 34915) activates ATP-dependent K^+ channels in isolated cardiac myocytes. *Biochemical and Biophysical Research Communications* **154**, 620–625.

Faivre, J-F. & Findlay, I. (1990) Action potential duration and activation of ATP-sensitive potassium current in isolated guinea-pig ventricular myocytes. *Biochimica et Biophysica Acta* **1029**, 167–172.

Fan, Z., Nakayama, K. & Hiraoka, H. (1990) Pinacidil activates the ATP-sensitive K^+ channel in inside-out and cell-attached patch membranes of guinea-pig ventricular myocytes. *Pflügers Archiv* **415**, 387–394.

Feld, G. K., Venkatesh, N. & Singh, B. N. (1986) Pharmacologic conversion and suppression of experimental canine atrial flutter: differing effects of D-sotalol, quinidine and lidocaine and significance of changes in refractoriness and conduction. *Circulation* **74**, 197–204.

Feld, G. K., Venkatesh, N. & Singh, B. N. (1988) Effects of *N*-acetylprocainamide and recainam in the pharmacologic conversion and suppression of experimental canine atrial flutter: significance of changes in refractoriness and conduction. *Journal of Cardiovascular Pharmacology* **11**, 573–580.

Follmer, C. H. & Colatsky, T. J. (1990) Block of delayed rectifier potassium current, I_K, by flecainide and E-4031 in cat ventricular myocytes. *Circulation* **82**, 289–293.

Follmer, C. H., Poczobutt, M. & Colatsky, T. J. (1989) Selective block of delayed rectification (I_K) in feline ventricular myocytes by Wy 48,986, a novel Class III antiarrhythmic agent. *Journal of Molecular and Cellular Cardiology* **21**, S185.

Fosset, M., DeWeille, J. R., Green, R. D., Schmid-Antomarchi, H. & Lazdunski, M. (1988) Antidiabetic sulfonylureas control action potential properties in heart cells via high affinity receptors that are linked to ATP-dependent K^+ channels. *Journal of Biological Chemistry* **263**, 7933–7936.

French, R. J. & Shoukimas, J. J. (1981) Blockage of squid axon potassium conductance by internal tetra-N-alkylammonium ions of various sizes. *Biophysical Journal* **34**, 271–291.

French, R. J. & Shoukimas, J. J. (1985) An ion's view of the potassium channel: the structure of the permeation pathway as sensed by a variety of blocking ions. *Journal of General Physiology* **85**, 669–698.

Friedman, P. L., Stewart, J. R. & Wit, A. L. (1973) Spontaneous and induced cardiac arrhythmias in subendocardial Purkinje fibers surviving extensive myocardial infarction in dogs. *Circulation Research* **33**, 612–626.

Furukawa, T., Tsujimura, Y., Kitamura, K., Tanaka, H. & Habuchi, Y. (1989) Time- and voltage-dependent block of the delayed K^+ current by quinidine in rabbit sinoatrial and atrioventricular nodes. *Journal of Pharmacology and Experimental Therapeutics* **251**, 756–763.

Gibson, J. K., Patterson, E. & Lucchesi, B. R. (1985) The antiarrhythmic actions of intravenous and oral UM424 in postinfarction canine myocardium. *Journal of Cardiovascular Pharmacology* **7**, 211–218.

Gibson, J. K., Patterson, E. & Lucchesi, B. R. (1986) Electrophysiologic, antiarrhythmic and cardiovascular actions of UM301, a quaternary ammonium compound. *Journal of Pharmacology and Experimental Therapeutics* **237**, 318–325.

Gibson, J. K., Stewart, J. R., Li, Y-P., & Lucchesi, B. R. (1983) Electrophysiologic effects of bretylium tosylate on the canine heart during coronary artery occlusion and reperfusion. *Journal of Cardiovascular Pharmacology* **5**, 517–524.

Giles, W. R. & Van Ginneken, A. C. G. (1985) A transient outward current in isolated cells from the crista terminalis of rabbit heart. *Journal of Physiology* **368**, 243–264.

Goldberg, M. R. (1988) Clinical pharmacology of pinacidil: a prototype for drugs that affect potassium channels. *Journal of Cardiovascular Pharmacology* **12**, S41–S47.

Gross, G., Pieper, G., Farber, N. E., Warltier, D. & Hardman, H. (1989) Effects of nicorandil on coronary circulation and myocardial ischemia. *American Journal of Cardiology* **63**, 11J–17J.

Grover, G. J., McCullough, J. R., Henry, D. E., Conder, M. L. & Sleph, P. G. (1989) Antiischemic effects of the potassium channel activators pinacidil and cromakalim and the reversal of these effects with the potassium channel blocker glyburide. *Journal of Pharmacology and Experimental Therapeutics* **251**, 98–104.

Grover, G. J., Sleph, P. G. & Dzwonczyk, S. (1990) Pharmacologic profile of cromakalim in the treatment of myocardial ischemia in isolated rat hearts and anaesthetized dog. *Journal of Cardiovascular Pharmacology* **16**, 853–864.

Gwilt, M., Arrowsmith, J. E., Blackburn, K. J., Burges, R. A., Cross, P. E., Dalrymple, H. W. & Higgins, A. J. (1991) UK-68,798: a novel, potent and highly selective class III antiarrhythmic agent which blocks potassium channels in cardiac cells. *Journal of Pharmacology and Experimental Therapeutics* **256**, 318–324.

Gwilt, M., Dalrymple, H. W., Blackburn, K. J., Burges, R. A. & Higgins, A. J. (1988)

UK-66,914: a novel class III antiarrhythmic agent which blocks potassium channels. *Circulation* **78**, II-150.

Gwilt, M., Dalrymple, H. W., Burges, R. A., Blackburn, K. J., Arrowsmith, J. E., Cross, P. E. & Higgins, A. J. (1989) UK-68,798 is a novel, potent and selective class III antiarrhythmic drug. *Journal of Molecular and Cellular Cardiology* **21**, S11.

Habuchi, Y., Nishimura, M. & Watanabe, Y. (1987) Electrophysiologic effects of nicorandil, a new antianginal agent, on action potentials and membrane currents of rabbit atrioventricular node. *Naunyn-Schmiedeberg's Archives of Pharmacology* **335**, 567–574.

Hall, D., Charocopos, F., Froer, K. L. & Rudolph, W. (1980) ECG changes during long term minoxidil therapy for severe hypertension. *Archives of Internal Medicine* **139**, 790–794.

Harrison, D. C. (1985) Antiarrhythmic drug classification: new science and practical applications. *American Journal of Cardiology* **56**, 185–187.

Harvey, R. D. & ten Eick, R. E. (1989) Voltage-dependent block of cardiac inward-rectifying potassium current by monovalent cations. *Journal of General Physiology* **94**, 349–361.

Haworth, R. A., Goknur, A. B. & Berkoff, H. A. (1989) Inhibition of ATP-sensitive potassium channels of adult rat heart cells by antiarrhythmic drugs. *Circulation Research* **65**, 1157–1160.

Hille, B. (1967) The selective inhibition of delayed potassium currents in nerve by tetraethylammonium ions. *Journal of General Physiology* **50**, 1287–1302.

Hille, B. (1977) Local anesthetics: hydrophilic and hydrophobic pathways for the drug-receptor interaction. *Journal of General Physiology* **69**, 497–515.

Hirano, Y. & Hiraoka, M. (1986) Changes in K^+ currents induced by Ba^{2+} in guinea pig ventricular muscles. *American Journal of Physiology* **251**, H24–H33.

Hiraoka, M. & Fan, Z. (1989) Activation of ATP-sensitive outward K^+ current by nicorandil (2-nicotinamidoethyl nitrate) in isolated ventricular myocytes. *Journal of Pharmacology and Experimental Therapeutics* **250**, 278–285.

Hiraoka, M., Sawada, K. & Kawano, S. (1986) Effects of quinidine on plateau currents of guinea pig ventricular myocytes. *Journal of Molecular and Cellular Cardiology* **18**, 1097–1106.

Hondeghem, L. M. & Katzung, B. G. (1977) Time- and voltage-dependent interactions of antiarrhythmic drugs with cardiac sodium channels. *Biochimica et Biophysica Acta* **472**, 373–398.

Hondeghem, L. M. & Katzung, B. G. (1984) Antiarrhythmic agents: the modulated receptor mechanism of action of sodium and calcium channel-blocking drugs. *Annual Review of Pharmacology and Toxicology* **24**, 387–423.

Hondeghem, L. M. & Snyders, D. J. (1990) Class III antiarrhythmics have a lot of potential but a long way to go: reduced effectiveness and dangers of reverse use dependence. *Circulation* **81**, 686–690.

Horie, M., Irisawa, H. & Noma, A. (1987) Voltage-dependent magnesium block of adenosine-triphosphate sensitive potassium channel in guinea-pig ventricular cells. *Journal of Physiology* **387**, 251–272.

Imaizumi, Y. & Giles, W. R. (1987) Quinidine-induced inhibition of transient outward current in cardiac muscle. *American Journal of Physiology* **253**, H704–H708.

Isenberg, G. (1976) Cardiac Purkinje fibers: cesium as a tool to block inwardly rectifying potassium currents. *Pflügers Archiv* **365**, 99–106.

Ishii, M., Katakami, T., Yokoyama, T., Banno, H., Hirayama, M. & Kamiya, J. (1990) Cardiac electrophysiologic effects of MS-551 a novel class III antiarrhythmic agent. *Japanese Journal of Pharmacology* **52**, 250P.

Jackman, W. M., Friday, K. J., Anderson, J. L., Aliot, E. M., Clark, M. & Lazzara,

R. (1988) The long QT syndromes: a critical review, new clinical observations and a unifying hypothesis. *Progress in Cardiovascular Diseases* **31**, 115–172.

Kakei, M., Yoshinaga, M., Saito, K. & Tanaka, H. (1986) The potassium current activated by 2-nicotinamidoethyl nitrate (nicorandil) in single ventricular cells of the guinea pig. *Proceedings of the Royal Society of London, Series B* **229**, 331–343.

Kameyama, M., Kakei, M., Sato, R., Shibasaki, T., Matsuda, H. & Irisawa, H. (1984) Intracellular Na^+ activates a K^+ channel in mammalian cardiac cells. *Nature* **309**, 354–356.

Kamiya, J., Banno, H., Yoshihara, I., Ishii, M. & Katakami, T. (1990) Antiarrhythmic effect and hemodynamic properties of MS-551, a new class III antiarrhythmic agent, in anesthetized dogs. *European Journal of Pharmacology* **183**, 1776.

Kantor, P. F., Coetzee, W. A., Carmeliet, E. E., Dennis, S. C. & Opie, L. H. (1990) Reduction of K^+ loss and arrhythmias in rat hearts: effect of glyburide, a sulfonylurea. *Circulation Research* **66**, 478–485.

Kass, R. S., Scheuer, T. & Malloy, K. J. (1982) Block of outward current in cardiac Purkinje fibers by injection of quaternary ammonium ions. *Journal of General Physiology* **79**, 1041–1063.

Katoh, H., Ogawa, S., Furuno, I., Sato, Y., Yoh, S., Saeki, K. & Nakamura, Y. (1990) Electrophysiologic effects of E-4031, a class III antiarrhythmic agent, on re-entrant ventricular arrhythmias in a canine 7-day-old myocardial infarction. *Journal of Pharmacology and Experimental Therapeutics* **253**, 1077–1082.

Kenyon, J. L. & Gibbons, W. R. (1979a) 4-Aminopyridine and the early outward current of sheep cardiac Purkinje fibers. *Journal of General Physiology* **73**, 139–157.

Kenyon, J. L. & Sutko, J. L. (1987) Calcium- and voltage-activated plateau currents of cardiac Purkinje fibers. *Journal of General Physiology* **89**, 921–958.

Kerr, M. J., Wilson, R. & Shanks, R. H. (1985) Suppression of ventricular arrhythmias after coronary artery ligation by pinacidil, a vasodilator drug. *Journal of Cardiovascular Pharmacology* **7**, 875–883.

Kim, D. & Clapham, D. E. (1989) Potassium channels in cardiac cells activated by arachidonic acid and phospholipids. *Nature* **244**, 1174–1176.

Kim, D., Lewis, D. L., Graziadei, L., Neer, E. J., Bar-Sagi, D. & Clapham, D. E. (1989) G-protein β g-subunits activate the cardiac muscarinic K^+-channel via phospholipase A_2. *Nature* **337**, 557–560.

Koerner, J. E. & Dage, R. C. (1990) Antiarrhythmic and electrophysiologic effects of MDL-11,939, a novel class III antiarrhythmic agent in anesthetized dogs. *Journal of Cardiovascular Pharmacology* **16**, 383–393.

Kohlhardt, M., Frobe, U. & Herzig, J. W. (1986) Modification of single cardiac sodium channels by DPI-201,106. *Journal of Membrane Biology* **89**, 163–172.

Kotake, H., Matsuoka, S., Ogino, O., Takami, T., Hasegawa, J. & Mashiba, H. (1987) Electrophysiological study of cibenzoline in voltage-clamped rabbit sinoatrial node preparations. *Journal of Pharmacology and Experimental Therapeutics* **241**, 982–986.

Kurachi, Y., Ito, H., Sugimoto, T., Schimizu, T., Miki, I. & Ui, M. (1987) Arachidonic acid metabolites as intracellular modulators of the G protein-gated cardiac K^+ channel. *Nature* **337**, 555–557.

Kus, T., Costi, P., Dubuc, M. & Shenasa, M. (1990) Prolongation of ventricular refractoriness by class Ia antiarrhythmic drugs in the prevention of ventricular tachycardia induction. *American Heart Journal* **120**, 855–863.

Lazzara, R. (1989) Amiodarone and toursade de pointes. *Annals of Internal Medicine* **31**, 549–551.

Lee, E. W., Mckay, M. C. & Lee, K. S. (1990) U-70226E, a novel class III antiarrhythmic compound activates a slow inward Na^+ and an outward K^+ current. *Journal of Molecular and Cellular Cardiology* **22**, S15.

Lewis, T. & Drury, A. N. (1926) Revised views of refractory period, in relation to drugs reputed to prolong it, and in relation to circus movement. *Heart* **13**, 95–100.

Li, T., Carr, A. A. & Dage, R. C. (1990) Effects of MDL-11,939 on action potential and contractile force in cardiac tissues: a comparison with bretylium, clofilium and sotalol. *Journal of Cardiovascular Pharmacology* **16**, 917–923.

Liu, B., Golyan, F., McCullough, J. R. & Vassalle, M. (1988) Electrophysiological and antiarrhythmic effects of the K-channel opener BRL 34915 in cardiac Purkinje fibers. *Drug Development Research* **14**, 123–139.

Lodge, N. J., Follmer, C. F., Mao, H. & Colatsky, T. J. (1990) Modulation of the delayed rectifier I_K by cadmium in cat ventricular myocytes. *Biophysical Journal* **57**, 506a.

Lumma, W. C. Jr (1989) Sematilide hydrochloride. *Drugs of the Future* **14**, 234–236.

Lumma, W. C. Jr, Wohl, R. A., Davey, D. D., Argentieri, T. M., DeVita, R. J., Gomez, R. P., Jain, V. K., Marisca, A. J., Morgan, T. K. Jr, Reiser, H. J., Sullivan, M. E., Wiggins, J. & Wong, S. S. (1987) Rational design of 4-[(methylsulfonylamino]benzamides as class III antiarrhythmic agents. *Journal of Medicinal Chemistry* **30**, 755–758.

Lynch, J. L. Jr, Heaney, L. A., Wallace, A. A., Gehret, J. R., Selnick, H. G. & Stein, R. B. (1990) Suppression of lethal ischemic ventricular arrhythmias by the class III agent E4031 in a canine model of previous infarction. *Journal of Cardiovascular Pharmacology* **15**, 764–775.

MacKinnon, R. & Yellen, G. (1990) Mutations affecting TEA blockade and ion permeation in voltage-activated channels. *Science* **250**, 276–279.

McPherson, G. A. & Angus, J. A. (1989) Phentolamine and structurally related compounds selectively antagonize the vascular actions of the K^+ channel opener cromakalim. *British Journal of Pharmacology* **97**, 941–949.

Marban, E. & Tsien, R. W. (1982) Effects of nystatin-mediated intracellular ion substitution on membrane currents in calf Purkinje fibers. *Journal of Physiology* **329**, 569–587.

Matsuda, H. (1988) Open-state substructure of inwardly rectifying potassium channels revealed by magnesium block in guinea-pig heart cells. *Journal of Physiology* **397**, 237–258.

Meier, C. F. Jr & Katzung, B. G. (1981) Cesium blockade of delayed outward currents and electrically induced pacemaker activity in mammalian ventricular myocardium. *Journal of General Physiology* **77**, 531–547.

Mestre, M., Escande, D. & Cavero, I. (1990) Antifibrillatory effects of RP 58866, a potassium channel blocker, in dog and micropig hearts subjected to ischemia and reperfusion. *European Journal of Pharmacology* **183**, 1239.

Meves, H. & Pinchon, Y. (1977) The effect of internal and external 4-aminopyridine on the potassium currents in intracellularly perfused squid giant axon. *Journal of Physiology* **268**, 511–532.

Mirro, M. J., Watanabe, A. M. & Bailey, J. C. (1981) Electrophysiological effects of the optical isomers of disopyramide and quinidine in the dog. Dependence on stereochemistry. *Circulation Research* **48**, 867–874.

Nademanee, K., Pacifico, A., Antimisiaris, M., Taylor, A., Taylor, R., Boahene, A., Chipin, L., O'Neill, P., Pruitt, C. & Singh, B. (1990) Electrophysiologic and antiarrhythmic effects of sematilide in humans. *Circulation* **82**, (Suppl. III), 198.

Nakaya, Y., Varro, A., Elharrar, V. & Surawicz, B. (1989) Effect of altered repolarization course induced by antiarrhythmic drugs and constant current pulses on duration of premature action potentials in canine cardiac Purkinje fibers. *Journal of Cardiovascular Pharmacology* **14**, 908–918.

Nishimura, M., Sato, N., Tanaka, H., Habuchi, Y. & Watanabe, Y. (1990) A novel class III antiarrhythmic agent E-4031 suppresses automaticity in the rabbit sinoatrial node by blocking the delayed rectifying K^+ current. *Circulation* **82**, (Suppl. III), 527.

Noble, D. & Tsien, R. W. (1969) Outward membrane currents activated in the plateau range of potentials in cardiac Purkinje fibers. *Journal of Physiology* **200**, 205–231.

Noma, A. & Shibasaki, T. (1985) Membrane current through adenosine-triphosphate regulated potassium channels in guinea pig ventricular cells. *Journal of Physiology* **363**, 463–480.

Oinuma, H., Miyake, K., Yamanaka, M., Nomoto, K., Kato, H., Sawada, K., Shino, M. & Hamano, S. (1990) 4'-[(4-Piperidyl) carbonyl]methanesulfonanilides as potent, selective, bioavailable class III antiarrhythmic agents. *Journal of Medicinal Chemistry* **33**, 903–905.

Osterreider, W. (1988) Modification of K^+ conductance of heart cell membrane by BRL 34915. *Naunyn-Schmiedeberg's Archives of Pharmacology* **337**, 93–97.

Osterreider, W., Young, Q. F. & Trautwein, W. (1982) Effects of barium on the membrane currents in the rabbit SA node. *Pflügers Archiv* **394**, 78–84.

Poizot, A., Balter, P. & Armstrong, J. M. (1990) Effect of D-sotalol and sematilide on action potentials generated in rabbit isolated Purkinje fibers bathed in normal and ischemic solutions. *Therapie* **45**, 446.

Pratt, C. M., Brater, D. C., Harrell, F. E., Kowey, P. R., Leier, C. V., Lowenthal, D. T., Messerli, F., Packer, M., Pritchett, E. L. C. & Ruskin, J. N. (1990) Clinical and regulatory implications of the Cardiac Arrhythmia Suppression Trial. *American Journal of Cardiology* **65**, 103–105.

Rasmussen, H. S., Kleinetmans, D., Walker, D. & Rapeport, W. G. (1990) Double blind, placebo controlled parallel group study of the effect of UK-68,798, a novel class III antiarrhythmic agent, on the pharmacokinetics and pharmacodynamics of digoxin. *European Heart Journal* **11**, 57.

Reichardt, B., Konzen, G. & Hauswirth, O. (1990) Pirmenol, a new antiarrhythmic drug with potassium- and sodium-channel blocking activity: a voltage clamp study in rabbit Purkinje fibers. *Naunyn-Schmiedeberg's Archives of Pharmacology* **341**, 462–471.

Rials, S. J., Sewter, J., Wu, Y., Marinchak, R. A. & Kowey, P. R. (1990) Comparative antifibrillatory activity of amiodarone versus risotilide in acute ischemia. *Clinical Research* **38**, 782A.

Ripoll, C., Lederer, W. J. & Nichols, C. G. (1990) Modulation of ATP-sensitive K^+ channel activity and contractile behavior in mammalian ventricle by the potassium channel openers cromakalim and RP 49356. *Journal of Pharmacology and Experimental Therapeutics* **255**, 429–435.

Robertson, D. W. & Steinberg, M. I. (1990) Potassium channel modulators: scientific applications and therapeutic promise. *Journal of Medicinal Chemistry* **33**, 1529–1541.

Roden, D. M., Bennett, P. B., Snyders, D. J., Balser, J. R. & Hondeghem, L. M. (1988) Quinidine delays I_K activation in guinea pig ventricular myocytes. *Circulation Research* **52**, 1055–1058.

Sakmann, B. & Trube, G. (1984) Conductance properties of single inwardly-rectifying potassium channels in ventricular cells from guinea pig heart. *Journal of Physiology* **347**, 641–657.

Sakmann, B., Noma, A. & Trautwein, W. (1983) Acetylcholine activation of single muscarinic K^+ channels in isolated pacemaker cells of the mammalian heart. *Nature* **303**, 250–253.

Salata, J. J. & Wasserstrom, J. A. (1988) Effects of quinidine on action potentials and ionic currents in isolated canine ventricular myocytes. *Circulation Research* **62**, 324–337.

Sanguinetti, M. C. & Jurkiewicz, N. K. (1990a) Two components of cardiac delayed rectifier K^+ current: differential sensitivity to block by class III antiarrhythmic agents. *Journal of General Physiology* **96**, 195–215.

Sanguinetti, M. C. & Jurkiewicz, N. K. (1990b) Lanthanum blocks a specific component of I_K and screens membrane surface charge in cardiac cells. *American Journal of Physiology* **259**, H1881–H1889.

Sanguinetti, M. C. & Jurkiewicz, N. K. (1991) I_K is comprised of two currents in guinea pig atrial cells. *Biophysical Journal* **59**, 281a.

Sanguinetti, M. C., Scott, A. L., Zingaro, G. J. & Siegl, P. K. S. (1988) BRL 34915 (cromakalim) activates ATP-sensitive K^+ current in cardiac muscle. *Proceedings of the National Academy of Sciences USA* **85**, 8360–8364.

Sano, T., Sugiyama, K., Hanaki, Y., Shimada, Y. & Ozawa, T. (1990) Effects of antiarrhythmic agents classified as class III group on ischemia-induced myocardial damage in canine hearts. *British Journal of Pharmacology* **99**, 577–581.

Sasyniuk, B. I., Valois, M. & Toy, W. (1989) Recent advances in understanding the mechanisms of drug-induced toursades de pointes arrhythmias. *American Journal of Cardiology* **62**, 29J–32J.

Scholtysik, G., Salzmann, R., Berthold, R., Herzig, J. W., Quast, U. & Markstein, R. (1985) DPI 201,106, a novel cardioactive agent. Combination of cAMP-independent positive inotropic, negative chronotropic, action potential prolonging coronary dilatory properties. *Naunyn-Schmiedeberg's Archives of Pharmacology* **329**, 316–325.

Schwartz, J. B. & Herre, J. M. (1989) The electrophysiological effects of alpha-chloralose anesthesia in the intact dog: (1) alone and (2) in combination with verapamil. *PACE* **12**, 283–293.

Sedgwick, M., Rasmussen, H. S. & Cobbe, S. M. (1990) The effect of intravenous UK-68798, a novel class III antiarrhythmic agent, on electrocardiographic parameters in patients with ischemic heart disease. An open study. *European Heart Journal* **11**, 240.

Sedgwick, M., Rasmussen, H. S., Walker, D. & Cobbe, S. M. (1991) Pharmacokinetic and pharmacodynamic effects of UK-68,798, a new potential class III antiarrhythmic drug. *British Journal of Clinical Pharmacology* **31**, 515–519.

Shah, A., Cohen, I. S. & Rosen, M. R. (1988) Stimulation of cardiac alpha receptors increases Na/K pump current and decreases g_k via a pertussis toxin-sensitive pathway. *Biophysical Journal* **54**, 219–225.

Sheldon, R. S., Rahmberg, M. & Duff, H. J. (1990) Quinidine/quinine: stereospecific electrophysiologic and antiarrhythmic effects in a canine model of ventricular tachycardia. *Journal of Cardiovascular Pharmacology* **16**, 818–823.

Shibasaki, T. (1987) Conductance and kinetics of delayed rectifier potassium channels in nodal cells of the rabbit heart. *Journal of Physiology* **387**, 227–250.

Shibata, E. F., Drury, T., Refsum, H., Aldrete, V. & Giles, W. (1989) Contributions of a transient outward current to repolarization in human atrium. *American Journal of Physiology* **257**, H1773–H1781.

Siegelbaum, S. A. & Tsien, R. W. (1980) Calcium-activated transient outward current in calf cardiac Purkinje fibers. *Journal of Physiology* **299**, 485–506.

Simmons, M. A., Creazzo, T. & Hartzell, H. C. (1986) A time-dependent and voltage-sensitive K^+ current in single cells from frog atrium. *Journal of General Physiology* **88**, 739–755.

Singh, B. N. & Vaughan Williams, E. M. (1970a) A third class of antiarrhythmic action. Effects on atrial and ventricular intracellular potentials, and other pharmacologic actions on cardiac muscle, of MJ1999 and AH3474. *British Journal of Pharmacology* **39**, 675–687.

Singh, B. N. & Vaughan Williams, E. M. (1970b) The effect of amiodarone, a new antianginal drug, on cardiac muscle. *British Journal of Pharmacology* **39**, 657–668.

Smallwood, J. K., Ertel, P. J. & Steinberg, M. I. (1990) Modification by glibenclamide of the electrophysiological consequences of myocardial ischemia in dogs and rabbits. *Naunyn-Schmiedeberg's Archives of Pharmacology* **342**, 214–220.

Spinelli, W., Follmer, C. F., Parsons, R. & Colatsky, T. J. (1990) Effects of cromakalim, pinacidil, and nicorandil on cardiac refractoriness and arterial pressure in open-chest dogs. *European Journal of Pharmacology* **179**, 243–252.

Standen, N. B. & Stanfield, P. R. (1978) A potential- and time-dependent blockade of inward rectification in frog skeletal muscle fibres by barium and strontium ions. *Journal of Physiology* **280**, 169–191.

Stanfield, P. R. (1970) The effect of the tetraethylammonium ion on the delayed currents of frog skeletal muscle. *Journal of Physiology* **209**, 209–229.

Starmer, C. F. & Grant, A. O. (1985) Phasic ion channel blockade: a kinetic model and parameter estimation procedure. *Molecular Pharmacology* **28**, 348–356.

Steinberg, M. I., Ertel, P., Smallwood, J. K., Wyss, V. & Zimmerman, K. (1988) The relation between vascular relaxant and cardiac electrophysiological effects of pinacidil. *Journal of Cardiovascular Pharmacology* **12**, S30–S40.

Steinberg, M. I., Lindstrom, T. D. & Fasola, A. F. (1984) Clofilium. In Scriabine, A. (ed.), *New Drugs Annual: Cardiovascular Drugs*, Raven Press, New York, pp. 103–121.

Steinberg, M. I., Wiest, S. A., Zimmerman, K. M., Ertel, P. J., Bemis, K. G. & Robertson, D. W. (1991) Chiral recognition of pinacidil and its 3-pyridyl isomer by canine cardiac and smooth muscle: antagonism by sulfonylureas. *Journal of Pharmacology and Experimental Therapeutics* **256**, 222–229.

Takano, M. & Noma, A. (1990) Selective modulation of the ATP-sensitive K^+ channel by nicorandil in guinea-pig cardiac cell membrane. *Naunyn-Schmiedeberg's Archives of Pharmacology* **342**, 592–597.

Tande, P. M., Bjornstad, H., Yang, T. & Refsum, H. (1990) Rate-dependent class III antiarrhythmic action, negative chronotropy, and positive inotropy of a novel I_K blocking drug, UK-68,798; potent in guinea pig but no effect in rat myocardium. *Journal of Cardiovascular Pharmacology* **16**, 401–410.

Task Force of the Working Group on Arrhythmias of the European Society of Cardiology (1990) CAST and beyond: implications of the Cardiac Arrhythmia Suppression Trial. *Circulation* **81**, 1123–1127.

Thuringer, D. & Escande, D. (1989) Apparent competition between ATP and the potassium channel opener RP 49356 on ATP sensitive K^+ channels of cardiac myocytes. *Molecular Pharmacology* **36**, 897–902.

Tohse, N., Nakaya, H., Hattori, Y., Endou, M. & Kanno, M. (1990) Inhibitory effect mediated by α_1-adrenoceptors on transient outward current in isolated rat ventricular cells. *Pflügers Archiv* **415**, 575–581.

Tourneur, Y., Mitra, R., Morad, M. & Rougier, R. (1987) Activation properties of the inward-rectifying potassium channel on mammalian heart cells. *Journal of Membrane Biology* **97**, 127–135.

Tseng, G-N. & Hoffman, B. F. (1989) Two components of transient outward current in canine ventricular myocytes. *Circulation Research* **64**, 633–647.

Tseng, G-N. & Hoffman, B. F. (1990) Actions of pinacidil on membrane currents in canine ventricular myocytes and their modulation by intracellular ATP and cAMP. *Pflügers Archiv* **415**, 414–424.

Tsuchihashi, K. & Curtis, M. J. (1990) Chemical defibrillation in ischemia and reperfusion by selective blockade of the transient outward current (I_{to}). *Circulation* **82**, (Suppl. III), 452.

Van Bogaert, P. P. & Snyders, D. J. (1982) Effects of 4-aminopyridine on inward rectifying and pacemaker currents of cardiac Purkinje fibers. *Pflügers Archiv* **394**, 230–238.

Van Ginneken, A. C. G. & Giles, W. (1991) Voltage clamp measurements of the hyperpolarization-activated inward current I_f in single cells from rabbit sino-atrial node. *Journal of Physiology* **434**, 57–83.

Varro, A., Elharrar, V. & Surawicz, B. (1985a) Effect of antiarrhythmic drugs on the premature action potential duration in canine cardiac Purkinje fibers. *Journal of Pharmacology and Experimental Therapeutics* **233**, 304–311.

Varro, A., Nakaya, Y., Elharrar, V. & Surawicz, B. (1985b) Effect of antiarrhythmic drugs on the cycle length-dependent action potential duration in dog Purkinje and ventricular muscle fibers. *Journal of Cardiovascular Pharmacology* **8**, 178–185.

Vaughan Williams, E. M. (1958) The mode of action of quinidine on isolated rabbit atria interpreted from intracellular potential records. *British Journal of Pharmacology* **13**, 276–287.

Vaughan Williams, E. M. (1970) Classification of antiarrhythmic drugs. In Sandoe, E., Flensted-Jansen, E. & Olesen, K. H. (eds), *Symposium on Cardiac Arrhythmias*. AB Astra, Sodertaljie, Sweden, pp. 449–472.

Vaughan Williams, E. M. (1984) A classification of antiarrhythmic actions reassessed after a decade of new drugs. *Journal of Clinical Pharmacology* **24**, 129–147.

Vleugels, A., Vereecke, J. & Carmeliet, E. (1980) Ionic currents during hypoxia in voltage-clamped cat ventricular muscle. *Circulation Research* **47**, 501–508.

Walker, M. J. A. & Beatch, G. N. (1988) Electrically-induced arrhythmias in the rat. *Proceedings of the Western Pharmacological Society*, **31**, 167–170.

Weidmann, S. (1955) Effects of calcium and local anesthetics on electrical properties of Purkinje fibers. *Journal of Physiology* **129**, 568–582.

Wilde, A. A. M., Escande, E., Schumacher, C. A., Thuringer, D., Mestre, M., Fiolet, J. W. T. & Janse, M. J. (1990) Potassium accumulation in the globally ischemic mammalian heart: a role for the ATP-sensitive potassium channel. *Circulation Research* **67**, 835–843.

Wit, A. L., Steiner, C. & Damato, A. N. (1970) Electrophysiologic effects of bretylium tosylate on single fibers of the canine specialized conducting system and ventricle. *Journal of Pharmacology and Experimental Therapeutics* **173**, 344–356.

Wolleben, C. D., Sanguinetti, M. C. & Siegl, P. K. S. (1989) Influence of ATP-sensitive potassium channel modulators on ischemia-induced fibrillation in isolated rat hearts. *Journal of Molecular and Cellular Cardiology* **21**, 783–788.

Wong, W., Birgersdotter, B., Turgeon, J. & Roden, D. (1990) Steady-state pharmacokinetics and pharmacodynamics of the class III antiarrhythmic sematilide. *Circulation* **82**, (Suppl. III), 198.

Wong, W., Pavlou, H. N. & Roden, D. M. (1989) Pharmacology of sematilide, a class III procainamide analog, in man. *Circulation* **80**, (Suppl. II), 326.

Yanagihara, K. & Irisawa, H. (1980) Inward current activated during hyperpolarization in the rabbit sinoatrial node. *Pflügers Archiv* **385**, 207–217.

Yeh, J. Z., Oxford, G. S., Wu, C. H. & Narahashi, T. (1976) Interactions of aminopyridines with potassium channels of squid axon membranes. *Biophysical Journal* **16**, 77–81.

Yue, D. T. & Marban, E. (1988) A novel cardiac potassium channel that is active and conductive at depolarized potentials. *Pflügers Archiv* **413**, 127–133.

Zuanetti, G. & Corr, P. B. (1991) Antiarrhythmic efficacy of a new class III agent, UK-68,798, during chronic myocardial infarction: evaluation using three-dimensional mapping. *Journal of Pharmacology and Experimental Therapeutics* **256**, 325–334.

Chapter 13
Potassium channel activators: structure–activity relationships

J. M. Evans, M. S. Hadley and G. Stemp

Introduction

Although the physiology of K-channels has been studied for several decades, a major contribution to the spectacular increase in the investigation of these ion channels in recent years can be ascribed to the discovery (Ashwood *et al.*, 1984, 1986; Evans & Stemp, 1991), and elucidation of the mode of action (Hamilton *et al.*, 1986) of cromakalim, BRL 34915. Cromakalim was the first antihypertensive agent to be shown to act by opening ATP-sensitive K-channels (K_{ATP}).* A considerable part of the ensuing endeavour has concerned the discovery and application of synthetic molecules which open K-channels, and is reflected by the published interest of over 20 pharmaceutical organizations worldwide. This interest includes certain older compounds for which the mode of action was determined after the emergence of cromakalim.

---

*It is still uncertain whether cromakalim opens K_{ATP} in smooth muscle. For a discussion of this point, *see* Chapters 7 and 14.

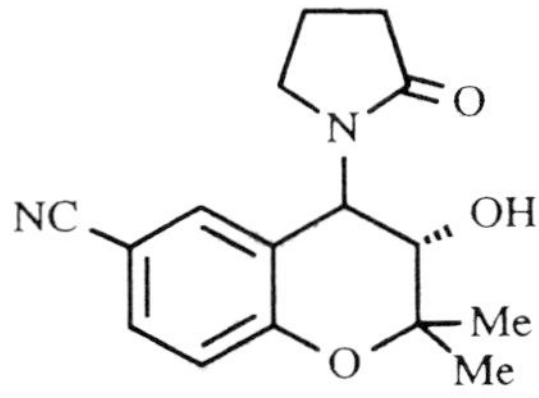

CROMAKALIM

A detailed description of structure–activity relationships (SARs) in K-channel activators (KCAs)* is complicated by the diverse range of compound structures, the plethora of indications for which they are claimed, and the use of different pharmacological models for any given disorder. Nevertheless, the major indication for which KCAs have been tested is hypertension and data are available, principally from rat models, to construct SARs. In addition, results primarily obtained from isolated guinea-pig trachealis, delineate further useful SARs for the airways smooth muscle relaxant abilities of KCAs, and, in some instances, correlations between different models have been made that enable a degree of extrapolation to be exercised. Also, certain studies compare cromakalim with other KCAs, some of which are structurally dissimilar to cromakalim, and so approximate rank orders of potency between the different types of KCAs can be established.

Preliminary accounts of SARs in KCAs have appeared (Edwards & Weston, 1989, 1990), and the topic has been partly covered in the excellent and comprehensive review on K-channels (Robertson & Steinberg, 1990a). This chapter seeks to expand on those previous publications, by reviewing the SARs of different series of KCAs that are grouped together according to a similarity of structure, within the constraints mentioned above. At the same time those compounds that are being progressed to clinical evaluation, or that are highlighted in their source publications, are identified.

Benzopyran KCAs

The series of KCAs based on the benzopyran, or chroman, structure, and typified by cromakalim, is the most extensively examined of all. The SARs in benzopyrans are most conveniently considered by a description of the structural modifications that have been made at each of the pyran ring positions, O(1)–C(4) of cromakalim, and those that have been made in the aromatic ring, both in terms of the nature and location of substituents, and the replacement of the benzene ring by other aromatic nuclei. In

---

*Activator is used here in a general rather than in an electrophysiological sense. It is not yet clear whether the opening of K-channels by agents like cromakalim is exerted by channel activation (*see* Hille, 1992).

cromakalim, the pyrrolidinone group at C(4) is *trans* to the hydroxyl group at C(3). It has been reported that *trans* compounds are approximately 10-fold more potent than the corresponding *cis* isomers (Ashwood *et al.*, 1986). Of the two enantiomers of cromakalim, BRL 38227 with the 3S,4R configuration is about 100-fold more potent than BRL 38226, the enantiomer with the 3R,4S configuration. In this review, racemates like cromakalim are shown with a normal bond at C(4) whereas, single enantiomers like BRL 38227 are depicted with a tapering bond at C(4). The data refer to lowering of blood pressure in the spontaneously hypertensive rat (SHR) unless indicated otherwise.

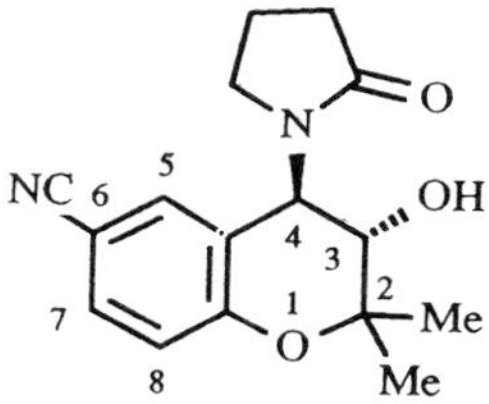

BRL 38227

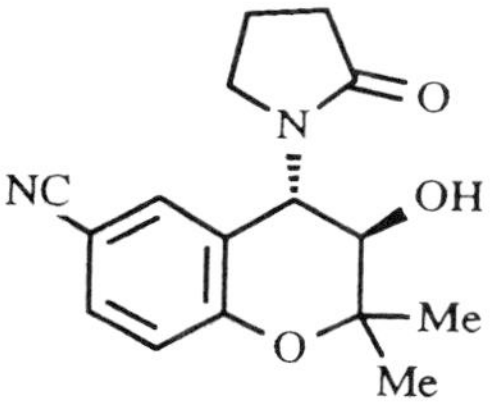

BRL 38226

Position 1

When the pyran ring oxygen atom of cromakalim was replaced by an amino (Evans & Stemp, 1985) or methylene group (Evans & Stemp, 1986) as in compounds (1a), potency was reduced 10-fold. In a related 6-methyl analogue (1b), replacement of the pyran oxygen atom by the sulphur atom maintained activity (Smith, 1990), but oxidation of the sulphur atom to sulphoxide or sulphone groups gave less potent compounds. Removal of the oxygen atom to give the 1,1-dimethylindanes (2), produced KCAs which were generally slightly less potent than their chroman counterparts in relaxing guinea-pig trachealis *in vitro* (Buckle *et al.*, 1991a).

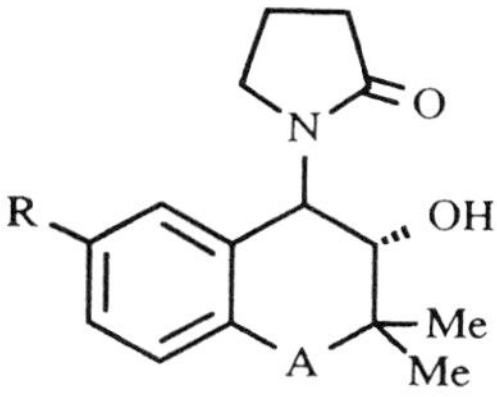

(1a) R = CN, A = NH, CH_2
(1b) R = Me, A = S, SO, SO_2

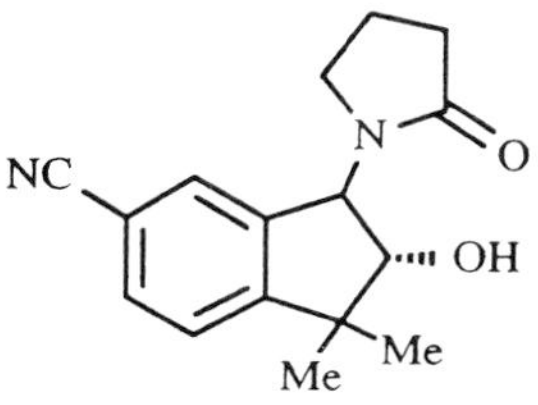

(2)

Position 2

The presence of a *gem*-dimethyl group at this position was found to be a critical feature for activity (Ashwood *et al.*, 1986) as the equivalent dihydro-chroman was virtually devoid of antihypertensive activity. The compound with a single methyl group of indeterminate stereochemistry had intermediate activity. The essential role of the *gem*-dimethyl group for activity is not easily understood, although it was proposed (Ashwood *et al.*, 1986) that it prevented an unwanted metabolic attack at this position. However, this seems an unlikely explanation as the activity differences are also seen *in vitro*. Conformational differences, or binding of the *gem*-dimethyl group to a hydrophobic site may be of importance. Interestingly, compounds containing spirocycloalkyl groups have been found to be much less potent than those possessing a dimethyl group (Lang & Wenk, 1988; Bergmann & Gericke, 1990).

Although the *gem*-dimethyl group is evinced to be a critical feature for high potency in both the benzopyran (Ashwood *et al.*, 1986) and indane (Buckle *et al.*, 1991a) series of KCAs, the nitrobenzoxepine (3) without this group retained about one-tenth the potency of the 6-nitro analogue of cromakalim (Webster & Cassidy, 1988).

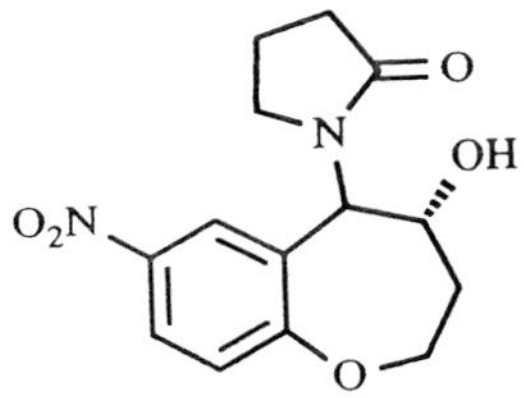

(3)

Position 3

The hydroxyl group at this position was shown to be a necessary feature for good activity, as replacement by a hydrogen atom lowered activity (Ashwood *et al.*, 1986). Esterification retained activity (Ashwood *et al.*, 1986; Houge-Frydrych & Evans, 1989; Bergmann & Gericke, 1990), as did oxidation to the ketone (Buckle *et al.*, 1991b), whereas replacement by a whole range of other substituents (Buckle *et al.*, 1991b) attenuated activity quite markedly. An approximate order of potency based on these reports is:

OH, OCOH, ONO_2 > OCOMe, =O, H $\gg$ CH_2OH, COOMe, F,

NO_2, CHO, CH_2OMe, CH_2F, pyrrolidinone

One of the most interesting developments at this position has been made (Stemp, 1990) by incorporating a substituted amide or urea group in combination with a *trans* hydroxyl group at C(4). Certain of these novel structures, such as (4), are reported to be about as potent as cromakalim. This transposition of the amide and hydroxyl groups has resulted in a series of benzopyrans with different SARs about the carbonyl-containing substituent to those found in the cromakalim series, and it remains to be seen whether these structural changes will result in any differences in profile compared to cromakalim.

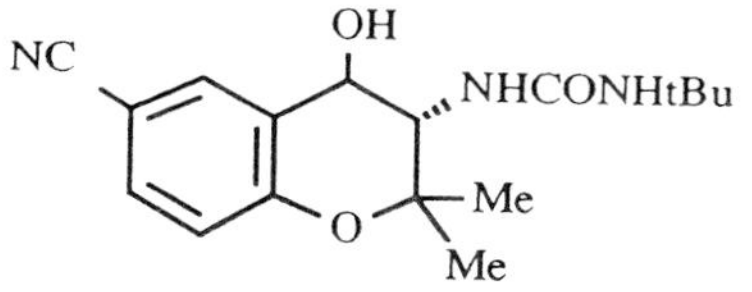

(4)

Position 4

Variation in the group attached to the benzopyran nucleus at this position has proved to be a fertile area of investigation, with several compounds bearing groups other than the pyrrolidinone of cromakalim, being progressed to the clinic.

Lactams (Ashwood *et al.*, 1986) were more than twice as potent as the original equivalent cyclic amines (Evans *et al.*, 1983). However, the amines showed only weak activity *in vitro* and it is possible that they are metabolized to the corresponding lactams *in vivo*. The size of the lactam ring was found to have an important effect on potency (Ashwood *et al.*, 1986; Buckle *et al.*, 1990), the approximate order being:

6-membered > 5-membered ≫ 4, 7 or 8-membered rings

Unsaturation has been introduced into the six-membered lactam (Bergmann & Gericke, 1990; Buckle *et al.*, 1990), the pyridone group conferring similar potency to the piperidinone group. Two examples of KCAs containing the former group, EMD 52692 and EMD 56431, are being progressed for angina pectoris and hypertension (Sombroek *et al.*, 1990). Unsaturation has also been introduced into the five-membered lactam ring, the enol ether (5) being described as the most potent of the series (Genain & Pinhas, 1990), but comparative data with cromakalim were not presented.

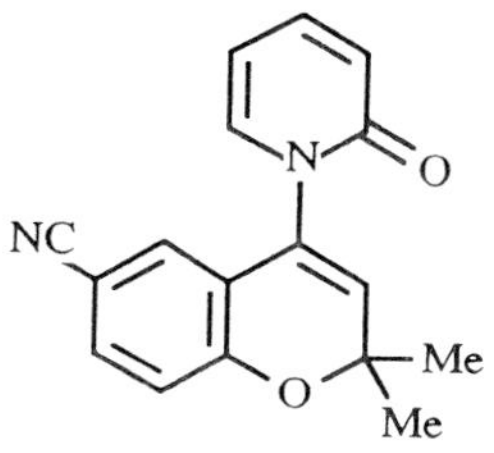

EMD 52692

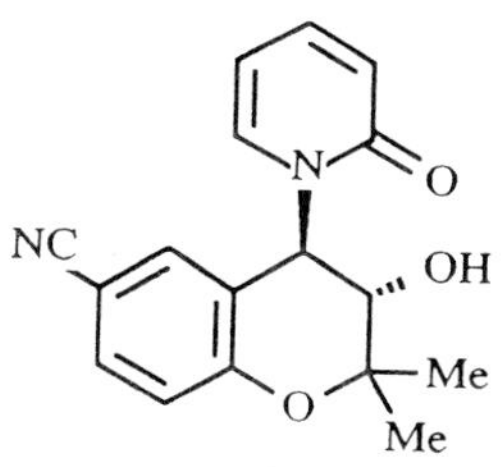

EMD 56431

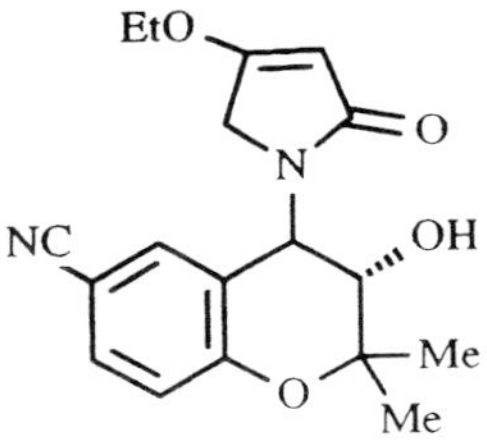

(5)

Incorporation of additional heteroatoms into the pyrrolidinone, piperidinone and pyridone groups tended to lower potency, although they still provide reasonably potent KCAs (Ashwood *et al.*, 1986; Bergmann & Gericke, 1990). Approximate orders of activity in the three series are presented in Fig. 13.1.

The position of the carbonyl group in the C(4) cyclic substituent has been varied (Bergmann & Gericke, 1990), and the 4-oxopiperidinyl analogue found to be virtually inactive compared with the 2-oxopiperidinyl compound, whereas in marked contrast, in the unsaturated series the 4-pyridonyl compound possessed significant activity (Fig. 13.2). No explanation for this interesting difference was given.

In general, substituents on the lactam ring do not enhance potency, the one notable exception being a methyl group at C(5') in the pyrrolidinone ring. The 3S,4R,5'R/3R,4S,5'S racemate (6) is reported (Englert *et al.*, 1988a; Bartmann, 1989) to be twice as potent as cromakalim in lowering blood pressure. As the activity of cromakalim resides predominantly in the 3S,4R enantiomer, it is presumed that the activity of (6) resides in the 3S,4R,5'R enantiomer. Thus the 5'R methyl substituent appears to be responsible for the doubling of activity. Interestingly, S 0121, the (−)-3R,4S,5'R enantiomer, which contains the 3R,4S-stereochemistry that might be expected not to confer blood pressure lowering activity, is reported to reduce the amplitude of spontaneous contractions of the guinea-pig isolated ureter smooth muscle. Hence S 0121 might have an application in easing the passage of kidney stones through the ureter.

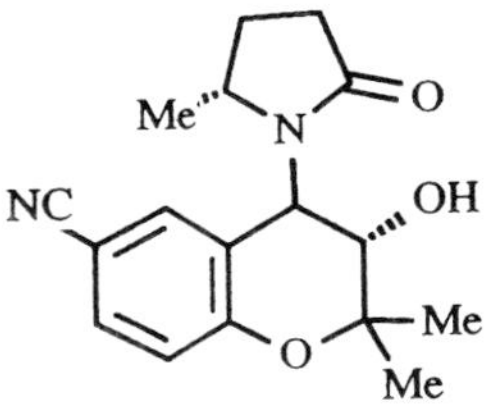

(6)

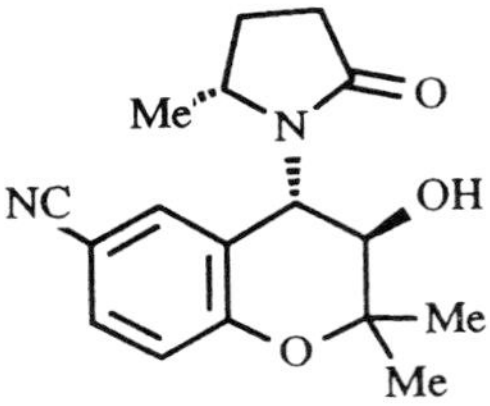

S 0121

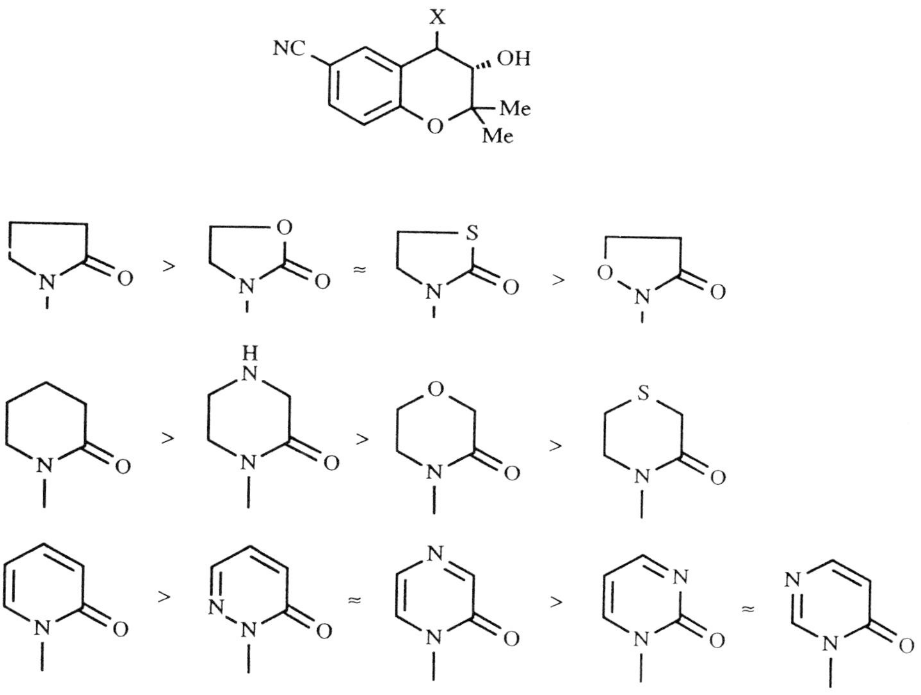

Fig. 13.1. Approximate orders of activity in substituted lactams.

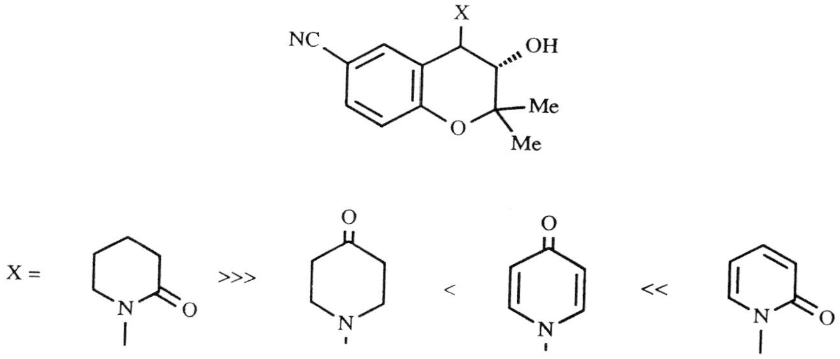

Fig. 13.2. Effect of lactam carbonyl position on activity.

Compounds have been described with a benzene ring fused to the lactam ring, as in for example, the isoindolone substituent in WAY-120 491 (celikalim). The homologous isoquinolone substituent in structure (7) was reported (Ashwood & Evans, 1986) to confer less activity than the piperidinone moiety.

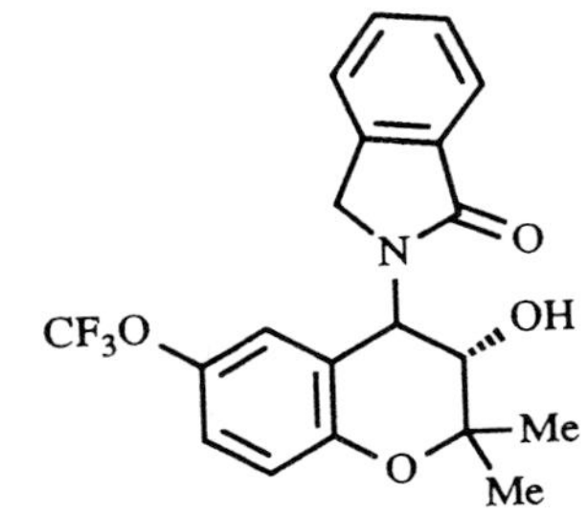

WAY-120 491 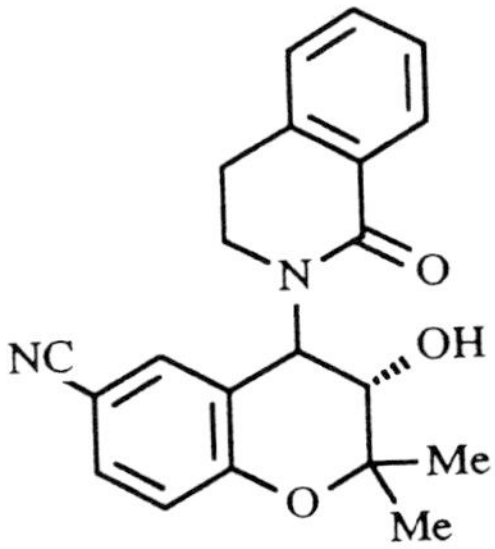   (7)

The lactam ring can be replaced by an acyclic amide group (8). Optimal activity, similar to that of cromakalim, was found for the acetamide (8, R_1 = H, R_2 = Me) (Ashwood et al., 1990). The corresponding formamide (8, R_1 = R_2 = H) and analogues with larger R_1 and R_2 alkyl groups were less potent. However, good activity was found for a series of benzamides such as compound (8, R_1 = H, R_2 = Ph). In the benzamide, the phenyl ring could be replaced by certain other heteroaryl rings, with optimal activity found for 2-, or 3-furyl and 2-pyrrolyl rings.

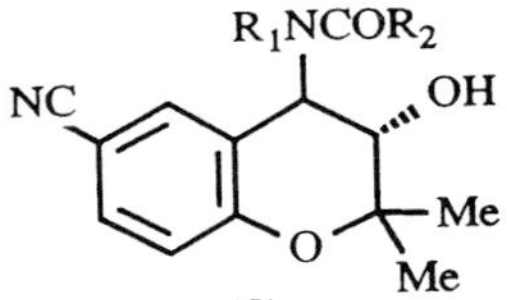

(8)

A urea (9) (Ashwood et al., 1990) or a cyanoguanidine (10) (Burrell et al., 1990b) group can be incorporated in place of an acyclic amide with retention of activity. Interestingly, a phenyl-substituted cyanoguanidine (11) was stated (Atwal et al., 1990a) to demonstrate little or no vasodilator activity, but to possess anti-ischaemic properties. A closely related cyclic analogue of the cyanoguanidine, a cyanoiminothiazolidine substituent has been incorporated into the benzopyran FR 119748, which is described as being about twice as potent as cromakalim (Shiokawa et al., 1989). Acylated hydrazines such as (12) have also been reported to be approximately equipotent to cromakalim (Yamanaka et al., 1989).

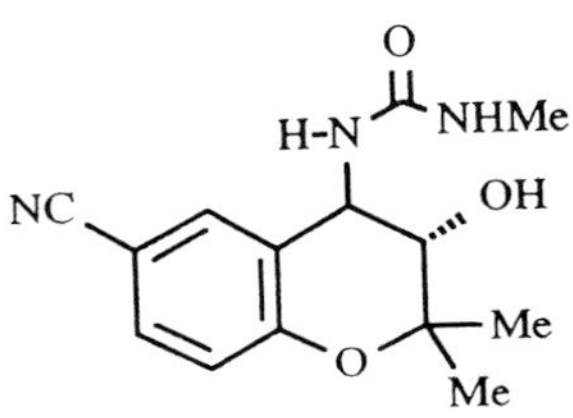

(9) 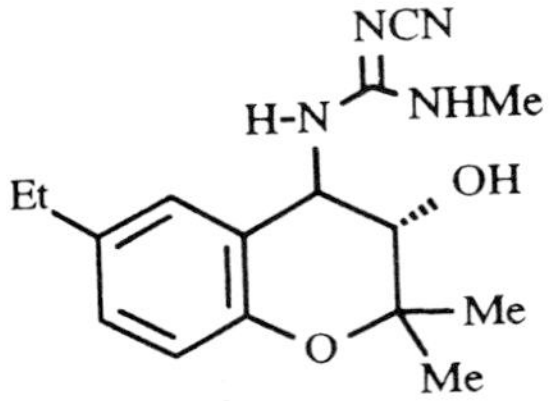   (10)

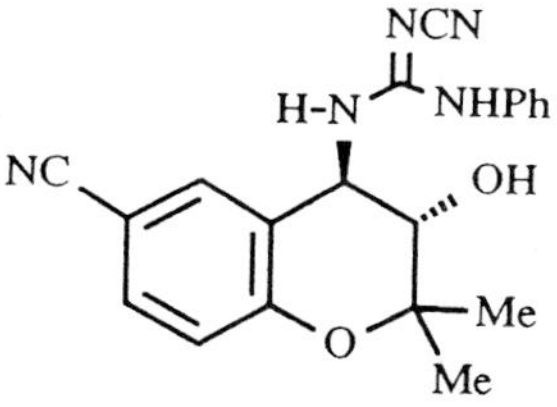

(11)

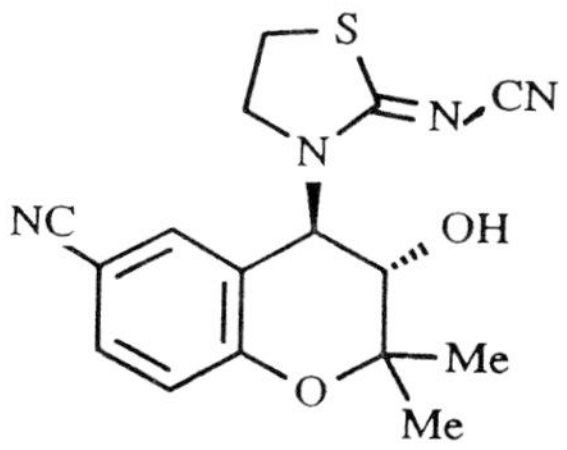

FR 119748

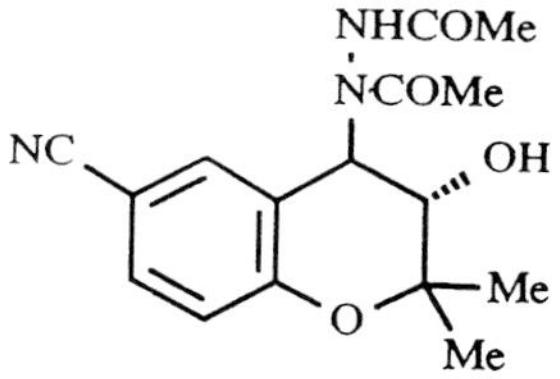

(12)

Conversion of amide carbonyl groups to thiocarbonyl groups gave thiapyrrolidinones and thioamides of equivalent potency, whereas thioureas were less potent (Ashwood *et al.*, 1990).

In certain compounds such as SDZ PCO 400 an oxygen link has been successfully employed. SDZ PCO 400 is reported to be equipotent with cromakalim, but with a longer half-life in a monkey model (Fozard *et al.*, 1990). Interestingly, SDZ PCO 400 has been reported (Dunne, 1990) to inhibit K_{ATP}-channels in pancreatic insulin secreting cells. Cromakalim, and other KCAs such as RP 49356 and pinacidil open such channels but only at very high concentrations ($> 100\,\mu\text{M}$), suggesting that at therapeutically administered doses these compounds will relax smooth muscle cells without having effects upon the regulation of insulin secretion. These observations indicate that there is a degree of structural diversity in ATP-sensitive channels from different tissues. The carbonyl groups in cromakalim and SDZ PCO 400 occupy different positions in space, and it is interesting to speculate that this structural difference may account for their different profile in pancreatic cells. Another ether, EMD 57283 was found to be more potent and longer acting than cromakalim in SHR (Bergmann *et al.*, 1990).

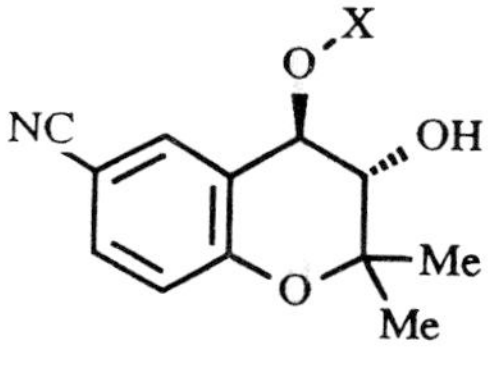

X =

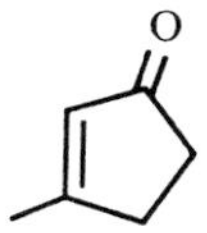

SDZ PCO 400

X =

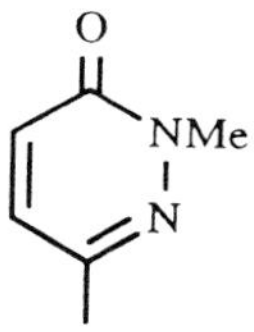

EMD 57283

EMD 57283 is an example of a tightly defined series of which the 6-oxo-1-methyl-3-pyridazinyloxy and 2-oxo-1-methyl-4-pyridyloxy groups (see Fig. 13.3) confer the optimal potency, possibly due to an inability to tautomerize.

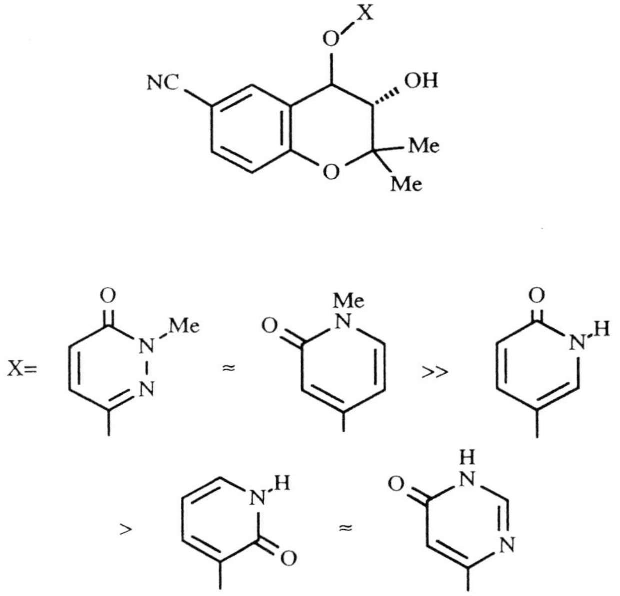

Fig. 13.3. Compounds linked by oxygen to benzopyran ring.

Besides the oxygen link to cyclic moieties, an amino-linked heterocycle has been successfully employed in a KCA, the aminotriazole (13) group causing an approximate threefold increase in potency over cromakalim (Burrell & Stemp, 1990). In contrast to the oxygen-linked compounds described above, it is intriguing to note that (13) does not contain a carbonyl group in the C(4) substituent. In addition, certain amino-linked substituted phenyl chromans and chromenes have been described, as in for example, SR 46276 (Garcia et al., 1990), as useful antidepressants, with little or no effect on the cardiovascular system.

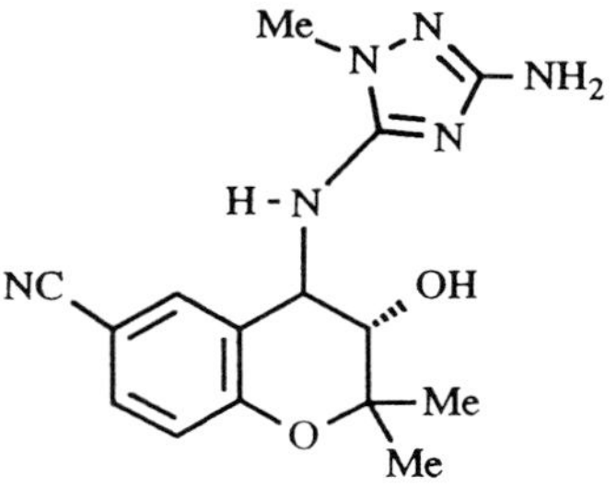

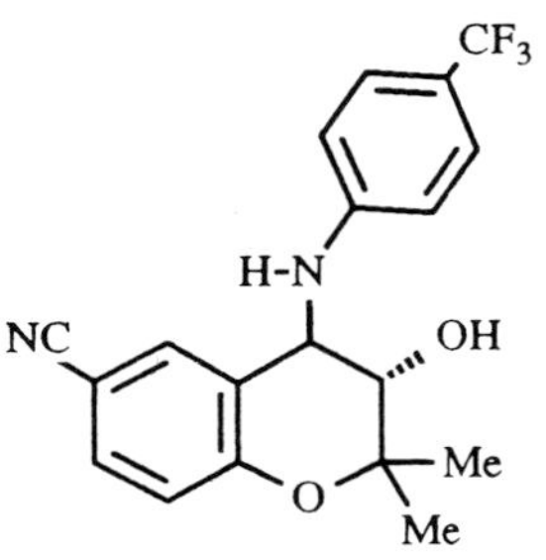

In a different approach, a 2-pyridyl N-oxide has been linked directly to the chromene nucleus in Ro 31-6930. This compound is reported to be an order of magnitude more potent than cromakalim in rat models, although, unlike cromakalim, it did not reduce renal vascular resistance in the anaesthetized dog (Paciorek *et al.*, 1990). In the anaesthetized rat, however, both compounds reduced renal vascular resistance but only cromakalim exerted a selective action on the renal vascular bed (Duty *et al.*, 1990). The importance of the *N*-oxide group is illustrated by its replacement by a phenolic hydroxy group which resulted in an approximate 100-fold decrease in potency. Presumably the *N*-oxide in this molecule is behaving as a carbonyl equivalent (Attwood *et al.*, 1988).

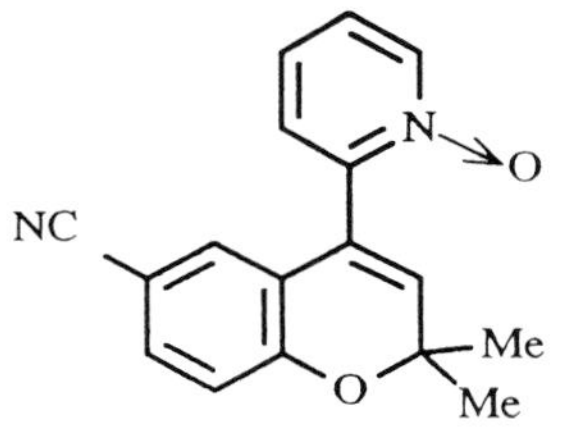

Ro 31-6930

Positions 3/4

The effects of varying the orientation of the substituents at C(3) and C(4) were discussed earlier.

Removal of the elements of water across these positions to give the achiral chromenes provides compounds of variable activity compared with the corresponding chroman-3-ols. Thus it was reported (Ashwood *et al.*, 1986) that the activity and SARs of chromenes of close analogues of cromakalim, for example compound (14), paralleled that of the chroman-3-ols, whereas in a single example of an acyclic amide, the 4-acetylamino derivative, the chromene was less potent than the chroman-3-ol (Ashwood *et al.*, 1990).

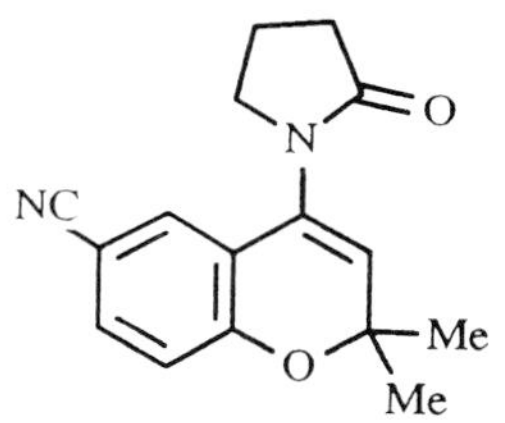

(14)

In contrast to these findings, the antihypertensive activity of chromenes related to EMD 52692 was significantly enhanced in most cases when compared with the corresponding racemic chromanols (Bergmann & Gericke, 1990; Buckle *et al.*, 1990), but in the O-linked series related to EMD 57283, chromene equivalents did not display any significant activity

(Bergmann *et al.*, 1990). It is also interesting to note that the tetra-hydronaphthalen-3-ol equivalent of cromakalim was less potent than the equivalent dihydronaphthalene (Ashwood *et al.*, 1990).

Aromatic substituents

The position and nature of substituents in the aromatic ring are of prime importance in influencing activity (Ashwood *et al.*, 1986). The optimal position for a substituent is at position C(6). Substitution at position C(7) can also result in potent compounds, but substitution at positions C(5) and C(8) generally results in little activity.

A propensity to high potency is associated with the presence of a strong electron withdrawing group at C(6) (Ashwood *et al.*, 1986), an approximate ranking for conferring activity being:

NO_2, CN > COMe > CO_2Me > CHO, Cl > H

More recently, the incorporation of the trifluoromethyl (Buckle *et al.*, 1990; Burrell *et al.*, 1990), and pentafluoroethyl groups (Smith *et al.*, 1990) has been reported to give KCAs of high potency. Another fluorine containing group, the trifluoromethoxy group, has been utilized in WAY-120,491 which is less potent than cromakalim (Morin *et al.*, 1990).

Surprisingly, it has been found (Burrell *et al.*, 1990) that chromanols containing alkyl groups at position C(6) are potent KCAs with the 6-ethyl analogue of cromakalim showing one-third of the latter's potency. Thus it appears that an electron-withdrawing substituent at C(6) is not obligatory. The dimensions of the alkyl group have some influence on the degree of activity, an approximate order of activity being:

ethyl, isopropyl, *t*-butyl > *n*-propyl, cyclopentyl > methyl > phenyl

Although attachment of the phenyl group at C(6) provided little activity (Burrell *et al.*, 1990), the interposition of a sulphonyl group, thus converting it to an electron-withdrawing substituent, gave compound (15) which was more potent than cromakalim as a coronary blood flow enhancer (Englert *et al.*, 1988b). In addition the 3S,4R enantiomer, HOE 234, of compound (15) has been shown (Klaus *et al.*, 1990a) to be a more potent vasodilator than cromakalim in a variety of *in vitro* smooth muscle preparations.

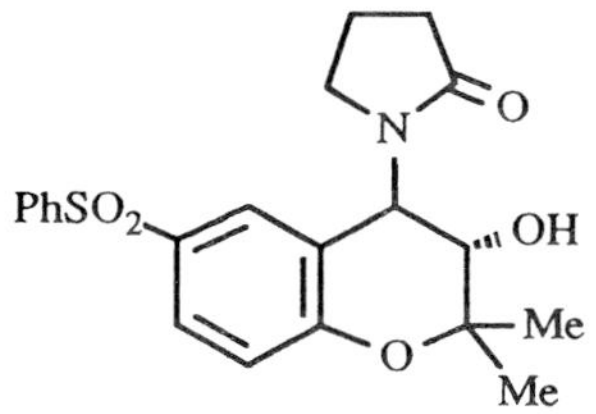

(15)

The finding that KCAs containing a substituent at C(6) or C(7) are the most potent has prompted limited investigations of examples of benzo-pyranols containing substituents at both these positions. Thus incorporation of an acetylamino, or amino substituent at C(7) in a 6-nitro compound enhanced potency, whereas the reverse combination demonstrated a reduced potency (Ashwood *et al.*, 1986). In contrast to the pairing of an electron-withdrawing and an electron-donating group, two examples, the 6-bromo-7-nitro-, and 6-cyano-7-nitro-benzopyrans showed that the combination of two electron-withdrawing groups is the most potent substitution pattern (Ashwood *et al.*, 1990). Although certain combinations of substituents clearly enhance antihypertensive activity, the addition of a C(7) methoxy group to the phenylsulphonyl KCA (15) lowered its coronary blood flow enhancing activity (Englert *et al.*, 1988b).

Aromatic replacements

Heteroaryl replacements for the phenyl ring of benzopyran based KCAs have been made. Thus pyranopyridine and pyranopyridine *N*-oxides have been prepared after a study of electrostatic potentials (Plates 13.1 & 13.2) indicated that the pyrano[3,2-c]pyridine (16), with the nitrogen atom at the key C(6) position, was a potential replacement for the 6-cyano benzopyran nucleus in KCAs of the cromakalim type (Burrell *et al.*, 1990).

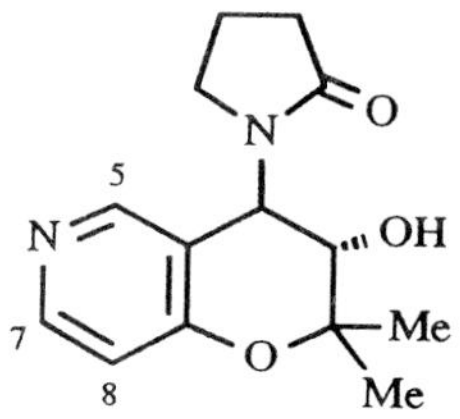

(16)

The position of the nitrogen atom was an important characteristic, as in parallel with the observation (previous section) that substituents in benzopyran KCAs must be located at certain positions for optimal activity, the order of activity in pyranopyridines was found to be:

(6-CN) = 6-N, 6-N → O > 7-N > 5-N, 8-N

This ranking may explain, in part, the lower potency of the 7-trifluoro-pyrano[2,3-b]pyridine (17) (Lang & Wenk, 1988) in comparison with cromakalim.

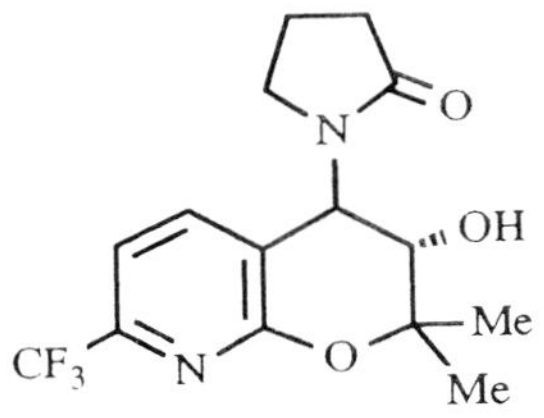

(17)

Substituted thiophene replacements have also been disclosed (Press *et al.*, 1990), particularly the 2-nitrothiophene analogue (18) in which the nitro substituent is required for high potency, as the compound lacking this feature is more than 100-fold less potent. Presumably, the 2-nitro substituent is performing a similar rôle to an electron-withdrawing substituent at C(6) or C(7) of a benzopyran KCA.

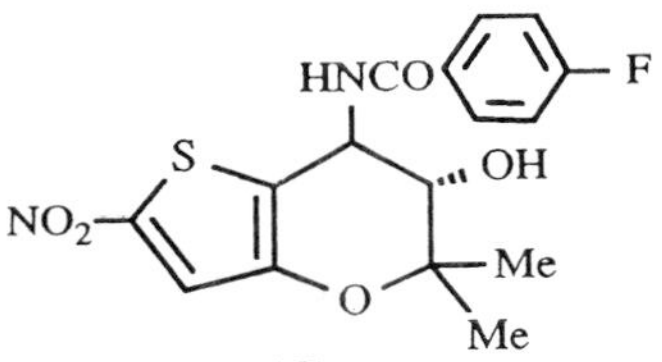

(18)

Replacement of the 6-cyanophenyl group of cromakalim with the benzoxadiazole ring system of NIP 121 (Arakawa *et al.*, 1990) enhances potency by an order of magnitude over cromakalim. It is interesting that the additional ring is fused at the important C(6) and C(7) positions of the benzopyran.

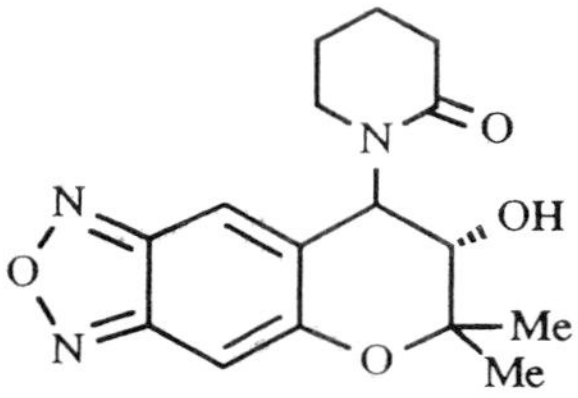

NIP 121

Pyridine/pyrimidine KCAs

Pinacidil

This compound, developed from a series of hypotensive thioureas (Petersen *et al.*, 1978), was shown to belong to the class of KCAs (Southerton *et al.*, 1988) after the discovery of the mode of action of cromakalim. Structure–activity relationship studies were concentrated on the position of attachment of the side chain to the pyridine ring, the nature of the group X, and the type of alkyl substituent R in general formula (19).

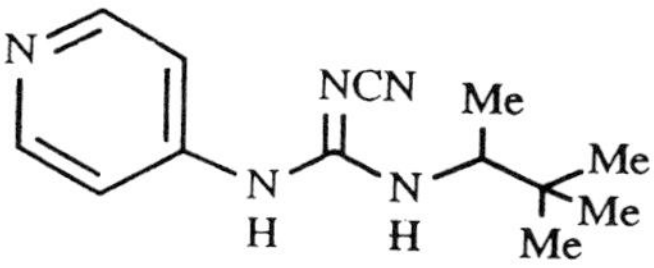

PINACIDIL

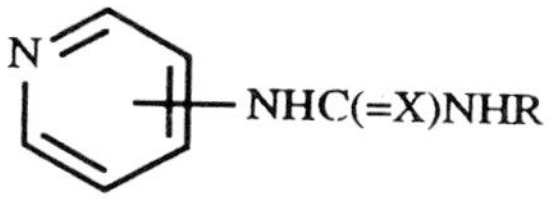

NHC(=X)NHR

(19)

The majority of the 3-pyridyl compounds were found to be up to 20-fold more potent than the 4-pyridyl analogues, and less toxic, with the exception of pinacidil itself which was defined as twice as potent as its corresponding 3-pyridyl isomer. Examples of 2-pyridyl compounds were at least 200 times less potent than their 3-pyridyl counterparts. Substitution in the 3-pyridyl ring generally caused a marked decline in activity, the one exception being a C(5) bromine atom insertion which only lowered potency about 5-fold.

In the 3-pyridyl series, the thiourea (X = S) was found to be more potent than the corresponding urea (X = O), while the cyanoguanidine (X = N—CN) was about 200 times as potent as the thiourea. Replacement of the cyano segment of the cyanoguanidine group by a variety of other groups such as OH, OMe, CO_2Et and $CONH_2$ only gave compounds of weak activity.

Optimal activity for the group R was found to be associated with a branched alkyl group of four or five carbon atoms. In contrast, unbranched alkyl, cycloalkyl, phenyl or benzyl group insertion gave weakly active compounds. An approximate ranking order of potency ascribed to the group R in the 3-pyridyl series is:

t-Bu, t-C_5H_{11} > CH(Me)CMe_3 > i-Pr, neo C_5H_{11} > Ph > CH_2Ph, n-Bu, cyclopentyl

Although pinacidil was described (Petersen et al., 1978) as approximately twice as potent as its 3-pyridyl analogue LY 222 675 as an antihypertensive agent, it was found (Weston et al., 1988) that the order of potency was reversed in inhibition of 20 μM KCl-induced contractions and in ^{86}Rb efflux studies in the isolated rat portal vein. Supporting data were presented (Robertson & Steinberg, 1990b) for this finding, on the basis of an ability to relax phenylephrine-induced contractions in the canine cephalic vein. In this test the (−)-enantiomer is reported to be about six times as potent as the racemate LY 222 675, and about eightfold more potent than (racemic) pinacidil. It is not known how these data compare with those for the (−)-R, biologically active, enantiomer of pinacidil which has recently been disclosed (Edwards & Weston, 1990).

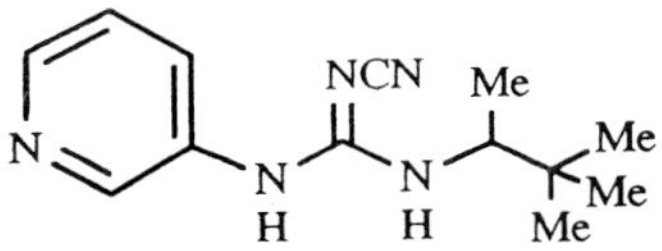

LY 222675

A noteworthy observation is that following the replacement of the substituted aromatic ring in cromakalim by an appropriately located pyridine ring, the converse has been achieved in both pinacidil and RP 49356 (see below). Thus a patent divulges (Atwal *et al.*, 1990b) compounds such as (20), but no data were presented to support any equivalence of the aromatic groups.

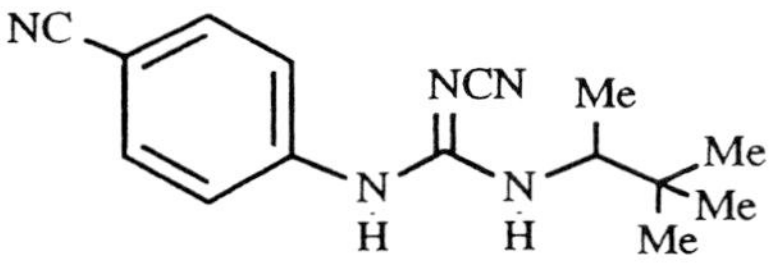

(20)

RP 49356

This KCA, derived from a series originally developed as potential inhibitors of K^+/H^+ ATPase is reported to be about as potent as cromakalim in SHR (Mondot *et al.*, 1989), but only one-third as potent in suppressing the spontaneous type of guinea-pig trachea (Berry *et al.*, 1991). Biological activity resides mainly in the $(-)$-1R,2R-enantiomer RP 52891 (Aloup *et al.*, 1990). Analogues of RP 49356 have been reported, and from the limited data available on their ability to inhibit 20 mм KCl-induced contractions in the rat isolated aorta preparation (Cook *et al.*, 1989a–c; Palfreyman *et al.*, 1990), some approximate SARs have been deduced. In those instances where *cis/trans* geometry in the thiopyran group can exist, the *trans* (as in RP 49356) isomers were the more potent.

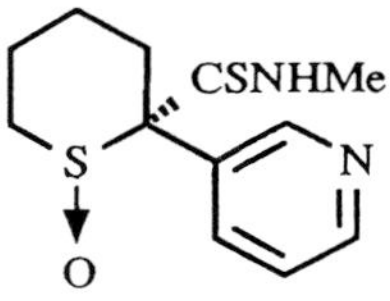

RP 49356

In a series of cyclohexane analogues (21) the sulphoxide group of RP 49356 has been replaced by carbonyl, oxime, methylene, imino, hydroxyl or substituted alkyl groups, but these substituents served only to attenuate activity.

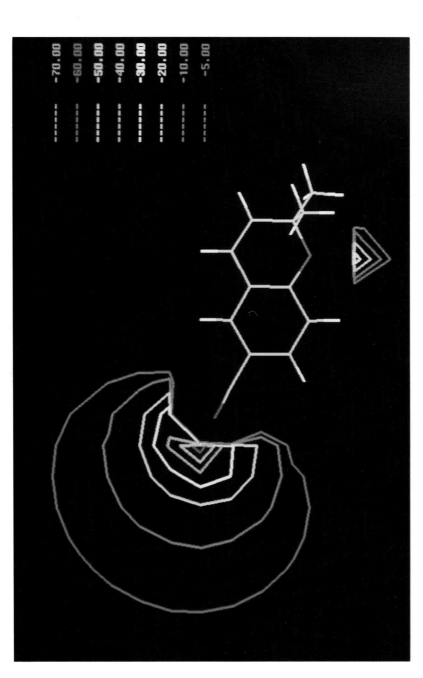

Plate 13.1. Two-dimensional electrostatic potential map of 6-cyano-2,2-dimethyl-2H-1-benzopyran (Plate 13 2 shows 2,2-dimethyl-2H-pyrano[3,2-c]pyridine). Both maps were generated using the *ab initio* program GAMESS and displayed on a Silicon Graphics Iris workstation. The contour levels are in kcal/mol and show the areas around each molecule that are attractive towards a point positive charge.

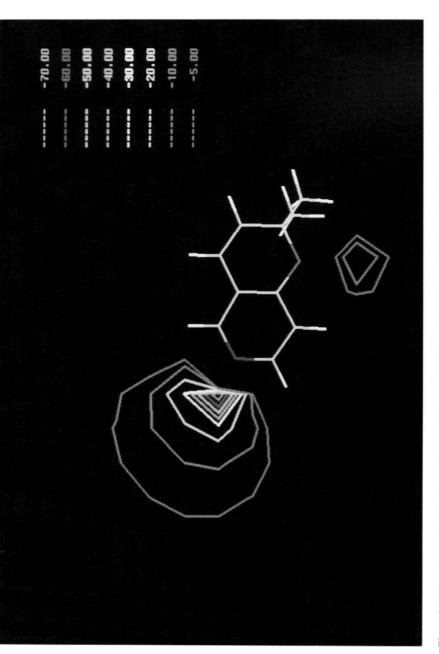

Plate 13.2. Two-dimensional electrostatic potential map of 2,2-dimethyl-2*H*-pyrano[3,2-c]pyridine. See caption to Plate 13.1 for further details.

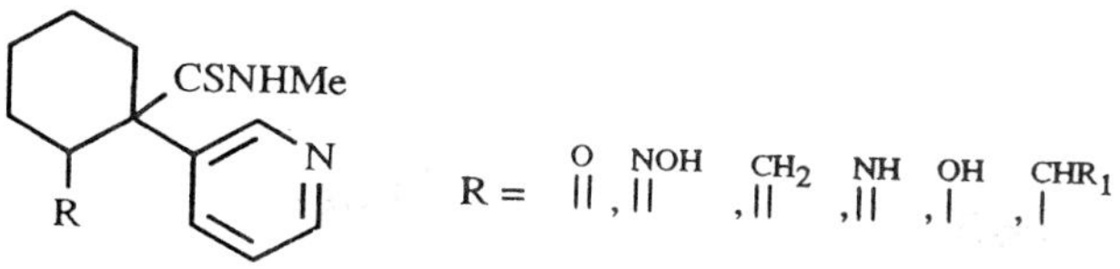

(21)

However, substitution on certain of these groups can enhance potency, thus the phenylthio methylene group in structure (22) confers almost a 1000-fold increase in potency compared with the methylene parent, and appears to be one of the most potent compounds in the series. Both O-methyl and O-benzyl oximes are more potent than the parent oxime.

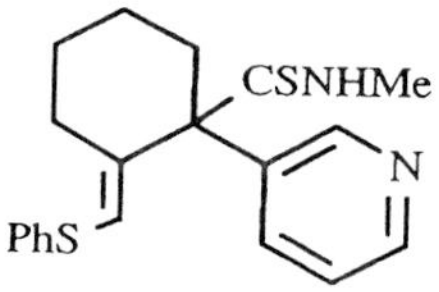

(22)

Replacement of the pyridine ring by a benzene ring results in a loss of potency, but incorporation of electron-withdrawing substituents can restore activity, an approximate ranking of substituents by activity being:

$3,4\text{-Cl}_2 > 3\text{-NO}_2, 3\text{-CF}_3 > 3\text{-CN} > 4\text{-Cl} > H$

Fusion of a second ring to the benzene or pyridine ring enhances activity. Thus a 2-naphthyl substituent provides for greater activity than does a phenyl group, while a 3-quinolyl group enhances activity over a 3-pyridyl group. Both ring contraction of the saturated ring to a five-membered ring, and extension of the alkyl group flanking the thioamide group maintain the activity of the series.

Minoxidil sulphate

The enzyme O-sulphotransferase converts minoxidil *in vivo* to the sulphate, which was recognized as a KCA after the elucidation of the mechanism of action of cromakalim. Some preliminary X-ray data and limited SAR data are available (McCall *et al.*, 1983) on modifications of the piperidine ring. Replacement by methylamino or dialkylamino groups results in a decline in potency, the latter being about 30-fold less potent. Ring contraction to pyrrolidine reduced potency by about a 100-fold, while its replacement by the morpholine group lowered potency some 50 times.

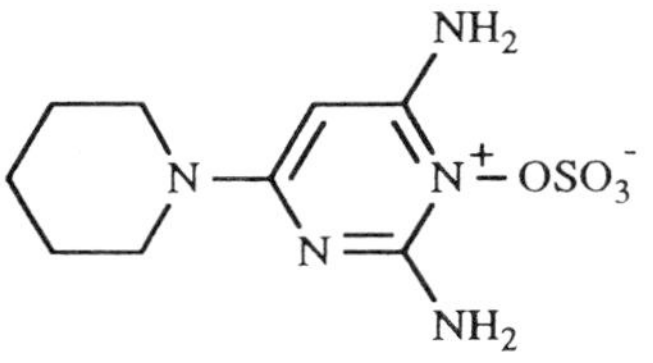

MINOXIDIL SULPHATE

Although minoxidil sulphate has been classed as a KCA, being about 30-fold less potent than cromakalim in abolishing spontaneous contractions in the rat portal vein (Winquist *et al.*, 1989), significant differences between it and cromakalim have emerged. Thus, for example minoxidil sulphate, unlike cromakalim did not relax oxytocin induced spasm in isolated rat uterus (Piper & Hollingsworth, 1991). In contrast (Newgreen *et al.* 1990), both KCAs relaxed 20 mM KCl-induced contractions in a rat thoracic aorta preparation, although it was shown that the K-channel opening action of minoxidil sulphate was not associated with the opening of an ^{86}Rb permeable K-channel.

Diazoxide

This compound, developed from a series of sulphamoyl-substituted 2H-1,2,4-benzothiadiazino 1,1-dioxide diuretics, was recently discovered (Quast & Cook, 1989) to be a KCA possessing about a hundredth the potency of cromakalim. Limited SAR data are available (Topliss *et al.*, 1963, 1964) from studies of i.v. administration to mongrel dogs, but precise correlations are not available due to the different methods of reporting the data in the two publications.

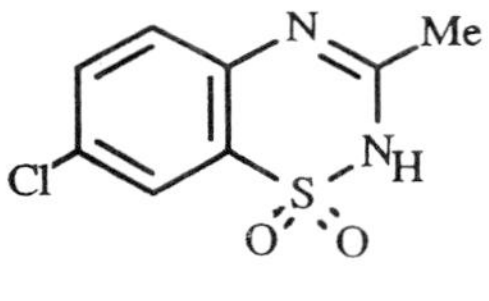

DIAZOXIDE

Substitution on the nitrogen atoms at positions 2 and 4 by alkyl groups attenuated activity. At C(3), however, variation of the methyl group produced a variable response. Its removal resulted in a reduction in potency, whereas the ethyl analogue was more potent. Further chain extension resulted in a reduction in potency, although strangely, potency was restored with the n-pentyl analogue. Branching of the alkyl group at the α-carbon atom enhanced potency. An approximate order of activity appears to be:

Et ⩾ Me, *n*-Pr, *n*-pentyl, *t*-Bu > *n*-Bu.

Alkenyl groups conferred either equal or less activity than their saturated counterparts. In general, substituents in alkyl chains at C(3) caused a decline in potency, as only the methoxymethyl group retained reasonable activity. Alkyl group replacement by aryl or heteroaryl moieties yielded compounds of negligible activity. Compounds containing the double bond at positions 3 and 4 were generally more potent than the corresponding saturated analogues. With regard to aromatic substitution it was established that a chlorine, bromine or trifluoromethyl substituent at C(6) or C(7) provided optimal activity.

Compounds with mixed actions

Nicorandil

This was the first compound to be shown to increase membrane K^+ ion conductance in vascular smooth muscle cells (Furukawa et al., 1981), although it was subsequently disclosed to have the additional property of activation of soluble guanylate cyclase (Holzmann, 1983).

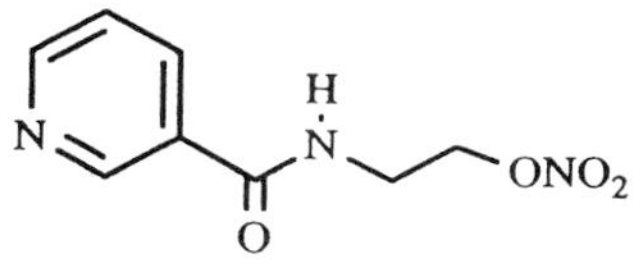

NICORANDIL

A small amount of structural variation has been described (Inoue et al., 1984) based on the ability of three additional analogues to inhibit K^+-induced contraction of the canine mesenteric artery. Basically, the parent alcohol, and a 3-pyridyl ester of the alcohol were inactive, while the additional side chain in SG 114 conferred higher potency than that observed for nicorandil.

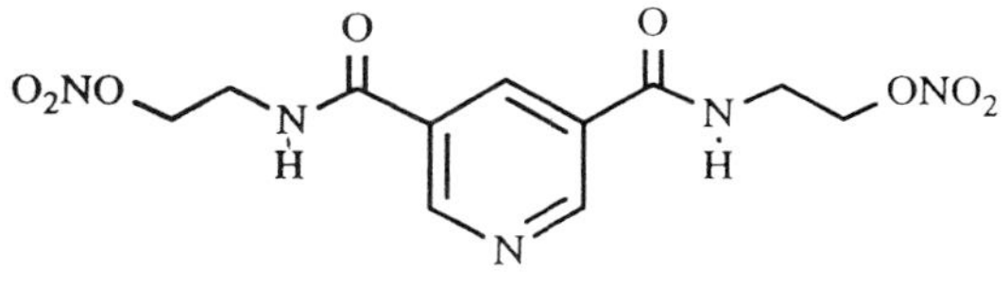

SG 114

KRN 2391

The structure of this compound bears a close resemblance to nicorandil. Nevertheless, KRN 2391 has a 30-fold potency advantage in lowering blood pressure, on i.v. administration to anaesthetized dogs. It is also claimed to be 3-fold more potent than cromakalim in the same model (Kaneta et al., 1990).

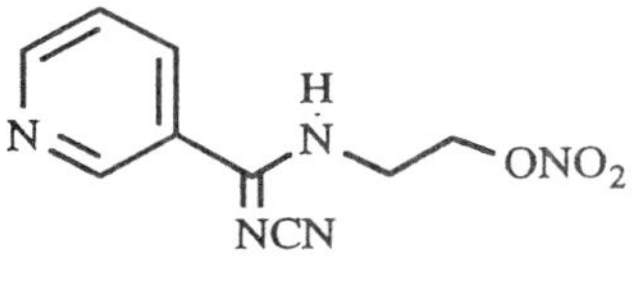

KRN 2391

Niguldipine

Low concentrations of this Ca- channel blocking agent were also reported to increase K^+ ion currents in isolated vascular smooth muscle cells, with the property being restricted to the (+)-enantiomer (Klöckner et al., 1989).

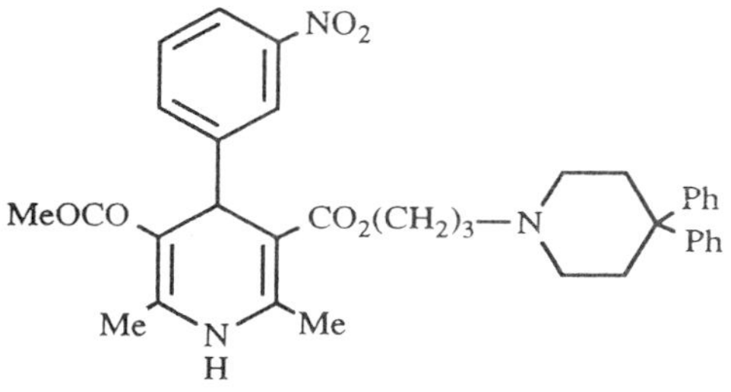

NIGULDIPINE

Forskolin

The relaxant effect of this compound in vascular smooth muscle has been ascribed to activation of adenylate cyclase and K-channel opening (Klaus et al., 1990b).

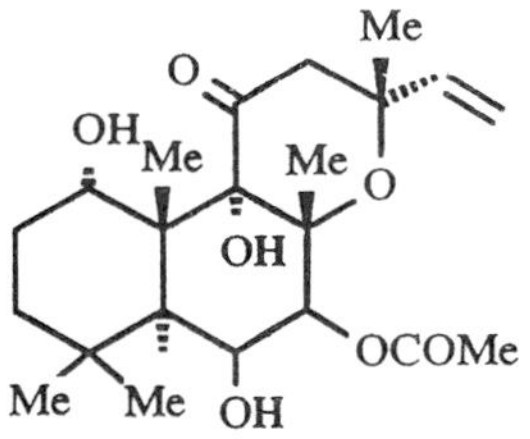

FORSKOLIN

E 4080

The vasodilating effect of this recently disclosed compound in isolated vascular smooth muscle of rat and guinea-pig, has been compared with cromakalim (Ogawa et al., 1990), and found to be an order of magnitude less potent. Studies using glibenclamide indicated the similarity of action of the two compounds.

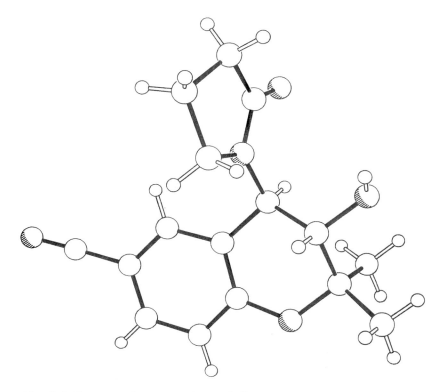

E 4080

Conformational studies on KCAs

Conformational analysis of drug molecules plays an important role in understanding their binding to receptors, and some preliminary reports on the conformational behaviour of the benzopyran class of KCA have recently appeared.

X-ray crystal analysis of cromakalim (Cassidy *et al.*, 1989) showed the conformation displayed in Fig. 13.4, where the pyrrolidinone ring is orthogonal to the benzopyran ring, and with the pyrrolidinone carbonyl group on the same side of the benzopyran ring as H(4).

The same conformation was found to predominate in solution in

Fig. 13.4. X-ray crystal structure of cromakalim.

CDCl$_3$ using nuclear magnetic resonance (NMR) techniques. Thus, from studies of nuclear Overhauser enhancement (NOE) differences and ^{13}C relaxation times, it was suggested that the pyrrolidinone ring was not rotating about the C(4)—N bond. The barrier to rotation about the bond was also investigated using semi-empirical molecular orbital calculations. The most stable structure corresponded to that determined by X-ray crystallography, although another minimum energy conformation was found at 210° from the X-ray structure. The difference in energy between these two minimum energy conformations was calculated to be 2.4 kcal/mol (10.1 kJ/mol), and it was concluded that with such a small energy difference either minimum could be close to the conformation adopted by cromakalim at its receptor.

A subsequent NMR study (Thomas & Whitcombe, 1990) at 400 MHz in CD$_3$OD confirmed the previously calculated energy difference between the two low energy conformers of cromakalim, and demonstrated their existence in solution at − 60°C. The barrier to rotation about the C(4)—N bond was also estimated from this experiment to be 11.5–13.5 kcal/mol (48.3–56.7 kJ/mol), indicating that fast rotation occurs about the C(4)—N bond at ambient temperature.

Similar NMR studies were also reported on compounds (23), the C(5′) methyl compound (6), and Ro 31-6930. For the piperidinone (23), two forms were observed in the ratio 88 : 12, with an energy difference of 1.2 kcal/mol (5 kJ/mol), and barrier to rotation about the C(4)—N bond of 16 kcal/mol (67.2 kJ/mol).

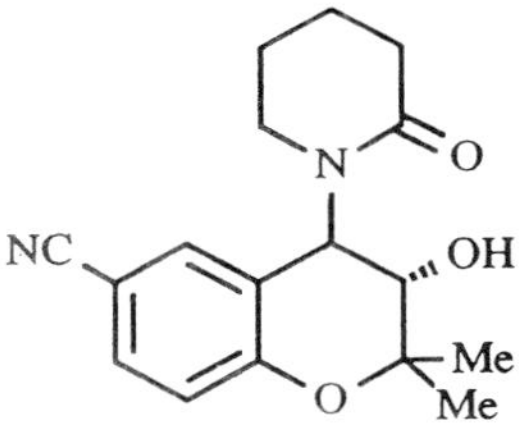

(23)

Incorporation of a 5′-methyl substituent in the pyrrolidinone ring of cromakalim (*see* benzopyran KCAs; position 4) as in compound (6) raised the barrier to rotation, but the NMR spectrum indicated that slow rotation was still occurring at room temperature.

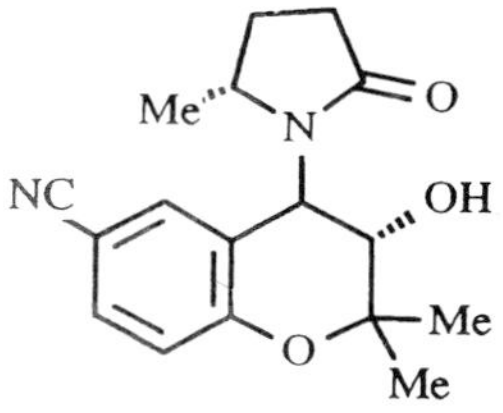

(6)

Low-temperature NMR studies on Ro 31-6930 indicated a barrier to rotation of 13 kcal/mol (54.5 kJ/mol) about the C(4)-pyridine N-oxide bond, but no further information was presented on rotamer populations in this molecule.

Limited evidence that the orientation of the amide carbonyl group at C(4) relative to the benzopyran ring is important in providing antihypertensive activity in this class of KCA has recently been presented (Ashwood et al., 1990). Compound (24) was found to be approximately threefold less potent than compound (25). Compound (24) showed two sets of signals in the ^{1}H NMR spectrum in dimethylsulphoxide, and variable temperature NMR showed that the signals coalesced at about 150°C, corresponding to an energy barrier to interconversion of 18–20 kcal/mol (75.5–84 kJ/mol). Since compound (25) showed only one set of signals in the NMR it was concluded that geometric isomerism about the tertiary amide bond in (24) was responsible for the effects observed in the NMR, and that the reduced potency of (24) was possibly due to the presence of an isomer lacking the required geometry about the amide bond.

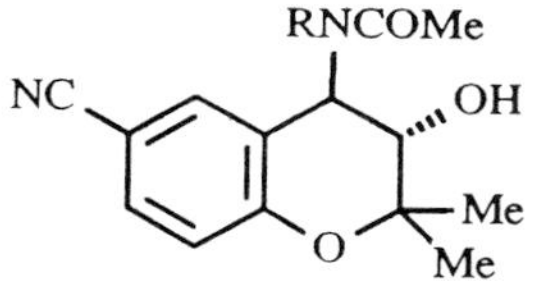

(24) R = Me

(25) R = H

Little information is available to date on the conformational analysis of non-benzopyran KCAs, although minimum energy conformations of pinacidil and cromakalim have been compared (Robertson & Steinberg, 1990a). Studies of this type are clearly underway with a view to identifying the features common to all KCAs, and ultimately the goal must be to use the information available from such studies to develop KCAs that are selective for a variety of different tissues.

Conclusions

This chapter has illustrated the advances in knowledge of SARs in KCAs made since the discovery of cromakalim. It has also described an increasingly diverse range of structural type in this class of compound, which encompasses not only novel molecules, but also some older drugs for which no mechanism had been previously assigned, as well as those compounds that rely on K-channel activation for a part of their pharmacological action. Finally, it has reviewed preliminary conformational studies that attempt to explain how KCA molecules may interact with their putative receptor(s).

Although a wide range of potential activities has been claimed for

KCAs, as yet only a few indications of selectivity have emerged. Extensive investigation is therefore required before useful selectivity is achieved, and SAR and conformational studies, as described in this chapter, are but a start in attaining such a goal.

References

Aloup, J. C., Farge, D., James, C., Mondot, S. & Cavero, I. (1990) 2-(3-Pyridyl)-tetra-hydrothiopyran-2-carbothioamide derivatives and analogues: a novel family of potent potassium channel openers. *Drugs of the Future* **15**, 1097–1108.

Arakawa, C., Yukinori, M., Yokoyama, T., Kawamura, N. & Tanaka, S. (1990) The antihypertensive effect of NIP 121, a novel potassium channel opener. *Japanese Journal of Pharmacology* **52** (suppl. 1), 311P.

Ashwood, V. A. & Evans, J. M. (1986) Chroman derivatives. *US Patent* 4,616,021 to Beecham.

Ashwood, V. A., Cassidy, F., Evans, J. M., Faruk, E. A. & Hamilton, T. C. (1984) *Trans*-4-cyclic-amido-3,4-dihydro-2H-1-benzopyran-3-ols as antihypertensive agents. In Dahlbom, R. & Nilsson, J. L. G. (eds), *VIIIth International Symposium on Medicinal Chemistry*, vol. 1. Swedish Pharmaceutical Press, Uppsala, Sweden, pp. 316–317.

Ashwood, V. A., Buckingham, R. E., Cassidy, F., Evans, J. M., Faruk, E. A., Hamilton, T. C., Nash, D. J. & Stemp, G. (1986) Synthesis and antihypertensive activity of 4-(cyclicamido)-2H-1-benzopyrans. *Journal of Medicinal Chemistry* **29**, 2194–2201.

Ashwood, V. A., Cassidy, F., Coldwell, M. C., Evans, J. M., Hamilton, T. C., Howlett, D. R., Smith, D. M. & Stemp, G. (1990) Synthesis and antihypertensive activity of 4-(substituted-carbonylamino)-2H-1-benzopyrans. *Journal of Medicinal Chemistry* **33**, 2667–2671.

Attwood, M. R., Jones, P. S. & Redshaw, S. (1988) New 4-aryl or heteroaryl benzo-pyran derivatives: used as potassium channel activators for controlling hypertension, angina, smooth muscle disorders etc. *European Patent Application* 298 452 to Hoffmann-La Roche.

Atwal, K. S., Grover, G. J. & Kim, K. S. (1990a) Pyranyl cyanoguanidine derivatives. *European Patent Application* 401 010 to Squibb.

Atwal, K. S., McCullogh, J. R. & Grover, G. J. (1990b) Aryl cyanoguanidines: potassium channel activators and methods of preparation. *European Patent Application* 354 553 to Squibb.

Bartmann, W. (1989) Hypertension — a problem solved. In van der Goot, H., Domány, G., Pallos, L. & Timmerman, H. (eds), *Trends in Medicinal Chemistry '88*. Elsevier, Amsterdam, pp. 629–657.

Bergmann, R. & Gericke, R. (1990) Synthesis and antihypertensive activity of 4-(1,2-dihydro-2-oxo-1-pyridyl)-2H-1-benzopyrans and related compounds, new potassium channel activators. *Journal of Medicinal Chemistry* **33**, 492–504.

Bergmann, R., Eiermann, V. & Gericke, R. (1990) 4-Heterocyclyloxy-2H-1-benzopyran potassium channel activators. *Journal of Medicinal Chemistry* **33**, 2759–2767.

Berry, J. L., Elliott, K. R. F., Foster, R. W., Green, K. A., Murray, M. A. & Small, R. C. (1991) Mechanical biochemical and electrophysiological studies of RP 49356 and cromakalim in guinea pig and bovine trachealis muscle. *Pulmonary Pharmacology* **4**, 91–98.

Buckle, D. R., Arch, J. R. S., Fenwick, A. E., Houge-Frydrych, C. S. V., Pinto, I. L.,

Smith, D. G., Taylor, S. G. & Tedder, J. M. (1990) Relaxant activity of 4-amido-3,4-dihydro-2H-1-benzopyrans in guinea pig isolated trachealis. *Journal of Medicinal Chemistry* **33**, 3028–3034.

Buckle, D. R., Arch, J. R. S., Foster, K. A., Houge-Frydrych, C. S. V., Pinto, I. L., Smith, D. G., Taylor, J. F., Taylor, S. G., Tedder, J. M. & Webster, R. A. B. (1991a) Synthesis and smooth muscle relaxant activity of a new series of potassium channel activators: 3-amido-1,1-dimethylindanols. *Journal of Medicinal Chemistry* **34**, 919–926.

Buckle, D. R., Houge-Frydrych, C. S. V., Pinto, I. L., Smith, D. G. & Tedder, J. M. (1991b) Structural modifications of the potassium channel activator cromakalim: the C-3 position. *Journal of the Chemical Society, Perkin Transactions 1*, 63–70.

Burrell, G. & Stemp, G. (1990) 1,2,4-Triazole derivatives, their preparation and their use for treating hypertension or respiratory tract disorders. *European Patent Application* 399 834 to Beecham.

Burrell, G., Cassidy, F., Evans, J. M., Lightowler, D. & Stemp, G. (1990) Variation in the aromatic ring of cromakalim: antihypertensive activity of pyranopyridines and 6-alkyl-2H-1-benzopyrans. *Journal of Medicinal Chemistry* **33**, 3023–3027.

Burrell, G., Stemp, G. & Smith, D. G. (1990) Preparation of N''-cyano-N-benzopyranyl-N'-methylguanidines and analogues as antihypertensives. *European Patent Application* 359 537 to Beecham.

Cassidy, F., Evans, J. M., Smith, D. M., Stemp, G., Edge, C. & Williams, D. J. (1989) Conformational analysis of the novel antihypertensive agent cromakalim (BRL 34915). *Journal of the Chemical Society, Chemical Communications* 377–378.

Cook, D. C., Hart, T. W., Mclay, I. M., Palfreyman, M. N. & Walsh, R. J. A. (1989b) Thioformamide derivatives. *European Patent Application* 321 273 to May & Baker.

Cook, D. C., Hart, T. W., Mclay, I. M., Palfreyman, M. N. & Walsh, R. J. A. (1989c) Derivatives of thioformamide. *European Patent Application* 321 274 to May & Baker.

Cook, D. C., Hart, T. W., Mclay, I. M., Palfreyman, M. N., Walsh, R. J. A. & Aloup, J-C. (1989a) Thioformamide derivatives. *European Patent Application* 326 297 to May & Baker.

Dunne, M. J. (1990) ATP-dependent potassium channels: their role and regulation. *Potassium Channels '90 — Structure, Modulation and Clinical Exploitation*, IBC Conference, London.

Duty, S., Paciorek, P. M., Waterfall, J. F. & Weston, A. H. (1990) A comparison of the haemodynamic profiles of Ro 31-6930, cromakalim and nifedipine in anaesthetised normotensive rats. *European Journal of Pharmacology* **185**, 35–42.

Edwards, G. & Weston, A. H. (1989) Potassium channel openers: their development and prospects. *Current Cardiovascular Patents* **1**, 1810–1823.

Edwards, G. & Weston, A. H. (1990) Potassium channel openers; structure activity relationships. *Trends in Pharmacological Sciences* **11**, 417–422.

Englert, C. H., Klaus, E., Lang, H.-J., Mania, D. & Scholkens, B. (1988a) New N-3-hydroxy-benzopyran-4-yl substituted lactam compounds — useful for reducing blood pressure and relaxing the ureter. *European Patent Application* 277 611 to Hoechst.

Englert, C. H., Lang, H.-J., Mania, D. & Scholkens, B. (1988b) New 6-arylsulphonyl-4-heterocyclyl-3-hydroxy-benzopyran derivatives — with cardiovascular activity, e.g. for treating hypertension, angina pectoris and cardiac insufficiency. *European Patent Application* 277 612 to Hoechst.

Evans, J. M. & Stemp, G. (1985) Di/Tetrahydroquinolines. *European Patent Application* 150 202 to Beecham.

Evans, J. M. & Stemp, G. (1986) N-Acylated di- or tetra-hydronaphthaleneamines, and antihypertensive compositions containing them. *European Patent Application* 168 619 to Beecham.

Evans, J. M. & Stemp, G. (1991) The discovery of cromakalim. *Chemistry in Britain* **27**, 439–442.

Evans, J. M., Fake, C. S., Hamilton, T. C., Poyser, R. H. & Watts, E. A. (1983) Synthesis and antihypertensive activity of substituted *trans*-4-amino-3,4-dihydro-2,2-dimethyl-2H-1-benzopyran-3-ols. *Journal of Medicinal Chemistry* **26**, 1582–1589.

Fozard, J. R., Menninger, K., Cook, N. S., Blarer, S. & Quast, U. (1990) The cardiovascular effects of SDZ PCO 400 *in vivo*: comparison with cromakalim. *British Journal of Pharmacology* **99**, 7P.

Furukawa, K., Itoh, T., Kajiwara, M., Kutamura, K., Suzuki, H., Ito, Y. & Kuruyama, H. (1981) Vasodilating actions of 2-nicotinamidoethyl nitrate on porcine and guinea pig coronary arteries. *Journal of Pharmacology and Experimental Therapeutics* **218**, 248–259.

Garcia, G., Di Malta, A. & Soubrie, P. (1990) 2,2-Dimethyl-6-substituted chromans and chromenes — having antidepressant activity. *European Patent Application* 370 901 to Sanofi.

Genain, G. & Pinhas, H. (1990) Novel benzopyranylpyrrolinone derivatives. *European Patent Application* 377 966 to Syntex.

Hamilton, T. C., Weir, S. W. & Weston, A. H. (1986) Comparison of the effects of BRL 34915 and verapamil on electrical and mechanical activity in rat portal vein. *British Journal of Pharmacology* **88**, 103–111.

Hille, B. (1992) Modifiers of gating. In *Ionic Channels of Excitable Membranes*. Sinauer, MA, pp. 445–471.

Holzmann, S. (1983) Cyclic GMP one possible mediator of coronary arterial relaxation by nicorandil (SG-75). *Journal of Cardiovascular Pharmacology* **5**, 364–370.

Houge-Frydrych, C. S. V. & Evans, J. M. (1989) New smooth muscle relaxant nitric acid esters. *Patent Cooperation Treaty Application* 8905–808 to Beecham.

Inoue, T., Kanimura, Y., Fujisawa, K., Itoh, T. & Kuriyama, H. (1984) Effects of 2-nicotinamidoethyl nitrate (nicorandil; SG-75) and its derivatives on smooth muscle cells of the canine mesenteric artery. *Journal of Pharmacology and Experimental Therapeutics* **229**, 793–802.

Kaneta, S., Jinno, Y., Harada, K., Ohta, H., Ogawa, N. & Nishikori, K. (1990) Cardiohaemodynamic effect of KRN 2391, a novel vasodilator, in anaesthetised dogs. *Japanese Journal of Pharmacology* **52**, 374P.

Klaus, E., Linz, W., Schölkens, B. & Englert, H. (1990a) Characterization of HOE 234, a novel K+-channel opener, in isolated vessels. *Naunyn-Schmiedeberg's Archives of Pharmacology* **342** (Suppl.), R17.

Klaus, E., Englert, H., Hropot, M., Metzger, H., Tilly, H. & Wiener, G. (1990b) K-channel opening contributes to the relaxant activity of forskolin in vascular smooth muscle. *Naunyn-Schmiedeberg's Archives of Pharmacology* **341** (Suppl.), R62.

Klöckner, U., Trieschmann, U. & Isenberg, G. (1989) Pharmacological modulation of calcium and potassium channels in isolated vascular smooth muscle cells. *Arzneimittelforschung* **39**, 120–126.

Lang, R. W. & Wenk, P. F. (1988) Synthesis of selectively trifluoromethylated pyridine derivatives as potential antihypertensives. *Helvetica Chimica Acta* **71**, 596–601.

McCall, J. M., Aiken, J. W., Chidester, C. G., Ducharme, D. W. & Wendling, M. G. (1983) Pyrimidine and triazine 3-oxide sulphates: a new family of vasodilators. *Journal of Medicinal Chemistry* **26**, 1791–1793.

Mondot, S., Caillard, C. G., James, C., Aloup, J-C. & Cavero, I. (1989) Antihypertensive and haemodynamic profile of 49356RP, a novel vasorelaxant agent with potassium channel activating properties. *Fundamental and Clinical Pharmacology* **3**, 158.

Morin, M. E., Wojdam, A., Oshiro, G., Colatsky, T. & Quagliato, D. (1990) Antihypertensive and hypotensive effects of the potassium channel activator, WAY-120,491 in spontaneously hypertensive, DOCA salt, 2K-1C Goldblatt Hypertensive, and Wistar–Kyoto normotensive rats. *FASEB Journal* **4**, A747.

Newgreen, D. T., Bray, K. M., McHarg, A. D. *et al.* (1990) The action of diazoxide and minoxidil sulphate on rat blood vessels: a comparison with chromakalim. *British Journal of Pharmacology,* **100**, 605–613.

Ogawa, T., Sawada, K. & Shoji, T. (1990) Vasodilating effects of E 4080 in isolated vascular smooth muscles: comparison with cromakalim and verapamil. *European Journal of Pharmacology* **183**, 1265.

Paciorek, P. M., Burden, D. T., Burke, Y. M., Cowlrick, I. S., Perkins, R. S., Taylor, J. C. & Waterfall, J. F. (1990) Preclinical pharmacology of Ro 31-6930, a new potassium channel opener. *Journal of Cardiovascular Pharmacology* **15**, 188–197.

Palfreyman, M. N., Vicker, N. & Walsh, R. J. A. (1990) Thioformamide derivatives. *European Patent Application* 377 532 to May & Baker.

Petersen, H. J., Nielsen, C. K. & Arrigoni-Martelli, E. (1978) Synthesis and hypotensive activity of N-alkyl-N″-cyano-N′-pyridylguanidines. *Journal of Medicinal Chemistry* **21**, 773–791.

Piper, I. & Hollingsworth, M. (1991) Cromakalim, RP49356, pinacidil and minoxidil sulphate in the rat uterus and their antagonism by glibenclamide. *British Journal of Pharmacology* **88**, 807P.

Press, J. B., Sanfilippo, P., McNally, J. J. & Falotico, R. (1990) Novel substituted thienopyrans as antihypertensive agents. *European Patent Application* 360 621 to Ortho.

Quast, U. & Cook, N. S. (1989) *In vitro* and *in vivo* comparison of two K$^+$ channel openers, diazoxide and cromakalim, and their inhibition by glibenclamide. *Journal of Pharmacology and Experimental Therapeutics* **250**, 261–271.

Robertson, D. W. & Steinberg, M. I. (1990a) Potassium channel modulators: Scientific applications and therapeutic promise. *Journal of Medicinal Chemistry* **33**, 1529–1541.

Robertson, D. W. & Steinberg, M. I. (1990b) Improvements in and relating to guanidine derivatives. *European Patent Application* 381 504 to Eli Lilly.

Shiokawa, Y., Takimoto, K., Takenaka, K. & Kato, T. (1989) Benzopyran derivatives and processes for preparation thereof. *European Patent Application* 344 747 to Fujisawa.

Smith, D. G. (1990) 4-Amido-3,4-dihydro-2H-1-benzothiopyran-3-ols and their sulphoxide and sulphone derivatives — cromakalim analogues. *Journal of the Chemical Society, Perkin Transactions 1* 3187–3191.

Smith, D. G., Buckle, D. R. & Pinto, I. L. (1990) New benzopyran, thiopyran and piperidine derivatives having smooth muscle relaxing activity, useful as bronchodilators and antihypertensives. *European Patent Application* 376 524 to Beecham.

Sombroek, J., Bergmann, R. & Gericke, R. (1990) Novel potassium channel activators. *XIth International Symposium on Medicinal Chemistry*, Jerusalem, Israel, abstracts, p. 27.

Southerton, J. S., Weston, A. H., Bray, K. M., Newgreen, D. T. & Taylor, S. G. (1988) The potassium channel opening action of pinacidil; studies using biochemical, ion flux and microelectrode techniques. *Naunyn Schmiedeberg's Archives of Pharmacology,* **338**, 310–318.

Stemp, G. (1990) New benzopyran-type compounds — having potassium channel activating, blood pressure lowering and bronchodilator activity, or being intermediates for active compounds. *European Patent Application* 375 449 to Beecham.

Thomas, W. A. & Whitcombe, I. W. A. (1990) Conformational behaviour of cromakalim and related potassium channel activators. *Journal of the Chemical Society, Chemical Communications*, 528–529.

Topliss, J. G., Sherlock, M. H., Reimann, H., Konzelman, L. M., Shapiro, E. P., Pettersen, B. W., Schneider, H. & Sperber, B. (1963) Antihypertensive agents. I. Non diuretic 2H-1,2,4-benzothiadiazine 1,1-dioxides. *Journal of Medicinal Chemistry* **6**, 122–127.

Topliss, J. G., Konzelman, L. M., Shapiro, E. P., Sperber, N. & Roth, F. E. (1964) Antihypertensive agents. II. 3-Substituted-2H-1,2,4-benzothiadiazine 1,1-dioxides. *Journal of Medicinal Chemistry* **7**, 269–273.

Webster, R. A. & Cassidy, F. (1988) New benzoxepine and related compounds — useful as smooth muscle relaxants. *Patent Cooperation Treaty Application* 8 911 477 to Beecham.

Weston, A. H., Southerton, J. S., Bray, K. M., Newgreen, D. T. & Taylor, S. G. (1988) The mode of action of pinacidil and its analogues P 1060 and P 1368: results of studies in rat blood vessels. *Journal of Cardiovascular Pharmacology* **12** (Suppl. 2), S10–S16.

Winquist, R. J., Heaney, L. A., Wallace, A. A., Baskin, E. P., Stein, R. B., Garcia, M. L. & Kaczorowski, G. J. (1989) Glyburide blocks the relaxation response to BRL 34915 (cromakalim), minoxidil sulphate, and diazoxide in vascular smooth muscle. *Journal of Pharmacology and Experimental Therapeutics* **248**, 149–156.

Yamanaka, T., Seki, T., Nakajima, T. & Yaoka, O. (1989) Benzopyran compound and its pharmaceutical use. *European Patent Application* 339 562 to Yoshitomi.

Chapter 14
Effects of potassium channel modulators on the cardiovascular system

G. Edwards, S. Duty, D. J. Trezise and A. H. Weston

Introduction

Studies on the effects of K-channel modulators on the cardiovascular system can be broadly divided into two areas. In one of these, K-channel blockers and openers are being evaluated for use in the treatment of a variety of cardiovascular diseases. Although some mention of this aspect of their action will be made in this chapter, the reader is referred to Chapters 12 and 17 for a more detailed discussion of these clinical aspects. In addition to their therapeutic potential, the K-channel modulators have also proved to be important tools in evaluating the role of K-channels in a variety of excitable cells. For the background to this, the reader is referred to Chapters 6–10. The purpose of this section is to consolidate and to expand upon the information given in the above-mentioned chapters and to present a broad picture of the consequences of modulating K-channels in the cardiovascular system. Earlier reviews of this area include Hamilton and Weston (1989), Cook and Quast (1990), Edwards and Weston (1990a,b), Friedel and Brogden (1990), Robertson and Steinberg (1990), Evans and Longman (1991) and Weston and Edwards (1991, 1992).

Cardiovascular actions of K-channel openers *in vivo*

Systemic haemodynamic effects

General characteristics

The prototype benzopyran K-channel opener cromakalim (*see* Chapter 13) was originally selected for development on the basis of its hypotensive action in rats (Ashwood *et al.*, 1986). Following the discovery of its K-channel opening properties *in vitro* (Hamilton *et al.*, 1986), retrospective analysis indicated that the action of a number of previously recognised antihypertensive agents such as pinacidil, minoxidil sulphate and diazoxide, were associated with the opening of plasmalemmal K-channels in vascular smooth muscle (Hamilton & Weston, 1989). To this list of K-channel openers can be added nicorandil, an antianginal drug originally described by Uchida *et al.* (1978). This agent both opens K-channels (Furukawa *et al.*, 1981) and activates guanylate cyclase (Holzmann, 1983), its *in vivo* and *in vitro* profile being derived from a combination of these two properties.

Many of the K-channel openers are racemic mixtures. When this is the case, their hypotensive properties reside with a single enantiomeric component suggesting a stereospecific interaction with the active site(s) (Buckingham *et al.*, 1986a; Hof *et al.*, 1988; Cavero *et al.*, 1991a). This finding is consistent with studies performed in isolated blood vessels which reveal that the vasorelaxant properties of racemic K-channel openers also reside in a single enantiomer (Buckingham *et al.*, 1986a; Bray *et al.*, 1987b).

The blood pressure lowering effects of K-channel openers have been reported in a variety of species including the rat (cromakalim: Buckingham *et al.*, 1986b; cromakalim and SR 44866: Richer *et al.*, 1989; cromakalim and Ro 31-6930: Duty *et al.*, 1990; SDZ PCO 400: Fozard *et al.*, 1990), rabbit (cromakalim: Cook & Hof, 1988), cat (cromakalim: Buckingham *et al.*, 1986b; cromakalim, nicorandil and pinacidil: Longman *et al.*, 1988; cromakalim and Ro 31-6930; Paciorek *et al.*, 1990) and dog (cromakalim: Dumez *et al.*, 1988; cromakalim and Ro 31-6930 (Paciorek *et al.*, 1990). The hypotensive effects result primarily from a fall in total peripheral resistance (*see* regional haemodynamic effects). Such effects of K-channel openers may last for several hours following single dose administration indicating the long duration of action of some of these compounds (Buckingham *et al.*, 1986b; Clapham & Longman, 1989; Paciorek *et al.*, 1990).

Aortic strips from spontaneously hypertensive (SH) rats were initially reported to be equisensitive to the relaxant effects of cromakalim as identical vessels obtained from normotensive animals (Falotico *et al.*,

1989). In contrast, a later study reported that vessels from SH rats were more sensitive than those from normotensive controls (Miyata *et al.*, 1990b). Several reports have indicated that the hypotensive efficacy of cromakalim is similar in both SH and normotensive cats (Clapham & Buckingham, 1988; Longman *et al.*, 1988; Clapham & Longman, 1989), although contradictory data showing greater efficacy in SH as opposed to normotensive rats has appeared (Falotico *et al.*, 1989). There seems to be little difference between the hypotensive effects of K-channel openers in conscious and anaesthetized animals (cromakalim: Clapham & Buckingham, 1988; Longman *et al.*, 1988; Clapham & Longman, 1989; cromakalim and SR44866; Richer *et al.*, 1990a).

Effects on the heart

Tachycardia accompanies the hypotensive response to all tested K-channel openers. For example, doses of cromakalim and Ro 31-6930 which produce maximal hypotensive effects in the anaesthetized rat are accompanied by a tachycardia of approximately 30–50 beats/min (Duty *et al.*, 1990). The cromakalim-induced tachycardia observed in the rat and rabbit is believed to be a sympathetic reflex since it is prevented by pretreatment with the β-adrenoceptor blocking agents propranolol and bopindolol, respectively (Buckingham *et al.*, 1986b; Cook & Hof, 1988). Adding further support to the proposed reflex nature of this tachycardia, Grosset and Hicks (1986) found that even high doses of cromakalim failed to modify the rate of spontaneously beating guinea-pig isolated atria, indicating a lack of direct cardiostimulatory effects of this compound.

In the anaesthetized cat, cromakalim increases the baroreceptor sensitivity to pressor agents such as phenylephrine while pinacidil has no effect on this parameter (Clapham & Cooper, 1988). In complete contrast, this same study revealed that pinacidil increased baroreceptor sensitivity to sodium nitroprusside whereas cromakalim was without effect. Clearly further work is needed with other K-channel openers to clarify these actions and to determine the overall effects of this group of agents on baroreceptor reflexes.

Little change in contractility of ventricular muscle is observed over the hypotensive dose range in either the cat, rabbit or dog (Clapham & Buckingham, 1988; Hof *et al.*, 1988; Paciorek *et al.*, 1990). These findings are consistent with reports *in vitro* in which cromakalim preferentially dilates vascular tissue and has little effect on tension in, for example, isolated rabbit papillary tissue (Longman *et al.*, 1988). In the dog, however, some depression of cardiac contractility has been reported with very high doses of both cromakalim and nicorandil (Yamada *et al.*, 1990).

Involvement of glibenclamide-sensitive K-channels

The hypotensive effects of all the K-channel openers so far tested are attenuated by the intravenous administration of glibenclamide (approximately 20 mg/kg). Such inhibitory effects have been described in the rat (Buckingham *et al.*, 1989; Cavero *et al.*, 1989, 1991b; Quast & Cook, 1989; Richer *et al.*, 1990b) and in the dog (Yamada *et al.*, 1990). In a particularly thorough study in the anaesthetized rat (Richer *et al.*, 1990b), glibenclamide (20 mg/kg) inhibited the hypotensive effects of a range of structurally dissimilar K-channel openers including nicorandil but had no effect on the blood pressure lowering produced by nitrendipine or papaverine. The ability of glibenclamide to inhibit the *in vivo* effects of nicorandil differs from the findings *in vitro*. Newgreen *et al.* (1990) showed that methylene blue (an inhibitor of guanylate cyclase) inhibited the relaxant effects of nicorandil in rat aorta while glibenclamide had little inhibitory effect against this agent. This minimal inhibitory effect of glibenclamide *in vitro* probably reflects the mixed action of nicorandil, i.e. its ability both to stimulate guanylate cyclase and to open K-channels. The *in vivo* efficacy of intravenous glibenclamide suggests that the *in vivo* effects of nicorandil may reflect more the K-channel opening properties of the dual-action agent. In contrast to its efficacy by the intravenous route, orally administered glibenclamide (100 mg/kg) failed to inhibit the hypotensive response to cromakalim in the rat (Buckingham *et al.*, 1989). This may indicate a reduced bioavailability of glibenclamide following oral administration.

In addition to inhibiting the hypotensive responses to K-channel openers, intravenously administered glibenclamide (20 mg/kg) also antagonizes (as would be expected) cromakalim-induced reflex tachycardia in rats (Buckingham *et al.*, 1989). The cardiodepressant effects of cromakalim and nicorandil in the dog are also inhibited (Yamada *et al.*, 1990). Glibenclamide itself has few cardiovascular effects, although in higher doses (30 mg/kg) a transient increase in blood pressure was detected following glibenclamide administration in the rat (Quast & Cook, 1989). The *in vivo* inhibitory effects of glibenclamide are consistent with its *in vitro* profile and suggest that both the *in vitro* and the *in vivo* changes produced by K-channel openers reflect their ability to open glibenclamide-sensitive K-channels. Such an action of these hypotensive agents *in vivo* is further supported by exclusion of other possible mechanisms; antagonists of several vascular receptors including those active at the α_2-adrenoceptor, the β_2-adrenoceptor, the dopamine-1 and serotonin receptors do not modify the actions of the K-channel openers (Cavero *et al.*, 1989). Furthermore, apamin, a selective blocker of a small Ca-dependent K-channel (SK_{Ca}) (*see* Chapter 11) does not inhibit the hypotensive effects of cromakalim in the anaesthetized rabbit, further suggesting that the effects of K-channel openers are selectively exerted at a glibenclamide-sensitive K-channel (Cook & Hof, 1988).

Inhibition of agonist-induced pressor responses

Potassium channel openers generally inhibit agonist-induced pressor responses. Early studies showed that pinacidil inhibited the increase in blood pressure produced by α-adrenoceptor agonists in the pithed rat (Thoolen et al., 1983). In a more recent study conducted in the anaesthetized rat, both cromakalim and SR 44866 attenuated the rise in blood pressure produced by the α_2-adrenoceptor agonist, UK14304 (Richer et al., 1990b). Similarly the regional vasoconstrictor responses of UK14304 were reduced by administration of these K-channel openers. Not all pressor responses are sensitive to inhibition by K-channel openers. Despite the marked antivasoconstrictor effects of K-channel openers against angiotensin II-induced contractions of isolated smooth muscle, cromakalim, nicorandil and pinacidil produced only minimal antagonism of the pressor responses to this peptide in the anaesthetized normotensive rat (Cook et al., 1988).

Regional haemodynamic changes

Several workers have examined the regional haemodynamic profile of a wide variety of K-channel openers. However, although a number of trends do appear, there is still a large degree of discrepancy between results obtained by the different groups. These differences, which persist even when comparing data within the same species, may reflect the differing protocols used to classify the profiles of selectivity for different beds. Some studies have considered the maximum effect of a single administered dose and have therefore examined the capacity for change in a particular bed (Longman et al., 1988; Cavero et al., 1989; Shoji et al., 1990). In contrast, other studies have involved a full dose-range protocol to examine the order of threshold potency in different regions of the vasculature (Hof et al., 1988; Duty et al., 1990).

Although only relatively few data are available it is clear that the K-channel openers reduce vascular resistance in a multiplicity of regional beds. The most commonly studied areas include the mesenteric, renal and hindquarter (iliac or femoral) vascular beds. The hindquarter vasculature is subject to marked falls in resistance. In the anaesthetized rat or dog, this amounts to a reduction of 40% or more with cromakalim, SR44866 and Ro 31-6930, although little change in actual blood flow is apparent (Richer et al., 1989; Duty et al., 1990; Paciorek et al., 1990). This is probably due to the marked systemic hypotensive effects found at the relatively high concentrations required to dilate the skeletal muscle vasculature in most species (Buckingham *et al.*, 1986b; Hof *et al.*, 1988; Richer *et al.*, 1989). However, some workers have described an increase in hindquarter blood flow in the rat (Cavero *et al.*, 1989; Shoji *et al.*, 1990). Mesenteric vascular resistance is also reduced by all K-channel openers so far studied. In the anaesthetized cat, rat or dog, falls in mesenteric vascular resistance of between 30 and 50% are produced by cromakalim, pinacidil, nicorandil or Ro 31-6930 (Longman *et al.*, 1988; Duty *et al.*, 1990; Paciorek *et al.*, 1990). As observed for the hindquarters, despite these marked reductions in vascular resistance, little or no actual increase in blood flow to the mesentery has been detected (Bang-Olsen & Arrigoni-Martelli, 1983; Buckingham *et al.*, 1986b; Richer *et al.*, 1989).

Although the K-channel openers exert similar effects in hindquarters and mesenteric beds, marked differences have been observed in studies on the renal vasculature. Using pulsed Doppler flowmetry in the anaesthetized cat, Longman *et al.* (1988) found that while renal vascular resistance was markedly decreased with cromakalim (approximately 40%) no such reduction was observed with either pinacidil or nicorandil. In the rat, cromakalim, SR 44866 and Ro 31-6930 each produced a reduction in renal vascular resistance (Richer *et al.*, 1989; Duty *et al.*, 1990). Other studies performed in the anaesthetized dog have shown that pinacidil, as well as cromakalim, reduces renal vascular resistance (Bang-Olsen & Arrigoni-Martelli, 1983; Paciorek *et al.*, 1990). Species differences in the sensitivity of the renal vasculature may explain these differences. Further support for interspecies variations is provided by the findings of Hof *et al.* (1988) in which cromakalim failed to reduce renal vascular resistance in the anaesthetized rabbit.

The effects of cromakalim on renal blood flow are variable. In the anaesthetized cat, cromakalim increases flow (Buckingham *et al.*, 1986b; Clapham & Buckingham, 1988; Clapham & Longman, 1989), while in the rat no such changes have been detected (Cavero *et al.*, 1989; Shoji *et al.*, 1990). Clearly further consolidatory work is required to clarify these renal effects. The effects of cromakalim on renal vascular parameters in humans are described in Chapter 17.

Effects on plasma hormone levels

Effects on the renin/angiotensin II system

Ferrier *et al.* (1989) demonstrated that cromakalim directly stimulated the release of renin from cultured juxtaglomerular cells. However, despite the large number of animal studies concerning the effects of K-channel openers on renal vascular resistance and blood flow (*see above*), relatively few data concerning changes in renal hormone levels have been published. In one early study performed in the conscious normotensive dog, pinacidil

(0.5 mg/kg) was found to increase plasma renin activity (PRA) approximately threefold (Arrigoni-Martelli *et al.*, 1980). Similarly, pinacidil (0.6 mg/kg) produced an approximate fourfold increase in the PRA in the conscious normotensive cat, whereas equihypotensive doses of cromakalim produced a smaller increase in PRA than pinacidil (twofold versus fourfold; Clapham & Longman, 1989). It is well established that an increase in renal blood flow opposes the secretion of renin (Davis & Freeman, 1976) and thus the ability of cromakalim to increase renal blood flow (Buckingham *et al.*, 1986b; Clapham & Longman, 1989) may form the basis for the less marked increase of PRA seen with cromakalim.

Richer *et al.* (1990b) have convincingly demonstrated that the increased PRA produced by both SR 44866 and cromakalim in anaesthetized rats is inhibited by glibenclamide. This finding provides further evidence that the underlying mechanism is related to K-channel opening although the relative contribution of an indirect action via vasodilation *per se* or of a direct action on the juxtaglomerular cells is unclear.

Effects on plasma insulin and glucose levels

A variety of agents is known to alter the membrane potential of the β-cell and thereby modify the rate of insulin secretion and subsequently the level of plasma glucose. In particular, the K-channel blocking agents such as the sulphonylureas tolbutamide, glipizide and glibenclamide are effective hypoglycaemic agents. They act partly by raising the level of plasma insulin and thereby lowering blood glucose level (Ashcroft & Ashcroft, 1990). Since these K-channel blockers lower blood glucose it is possible that K-channel openers might increase blood glucose levels by promoting β-cell membrane hyperpolarization resulting in reduced insulin secretion. The hyperglycaemic effects of the antihypertensive agent diazoxide are known to involve inhibition of insulin secretion (Seltzer & Allen, 1965) and this effect is now believed to involve the opening of K-channels inhibited by intracellular adenosine triphosphate (K_{ATP}) within the β-cell membrane resulting in hyperpolarization (*see* Chapter 6). Inhibition of insulin secretion by hormonal stimuli, such as the peptides galanin and somatostatin, is also believed to involve opening of glibenclamide-sensitive K-channels (De Weille *et al.*, 1988; Dunne *et al.*, 1989).

A wide selection of K-channel opening agents including cromakalim, pinacidil and RP 49356 is now known to open K_{ATP} in insulin-secreting cell lines. Such an effect (Dunne, 1990; Dunne *et al.*, 1990; *see also* Chapter 6), reduces insulin secretion *in vitro* although the concentrations required to produce this effect are extremely high (Garrino *et al.*, 1989; Dunne, 1990). *In vivo*, hypotensive doses of K-channel openers, with the exception of diazoxide have negligible effects on blood glucose (Quast & Cook, 1989) or plasma insulin levels (Wilson *et al.*, 1988a; Richer *et al.*, 1990b; Pratz *et al.*, 1991).

Effects of K-channel modulators on the heart

General background

The cardiac effects of K-channel blockers are extensively described in Chapters 8 and 12. In this section the effects of K-channel openers on the heart are detailed and the effects of K-channel blockers are only included where necessary. The reader is referred to Chapter 8 for a detailed description of cardiac K-channels.

Any increase in the frequency or duration of K-channel opening, for example by K-channel openers, produces an increase in the outward current, opposing the depolarizing effects of the inward movements of Ca^{2+} in nodal cells or of Na^+ and Ca^{2+} in non-nodal tissue. Thus, K-channel openers produce an earlier termination of the action potential, shortening the action potential duration (APD) and perhaps also reducing the action potential frequency without affecting the rate at which Na^+ enters (V_{max}). Many K-channel openers exert a direct inhibitory effect on cardiac muscle, e.g. cromakalim ($>1\ \mu M$; guinea-pig ventricles, ferret and guinea-pig papillary muscle, dog and sheep Purkinje fibres: Liu *et al.*, 1988; Osterrieder, 1988; Sanguinetti *et al.*, 1988; Bril & Man, 1990), pinacidil ($>3\ \mu M$; canine Purkinje fibres, guinea-pig papillary muscle, rabbit sinoatrial node: Smallwood & Steinberg, 1988; Hirai *et al.*, 1990; Martin & Chinn, 1990), nicorandil ($>10 \mu M$; canine Purkinje fibres: Imanishi *et al.*, 1983), SR 44866 ($>10\ \mu M$; guinea-pig ventricles, guinea-pig papillary muscle: Findlay *et al.*, 1989; Faivre & Findlay, 1990) and both the racemate RP 49356 and its active enantiomer RP 52891 ($30\ \mu M$; guinea-pig papillary muscle: Mondot *et al.*, 1988; Cavero *et al.*, 1991a).

In vitro effects on cardiac muscle and conducting tissue

Cromakalim, pinacidil and nicorandil produce marked shortening of APD of ventricular and Purkinje fibres and reduce automaticity (Imanishi *et al.*, 1983, 1984; Cain & Metzler, 1985; Kakei *et al.*, 1986b; Scholtysik, 1987; Sanguinetti *et al.*, 1988; Smallwood & Steinberg, 1988). The effect of the K-channel openers on both channel opening and APD shortening is temperature-dependent, being more pronounced at 37°C than at room temperature (Sanguinetti *et al.*, 1988; Findlay *et al.*, 1989; Thuringer & Escande, 1989; Martin & Chinn, 1990). In isolated preparations, K-channel openers also decrease the sinus rate and cardiac contractility (Cohen & Colbert, 1986; Longman *et al.*, 1988; Steinberg *et al.*, 1988; Yanagisawa *et al.*, 1988; Nielsen *et al.*, 1989; Grover *et al.*, 1990a). The reduction in contractility is thought to be secondary to the shortening of the APD which reduces the time available for Ca^{2+} influx and hence the maximum intracellular Ca^{2+} concentration (Yanagisawa et al., 1988). The marked negative inotropic effect produced by K-channel openers in vitro is not seen in vivo (Kawashima & Liang, 1985), possibly because of the lower concentration of K-channel openers used in vivo or because of reflex sympathetic activation.

Effects of K-channel modulators in hypoxia and ischaemia

Accumulation of extracellular potassium, $[K^+]_o$, associated with myocardial ischaemia (Weiss & Shine, 1982) is thought to be involved in the generation of ischaemia-induced arrhythmias (Kramer & Corr, 1984; Janse & Wit, 1989). However, the cause of the increase in $[K^+]_o$ remains to be conclusively determined. During hypoxia, the depression of oxidative metabolism may cause an inhibition of the Na : K pump with depolarization resulting from a reduction in the transmembrane K^+-gradient (Ruiz-Petrich et al., 1991). To oppose the depolarization, K^+-efflux through the inward rectifier channel, K_{IR}, is increased and the subsequent extracellular accumulation of K^+ probably contributes to the APD-shortening associated with hypoxia (Ruiz-Petrich et al., 1991).

In addition, some ischaemia-induced loss of intracellular K^+ (and consequent extracellular accumulation) may be due to a fall in the intracellular ATP concentration, $[ATP]_i$, and the opening of K-channels (K_{ATP}) sensitive to intracellular ATP (Trube & Hescheler, 1984; Noma & Shibasaki, 1985; Fosset et al., 1988; Sanguinetti et al., 1988). Epicardial cells are more sensitive to ischaemia-induced electrophysiological changes than endocardial cells and this heterogeneity is thought to possibly facilitate re-entrant arrhythmias (Gilmour & Zipes, 1980; Kimura et al., 1986). An explanation for the different regional sensitivities to the metabolic effects of ischaemia was recently provided by Furukawa and coworkers (1991) who found that the sensitivity of K_{ATP} to a fall in $[ATP]_i$ was greater in epicardial than endocardial cells. Thus glibenclamide, a selective blocker of K_{ATP} in the heart (Escande et al., 1988; Sanguinetti et al., 1988) would be expected to oppose the APD shortening and reduce the incidence of arrhythmias. Such an effect has been demonstrated in the guinea-pig heart in vitro (Fosset et al., 1988; Sanguinetti et al., 1988). Although glibenclamide was effective in the rabbit in vivo, a similar effect was not produced in the dog (Smallwood et al., 1990). Similarly, these workers were unable to detect any protective effect of glibenclamide against electrically induced ventricular fibrillation in dogs subject to acute ischaemia. In the rabbit heart, glibenclamide does not oppose the APD shortening until about 30 min after hypoxia induction (de Lorenzi et al., 1990) suggesting that K_{ATP} may not play an important role until this time. However, Venkatesh et al. (1991)

have recently demonstrated that the concentration of adenosine diphosphate (ADP) likely to be achieved intracellularly during myocardial ischaemia inhibits the blocking effect of sulphonylureas on K_{ATP}. Thus, the inability of the sulphonylureas to inhibit K^+-efflux during ischaemic episodes does not exclude the possibility that outward K-current through K_{ATP} is enhanced. The antiarrhythmic effects of K-channel blockers will be dependent on the relative contributions of K_{ATP} or other K-channels to ischaemia-induced K^+-efflux in different species.

It is currently uncertain whether the loss of K^+ during hypoxia or ischaemia is beneficial or detrimental to the tissue. One consequence of such K^+ loss is that the cell becomes hyperpolarized and cellular activity is reduced. This could be important in conserving intracellular ATP, preventing the intracellular concentration from falling to a critically low level (Noma & Shibasaki, 1985). Furthermore, the cellular hyperpolarization would reduce Ca^{2+}-entry, an event which is associated with reperfusion damage (Shen & Jennings, 1972; Henry et al., 1977). However, the accumulation of extracellular K^+ (originating from the ischaemic region) would also cause depolarization of other cells in adjacent non-ischaemic areas, and the increased entry of Ca^{2+} through voltage-regulated Ca-channels would stimulate cellular activity. Since the APD of cells in ischaemic and non-ischaemic areas would differ, re-entrant arrhythmias could be provoked. Blockers of K_{ATP}, e.g. glibenclamide or tolbutamide, prevent such arrhythmias by maintaining APD in hypoxic cells (Wolleben et al., 1989). The K-channel openers are currently under development as antihypertensive agents. Since the hypertensive patient is also at risk from heart disease, it is important that the effect of K-channel opening during myocardial ischaemia is known.

Pro- and antiarrhythmic effects of K-channel modulators

Hypoxia and myocardial ischaemia are each associated with marked depolarization of the diastolic resting membrane potential (Ruiz-Ceretti et al., 1983; Grover et al., 1989). Cromakalim (7 μM) was capable of reversing this depolarization in a rat model of ischaemia and the effect of cromakalim itself was reversed by glibenclamide (Grover et al., 1989). The hyperpolarizing effect of K-channel openers on abnormally depolarized cells may be antiarrhythmic (Cain & Metzler, 1985; Kerr et al., 1985). During ischaemia the shortening of APD, which may be a contributory factor in the generation of ischaemia-induced arrhythmias, could conceivably be aggravated by K-channel openers which have a similar effect. However, protective effects of cromakalim and pinacidil against arrhythmias induced either by ischaemia or abnormal repolarization were found to occur with concentrations lower than those which are necessary to reduce APD (Grover et al., 1989; Fish et al., 1990). In addition, cromakalim was found to inhibit both spontaneous activity and oscillatory activity induced by high extracellular Ca^{2+}, $[Ca^{2+}]_o$, in isolated Purkinje fibres at both high and low membrane potentials (Liu *et al.*, 1988). Pinacidil also reduced arrhythmias produced 22–24 h after coronary artery ligation in dogs. The arrhythmias arising approximately 24 h after coronary artery occlusion are due to abnormal automaticity in subendocardial Purkinje fibres (Friedman *et al.*, 1973; Horowitz *et al.*, 1976). Such arrhythmias are not improved by class III (K-channel blockers) or class IV (Ca-channel blockers) antidysrhythmic agents (Kerr *et al.*, 1985). However, conflicting reports about the antiarrhythmic effects of K-channel openers exist. Both Siegl *et al.* (1989) and Grover *et al.* (1990c) found that cromakalim increased the incidence of fibrillation during reperfusion of globally ischaemic rat isolated hearts, and *in vivo*, Chi *et al.* (1989) found that pinacidil increased the likelihood of ventricular fibrillation in infarcted dogs subjected to ischaemia. In normal hearts reports are also equivocal. Nielsen *et al.* (1989) found no proarrhythmic effect of this concentration of pinacidil in the rabbit perfused heart although Wolleben *et al.* (1989) found that pinacidil reduced the time to ventricular fibrillation in the rat isolated heart preparation. Nevertheless, it must be pointed out that the proarrhythmic concentration of pinacidil far exceeds the hypotensive therapeutic concentration (Carlsen *et al.*, 1983). Thus both K-channel openers and K-channel blockers have proved to be potentially useful for the treatment of cardiac arrhythmias. The protection afforded by each agent would be dependent upon the underlying cause of the arrhythmia.

Protection against ischaemic damage

The problems of ischaemia are not only related to restricted blood flow, but are also compounded by blood reperfusion. Thus, after a successful coronary artery bypass, reperfusion damage may result in myocardial necrosis (Bulkley & Hutchins, 1977), an effect similar to that produced by temporary coronary artery occlusion in dogs (Jennings *et al.*, 1960). In animal models, damage subsequent to ischaemia can been assessed *in vivo* by determination of lactate dehydrogenase release (which is closely correlated with cardiac necrosis; Van der Laarse *et al.*, 1979) or by measurement of end diastolic pressure (EDP) which reflects compliance of the heart (and is inversely proportional to the extent of ischaemic damage; Tilton *et al.*, 1985; Vogel *et al.*, 1986). Both of these parameters are favourably affected by K-channel openers (pinacidil, cromakalim, nicorandil, RP 52891 and KRN2391) administered directly into the coronary circulation (Grover *et al.*, 1989, 1990a,b; Cavero *et al.*, 1991a; Ohta *et al.*, 1991). Myocardial ischaemia is associated with metabolic acidosis due to hydrolysis of ATP and lactate accumulation (Ichihara *et al.*, 1984). Using myocardial acidosis as an indicator of ischaemia the anti-ischaemic properties of both nicorandil and the K-channel opener LP-805 have been demonstrated (Ichihara *et al.*, 1991). The anti-ischaemic effects of cromakalim, pinacidil and RP 52891 were inhibited by glibenclamide and also by 5-hydroxydecanoate (Grover *et al.*, 1990a,b; McCullough *et al.*, 1991), blockers which are apparently selective for K_{ATP} in the heart (Escande *et al.*, 1988; Sanguinetti *et al.*, 1988; Notsu *et al.*, 1992) indicating the involvement of such K-channels in the cardiac protective effect of K-channel openers. Interestingly, Grover and coworkers found that, unlike glibenclamide, 5-hydroxydecanoate did not antagonize the pre-ischaemic cardiodepressant effect of cromakalim or RP 52891, suggesting a preferential effect of 5-hydroxydecanoate in ischaemic tissue (Grover *et al.*, 1990b; McCullough *et al.*, 1991).

Intracoronary infusion of cromakalim, pinacidil or RP 52891 in dogs (administered both before occlusion and during the experiment) produced up to a 50% reduction (in comparison to controls) in the infarct size resulting from 90 min occlusion of the left circumflex artery (Grover *et al.*, 1989, 1990a; Auchampach *et al.*, 1990). This effect was associated with a reduced incidence of ventricular fibrillation during reperfusion (Grover *et al.*, 1990a). A similar protection is not provided by systemic administration of K-channel openers perhaps because of coronary steal (Imai *et al.*, 1988). In fact, the use of K-channel openers systemically may be detrimental since any hypotensive effect will reduce blood flow to the ischaemic zone. This has been demonstrated in dogs with a coronary artery stenosis in which pinacidil increased the infarct size produced by occlusion of the left anterior descending coronary artery (Sakamoto *et al.*, 1989).

The cardioprotective action of the K-channel openers is due to an enhanced coronary blood flow together with a reduced myocardial function (Rademacher *et al.*, 1990). Any reduction in infarct size by K-channel openers should also be beneficial in reducing the incidence of fatal ventricular arrhythmias. In addition, cromakalim provides some protection against the fall in intracellular ATP resulting from ischaemia, although this was not significant until about 10 min into the ischaemic period (Grover, 1991). Such protection could be linked to hyperpolarization which, by reducing influx of Ca, would also reduce the activity of Na : K ATPase.

In the normal dog heart, a low dose of pinacidil or nicorandil increases blood flow uniformly across the left ventricular wall. Although higher doses favour an increase in the blood flow to the subepicardium, the blood flow to the subendocardium is also increased (Lamping & Gross, 1984, 1985; Bache *et al.*, 1990a,b). However, the ability to increase coronary blood flow in a normal heart almost certainly does not reflect the potential actions of K-channel openers in patients with ischaemic heart disease in which the coronary arteries are probably maximally dilated. Indeed, it is possible that, by dilating vessels in non-ischaemic areas, these drugs may reduce blood flow to ischaemic areas and thus be detrimental in the treatment of myocardial ischaemia. In dogs with a coronary artery stenosis, a low dose of pinacidil caused a redistribution of coronary flow towards the subepicardium (Bache et al., 1990a). Despite the low probability that pinacidil would actually reduce the subendocardial flow, Bache and coworkers concluded that 'pinacidil could have the potential to aggravate subendocardial ischaemia in severe coronary occlusive disease'. In the hypertrophied left ventricle there is already a reduced flow to the subendocardium which increases the tendency for myocardial ischaemia (Vrobel et al., 1980; Bache et al., 1984). Although K-channel openers might be expected to aggravate this condition, and indeed, pinacidil does produce a greater increase in the subepicardial blood flow of the hypertrophied ventricle, the flow to the subendocardium is still increased by pinacidil in comparison to controls (Bache et al., 1990b).

Both nicorandil and pinacidil are potent coronary vasodilators, producing a marked increase in coronary blood flow (Taira et al., 1979; Kawashima & Liang, 1985). Although their action is associated with a reflex increase in heart rate and contractility, which increases O_2 consumption, they decrease systemic blood pressure which reduces afterload on the heart and therefore the myocardial O_2 demand. It has been shown that the pinacidil-induced flow increase far exceeds the increased myocardial O_2 demand (Kawashima & Liang, 1985). These effects suggest that K-channel openers might be useful in the treatment of angina pectoris (Kawashima & Liang, 1985).

Potassium channels involved in the cardiac effects of K-channel openers

The K-channel(s) involved in the action of the K-channel openers in the heart is uncertain. Since most K-channel openers are 10–300 times less potent in the heart than in blood vessels (De Peyer et al., 1989; Osterrieder & Waterfall, 1989), the target K-channel may differ from that in vascular smooth muscle. Supporting this is the finding that diazoxide, which opens K_{ATP} in pancreatic β-cells (Trube et al., 1986) and shows the characteristics of a K-channel opener in vascular smooth muscle (Newgreen et al., 1990) inhibits K_{ATP} and prolongs APD in ventricular cells (Faivre & Findlay, 1989). Furthermore, LY222675, which has a potency comparable to that of pinacidil in relaxing canine cephalic veins is more than six times more potent than pinacidil in shortening APD of canine Purkinje fibres (Steinberg et al., 1989).

The delayed rectifier channel (K_{dr}: see Chapter 8) is an unlikely site of action of the K-channel openers since the current induced by these agents is both time- and voltage-independent (Arena & Kass, 1989). A role for Ca-sensitive K-channels (K_{Ca}) is similarly improbable since these are associated with only a relatively small current in either the atrium or ventricle (Hiraoka & Kawano, 1986; Giles & Imaizumi, 1988), although they may be more important in Purkinje fibres (Callewaert et al., 1986). In addition, the characteristic effects of pinacidil are produced in Ca-free conditions (Martin & Chinn, 1990). The presence of a K-channel opened by high (20 mM) intracellular $[Na^+]$ in the heart (K_{Na}) has been described (Kameyama et al., 1984), but its role, if any, has not yet been determined. The requirement for extremely high $[Na^+]$ to activate the channel suggests that it may not have a normal physiological role (Wang et al., 1991). The effects of K-channel openers on these channels have not yet been fully determined although the effect of pinacidil occurs even in the absence of Na^+ (Arena & Kass, 1989) and nicorandil has no effect on K_{Na} (Takano & Noma, 1990). A further group of K-channels upon which any effects of K-channel openers remain to be established comprises those which carry currents of the $I_{K(to)}$ type (see Chapter 8). Thus the two main types of K-channel currently believed to be involved in the direct effects of the K-channel openers on the heart are the K_{ATP}-channel and the inward rectifier K-channel, K_{IR}. The reader is referred to Chapter 8 for a detailed discussion of the properties of the cardiac K_{ATP} and K_{IR}.

Role of K_{IR} and K_{ATP}

In isolated guinea-pig ventricular cells, pinacidil increases the current through K_{IR} by reducing rectification, but has no effect on the delayed (outward) rectifier, K_{dr} (Iijima & Taira, 1987). Bril and Man (1990) similarly concluded that the K-channel openers were acting on K_{IR} (and possibly also on delayed rectifiers) in canine Purkinje fibres. However, K_{IR} is not thought to be involved in the action of nicorandil (Kakei et al., 1986b; Takano & Noma, 1990).

Several reports indicate a reduction by K-channel openers of the outward K^+-current through K_{IR}. Thus, under hyperpolarizing conditions, pinacidil (500 μM), cromakalim (10 μM) and nicorandil (200 μM) block K_{IR} (Kakei et al., 1986b; Osterrieder, 1988; Martin & Chinn, 1990). A low concentration of pinacidil (10–50 μM) blocks K_{IR} in guinea-pig and canine ventricular myocytes (Nakayama et al., 1990; Tseng & Hoffman, 1990). Pinacidil probably blocks K_{IR} from the outer surface, because internal application had no effect (Fan et al., 1990a). Interestingly, in the absence of ATP, although pinacidil (100 μM) abolishes rectification, its inhibitory effect on the inward rectifier current is lost (Martin & Chinn, 1990).

The K_{ATP}, first described in heart cells by Noma (1983), is normally closed under physiological conditions. If the $[ATP]_i$ is reduced, in response to hypoxia or anoxia (Noma & Shibasaki, 1985), or if the cell is metabolically compromised (Noma, 1983; Trube & Hescheler, 1984), the K_{ATP}-channels open. Nevertheless, it is not certain that the $[ATP]_i$ in the heart could fall sufficiently to trigger the opening of K_{ATP} (Elliot et al., 1989). Indirect evidence presented by Allen and Orchard (1987) suggests that ischaemia- or hypoxia-induced action potential shortening can occur when the [ATP]$_i$ is only marginally reduced. In addition, Faivre and Findlay (1990) have recently shown that an increase in the open probability of only 1% would be sufficient to cause a 50% reduction in action potential duration. Furthermore, adenosine accumulates in ischaemic muscle (Rubio et al., 1969; Olsson, 1970). Although adenosine had apparently no effect on intact ventricular cells or on pancreatic β-cells (Isenberg & Belardinelli, 1984; Kakei et al., 1986a), it was found to open K_{ATP} in outside-out patches from rat ventricular myocytes (Kirsch et al., 1990). In the coronary artery, activation of K_{ATP} is thought to be responsible for both hypoxia- and adenosine-induced effects (Daut et al., 1990).

Direct effects of cromakalim on K_{ATP} in the heart were first described by Escande et al. (1988), Sanguinetti et al. (1988) and Osterrieder (1988). Cromakalim ($> 3\,\mu M$) or hypoxia produced a shortening of APD in guinea-pig papillary muscle which was reversed by glibenclamide ($3\,\mu M$), although glibenclamide alone had no effect. In isolated patches of guinea-pig ventricular myocytes, glibenclamide ($10\,\mu M$) was similarly without effect on whole-cell current, but abolished the marked increase induced by cromakalim ($10\,\mu M$). The inability of glibenclamide to reduce the whole-cell K-current in the absence of cromakalim, and the similar effects of glibenclamide on hypoxia- and cromakalim-induced APD-shortening led Sanguinetti and coworkers (1988) to conclude that cromakalim was acting on K_{ATP}. Almost simultaneously, Escande et al. (1988) demonstrated that the channel opened by cromakalim and inhibited by glibenclamide was also inhibited by ATP ($3\,mM$). The lack of effect of glibenclamide in the absence of a K-channel opener suggests that the channel opened by the K-channel opener is closed under normal physiological conditions. However, the extent to which the glibenclamide-sensitive K-channel(s) is normally open might be species-dependent, since glibenclamide ($10\,\mu M$) had no effect on guinea-pig ventricles (Sanguinetti et al., 1988) whereas a concentration of $1\,\mu M$ increased APD in canine isolated Purkinje fibres (Smallwood et al., 1990) and $10\,\mu M$ had a similar effect in rat ventricular muscle (Faivre & Findlay, 1989).

Although K-channel openers are effective whether applied at the intracellular (Escande et al., 1989) or extracellular side of an isolated membrane patch (Pilsudski et al., 1990a), a higher concentration of pinacidil (100–$200\,\mu M$) was required to enhance whole-cell currents (Fan et al., 1990b). This implies that the K-channel openers do not bind at an external site. Potassium-channel openers are effective in the absence of ATP, and thus they do not seem simply to interfere with the binding of ATP to its site of interaction at the channel. However, channels can only be opened by K-channel openers if 'run-down' has not occurred. It is thought that the

K_{ATP}-channels must be phosphorylated to be capable of opening, and that 'run down' is due to dephosphorylation (Findlay & Dunne, 1986; Findlay, 1987; Ohno-Shosaku *et al.*, 1987). Thus ATP has two opposing effects on the channel; although ATP itself causes inhibition of channel opening, a low concentration is required to maintain the channel in a phosphorylated state to permit opening (*see* Chapter 6). The 'run-down' channel is more sensitive to ATP than the 'non-inactivated' channel (Ashcroft, 1988; Thuringer & Escande, 1989). It has been proposed that K-channel openers normalize the channel responsiveness to ATP (Thuringer & Escande, 1989).

There are several reports of apparent antagonism between ATP and the K-channel openers. In the presence of a low concentration of ATP at the intracellular side of the membrane ($[ATP]_i$; 0.1 mM), nicorandil increases the open probability of K_{ATP} (Takano & Noma, 1990). The enhanced opening induced by nicorandil was opposed by increasing $[ATP]_i$ (Takano & Noma, 1990). In the absence of ATP, nicorandil (1 mM) produced some increase in the opening of K_{ATP}, but to a lesser extent than pinacidil (300 μM; Takano & Noma, 1990). Thuringer and Escande (1989) found that ATP produced a parallel rightward shift of the channel activation dose–response curve to RP 49356, and similarly, RP 49356 produced a parallel shift in the inhibitory dose–response curve to ATP. Although this is consistent with inhibition of ATP binding by RP 49356 as suggested by Thuringer and Escande (1989), the inability of high concentrations of the K-channel opener pinacidil to overcome the inhibitory effect of ATP led Fan and coworkers (1990b) to suggest that this compound binds to a different site but modulates the affinity of the receptor for ATP. Takano and Noma (1990) found that the binding rate of ATP was reduced by nicorandil without any effect of this agent on the rate of unbinding. Pinacidil (30 μM) increases the open state probability of a K_{ATP}-channel in isolated patches prepared from guinea-pig ventricles. The pinacidil-induced openings are inhibited by increasing the concentration of ATP at the intracellular side of the patch to 5 mM (Fan *et al.*, 1990a).

Effects on coronary blood flow

Coronary artery occlusion results in myocardial ischaemia, a condition in which the blood supply to the myocardium is insufficient to meet the metabolic demands. However, the rate at which occlusion occurs determines the effects produced. A slowly developing occlusion, e.g. atherosclerosis, allows the development of a collateral circulation which attenuates the effect of the restricted flow through the coronary arteries. The main condition associated with restricted coronary blood flow is angina pectoris. Complete occlusion of the coronary artery results in myocardial infarction. Most of the deaths following infarction are associated with arrhythmias, the incidence of which is related to the infarct size. Thus, pharmacological intervention to restrict the size of the infarct or to control the arrhythmias should be beneficial in reducing mortality.

In vivo, RP 52891 is a selective coronary vasodilator. In anaesthetized dogs this compound produced a large increase in coronary blood flow with a dose (1 μg/kg, i.v.) which had no effect on either blood pressure or heart rate (Cavero *et al.*, 1991a). Certain other K-channel openers produce a similar effect (Gross, 1991). This suggests that the K-channel openers might prove to be useful in the treatment of myocardial ischaemia. They may also prove to be beneficial in the treatment of coronary vasospasm which is thought to be due to a decreased K-conductance in large epicardial coronary arteries (Iwaki *et al.*, 1987).

In vitro, the response to K-channel openers in rat or rabbit aorta is independent of an intact endothelium (Taylor *et al.*, 1988; Cook, 1989). In contrast, *in vivo*, part of the coronary artery response to K-channel openers is possibly endothelium-dependent. Large arteries respond to a rapid increase in blood flow by dilation (Gerova *et al.*, 1979). The ability of cromakalim and pinacidil to increase blood flow through the circumflex artery is reduced by a flow-limiting stenosis suggesting that part of the relaxant effect of these agents is initiated by the endothelium in response to the increased coronary blood flow (Giudicelli *et al.*, 1990).

During periods when blood flow through coronary arteries is restricted the flow through collateral vessels becomes important. The development of a good collateral circulation in response to exercise or to slowly developing atherosclerosis is thought to be protective against ischaemic heart disease. Any compound which could selectively relax collateral blood vessels would increase blood flow to ischaemic tissue and therefore be useful therapeutically. There is some evidence that cromakalim may preferentially dilate collateral vessels in skeletal muscle (Angersbach & Nicholson, 1988). A similar early finding that nicorandil was selective for collateral vessels in a model of acute coronary occlusion in dogs was difficult to attribute directly to an effect via K-channel opening since this compound has a mixed vasorelaxant action, part of which, i.e. activation of guanylate cyclase, is due to the presence of its nitro-group (Holzmann, 1983). However, a similar effect of the non-chiral benzopyran EMD 52692 suggests that this action may be typical of K-channel openers. The concentration of EMD 52692 which increased coronary collateral blood flow in dogs had no effect on either blood pressure or blood flow to non-ischaemic myocardium (Gross, 1991). This, together with the low concentration of EMD 52692 required to relax isolated canine collateral blood vessels ($EC_{50} = 20$ nM; Gross, 1991) might indicate a selective effect of the K-channel openers on coronary blood flow. To be therapeutically useful, it would be essential for the K-channel openers to relax preferentially the collateral vessels, since the beneficial effect of nicorandil was not obtained if the systemic blood pressure was reduced (Lamping & Gross, 1984).

Effects of K-channel openers on isolated blood vessels

Effects on spontaneous mechanical activity

Portal veins of several species (e.g. rat, guinea-pig) exhibit spontaneous mechanical activity *in vitro*. In rat portal vein Hamilton *et al*. (1986) first demonstrated that cromakalim reduced the amplitude and frequency of spontaneous tension waves, and at sufficiently high concentrations (i.e. 1 μM) abolished mechanical activity. Subsequently, similar inhibitory effects of pinacidil, minoxidil sulphate and diazoxide have been described (Bray *et al*. 1987a; Southerton *et al*., 1988; Newgreen *et al*., 1990).

Relaxation of KCl-induced contractile responses

Increasing the $[K^+]$ of physiological salt solutions (PSS) is a widely used technique for the initiation of mechanical responses in isolated blood vessels. The depolarization of smooth muscle cells in this way permits the opening of voltage-dependent Ca-channels and hence the influx of Ca^{2+} into the cytosol (Hof & Vuorela, 1983). Depending on the nature of the vessel these mechanical responses comprise either a series of transient oscillations in tension (e.g. rat portal vein) or a sustained, tonic contraction (e.g. rabbit aorta). The magnitude of the response is directly related to the concentration of K^+ in the PSS, between the ranges 10–80 mM. A recent study has shown the importance of maintaining normal osmolarity when using high K-solutions (Nielsen-Kudsk *et al*., 1992).

If a tissue is exposed to a putative K-channel opening drug in sufficient concentration the K-permeability of the cell membrane will dominate all other ion permeabilities, provided that the K-channel does not inactivate and can remain open under conditions of raised membrane potential. The cells will assume a membrane potential at or close to the theoretical K-equilibrium potential (E_K) value provided no compensatory mechanism is activated. Addition of K^+ to the PSS will lower the membrane potential to a new E_K but a contraction will only be produced when the new E_K is less negative than the potential at which voltage-operated Ca-channels open. This potential is not known for certain in intact tissues but probably lies between -40 and -50 mV (Bolton *et al*., 1984; Hamilton *et al*., 1986). Thus a K-channel opener should be able to relax a contraction produced by addition of 20 mM K^+ (E_K approximately -50 mV), but have no effect on a contraction produced by 80 mM K^+ (E_K approximately -20 mV).

The relaxation of low (<30 mM) but not high (>80 mM) K^+-induced contractile responses is now considered diagnostic of a K-channel opening action. Weir and Weston (1986b) first showed that cromakalim inhibited the development of the contractile response to concentrations of K^+ lower than 30mM but had little effect against higher concentrations in both rat portal vein and aorta. Established contractions of rat aorta to low (< 30 mM) but not high (80 mM) K^+ were completely relaxed by cromakalim (e.g. Newgreen et al., 1990). Similar observations have been made with cromakalim and other K-channel openers in rabbit aorta, mesenteric and cerebral arteries, and dog coronary and middle cerebral artery (Kreye et al., 1987; Cook et al., 1988b; Masuzawa et al., 1990a,b; Parsons et al., 1991a; Trezise & Weston, 1991).

In all blood vessels studied cromakalim has no inhibitory effects on high K^+-induced contractile responses suggesting that this agent acts solely by opening K-channels. Pinacidil, at high concentrations (i.e. $> 10 \mu M$), clearly has an additional vasorelaxant mode of action since it relaxes high K^+-induced spasm of rabbit and cat basilar arteries (Parsons et al., 1991a; Trezise & Weston, 1991a). Similar observations have been made with diazoxide in rat aorta (Newgreen et al., 1990). One of the earliest recognized K-channel opening compounds, nicorandil, produces substantial relaxation of high K^+-induced contractions; evidence exists to suggest that this additional inhibitory action is probably associated with stimulation of guanylate cyclase (Holzmann, 1983; Sumimoto et al., 1987).

Effects on $^{42}K^+$/$^{86}Rb^+$-efflux

Measurement of the efflux of radiolabelled K^+ or Rb^+ from isolated blood vessels is a widely used technique in the assessment of vascular K-channel opening properties of drugs (Fig. 14.1). In early experiments $^{86}Rb^+$ was used as a marker for K^+, principally because of its higher specific activity and longer half-life. Several reports show that cromakalim enhances the rate of ^{86}Rb exchange in rat aorta and portal vein (Hamilton et al., 1986; Weir & Weston, 1986b; Newgreen et al., 1990). Similar observations have been made in other vascular preparations, for example guinea-pig portal vein (Quast, 1987), rabbit mesenteric artery (McHarg et al., 1990) and dog coronary and middle cerebral artery (Masuzawa et al., 1990a,b). Pinacidil, minoxidil sulphate, nicorandil and diazoxide also increase the rate $^{86}Rb^+$ exchange in isolated blood vessels (Weir & Weston, 1986b; Bray & Weston, 1987; Videbaek et al., 1988; Masuzawa et al., 1990a,c; Newgreen et al., 1990). More recently, simultaneous measurements of the efflux of ^{42}K and ^{86}Rb from vascular smooth muscle have been made. In these studies the absolute increases in ^{42}K-efflux evoked by K-channel opening drugs consistently exceed the absolute ^{86}Rb-efflux changes (e.g. Bray & Weston, 1987; Quast & Baumlin, 1988; Newgreen et al., 1990) reflecting the fact that measurement of ^{86}Rb-flux generally underestimates the flux of K^+ (Smith et al., 1986). Recent data suggest that some K-channels may

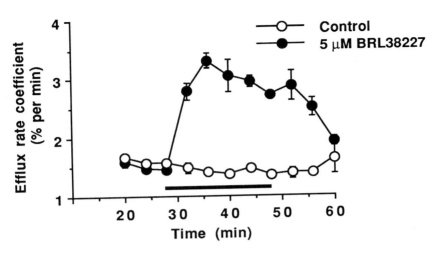

Fig. 14.1. Typical effects of BRL 38227 on ^{42}K-exchange in segments of rat isolated aorta (mean $\pm$ SEM values, $n = 5$ are shown). The marked increase in ^{42}K-efflux is a feature characteristic of all known K-channel openers. (G. Edwards, unpublished observations.)

be very impermeable to ^{86}Rb, a factor which contributes to the ^{42}K$/^{86}$Rb-flux differences (Newgreen *et al.*, 1990). Furthermore, in rat aorta and portal vein, minoxidil sulphate may exert a selective opening action on ^{86}Rb-impermeable K-channels (Newgreen *et al.*, 1990).

Interestingly, cromakalim evokes larger increases in ^{86}Rb-efflux under partially depolarized (i.e. 20 mM K$^+$), when compared with unstimulated conditions (Cox, 1990; Masuzawu *et al.*, 1990a). Indeed, in blood vessels in which in normal PSS it is difficult to detect effects of cromakalim on ^{86}Rb-flux (e.g. rat tail artery and mesenteric branches, dog middle cerebral artery), elevating extracellular K$^+$ reveals that cromakalim can evoke efflux of ^{86}Rb (Cox, 1990; Masuzawa *et al.*, 1990a).

Electrophysiological effects

Intra- and extracellular recording

The effects of K-channel openers on the electrical activity of isolated blood vessels have been studied using conventional techniques for both extra-cellular and intracellular recording. In spontaneously-contracting portal veins associated electrical discharges are first shortened and then abolished by cromakalim (Hamilton *et al.*, 1986), pinacidil (Bray *et al.*, 1987a; Southerton *et al.*, 1988), nicorandil (Karashima *et al.*, 1982), diazoxide and minoxidil sulphate (Newgreen *et al.*, 1990). Subsequently, a con-centration-dependent hyperpolarization develops and this usually persists for the duration of the recording (at least up to 30 min; Fig. 14.2). In a

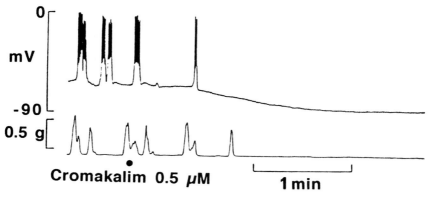

Fig. 14.2. Effect of cromakalim on membrane potential and spontaneous mechanical activity (upper trace) and membrane potential in rat portal vein. Note the marked membrane hyperpolarization which is sustained in the continuing presence of cromakalim. (From Hamilton *et al.*, 1986, with permission.)

single intracellular recording from a smooth muscle pacemaker cell in rat portal vein, minoxidil sulphate slowed the rate of rise of the pacemaker potential, thus delaying the firing of the action potential (Newgreen *et al.*, 1990). This action is probably responsible for the decrease in the frequency of spontaneous activity observed with minoxidil sulphate and other K-channel opening agents in this tissue.

In blood vessels that are electrically and mechanically quiescent at rest, K-channel openers typically evoke membrane hyperpolarization. This has been demonstrated in rat and rabbit aorta (Taylor *et al.*, 1988; Bray *et al.*, 1991), rabbit pulmonary artery (Kreye *et al.*, 1987), rat and rabbit mesenteric resistance arteries (Videbaek *et al.*, 1988; McHarg *et al.*, 1990) and guinea-pig mesenteric artery and vein (Nakao *et al.*, 1988). In each case the final membrane potential achieved in the presence of the K-channel opening drug approached the theoretical value for E_K (i.e. -80 to -90 mV). With the exception of the study in guinea-pig mesenteric vasculature (Nakao *et al.*, 1988) in which membrane potential changes evoked by cromakalim were transient, membrane hyperpolarization is generally sustained in the continual presence of a K-channel opening drug. In rabbit mesenteric arterioles, glibenclamide inhibited the hyperpolarizing action of cromakalim (McHarg *et al.*, 1990).

Few data exist describing the electrical effects of K-channel openers under depolarized conditions. This probably reflects the difficulty in impaling contracted smooth muscle cells with sharp glass microelectrodes. However, in guinea-pig mesenteric artery Nakashima *et al.* (1990) showed that pinacidil caused membrane hyperpolarization (toward the new E_K) in preparations depolarized by concentrations of up to 20 mM K$^+$. In higher concentrations of K$^+$ (above 20 mM), pinacidil had no effect on membrane potential. In the presence of pinacidil the slope of the recorded membrane potential line at different $[K^+]_o$ was similar to that predicted by the Nernst equation for a K-selective membrane. Clearly these measurements demonstrate the K-channel opening effects of pinacidil. In the same study pinacidil inhibited noradrenaline-induced depolarization (Nakashima *et al.*, 1990). Similarly, the depolarizing actions of noradrenaline in rabbit mesenteric resistance arteries and portal veins are reduced in the presence of K-channel openers (Leblanc *et al.*, 1989; McHarg *et al.*, 1990).

Inhibition by K-channel blockers

The mechanoinhibitory effects of K-channel openers in isolated blood vessels are attenuated by the sulphonylurea glibenclamide (Wilson *et al.*, 1988b; Winquist *et al.*, 1989; Masuzawa *et al.*, 1990b,c; Newgreen *et al.*, 1990; Parsons *et al.*, 1990b; Wickenden *et al.*, 1991), a selective inhibitor of K_{ATP} in pancreatic β-cells (Ashford, 1990), and by tetraethylammonium (TEA), 4-aminopyridine (4-AP) and procaine, less selective K-channel blocking agents (Quast, 1987; Southerton & Weston, 1987; Wilson *et al.*, 1988b; Winquist *et al.*, 1989). Charybdotoxin, apamin and noxiustoxin, blockers of large and small conductance Ca-dependent, and K_{dr}-channels respectively, did not antagonize responses to K-channel openers (Weir & Weston, 1986a; Strong *et al.*, 1989; Winquist *et al.*, 1989; Wickenden *et al.*, 1991). Interestingly a purified fraction (termed leiurotoxin by Chicci *et al.*, 1988) of the crude venom from which charybdotoxin is obtained (*Leiurus quinquestriatus var. herbraeus* venom), inhibits cromakalim-evoked Rb^+-efflux from rabbit aortic smooth muscle (Strong *et al.*, 1989) (*see* Chapter 11).

Effects on specific K-channels

Involvement of K_{ATP}

No clear picture has yet emerged of the nature of the K-channel opened by cromakalim and related drugs in vascular smooth muscle cells. It is tempting to suggest that the induced K-current is carried by K_{ATP}, since both K-channel opener-induced vasorelaxation and K_{ATP} in pancreatic β-cells are blocked by glibenclamide. Moreover, in rabbit mesenteric artery Standen *et al.* (1989) identified a K-selective channel that was opened by a reasonably low concentration of cromakalim (1 μM), closed by ATP and inhibited by glibenclamide (20 μM). The high conductance of the channel in these experiments (135 pS at 0 mV with 60 mM extracellular K^+ and 120 mM intracellular K^+) contrasts with the much lower conductance of K_{ATP} in the pancreatic β-cell (Ashford, 1990). In addition, the concentration of glibenclamide used (20 μM) was in excess of that required to either inhibit the relaxant effects of cromakalim in the same study (i.e. 250 nM) or to block K_{ATP} selectively in the β-cell (*see* Chapter 6). Indeed the selectivity of such a high concentration of glibenclamide for a single channel type is questionable, casting doubts over whether the effect of such concentrations of glibenclamide on vascular smooth muscle really indicates the involvement of a K_{ATP}-channel similar to that described in the pancreatic β-cell.

Involvement of large conductance Ca-sensitive K-channels (BK_{Ca})

Potassium-channel openers have also been shown to increase the open probability of charybdotoxin (ChTX)-sensitive BK_{Ca} in membrane patches from rat portal vein cells (Hu *et al.*, 1990) and coronary artery cells (Gelband *et al.*, 1989, 1990; Silberberg & van Breemen, 1990) or after incorporation of BK_{Ca} (isolated from rabbit aorta) into planar lipid bilayers (Gelband *et al.*, 1990). Consistent with findings that the effects of K-channel openers both *in vivo* and *in vitro*, are inhibited by glibenclamide, the ability of the K-channel openers to increase the open probability of the BK_{Ca} was also antagonized by glibenclamide. However, other reports have failed to detect inhibition of whole cell cromakalim-stimulated currents by ChTX (Beech & Bolton, 1989a; Nakao & Bolton, 1991). This, together with the inability of ChTX to modify either the mechano-inhibitory effects of cromakalim in the rat or rabbit portal vein (Winquist *et al.*, 1989; Wickenden *et al.*, 1991) or the ^{86}Rb-efflux-stimulating effects of cromakalim in rabbit aorta (Strong *et al.*, 1989), suggests that an effect on BK_{Ca} is unlikely to contribute to the physiologically relevant actions of the K-channel openers.

Role of small conductance K-channels

There have been numerous reports describing effects of K-channel openers on small conductance K-channels in isolated membrane patches from vascular smooth muscle. The channels reported by different laboratories apparently differ in their sensitivity to calcium or to ATP. It remains to be determined whether the various groups have identified distinct K-channel types or whether the differences may be attributed to species or tissue variations or to the different experimental conditions (e.g. pipette solutions) utilized by each laboratory. In general, the concentrations of the K-channel openers which have been utilized to demonstrate an increased opening of K-channels in isolated patches (10–500 μM; Gelband *et al.*, 1990; Kajioka *et al.*, 1990) is far higher than would be predicted from their potency as vasorelaxants *in vitro* (Southerton *et al.*, 1988; Newgreen *et al.*, 1990). Thus, Kajioka *et al.* (1990) found a 10 pS ATP- and Ca-sensitive K-channel in rat portal vein was opened by nicorandil (> 30 μM). In contrast, in the rabbit portal vein the low conductance (15 pS) K-channel activated by pinacidil (100 μM) was ATP-sensitive but not Ca-sensitive (Kajioka *et al.*, 1991).

Nakao and Bolton (1991) have described a 7.5 pS K-channel in membrane patches isolated from rabbit portal vein and mesenteric artery cells. Relatively high concentrations of cromakalim ($20\,\mu$M) and glibenclamide ($30\,\mu$M) were required to modify the channel open probability in the isolated patch, contrasting with the relatively low concentrations which were used to induce a K-current in the whole cell (cromakalim, $> 0.3\,\mu$M; glibenclamide, $> 1\,\mu$M). This raises the possibility that removal of membrane patches (and perhaps intracellular regulatory factors) might alter the sensitivity of channels to modulators. Such an effect was indeed recently reported by Kajioka et al. (1991). These authors found that the activity of a small conductance (15 pS) K-channel, evident in cell-attached recordings, was lost on excision of a patch. This channel, which was sensitive to ATP but not calcium could be activated by pinacidil ($> 3\,\mu$M) in the cell-attached patch configuration but was insensitive to concentrations as high as $100\,\mu$M pinacidl after patch excision. Guanosine diphosphate (GDP; $> 100\,\mu$M) was able to reactivate the channel in isolated patches only in the presence of pinacidil ($100\,\mu$M) (Kajioka et al., 1991).

Since, in isolated membrane patches, many K-channel types are apparently modified by the K-channel openers, examination of the effects of these agents on whole-cell currents may allow a better characterization of the main channel responsible for the effects of the K-channel openers in whole tissues. Both Beech and Bolton (1989a) and Noack et al. (1992b) concluded that a K-channel with a relatively small single channel conductance carried the current induced by cromakalim or BRL 38227, respectively. Based on the relative sensitivity of the current stimulated by cromakalim to inhibition by a series of K-channel blockers, and after the elimination of other major K-channels as potential sites of action, Beech and Bolton (1989a) concluded that the most likely channel to have been modulated by cromakalim was that which underlies the delayed rectifier current ($I_{K(V)}$). Although the current induced by cromakalim was apparently non-inactivating (in contrast to $I_{K(V)}$), it was proposed that cromakalim could have altered the voltage sensitivity of the delayed rectifier channel (K_V). A discrepancy in this proposal was the inability of glibenclamide ($50\,\mu$M) to inhibit $I_{K(V)}$ although the K-current stimulating effects of cromakalim ($10\,\mu$M) were clearly fully antagonized.

Noack and coworkers (1992a,b) have described a BRL 38227-induced current carried by channels with a relatively small single channel conductance and which is similar to that of Beech and Bolton (1989b). Under conditions of low calcium in the pipette and bath, a non-inactivating current was stimulated by BRL 38227 ($100\,$nM–$10\,\mu$M; Fig. 14.3) and this could be inhibited by either ciclazindol (1–$10\,\mu$M) or glibenclamide (1–$10\,\mu$M; Noack et al., 1992a,b). After application of BRL 38227, a slowly-developing increase in outward current associated with an increase in current noise was observed. Stationary fluctuation analysis revealed

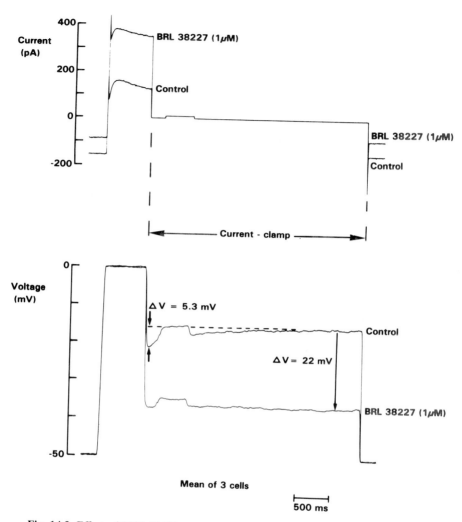

Fig. 14.3. Effect of BRL 38227 on membrane currents and membrane potential in rat portal vein using a combined voltage-clamp/current-clamp protocol. *Upper panel*: effects of BRL 38227 on membrane currents when the holding potential was stepped from − 50 to 0 mV. *Lower panel*: voltage protocol and membrane potential corresponding to the upper current traces. Note the magnitude of the membrane hyperpolarization (22 mV) associated with the BRL 38227-induced current. Data are the mean of 10 successive voltage/current-clamp protocols in each of three different cells. (From Noack *et al.*, 1992a, with permission.)

that the current induced by BRL 38227 had an underlying single channel conductance of 17 pS (Noack *et al.*, 1992a).

A relatively low conductance K-channel ($\gamma = 30$ pS) which is sensitive to extracellular calcium is present in the porcine coronary artery (Inoue *et al.*, 1989). This channel is opened by nicorandil (20–100 μM) under conditions in which it would normally be closed ($[Ca^{2+}]_o = 50\,\text{nM}$). It remains to be determined whether the K-channel opener-induced current described by Noack *et al.* (1992a,b) is similarly sensitive to $[Ca^{2+}]_o$. However, in simultaneous current- and voltage-clamp experiments the magnitude of the hyperpolarization produced by 1 μM BRL 38227 under low calcium conditions (via a 17 pS channel) was sufficient to explain all the vasorelaxant effects of this agent (Noack *et al.*, 1992a).

Further studies to clarify the present confusion concerning the K-channel type(s) opened to cromakalim and related drugs are clearly required. Indeed some evidence suggests that the relaxant effects of K-channel openers may not even be restricted to an action on K-channels. For example, cromakalim ($> 3\,\mu$M) inhibits Ca-currents typical of those carried by L-type Ca-channels in whole cells isolated from rat portal vein (Okabe *et al.*, 1990), and pinacidil reduces Cl^--conductance in rat mesenteric resistance arterioles (Videbaek *et al.*, 1990). However, the ability of cromakalim to inhibit Ca-current in single cells (Okabe *et al.*, 1990) probably has little relevance in whole tissues. In these, cromakalim fails to inhibit 80 mM KCl-induced contractions (Weir & Weston, 1986b) or the increase in $[Ca^{2+}]_i$ produced by either 45 or 90 mM KCl (Yanagisawa *et al.*, 1990).

Mechanisms of vasorelaxation

At the cellular level, K-channel opening moves the plasmalemmal membrane potential away from voltages at which ion channels involved in cell excitation open (Hamilton *et al.*, 1986). K-channel opening drugs thus exert a form of chemical voltage-clamping of the plasmalemma, thereby short-circuiting the depolarizing actions of excitatory stimuli. The primary consequence of this is considered to be the inhibition of Ca^{2+} entry via the indirect closure of voltage-dependent Ca-channels. Indeed, simultaneous tension recording and Ca^{2+} imaging techniques (fura-2) have shown that cromakalim inhibits both the increase in force and the increase in $[Ca^{2+}]_i$ evoked by 5–30 mM KCl in dog coronary artery and rabbit aorta (Yanagisawa *et al.*, 1990; Yoshitake *et al.*, 1991). The observation that cromakalim does not inhibit verapamil-sensitive increases in force and $[Ca^{2+}]_i$ induced by 90 mM KCl suggests that relaxant effects of cromakalim involve the opening of K-channels rather than the direct blockade of Ca-channels. Cromakalim has no effect on the $[Ca^{2+}]_i$-force relationship although both nicorandil and pinacidil shift this relationship to the right. This provides evidence that mechanisms unrelated to K-channel opening are also involved in the vasodilator effects of nicorandil and pinacidil (Yanagisawa *et al.*, 1990). In the case of pinacidil this phenomenon has been studied in detail. From experiments in skinned vascular smooth muscle, Itoh *et al.* (1991) concluded that pinacidil inhibits Ca^{2+}-induced contraction via a direct action on the contractile machinery, possibly at a site between Ca^{2+}-calmodulin complex formation and phosphorylation of the myosin light chain.

It is clear, however, from several studies that the vasorelaxant properties of K-channel openers cannot be explained solely by the indirect closure of dihydropyridine-sensitive voltage-dependent Ca-channels. Other putative mechanisms of vasorelaxation have thus been the subject of recent investigations.

Effects on intracellular Ca^{2+} stores

In rabbit aortic rings, a vascular preparation in which contraction can be elicited by agents that are either sensitive (e.g. KCl depolarization) or relatively insensitive (e.g. noradrenaline) to inhibition by dihydropyridine calcium antagonists, cromakalim exerts far greater antivasoconstrictor activity than Ca-entry blocking drugs (Cook et al., 1988b; Bray et al., 1991). Different inhibitory profiles of K-channel openers and Ca-antagonists versus agonist-induced contractile responses have also been observed in other blood vessels including rat aorta (Turner et al., 1989) and pig coronary artery (Cain & Nicholson, 1989).

The additional inhibitory effects of K-channel openers appear, on the whole, to be mediated via the opening of K-channels since they are both sensitive to glibenclamide and high extracellular K^+ (Cook et al., 1988b; Bray et al., 1991). It is possible that these agents do indirectly inhibit Ca^{2+}-influx through dihydropyridine-insensitive Ca-channels, which have been identified in vascular smooth muscle (Bean et al., 1986). However, the observation that noradrenaline-induced contraction is not associated with depolarization in tissues like rabbit aorta would argue against this proposal (Bray et al., 1991). Several lines of evidence however, suggest that it is more likely that effects on intracellular calcium stores are involved. In tissue-bath experiments, Bray et al. (1991) first showed that cromakalim inhibits both the refilling and release of Ca^{2+} from noradrenaline-sensitive intracellular stores in rabbit aorta by a glibenclamide-sensitive mechanism. These authors speculated that if in vascular smooth muscle, as in skeletal muscle, filling of intracellular Ca^{2+} stores involves an intracellular Ca : K exchange mechanism (Fink & Stephenson, 1987) such a mechanism could be the target for cromakalim and related drugs. A later study in the rat mesenteric arterial bed confirmed the inhibitory effects of cromakalim on noradrenaline-induced Ca^{2+} release and further showed that caffeine-induced Ca^{2+} release was unaffected by this K-channel opener (Quast & Baumlin, 1991).

Although an early study suggested that cromakalim did not interfere with the turnover of inositol phosphate (Coldwell & Howlett, 1987), Ito et al. (1991) demonstrated that BRL 38227 inhibits the synthesis of inositol 1,4,5-triphosphate (IP_3), and the associated increases in $[Ca^{2+}]_i$

and tension evoked by noradrenaline in rabbit mesenteric arteries bathed in Ca^{2+}-free bathing solution. These effects of BRL 38227 were attenuated by glibenclamide, high extracellular K^+, or by skinning the preparation suggesting that membrane hyperpolarization is essential for these inhibitory effects of BRL 38227 on the noradrenaline-induced Ca^{2+}-releasing mechanism. Pinacidil exerts similar inhibitory effects in rabbit mesenteric arteries (Itoh *et al.*, 1992). Taken together with similar observations in tracheal smooth muscle (Challiss *et al.*, 1992), these data suggest that opening of glibenclamide-sensitive plasmalemmal K-channels may negatively control the hydrolysis of phosphatidylinositol 4,5-biphosphate (PIP_2) induced by certain spasmogens. The overall picture of the vasorelaxant profile of K-channel openers in smooth muscle has become further complicated by a recent study showing that in airways smooth muscle cells BRL 38227 inhibits the refilling of an IP_3-sensitive Ca^{2+} pool via a mechanism that is independent of the plasmalemma (Chopra *et al.*, 1992). Whether such a mechanism also applies in vascular smooth muscle remains to be determined.

These studies clearly suggest that the K-channel openers inhibit vascular smooth muscle contraction not only by the indirect closure of L-type Ca-channels but also by compromising the intracellular Ca^{2+} release and storage mechanisms. Both effects are glibenclamide-sensitive, abolished in high K^+ solution and by removal of the plasmalemma suggesting that an interaction between the K-channel openers and a K-channel is the common underlying factor. The relative importance of these two vasorelaxant mechanisms may be agonist- and vessel-dependent.

Effects on transmitter release

Studies on a variety of non-vascular systems have shown that cromakalim, albeit at high concentrations ($> 10\,\mu M$), can inhibit neuronal excitability and neurotransmission (Alzheimer & ten Bruggencate, 1988; Schwörer & Kilbinger, 1989). In vascular tissues however, although neurotransmission is impaired by K-channel openers, no direct inhibition of transmitter release by these agents is involved. Thus McHarg *et al.* (1990) found that cromakalim reduced the amplitude and duration of excitatory junction potentials (EJPs) evoked by field stimulation in rabbit mesenteric artery, but concluded that such an effect was caused by an action on the smooth muscle itself. Similar findings have been obtained using pinacidil and in two studies, in guinea-pig and rabbit blood vessels, no inhibitory effect of this agent on labelled noradrenaline release was detected, although EJP amplitude and duration were reduced (Nedergaard, 1989; Nakashima *et al.*, 1990).

Effects on cyclic nucleotides and G proteins

The vasorelaxant effects of K-channel openers appear to be independent of changes in cyclic nucleotides, since neither diazoxide, minoxidil sulphate, nor cromakalim alter intracellular cyclic adenosine monophosphate (cAMP) or cyclic guanosine monophosphate (cGMP) concentrations in rat aorta (Southerton et al., 1988; Taylor et al., 1988; Newgreen et al., 1990). At high concentrations (100 μM) pinacidil significantly elevates cAMP levels (Kauffmann et al., 1986). Although nicorandil increases cGMP concentrations in bovine coronary artery (Holzmann, 1983) and rat and rabbit aorta (Miyata et al., 1990a & Ishibashi et al., 1991) this action is probably unrelated to its K-channel opening action (Newgreen et al., 1988). Cromakalim does not open K-channels via an intermediate action on a pertussis toxin-sensitive G protein (Quast et al., 1988).

Miscellaneous effects

In Ca-free PSS, cromakalim and other K-channel openers evoke an anomalous, delayed onset, slowly developing sustained contractile response in rabbit aorta (Bray et al., 1989; Duty & Weston, 1990). This phenomenon would seem to be a consequence of K-channel opening since it is attenuated by both glibenclamide and depolarizing conditions. The importance of this with relevance to the role of K-channels in regulating intracellular calcium handling and the relaxant properties of K-channel openers remains to be determined.

Effects of K-channel blockers on isolated blood vessels

Molecules as structurally diverse as simple inorganic cations (e.g. Ba^{2+}) and long chain polypeptides (e.g. charybdotoxin) demonstrate K-channel blocking properties (see Castle et al., 1989 and Cook and Quast, 1990 for reviews). A detailed description of the electrophysiology and function of K-channels in smooth muscle can be found in Chapter 7. In this section the mechanical effects of K-channel blockers in vascular smooth muscle are overviewed.

Mechanical effects

Simplistically, blockade of K-channels should decrease membrane K-conductance, cause membrane depolarization and hence increase smooth muscle cell excitability, assuming that the relevant K-channels are open under the experimental conditions. In vitro studies in vascular tissues generally show this to be the case.

Effects on resting tone in electrically quiescent blood vessels

In vessels which do not exhibit spontaneous mechanical activity several K-channel blockers have been shown to cause contraction. In high concentrations (10–100 mM) TEA evokes a biphasic contractile response of rabbit main pulmonary artery comprising an initial tonic phase followed by a phasic contractile response after prolonged incubation (> 30 min; Haeusler & Thorens, 1980). The initial event is accompanied by membrane depolarization, an increase in membrane resistance, anomalous (inward) rectification and occasionally spike potentials in response to externally applied depolarizing current pulses. At similar concentrations, TEA evokes action potentials and phasic tension waves in several other blood vessels, e.g. rabbit pulmonary artery (Casteels *et al.*, 1977), rabbit ear artery (Droogmans *et al.*, 1977), rabbit superior mesenteric artery (Harder & Sperelakis, 1979) and guinea-pig basilar artery (Fujiwara & Kuriyama, 1983). The ability of TEA to induce action potentials in normally electrically quiescent blood vessels has been attributed to the blockade of K-channels, thereby suppressing outward K-currents and thus permitting a net inward Ca-current that carries the action potential. At lower concentrations (< 5 mM), at which TEA shows some selectivity for BK_{Ca}-channels (Benham *et al.*, 1985; Beech & Bolton, 1989b), Cook (1989) found no direct contractile effect of TEA in rabbit aorta at concentrations below 1 mM. 3,4-diaminopyridine (3,4-DAP), however, at a concentration of 1 mM, contracted rabbit aorta (Cook, 1989) leading to the proposal that in this tissue the resting tension may be regulated by a population of K-channels which are more sensitive to 3,4-DAP than to TEA. Aminopyridines also evoke phasic contractions of human coronary artery (Uchida *et al.*, 1986) and guinea-pig pulmonary artery (Hara *et al.*, 1980), although these effects may not reflect a direct action on the smooth muscle itself. Inorganic cations such as Ba^{2+} and Cs^+ have been shown to block several different types of K-channel (Adams & Nonner, 1990). *In vitro*, Ba^{2+} induces contraction of vascular smooth muscle (Somlyo *et al.*, 1974; Karaki *et al.*, 1986) but its lack of specificity for any particular channel type does not allow the nature of the K-channels involved to be determined. Procaine and strychnine, blockers of both Na- and K-channels, also contract vascular smooth muscle (Shapiro, 1977; Louttit *et al.*, 1984; Ahn & Karaki, 1988).

More recently, isolated vascular tissue studies utilizing K-channel blockers with selectivity for specific channel types have been performed in attempts to clarify the role of K-channels in the control of vascular smooth muscle contractility. Charybdotoxin, a blocker of BK_{Ca} in vascular smooth muscle (Beech *et al.*, 1987), causes contraction of rabbit isolated aorta (Cook, 1989). It is unclear, however, if BK_{Ca}-channels, which are relatively insensitive to $[Ca]_i$, would be open at resting membrane potentials, thus leaving open the question whether ChTX contraction of vascular smooth muscle is due to blockade of these channels. An alternative explanation for these observations is that ChTX suppresses a resting (leak) K-conductance similar to that described in *Aplysia* neurones (Hermann & Erxleben, 1987). Neither apamin nor leiurotoxin I, blockers of SK_{Ca}-type channels contracts smooth muscle, suggesting that this type of channel does not contribute significantly to the control of resting tone (Chicchi *et al.*, 1988). Interestingly, glibenclamide causes endothelium-independent depolarization of rat, but not rabbit, small mesenteric artery (McHarg *et al.*, 1990; McPherson & Angus, 1991). Other less selective, putative blockers of K_{ATP} (i.e. phentolamine and alinidine) also depolarize rat mesenteric arteries (McPherson & Angus, 1991). However, apart from the rat coronary artery (Wolleben *et al.*, 1989), glibenclamide does not routinely contract vascular smooth muscle (e.g. Newgreen *et al.*, 1990; Masuzawa *et al.*, 1990b). It would thus seem that, at least in electrically quiescent blood vessels, glibenclamide-sensitive K-channels are not involved in the regulation of resting tension. This is supported by the observation that glibenclamide itself does not alter blood pressure *in vivo* (Smallwood *et al.*, 1990).

Effects on spontaneously active tissues

In spontaneously active blood vessels (e.g. portal veins of several species) many workers have described effects of K-channel blockers on mechanical activity. Interpretation of these data is difficult, however, since the electrical activity within the tissue is under constant modulation by pacemaker cells (Longmore & Weston, 1990). Drug-induced changes in mechanical activity may be the result of actions either at the pacemaker sites, or the contractile smooth muscle cells themselves. Tetraethylammonium, 4-AP, 3,4-DAP, procaine, noxiustoxin, ChTX and glibenclamide, but not apamin, increase spontaneous mechanical activity in rat portal vein (Southerton *et al.*, 1988; Winquist *et al.*, 1989; Longmore *et al.*, 1990; Wickenden *et al.*, 1991). Both TEA and procaine increase the amplitude and duration of phasic tension waves, with little effect on baseline tension, while 3,4-DAP increases baseline tension and contractile frequency, with little effect on the amplitude of contraction (Southerton *et al.*, 1988). In the case of TEA and procaine these mechanical effects probably reflect the blockade of a group of K-channels involved in membrane repolarization (resulting in elevation and prolonged duration of the rise in $[Ca^{2+}]_i$). The mechanical effects of 3,4-DAP are probably due to (i) the blockade of K-channels open at resting membrane potential resulting in membrane depolarization accompanied by an increase in baseline tension, and (ii) the blockade of K-channels involved in the modulation of the frequency of bursts of action potential discharge resulting in increased frequencies of both multispike complexes and contraction. The detailed effects of the other K-channel blockers on baseline tension, and frequency and amplitude of contraction have not been described.

Effects on agonist-evoked responses

In general, K-channel blockers augment contractile responses to exogenous vasoconstrictors. This phenomenon is most probably a consequence of two effects: (i) an increase in resting tone due to K-channel blockade, and (ii) a prolongation and increase in agonist-evoked rises in $[Ca^{2+}]_i$, by preventing K-efflux through K_V-type and/or K_{Ca}-type channels. In rabbit isolated aorta, TEA, 3,4-DAP and a ChTX-like toxin, but not apamin, augmented contractions due to low but not high KCl concentrations, and increased the maximum response to angiotensin II (Cook, 1989). Interestingly, TEA enhanced responses to angiotensin II at concentrations that did not cause contraction *per se*. Similar effects of TEA and aminopyridines on agonist-evoked contractions of rabbit main pulmonary artery and ear artery have also been observed (Glover, 1978; Haeusler & Thorens, 1980).

Other investigations into the effects of K-channel blockers on agonist-evoked responses have revealed more about the lack of specificity of some of these drugs for K-channels than they have concerning the role of K-channels in modulating vascular contractility. For example, glibenclamide inhibits contractions of vascular smooth muscle to prostaglandin $F_{2\alpha}$ and to the thromboxane A_2 mimetic U46619 (Cocks *et al.*, 1990; Zhang *et al.*, 1991). Furthermore, glibenclamide attenuates contractions to 30 mM KCl in rabbit coronary arteries (Nielsen-Kudsk & Thirstrup, 1991). It is thus clear that glibenclamide has an antagonist profile not restricted to K-channel blockade. In addition both quinine and procaine exhibit profiles of action in rabbit aorta which resemble Ca-entry blockers rather than K-channel blockers, in that they inhibit rather than augment KCl-evoked contractions (Ahn & Karaki, 1988; Cook & Quast, 1990).

Effects on neuronally evoked responses

The ultimate effect of K-channel blockers on neuronally evoked responses of blood vessels is a complex response resulting from interactions with both neuronal and smooth muscle K-channels. For example, 4-AP increases the contractile response of rabbit isolated ear artery to both transmural nerve stimulation and exogenous noradrenaline (Glover, 1978). The effect on nerve stimulation is greater than that on noradrenaline. One interpretation of these data is that 4-AP enhances vascular contractility directly (presumably by blocking smooth muscle K-channels) and increases transmitter release from sympathetic nerves. Indeed, Hara *et al.* (1980) speculated that in guinea-pig pulmonary artery and vein the contractile effect of 4-AP is a consequence of both noradrenaline release from sympathetic nerves and, at higher concentrations, of a direct action on the smooth muscle. The observation that 4-AP enhances neuronally stimulated [^{3}H]-noradrenaline release from dog saphenous vein adds strength to this supposition (Kato & Takata, 1987).

To date there are no detailed reports of effects of other K-channel blockers on neuronally evoked responses of isolated blood vessels. This type of experiment with TEA is complicated by the fact that TEA exerts several 'non-specific' actions including inhibition of muscarinic receptors (Adams et al., 1982) and inhibition of choline uptake by nerve terminals (Stanfield, 1983).

Endogenous K-channel openers: cardiovascular effects

Endothelium-derived hyperpolarizing factor (EDFH)

The role played by the vascular endothelium in acetylcholine-induced vasodilation was first recognized by Furchgott and Zawadski (1980). Using a variety of techniques, these workers showed that the *in vitro* relaxation of blood vessels produced by acetylcholine was largely associated with the release of an endogenous agent—endothelium-derived relaxing factor (EDRF)—from the vascular endothelium. Further details, including activation of smooth muscle soluble guanylate cyclase by EDRF and its probable identity as nitric oxide (NO) or a labile NO-containing moiety can be found in reviews by Furchgott (1984), Furchgott and Vanhoutte (1989) and Moncada et al. (1989).

In addition to muscarinic agonists, several agents including histamine and substance P produce endothelium-dependent relaxation of vascular smooth muscle (Furchgott, 1984). Microelectrode experiments in blood vessels showed that carbachol and substance P were also capable of generating endothelium-dependent membrane hyperpolarization (Bolton et al., 1984; Bolton & Clapp, 1986) and it was tacitly assumed by many that such changes were produced indirectly by EDRF release from the vascular endothelium. However, experiments involving both electrophysiological and ion flux techniques indicated that acetylcholine-induced hyperpolarization was associated with the release of a K-channel opening factor from the vascular endothelium (Southerton et al., 1987; Chen et al., 1988; Feletou & Vanhoutte, 1988; Taylor et al., 1988; Rand & Garland, 1990; Bray & Quast, 1991; Chen et al., 1991). Furthermore, experiments using NO-synthase inhibitors and the modifying agents oxyhaemoglobin and methylene blue strongly suggested that the K-channel opening factor was different from EDRF (Chen et al., 1988, 1991; Nagao & Vanhoutte, 1992).

Recent studies have indicated that NO itself can hyperpolarize vascular smooth muscle. This phenomenon, first reported by Tare *et al.* (1990) in uterine arteries, has also been observed by Garland and McPherson (1992) in rat small mesenteric artery and by Rand and Garland (1992) in rabbit basilar artery. In general, however, the hyperpolarizations produced by NO are relatively small and are only seen at near maximally-effective mechano-inhibitory concentrations of NO. The ability of NO to exert membrane potential changes contrasts with studies in a variety of tissues in which no such changes were detected (Beny & Brunet, 1988; Komori *et al.*, 1988; Brayden, 1990). Sodium nitroprusside also exerts little effect on vascular smooth muscle cell membrane potential (Ito *et al.*, 1978; Cheung & MacKay, 1985; Huang *et al.*, 1988; Southerton *et al.*, 1988) suggesting that elevation of cytosolic cGMP does not evoke hyperpolarization.

The observations on endothelium-dependent hyperpolarization collectively suggest that an entity distinct from EDRF is largely responsible for this phenomenon, and this factor has been designated 'endothelium-derived hyperpolarizing factor' (EDHF; Chen *et al.*, 1988). Further details on EDHF can be found in reviews by Taylor and Weston (1988) and Suzuki and Chen (1990), although the nature of this agent has still not been identified.

Although the ability of EDHF to open smooth-muscle K-channels is not in doubt (Chen *et al.*, 1988; Bray & Quast, 1991), the identity of the K-channel involved has not been clarified. In rabbit middle cerebral artery Standen *et al.* (1989) and Brayden (1990) reported that acetylcholine-evoked endothelium-dependent hyperpolarization was glibenclamide-sensitive. However, in guinea-pig coronary artery and rat small mesenteric artery, acetylcholine-induced hyperpolarization is unaffected by glibenclamide (Chen *et al.*, 1991; McPherson & Angus, 1991; Eckman *et al.*, 1992; Garland & McPherson, 1992). Furthermore, although acetylcholine-stimulated $^{42}K^+$-efflux is attenuated by TEA it is not inhibited by glibenclamide (Bray & Quast, 1991). These observations suggest that the released hyperpolarizing factor may not be identical in all tissues but further studies, particularly in cerebral arteries, are required before the situation can be clarified. In many tissues the endothelium-dependent membrane hyperpolarization produced by acetylcholine or histamine is more or less transient. Further, tachyphylaxis of the response often develops, an effect associated with receptor desensitization rather than with a lack of available EDHF (Chen *et al.*, 1988; Chen & Suzuki, 1989).

No clear picture regarding the relative contributions made by EDRF and EDHF to relaxation of isolated blood vessels in response to endothelium-dependent vasodilators has emerged. Using agents known to block the effects of EDRF (e.g. methylene blue, N^G-nitro-L-arginine), and in some cases inhibitors of the actions of EDHF (e.g. glibenclamide), has revealed that up to 30% of a given endothelium-dependent relaxation may be produced by EDHF. For example, in rat aorta a significant endothelium-dependent relaxation to histamine was still observed in the presence of methylene blue (Suzuki & Chen, 1990). Similarly, Brayden (1990) reported that in rabbit middle cerebral artery acetylcholine-evoked relaxation was only partially attenuated by methylene blue, yet abolished by a combination of both methylene blue and glibenclamide. In contrast, Parsons et al. (1991b) could find no effect of glibenclamide on acetylcholine evoked relaxation of this vessel, and observed that N^G-nitro-L-arginine completely abolished this response.

Such findings (sometimes minor contributions to relaxation, relative transience, tachyphylaxis) question the functional importance of EDHF in vivo (compared to EDRF). Perhaps the simplest explanation is that the relative contributions which EDHF and EDRF make to endothelium-dependent relaxations varies from vessel to vessel. Thus in rabbit basilar artery (Rand & Garland, 1992) acetylcholine-induced relaxations seem to involve little EDHF. In contrast, vessels like the rat small mesenteric artery develop large hyperpolarizations on exposure to acetylcholine and these are closely linked to relaxation (Garland & McPherson, 1992).

Little is known about those factors which induce EDHF release in vivo. Speculatively, haemodynamic shear stress (Olesen et al., 1988) could be one factor which triggers the production of this agent. Such stress hyper-polarizes vascular endothelial cells (Olesen et al., 1988) and the resulting influx of Ca^{2+} ions into the endothelium (Busse et al., 1988) could be the stimulus for EDHF release.

Calcitonin gene-related peptide (CRGP)

The polypeptide calcitonin gene-related peptide (CGRP) is found in neurones closely associated with central and peripheral blood vessels. It exerts potent vasodilator effects, some of which are endothelium-depen-dent (Brain et al., 1985; Bevan & Brayden, 1986; Prieto et al., 1991), a factor which complicates studies on the mode of action of CGRP. In rat aorta, in which the effects of CGRP are endothelium-dependent, the peptide failed to produce an increase in smooth muscle cGMP levels (Grace et al., 1987). Thus, in this tissue, the involvement of EDHF or another endogenous agent seems more likely than EDRF although this has not been established.

Recently, in a study which did not distinguish between endothelium-dependent and direct effects of CGRP, it was reported that CGRP hyper-polarized vascular smooth muscle. Furthermore this effect, together with part of the associated mechanical relaxation, was glibenclamide-sensitive (Nelson et al., 1990). In the same series of experiments, patch-clamp measurements showed that CGRP also activated a glibenclamide-sensitive smooth muscle K-channel. The implication that CGRP can directly open

K_{ATP} is clearly interesting although this was not established by Nelson *et al.* (1990) and further experiments are required to confirm this possibility.

In most types of mammalian heart, CGRP increases both rate and force of contraction. Such effects, together with the observation that Ca-currents and cAMP levels are increased (Ono *et al.*, 1989; Wang & Fiscus, 1989) suggest that the effects of CGRP may be basically similar to those of β-adrenoceptor agonists. In cardiac muscle, an increase in cAMP levels is associated with an increase in both Ca- and K-currents (Duchatelle-Gourdon *et al.*, 1989; Walsh *et al.*, 1989) and recently Kim (1991) reported that in rat heart, CGRP activated a K-channel with characteristics similar to that of K_{ACh}. No evidence for the activation of K_{ATP} by CGRP was detected in these studies.

Other vasodilators

Preliminary studies suggest that certain other endogenous agents may open K-channels in the cardiovascular system. For example, both prostacyclin and its stable analogue iloprost hyperpolarize vascular smooth muscle, an effect which is associated with the opening of K-channels (Siegel *et al.*, 1990). Prostacyclin or other cyclooxygenase products are not however, candidates for EDHF since the effects of the latter are not antagonized by indomethacin (Chen *et al.*, 1988). In rabbit middle cerebral arteries, there is some evidence that vasoactive intestinal polypeptide (VIP) opens glibenclamide-sensitive K-channels (Standen *et al.*, 1989). However, this phenomenon has yet to be systematically investigated and it is not yet clear whether VIP acts directly on the smooth muscle or exerts its effects via the release of EDHF.

References

Adams, D. J. & Nonner, W. (1990) Voltage-dependent potassium channel: gating, ion permeation and block. In Cook, N.S. (ed.), *Potassium Channels: Structure, Classification, Function and Therapeutic Potential*. Ellis Horwood Ltd, Chichester, pp. 40–69.

Adams, P. R., Brown, D. A. & Constanti, A. (1982) Pharmacological inhibition of the M-current. *Journal of Physiology* **322**, 233–262.

Ahn, H. Y. & Karaki, H. (1988) Inhibitory effects of procaine on contraction and calcium movement in vascular and intestinal smooth muscles. *British Journal of Pharmacology* **94**, 189–196.

Allen, D. G. & Orchard, C. H. (1987) Myocardial cell function during ischemia and hypoxia. *Circulation Research* **60**, 153–168.

Alzheimer, C. & ten Bruggengate, G. (1988) Actions of BRL 34915 (cromakalim) upon convulsive discharges in guinea-pig hippocampal slices. *Naunyn-Schmiedeberg's Archives of Pharmacology* **337**, 429–434.

Angersbach, D. & Nicholson, C. D. (1988) Enhancement of muscle blood cell flux and pO$_2$ by cromakalim (BRL34915) and other compounds enhancing membrane K$^+$ conductance, but not by Ca^{2+} antagonists or hydralazine, in an animal model of occlusive arterial disease. *Naunyn-Schmiedeberg's Archives of Pharmacology* **337**, 341–346.

Arena, J. P. & Kass, R. S. (1989a) Enhancement of potassium-sensitive current in heart cells by pinacidil: Evidence for modulation of the ATP-sensitive potassium channel. *Circulation Research* **65**, 436–445.

Arrigoni-Martelli, E., Kaergaard-Nielsen, Chr., Bang Olsen, U. & Petersen, H. J. (1980) N''-cyano-N-4-pyridyl-N'-1,2,2-trimethylpropylguanidine monohydrate (P1134); a new, potent vasodilator. *Experientia* **36**, 445–447.

Ashcroft, F. M. (1988) Adenosine 5′-triphosphate-sensitive potassium channels. *Annual Review of Neuroscience* **11**, 97–118.

Ashcroft, S. J. H. & Ashcroft F. M. (1990) Properties and functions of ATP-sensitive K-channels. *Cellular Signalling* **2**, 197–214.

Ashford, M. J. (1990) Potassium channels and modulation of secretion. In Cook, N. S. (ed.), *Potassium Channels, Structure, Classification, Function and Therapeutic Potential*. Ellis Horwood Ltd, Chichester, pp. 300–325.

Ashwood, V. A., Buckingham, R. E., Cassidy, F., Evans, J. N., Faruk, E. A., Hamilton, T. C., Nash, D. J., Stemp, G. & Willcocks, K. (1986) Synthesis and antihypertensive activity of 4-(cyclic amido)-2H-1-benzopyrans *Journal of Medicinal Chemistry* **29**, 2194–2201.

Auchampach, J. A., Maruyama, M., Cavero, I. & Gross, G. J. (1990) The potassium channel agonist RP 52891 reduces infarct size in the anesthetized dog. *The Pharmacologist* **32**, 147.

Bache, R. J., Arentzen, C. E., Simon, A. B. & Vrobel, T. R. (1984) Myocardial perfusion abnormalities during tachycardia in dogs with left ventricular hypertrophy: metabolic evidence for myocardial ischemia. *Circulation* **69**, 409–417.

Bache, R. J., Dai, X. Z. & Baran, K. W. (1990a) Effect of pinacidil on myocardial blood flow in the presence of a coronary artery stenosis. *Journal of Cardiovascular Pharmacology* **15**, 618–625.

Bache, R. J., Dai, X. Z. & Baran, K. W. (1990b) Effect of pinacidil on myocardial blood flow in the chronically pressure overloaded hypertrophied left ventricle. *Journal of Cardiovascular Pharmacology* **16**, 890–895.

Bang-Olsen, U. & Arrigoni-Martelli, E. (1983) Vascular effects in dogs of pinacidil (P1134), a novel vasoactive antihypertensive agent. *European Journal of Pharmacology* **88**, 389–392.

Bean, B. P., Sturek, M., Puga, A. & Hermsmeyer, K. (1986) Calcium channels in muscle cells from rat mesenteric arteries: modulation by dihydropyridines. *Circulation Research* **59**, 229–235.

Beech, D. J. & Bolton, T. B. (1989a) Properties of the cromakalim-induced potassium conductance in smooth muscle cells isolated from the rabbit portal vein. *British Journal of Pharmacology* **98**, 851–864.

Beech, D. J. & Bolton, T. B. (1989b) Two components of potassium current activated by depolarization of single smooth muscle cells from the rabbit portal vein. *Journal of Physiology* **418**, 293–309.

Beech, D. J., Bolton, T. B., Castle, N. A. & Strong, P. N. (1987) Characterisation of a toxin from scorpion (*Leiurus quinquestriatus*) venom that blocks *in vitro* both large (BK) K^+ channels in rabbit vascular smooth muscle and intermediate (IK) conductance Ca^{2+}-activated K^+ channels in human red cells. *Journal of Physiology* **387**, 32P.

Benham, C. D., Bolton, T. B., Lang, R. J. & Takewaki, T. (1985) The mechanism of action of Ba^{2+} and TEA on single Ca^{2+}-activated K^+ channels in arterial and intestinal smooth muscle cell membranes. *Pflügers Archiv* **403**, 120–127.

Beny, J. L. & Brunet, P. C. (1988) Neither nitric oxide nor nitroglycerin accounts for all the characteristics of endothelially-mediated vasodilatation of pig coronary arteries. *Blood Vessels* **25**, 308–311.

Bevan, J. A. & Brayden, J. E. (1986) Noradrenergic neural vasodilator mechanisms. *Circulation Research* **60**, 309–326.

Bolton, T. B. & Clapp, L. H. (1986) Endothelial-dependent relaxant actions of carbachol and substance P in arterial smooth muscle. *British Journal of Pharmacology* **87**, 713–723.

Bolton, T. B., Lang, R. J. & Takewaki, T. (1984) Mechanism of action of noradrenaline and carbachol on smooth muscle of guinea-pig anterior mesenteric artery. *Journal of Physiology* **351**, 549–572.

Brain, S. D., Williams, T. J., Tippins, J. R., Morris, H. R. & MacIntyre, I. (1985) Calcitonin gene related peptide is a potent vasodilator. *Nature* **313**, 54–56.

Bray, K. M. & Quast, U. (1991) Differences in the K^+-channels opened by cromakalim, acetylcholine and substance-P in rat aorta and porcine coronary artery. *British Journal of Pharmacology* **102**, 585–594.

Bray, K. M. & Weston, A. H. (1987) Differential concentration-dependent effects of K-channel openers on ^{42}K and ^{86}Rb efflux in rabbit isolated aorta. *British Journal of Pharmacology* **98**, 885P.

Bray, K. M., Duty, S. & Weston, A. H. (1989) Analysis of the spasmogenic effect of cromakalim in rabbit isolated aorta. *Journal of Physiology* **417**, 67P.

Bray, K. M., Newgreen, D. T., Small, R. C., Southerton, J. S., Taylor, S. G., Weir, S. W. & Weston, A. H. (1987a) Evidence that the mechanism of the inhibitory action of pinacidil in rat and guinea-pig smooth muscle differs from that of glyceryl trinitrate. *British Journal of Pharmacology* **91**, 421–429.

Bray, K. M., Newgreen, D. T. & Weston, A. H. (1987b) Some effects of the enantiomers of the potassium channel openers, BRL 34915 and pinacidil, on rat blood vessels. *British Journal of Pharmacology* **91**, 357P.

Bray, K. M., Weston, A. H., Duty, S., Newgreen, D. T., Longmore, J., Edwards, G. & Brown, T. J. (1991) Differences between the effects of cromakalim and nifedipine on agonist-induced responses in rabbit aorta. *British Journal of Pharmacology* **102**, 337–344.

Brayden, J. E. (1990) Membrane hyperpolarization is a mechanism of endothelium-dependent cerebral vasodilation. *American Journal of Physiology* **259**, H668–H673.

Bril, A. & Man, R. Y. K. (1990) Effects of the potassium channel activator, BRL 34915, on the action potential characteristics of canine cardiac Purkinje fibres. *Journal of Pharmacology and Experimental Therapeutics* **253**, 1090–1096.

Buckingham, R. E., Clapham, J. C., Hamilton, T. C., Longman, S. D., Norton, J. & Poyser, R. H. (1986a) Stereospecific mechanism of action of the novel anti-hypertensive agent, BRL 34915. *British Journal of Pharmacology* **87**, 78P.

Buckingham, R. E., Clapham, J. C., Hamilton, T. C., Longman, S. D., Norton, J. & Poyser, R. H. (1986b) BRL 34915, a novel antihypertensive agent: comparison of effects on blood pressure and other haemodynamic parameters with those of nifedipine in animal models. *Journal of Cardiovascular Pharmacology* **8**, 798–804.

Buckingham, R. E., Hamilton, T. C., Howlett, D. R., Mootoo, S. & Wilson, C. (1989) Inhibition by glibenclamide of the vasorelaxant action of cromakalim in the rat. *British Journal of Pharmacology* **97**, 57–64.

Bulkley, B. H. & Hutchins, G. M. (1977) Myocardial consequences of coronary artery bypass graft surgery: the paradox of necrosis in areas of revascularization. *Circulation* **56**, 906–913.

Busse, R., Fichtner, H., Luckhoff, A. & Kohlhardt, M. (1988) Hyperpolarization and increased free calcium in acetylcholine-stimulated endothelial cells. *Journal of Physiology* **255**, H965–H969.

Cain, C. R. & Metzler, V. (1985) Electrophysiological effects of the antihypertensive agent BRL 34915 in guinea-pig papillary muscle. *Naunyn-Schmiedeberg's Archives of Pharmacology* **329**, R53.

Cain, C. R. & Nicholson, C. D. (1989) Comparison of the effects of cromakalim, a potassium conductance enhancer, and nimodipine, a calcium antagonist, on 5-hydroxytryptamine responses in a variety of vascular smooth muscle. *Naunyn-Schmiedeberg's Archives of Pharmacology* **340**, 293–299.

Callewaert, G., Vereecke, J. & Carmeliet, E. (1986) Existence of a calcium-dependent potassium channel in the membrane of cow cardiac Purkinje fibres. *Pflügers Archiv* **406**, 424–426.

Carlsen, J. E., Kandel, T., Jensen, H. E., Tango, M. & Trap-Jensen, J. (1983) Pinacidil a new vasodilator: pharmacokinetics of a new retarded release tablet in essential hypertension. *European Journal of Pharmacology* **25**, 557–561.

Casteels, R., Kitamura, K., Kuriyama, H. & Suzuki, H. (1977) Excitation-coupling in the smooth muscle cells of the rabbit pulmonary artery. *Journal of Physiology* **271**, 63–79.

Castle, N. A., Haylet, D. G. & Jenkins, D. H. (1989) Toxins in the characterisation of potassium channels. *Trends in Neurosciences* **12**, 59–65.

Cavero, I., Aloup, J-C., Mondot, S., James, C., Le Monnier de Gouville, A-C. & Mestre, M. (1991a) Cardiovascular pharmacology of the carbothioamide K^+ channel opener RP 49356 and its active enantiomer, aprikalim, RP 52891. *Current Drugs: Potassium Channel Modulators* **1**, B70–B81.

Cavero, I., Mondot, S. & Mestre, M. (1989) Vasorelaxant effects of cromakalim in rats are mediated by glibenclamide-sensitive potassium channels. *Journal of Pharmacology and Experimental Therapeutics* **248**, 1261–1268.

Cavero, I., Pratz, P. & Mondot, S. (1991b) K^+ channel opening mediates the vasorelaxant effects of nicorandil in the intact system. *Zeitschrift für Kardiologie* **80** (Suppl. 7), 35–41.

Challiss, R. A. J., Patel, N., Adams, D. & Arch, J. R. S. (1992) Inhibitory action of the potassium channel opener BRL 38227 on agonist-stimulated phosphoinositide metabolism in bovine tracheal smooth muscle. *Biochemical Pharmacology* **43**, 17–20.

Chen, G. & Suzuki, H. (1989) Some electrical properties of the endothelium-dependent hyperpolarisation recorded from rat arterial smooth muscle cells. *Journal of Physiology* **410**, 91–106.

Chen, G., Suzuki, H. & Weston, A. H. (1988) Acetylcholine releases endothelium-derived hyperpolarising factors and EDRF from rat blood vessels *British Journal of Pharmacology* **95**, 1165–1174.

Chen, G., Yamamoto, Y., Miwa, K. & Suzuki, H. (1991) Hyperpolarization of arterial smooth muscle induced by endothelial humoral substances. *American Journal of Physiology* **260**, H1888–H1892.

Cheung, D. W. & Mackay, M. J. (1985) The effects of sodium nitroprusside on smooth muscle cells of rabbit pulmonary artery and portal vein. *British Journal of Pharmacology* **86**, 117–124.

Chi, L., Uprichard, A. G. & Lucchesi, B. R. (1989) Failure of glibenclamide to protect against ischemic ventricular fibrillation in a canine model of myocardial infarction. *Journal of Molecular and Cellular Cardiology* **21** (Suppl. II), S89.

Chicchi, G. G., Gimenz-Gallego, G., Ber, E., Garcia, M. L., Winquist, R. & Cascieri, M. A. (1988) Purification and characterisation of a unique, potent inhibitor of apamin binding from *Leiurus quinquestriatus hebraeus* venom. *Journal of Biological Chemistry* **263**, 10 192–10 197.

Chopra, L. C., Twort, C. H. C. & Ward, J. P. T. (1992) Direct action of BRL 38227 and glibenclamide on intracellular calcium stores in cultured airway smooth muscle of rabbit. *British Journal of Pharmacology* **105**, 259–260.

Clapham, J. C. & Buckingham, R. E. (1988) The haemodynamic profile of cromakalim in the cat. *Journal of Cardiovascular Pharmacology* **12**, 555–561.

Clapham, J. C. & Cooper, S. M. (1988) Effect of cromakalim (BRL 34915) and pinacidil on baroreceptor sensitivity in the anaesthetised cat. *British Journal of Pharmacology* **93** (Suppl.), 200P.

Clapham, J. C. & Longman, S. D. (1989) Haemodynamic differences between cromakalim and pinacidil: comparison with nifedipine. *European Journal of Pharmacology* **171**, 109–117.

Cocks, T. M., King, S. J. & Angus, J. A. (1990) Glibenclamide is a competitive antagonist of the thromboxane A_2 receptor in dog coronary artery *in vitro*. *British Journal of Pharmacology* **100**, 375.

Cohen, M. L. & Colbert, W. E. (1986) Comparison of the effects of pinacidil and its metabolite pinacidil-N-oxide in isolated smooth and cardiac muscle. *Drug Development Research* **7**, 111–124.

Coldwell, M. C. & Howlett, D. R. (1987) Specificity of action of the novel antihypertensive agent, BRL 34915, as a potassium channel activator. Comparison with nicorandil. *Biochemical Pharmacology* **36**, 3663–3669.

Cook, N. S. (1989) Effect of some potassium channel blockers on contractile responses of the rabbit aorta. *Journal of Cardiovascular Pharmacology* **13**, 299–306.

Cook, N. S. & Hof, R. P. (1988) Cardiovascular effects of apamin and BRL 34915 in rats and rabbits. *British Journal of Pharmacology* **93**, 121–131.

Cook, N. S. & Quast, U. (1990) Potassium channel pharmacology. In Cook, N.S. (ed.), *Potassium Channels: Structure, Classification, Function and Therapeutic Potential.* Ellis Horwood Ltd, Chichester, pp. 181–258.

Cook, N. S., Weir, S. W. & Danzeisen, M. C. (1988) Anti-vasoconstrictor effects of the K^+ channel opener cromakalim on the rabbit aorta—comparison with the Ca^{2+}-antagonist isradipine. *British Journal of Pharmacology* **95**, 741–752.

Cox, R. H. (1990) Effects of putative K^+ channel activator BRL-34915 on arterial contraction and ^{86}Rb efflux. *Journal of Pharmacological and Experimental Therapeutics* **252**, 51–59.

Daut, J., Maier-Rudolph, W., von Beckerath, N., Mehrke, G., Gunther, K. & Goedel-Meinen, L. (1990) Hypoxic dilation of coronary arteries is mediated by ATP-sensitive potassium channels. *Science* **247**, 1341–1344.

Davis, J. O. & Freeman, R. H. (1976) Mechanisms regulating renin release. *Physiological Reviews* **56**, 1–56.

de Lorenzi, F., Allard, Y. E., Chartier, D. & Ruiz-Petrich, E. (1990) Blockers of ATP-sensitive K-channels and the action potential of hypoxic rabbit myocardium. *Federation Proceedings* **4** (Abstr.), A559.

De Peyer, J. E., Lues, I., Gericke, R. & Hausler, G. (1989) Characterization of K^+ channel activator, EMD 52692, in electrophysiological and pharmacological experiments. *Pflügers Archiv* **414** (Suppl. 1), S191.

De Weille, J., Schmidt-Antomarchi, H., Fosset, M. & Lazdunski, M. (1988) ATP-sensitive K^+ channels that are blocked by hypoglycemia-inducing sulfonylureas in insulin secreting cells are activated by galanin, a hyperglycemia-inducing hormone. *Proceedings of the National Academy of Sciences USA* **85**, 1312–1316.

Droogmans, G., Raeymakers, L. & Casteels, R. (1977) Electro- and pharmacomechanical coupling in the smooth muscle cells of the rabbit ear artery. *Journal of General Physiology* **70**, 129–148.

Duchatelle-Gourdon, I., Hartzell, H. C. & Lagrutta, A. A. (1989) Modulation of the delayed rectifier potassium current in frog cardiomyocytes by β-adrenergic agonists and magnesium. *Journal of Physiology* **415**, 251–274.

Dumez, D., Zazzi-Sudriez, E., Pautrel, C., Armstrong, J. M. & Hicks, P. E. (1988) Comparison of the cardiovascular and renal effects of BRL 34915 with those of nitrendipine in dogs and spontaneously hypertensive rats. *British Journal of Pharmacology* **93**, 201P.

Dunne, M. J. (1990) Effects of pinacidil, RP 49356 and nicorandil on ATP-sensitive potassium channels in insulin-secreting cells. *British Journal of Pharmacology* **99**, 487–492.

Dunne, M. J., Aspinall, R. J. & Petersen, O. H. (1990) The effects of cromakalim on ATP-sensitive potassium channels in insulin-secreting cells. *British Journal of Pharmacology* **99**, 169–175.

Dunne, M. J., Bullett, M. J., Li, G., Wollheim, C. B. & Petersen, O. H. (1989) Galanin activates nucleotide-dependent K$^+$-channels in insulin-secreting cells via a pertussis toxin-sensitive G-protein. *EMBO Journal* **8**, 418–420.

Duty, S. & Weston, A. H. (1990) Analysis of the mechanisms involved in the contractile response to cromakalim in isolated strips of rabbit aorta under Ca^{2+}-free conditions. *British Journal of Pharmacology* **99**, 2P.

Duty, S., Paciorek, P. M., Waterfall, J. F. & Weston, A. H. (1990) A comparison of the haemodynamic profiles of Ro 31-6930, cromakalim and nifedipine in anaesthetised normotensive rats. *European Journal of Pharmacology* **185**, 35–42.

Eckman, D. M., Frankovich, J. D. & Keef, K. D. (1992) Comparison of the actions of acetylcholine and BRL 38227 in the guinea pig coronary artery. *British Journal of Pharmacology* **106**, 9–16.

Edwards, G. & Weston, A. H. (1990a) Structure–activity relationships of K$^+$ channel openers. *Trends in Pharmacological Sciences* **11**, 417–422.

Edwards, G. & Weston, A. H. (1990b) Potassium channel openers and vascular smooth muscle relaxation. *Pharmacology and Therapeutics* **48**, 237–258.

Elliot, A. C., Smith, G. L. & Allen, D. G. (1989) Simultaneous measurements of action potential duration and intracellular ATP in isolated ferret hearts exposed to cyanide. *Circulation Research* **64**, 583–591.

Escande, D., Thuringer, D., LeGuern, S. & Cavero, I. (1988) The potassium channel opener cromakalim (BRL 34915) activates ATP-dependent K$^+$ channels in isolated cardiac myocytes. *Biochemical and Biophysical Research Communications* **154**, 620–625.

Escande, D., Thuringer, D., Le Guern, S., Courteix, J., Laville, M. & Cavero, I. (1989) Potassium channel openers through an activation of ATP-sensitive K$^+$ channels in guinea-pig cardiac myocytes. *Pflügers Archiv* **414**, 669–675.

Evans, J. M. & Longman, S. D. (1991) Potassium channel activators. *Annual Reports in Medicinal Chemistry* **26**, 73–82.

Faivre, J-F. & Findlay, I. (1989) Effects of tolbutamide, glibenclamide and diazoxide upon action potentials recorded from rat ventricular muscle. *Biochimica et Biophysica Acta* **984**, 1–5.

Faivre, J. F. & Findlay, I. (1990) Action potential duration and activation of ATP-sensitive potassium current in isolated guinea-pig ventricular myocytes. *Biochimica et Biophysica Acta* **1029**, 167–172.

Falotico, R., Keiser, J., Haertein, B., Cheung, W-M. & Tobia, A. (1989) Increased vasodilator responsiveness to BRL34915 in spontaneous hypertensive versus normotensive rats: contrast with nifedipine. *Proceedings of the Society for Experimental Biology and Medicine* **190**, 179–185.

Fan, Z., Nakayama, K. & Hiraoka, M. (1990a) Pinacidil activates the ATP-sensitive K$^+$ channel inside-out and cell-attached patch membranes of guinea-pig ventricular myocytes. *Pflügers Archiv* **415**, 387–394.

Fan, Z., Nakayama, K. & Hiraoka, M. (1990b) Multiple actions of pinacidil on adenosine triphosphate-sensitive potassium channels in guinea-pig ventricular myocytes. *Journal of Physiology* **430**, 273–295.

Feletou, M. & Vanhoutte, P. M. (1988) Endothelium-dependent hyperpolarization of canine coronary artery muscle. *British Journal of Pharmacology* **93**, 512–524.

Ferrier, C. P., Kurtz, A., Lehner, P., Shaw, S. G., Pusterla, C., Saxenhofer, H. &

Weidmann, P. (1989) Stimulation of renin secretion by potassium channel activation with cromakalim. *European Journal of Clinical Pharmacology* **36**, 443–447.

Findlay, I. (1987) ATP-sensitive K^+ channels in rat ventricular myocytes are blocked and inactivated by internal divalent cations. *Pflügers Archiv* **410**, 313–320.

Findlay, I & Dunne, M. J. (1986) ATP maintains ATP-inhibited K^+ channels in an operational state. *Pflügers Archiv* **407**, 238–240.

Findlay, I., Deroubaix, E., Guiraudou, P. & Coraboeuf, E. (1989) Effects of activation of ATP-sensitive K^+ channels in mammalian ventricular myocytes. *American Journal of Physiology* **257**, H1551–H1559.

Fink, R. H. A. & Stephenson, D. G. (1987) Ca^{2+} movements in muscle modulated by the state of K^+-channels in the sarcoplasmic reticulum membranes. *Pflügers Archiv* **409**, 374–380.

Fish, F. A., Prakash, C. & Roden, D. M. (1990) Suppression of repolarization-related arrhythmias *in vitro* and *in vivo* by low-dose potassium channel activators. *Circulation* **82**, 1362–1369.

Fosset, M., De Weille, J. R., Green, R. D., Schmid-Antomarchi, H. & Lazdunski, M. (1988) Antidiabetic sulphonylureas control action potential properties in heart cells via high affinity receptors that are linked to ATP-dependent K^+ channels. *Journal of Biological Chemistry* **263**, 7933–7936.

Fozard, J. R., Menninger, K., Cook, N. S., Blarer, S. & Quast, U. (1990) The cardiovascular effects of SDZ PCO 400 *in vivo*: a comparison with cromakalim. *British Journal of Pharmacology* **99**, 7P.

Friedel, H. A. & Brogden, R. N. (1990) Pinacidil: a review of its pharmacodynamic and pharmacokinetic properties and therapeutic potential in the treatment of hypertension. *Drugs* **40**, 929–967.

Friedman, P. L., Stewart, J. R. & Wit, A. L. (1973) Spontaneous and induced cardiac arrhythmias in subendocardial Purkinje fibres surviving extensive myocardial infarction in dogs. *Circulation Research* **33**, 612–626.

Fujiwara, S. & Kuriyama, H. (1983) Effects of agents that modulate potassium permeability on smooth muscle cells of the guinea-pig basilar artery. *British Journal of Pharmacology* **79**, 23–25.

Furchgott, R. F. (1984) The role of endothelium in the responses of vascular smooth muscle to drugs. *Annual Review of Pharmacology and Toxicology* **24**, 175–197.

Furchgott, R. F. & Vanhoutte, P. M. (1989) Endothelium-derived relaxing and contracting factors. *FASEB Journal* **3**, 2007–2018.

Furchgott, R. F. & Zawadski, J. V. (1980) The obligatory role of endothelial cells in the relaxation of arterial smooth muscle by acetylcholine. *Nature* **288**, 373–376.

Furukawa, T., Kimura, S., Furukawa, N., Bassett, A. L. & Myerburg, R. J. (1991) Role of cardiac ATP-regulated potassium channels in differential responses of endocaardial and epicardial cells to ischemia. *Circulation Research* **68**, 1693–1702.

Garland, C. J. & McPherson, G. A. (1992) Evidence that nitric oxide does not mediate the hyperpolarization and relaxation to acetylcholine in the rat small mesenteric artery. *British Journal of Pharmacology* **105**, 429–435.

Garrino, M. G., Plant, T. D. & Henquin, J. C. (1989) Effects of putative activators of K^+ channels in mouse pancreatic β-cells. *British Journal of Pharmacology* **98**, 957–965.

Gelband, C. H., Lodge, N. J. & van Breemen, C. (1989) A Ca^{2+}-activated K^+ channel from rabbit aorta: modulation by cromakalim. *European Journal of Pharmacology* **167**, 201–210.

Gelband, C. H., Silberberg, S. D., Gröschner, K. & van Breemen, C. (1990) ATP inhibits smooth muscle Ca^{2+}-activated K^+ channels. *Proceedings of the Royal Society London Series B* **242**, 23–28.

Gerova, M., Barta, E. & Gero, J. (1979) Sympathetic control of major coronary artery diameter in the dog. *Circulation Research* **44**, 459–467.

Giles, W. R. & Imaizumi, Y. (1988) Comparison of potassium currents in rabbit arterial and ventricular cells. *Journal of Physiology* **405**, 123–145.

Gilmour, R. F. & Zipes, D. P. (1980) Different electrophysiological responses of canine endocardium and epicardium to combined hyperkalemia, hypoxia, and acidosis. *Circulation Research* **46**, 814–825.

Giudicelli, J-F., La Rochelle, C. D. & Berdeaux, A. (1990) Effects of cromakalim and pinacidil on large epicardial and small coronary arteries in conscious dogs. *Journal of Pharmacology and Experimental Therapeutics* **255**, 836–842.

Glover, W. E. (1978) Potentiation of vasoconstrictor responses by 3- and 4-aminopyridine. *British Journal of Pharmacology* **63**, 577–585.

Grace, G. C., Dusting, G. J., Kemp, B. E. & Martin, T. J. (1987) Endothelium and the vasodilator action of rat calcitonin gene-related peptide (CGRP). *British Journal of Pharmacology* **91**, 729–733.

Gross, G. J. (1991) Coronary blood flow studies with potassium channel openers. *Current Drugs: Potassium Channel Modulators* B82–B92.

Grosset, A. & Hicks, P. E. (1986) Evidence for blood vessel selectivity of BRL 34915. *British Journal of Pharmacology* **89**, 500P.

Grover, G. J. (1991) Potassium channel openers and the treatment of myocardial ischaemia. *Current Drugs: Potassium Channel Modulators* B29–B38.

Grover, G. J., Dzwonczyk, S., Parham, C. S. & Sleph, P. G. (1990a) The protective effects of cromakalim and pinacidil on reperfusion function and infarct size in anesthetized dogs. *Cardiovascular Drugs* **4**, 465–474.

Grover, G. J., Dzwonczyk, S. & Sleph, P. G. (1990b) Reduction of ischemic damage in isolated rat hearts by the potassium channel opener, RP-52891. *European Journal of Pharmacology* **191**, 11–18.

Grover, G. J., McCullough, J. R., Henry, D. E., Conder, M. L. & Sleph, P. G. (1989) Anti-ischemic effects of the potassium channel activators pinacidil and cromakalim and the reversal of these effects with the potassium channel blocker glyburide. *Journal of Pharmacology and Experimental Therapeutics* **251**, 98–104.

Grover, G. J., Sleph, P. G. & Dzwonczyk, S. (1990c) Pharmacologic profile of cromakalim in the treatment of myocardial ischemia in isolated rat hearts and anesthetized dogs. *Journal of Cardiovascular Pharmacology* **16**, 853–864.

Grover, G. J., Sleph, P. G. & Parham, C. S. (1990d) Nicorandil improves postischemic contractile function independently of direct myocardial effects. *Journal of Cardiovascular Pharmacology* **15**, 698–705.

Haeusler, G. & Thorens, S. (1980) Effects of tetraethylammonium chloride on contractile, membrane and cable properties of rabbit artery muscle. *Journal of Physiology* **303**, 203–224.

Hamilton, T. C. & Weston, A. H. (1989) Cromakalim, nicorandil and pinacidil: novel drugs which open potassium channels in smooth muscle. *General Pharmacology* **20**, 1–9.

Hamilton, T. C., Weir, S. W. & Weston, A. H. (1986) Comparison of the effects of BRL 34915 and verapamil on electrical and mechanical activity in rat portal vein. *British Journal of Pharmacology* **88**, 103–111.

Hara, Y., Kitamura, K. & Kuriyama, H. (1980) Actions of 4-aminopyridine on vascular smooth muscle tissues of the guinea-pig. *British Journal of Physiology* **68**, 99–106.

Harder, D. R. & Sperelakis, N. (1979) Action potentials induced in guinea-pig arterial smooth muscle by tetraethylammonium. *American Journal of Physiology* **237**, C75–C80.

Henry, P. D., Schuchlieb, R., Davis, T., Weiss, E. S. & Sobel, B. E. (1977) Myocardial contracture and accumulation of mitochondrial calcium in ischaemic rabbit heart. *American Journal of Physiology* **233,** 677–684.

Hermann, A. & Erxleben, C. (1987) Charybdotoxin selectively blocks small Ca-activated channels in *Aplysia* neurons. *Journal of General Physiology* **90,** 24–47.

Hirai, S., Kotake, H., Kurata, Y., Hisatome, I., Hasegawa, J. & Mashiba, H. (1990) Effect of pinacidil on the electrophysiological properties in guinea-pig papillary muscle and rabbit sino-atrial node. *Journal of Pharmacy and Pharmacology* **42,** 339–343.

Hiraoka, M. & Kawano, S. (1986) Contribution of the transient outward current to the repolarization of rabbit ventricular cells. *Japanese Heart Journal* **27,** 77–83.

Hof, R. P. & Vuorela, H. J. (1983) Assessing calcium antagonism on vascular smooth muscle: a comparison of three methods. *Journal of Pharmacological Methods* **9,** 41–52.

Hof, R. P., Quast, U., Cook, N. S. & Blarer, S. (1988) Mechanism of action and systemic and regional hemodynamics of the potassium channel activator BRL 34915 and its enantiomers. *Circulation Research* **62,** 679–686.

Holzmann, S. (1983) Cyclic GMP as possible mediator of coronary arterial relaxation by nicorandil (SG-75) *Journal of Cardiovascular Pharmacology* **5,** 364–370.

Horowitz, L. N., Spear, J. F. & Moore, E. N. (1976) Subendocardial origin of ventricular arrhythmias in 24-hour-old experimental myocardial infarction. *Circulation* **53,** 56–63.

Hu, S., Kim, H. S., Okoli, P. & Weiss, G. B. (1990) Alterations by glyburide of effects of BRL 34915 and P1060 on contraction, ^{86}Rb efflux and maxi-K$^+$ channel in rat portal vein. *Journal of Pharmacology and Experimental Therapeutics* **253,** 771–777.

Huang, A. H., Busse, R. & Bassenge, E. (1988) Endothelium-dependent hyperpolarization of smooth muscle cells in rabbit femoral arteries is not mediated by EDRF (nitric oxide) *Naunyn-Schmiedeberg's Archives of Pharmacology* **338,** 438–442.

Ichihara, K., Haga, N. & Abiko, Y. (1984) Is ischaemia-induced pH decrease of dog myocardium respiratory or metabolic acidosis? *American Journal of Physiology* **246,** H652.

Ichihara, K., Morimoto, T., Shiba, T., Tsujitani, M. & Abiko, Y. (1991) Attenuation of ischemia-induced regional myocardial acidosis by LP-805, a newly developed vasodilator, in dogs. *European Journal of Pharmacology* **204,** 127–133.

Iijima, T. & Taira, N. (1987) Pinacidil increases the background current in single ventricular cells. *European Journal of Pharmacology* **141,** 139–141.

Imai, N., Liang, C., Stone, C. K., Sakamoto, S. & Hood, B. (1988) Comparative effects of nitroprusside and pinacidil on myocardial blood flow and infarct size in awake dogs with acute myocardial infarction. *Circulation* **77,** 705–711.

Imanishi, S., Arita, M., Aomine, M. & Kiyosue, T. (1984) Antiarrhythmic effects of nicorandil on canine cardiac Purkinje fibres. *Journal of Cardiovascular Pharmacology* **6,** 772–779.

Imanishi, S., Arita, M., Kiyosue, T. & Aomini, M. (1983) Effects of SG-75 (nicorandil) on electrical activity of canine cardiac Purkinje fibres. *Journal of Pharmacology and Experimental Therapeutics* **225,** 198–205.

Inoue, I., Nakaya, Y., Nakaya, S. & Mori, H. (1989) Extracellular Ca^{2+}-activated K channel in coronary artery smooth muscle cells and its role in vasodilation. *FEBS Letters* **255,** 281–284.

Isenberg, G. & Belardinelli, L. (1984) Ionic basis for the antagonism between adenosine and isoproterenol on isolated mammalian ventricular myocytes. *Circulation Research* **55,** 309–325.

Ishibashi, T., Hamaguchi, M. & Imai, S. (1991) 2-nicotinamidoethyl acetate (SG-209) is a potassium channel opener: structural activity relationship among nicorandil derivatives. *Naunyn-Schmiedeberg's Archives of Pharmacology* **344,** 235–239.

Ito, S., Kajikuri, J., Itoh, T. & Kuriyama, H. (1991) Effects of lemakalim on changes in Ca^{2+} concentration and mechanical activity induced by noradrenaline in the rabbit mesenteric artery. *British Journal of Pharmacology* **104**, 227–233.

Ito, Y., Suzuki, H. & Kuriyama, H. (1978) Effects of sodium nitroprusside on smooth muscle cells of rabbit pulmonary artery and portal vein. *Journal of Pharmacology and Experimental Therapeutics* **207**, 1022–1031.

Itoh, T., Seki, N., Suzuki, S., Ito, S., Kajikuri, J. & Kuriyama, H. (1992) Membrane hyperpolarization inhibits agonist-induced synthesis of inositol 1,4,5-triphosphate in rabbit mesenteric artery. *Journal of Physiology* **451**, 307–328.

Itoh, T., Suzuki, S. & Kuriyama, H. (1991) Effects of pinacidil on contractile proteins in high K^+-treated intact, and in β-escin-treated skinned smooth muscle of the rabbit mesenteric artery. *British Journal of Pharmacology* **103**, 1697–1702.

Iwaki, M., Mizobuchi, S., Nakaya, Y., Kawano, K., Niki, T. & Mori. H. (1987) Tetraethylammonium induced coronary spasm in isolated perfused rabbit heart: a hypothesis for the mechanism of coronary spasm. *Cardiovascular Research* **21**, 130–139.

Janse, M. J. & Wit, A. L. (1989) Electrophysiological mechanisms of ventricular arrhythmias resulting from myocardial ischemia and infarction. *Physiological Reviews* **69**, 1049–1168.

Jennings, R. B., Sommers, H. M., Smyth, G. A., Flack, H. A. & Linn, H. (1960) Myocardial necrosis induced by temporary occlusion of a coronary artery in the dog. *Pathology* **70**, 68–78.

Kajioka, S., Kitamura, K. & Kuriyama, H. (1991) Guanosine diphosphate activates an adenosine 5'-triphosphate-sensitive K^+ channel in the rabbit portal vein. *Journal of Physiology* **444**, 397–418.

Kajioka, S., Oike, M. & Kitamura, K. (1990) Nicorandil opens a calcium-dependent potassium channel in smooth muscle cells of the rat portal vein. *Journal of Pharmacology and Experimental Therapeutics* **254**, 905–913.

Kakei, M., Kelly, R. P., Ashcroft, S. J. H. & Ashcroft, F. M. (1986a) The ATP-sensitivity of K^+ channels in rat pancreatic β-cells is modulated by ADP. *FEBS Letters* **208**, 63–66.

Kakei, M., Yoshinaga, M., Saito, K. & Tanaka, H. (1986b) The potassium current activated by 2-nicotinamidoethyl nitrate (nicorandil) in single ventricular cells of guinea pigs. *Proceedings of the Royal Society London, Series B* **229**, 331–343.

Kameyama, M., Kakei, M., Sato, R., Shibasaki, T., Matsuda, H. & Irisawa, H. (1984) Intracellular Na^+ activates a K^+ channel in mammalian cardiac cells. *Nature* **309**, 354–356.

Karaki, H., Satake, N. & Shibata, S. (1986) Mechanism of barium-induced contraction in the vascular smooth muscle of rabbit aorta. *British Journal of Pharmacology* **88**, 821–826.

Karashima, T., Itoh, T. & Kuriyama, H. (1982) Effects of 2-nicotinamidoethyl nitrate on smooth muscle cells of the guinea-pig mesenteric and portal veins. *Journal of Pharmacology and Experimental Therapeutics* **221**, 472–480.

Kato, H. & Takata, Y. (1987) Differential effects of Ca antagonists on the noradrenaline release and contraction evoked by nerve stimulation in the presence of 4-aminopyridine. *British Journal of Pharmacology* **90**, 191–201.

Kauffman, R. F., Schenk, K. W., Conery, B. G. & Cohen, M. L. (1986) Effects of pinacidil on serotonin-induced contractions and cyclic nucleotide levels in isolated rat aorta: comparison with nitroglycerin, minoxidil and hydralazine. *Journal of Cardiovascular Pharmacology* **8**, 1195–1200.

Kawashima, S. & Liang, C. S. (1985) Systemic and coronary hemodynamic effects of pinacidil, a new anti-hypertensive agent, in awake dogs: comparison with hydralazine. *Journal of Pharmacology and Experimental Therapeutics* **232**, 369–375.

Kerr, M. J., Wilson, R. & Shanks, R. G. (1985) Suppression of ventricular arrhythmias after coronary artery ligation by pinacidil, a vasodilator drug. *Journal of Cardiovascular Pharmacology* **7**, 875–883.

Kim, D. H. (1991) Calcitonin-gene-related peptide activates the muscarinic-gated K^+ current in atrial cells. *Pflügers Archiv* **418**, 338–345.

Kimura, S., Basset, A. L., Kohya, T., Kozlovskis, P. L. & Myerburg, R. J. (1986) Simultaneous recording of action potentials from endocardium and epicardium during ischaemia in the isolated cat ventricle: Relation of temporal electrophysiologic heterogeneities to arrhythmias. *Circulation* **74**, 401–409.

Kirsch, G. E., Codina, J., Birnbaumer, L. & Brown, A. M. (1990) Coupling of ATP-sensitive K^+ channels to A_1-receptors by G-proteins in rat ventricular myocytes. *American Journal of Physiology* **259**, H820–H826.

Komori, K., Lorenz, R. R. & Vanhoutte, P. M. (1988) Nitric oxide, ACh and electrical and mechanical properties of canine arterial smooth muscle. *American Journal of Physiology* **255**, H207–H212.

Kramer, J. B. & Corr, P. B. (1984) Mechanisms contributing to arrhythmias during ischaemia and infarction. *European Heart Journal* **5**, (Suppl. B), 11–18.

Kreye, V. A. W., Gerstheimer, F. & Weston, A. H. (1987) Effects of BRL34915 on resting membrane potential and ^{86}Rb efflux in rabbit tonic vascular smooth muscle. *Naunyn-Schmiedeberg's Archives of Pharmacology* **335**, R64.

Lamping, K. A. & Gross, G. J. (1984) Comparative effects of a new nicotinamide nitrate derivative nicorandil SG-75 with nifedipine and nitroglycerin on tissue collateral blood flow following an acute coronary occlusion in dogs. *Journal of Cardiovascular Pharmacology* **6**, 601–608.

Lamping, K. A. & Gross, G. J. (1985) Improved recovery of myocardial segment function following a short coronary occlusion in dogs by nicorandil, a potential new antianginal agent, and nifedipine. *Journal of Cardiovascular Pharmacology* **7**, 158–166.

Leblanc, N., Wilde, D. W., Keef, K. D. & Hume, J. R. (1989) Electrophysiological mechanisms of minoxidil sulfate-induced vasodilation of rabbit portal vein. *Circulation Research* **65**, 1102–1111.

Liu, B., Golyan, F., McCullough, J. R. & Vassalle, M. (1988) Electrophysiological and antiarrhythmic effects of the K-channel opener, BRL 34915, in cardiac Purkinje fibres. *Drug Development Research* **14**, 123–139.

Longman, S. D., Clapham, J. C., Wilson, C. & Hamilton, T. C. (1988) Cromakalim, a potassium channel activator: a comparison of its cardiovascular haemodynamic profile and tissue specificity with those of pinacidil and nicorandil. *Journal of Cardiovascular Pharmacology* **12**, 535–542.

Longmore, J. & Weston, A. H. (1990) The role of K^+ channels in the modulation of vascular smooth muscle tone. In Cook, N. S. (ed.), *Potassium Channels: Structure, Classification, Function and Therapeutic Potential*. Ellis Horwood Ltd, Chichester, pp. 259–278.

Longmore, J., Newgreen, D. T. & Weston, A. H. (1990) Effects of cromakalim, RP-49356, diazoxide, glibenclamide and galanin in rat portal vein. *European Journal of Pharmacology* **190**, 75–84.

Louttit, J. B., Downing, O. A. & Wilson, K. A. (1984) Differential effects of strychnine on two types of vascular smooth muscle. *European Journal of Pharmacology* **98**, 249–253.

McCullough, J. R., Normandin, D. E., Conder, M. L., Sleph, P. G., Dzwonczyk, S. & Grover, G. J. (1991) Specific block of the anti-ischemic actions of cromakalim by sodium 5-hydroxydecanoate. *Circulation Research* **69**, 949–958.

McHarg, A. D., Southerton, J. S. & Weston, A. H. (1990) A comparison of the actions of cromakalim and nifedipine on rabbit isolated mesenteric artery. *European Journal of Pharmacology* **185**, 137–146.

McPherson, G. A. & Angus, J. A. (1991) Evidence that acetylcholine-mediated hyperpolarization of the rat small mesenteric artery does not involve the K^+ channel opened by cromakalim. *British Journal of Pharmacology* **103**, 1184–1190.

Martin, C. L. & Chinn, K. (1990) Pinacidil opens ATP-dependent K^+ channels in cardiac myocytes in an ATP- and temperature-dependent manner. *Journal of Cardiovascular Pharmacology* **15**, 510–514.

Masuzawa, K., Asano, M., Matsuda, T., Imaizumi, Y. & Watanabe, M. (1990a) Comparison of effects of cromakalim and pinacidil on mechanical activity and $^{86}Rb^+$ efflux in dog coronary arteries. *Journal of Pharmacology and Experimental Therapeutics* **253**, 586–593.

Masuzawa, K., Asano, M., Matsuda, T., Imaizumi, Y. & Watanabe, M. (1990b) Possible involvement of ATP-sensitive K^+ channels in the relaxant response of dog middle cerebral artery to cromakalim. *Journal of Pharmacology and Experimental Therapeutics* **255**, 818–825.

Masuzawa, K., Matsuda, T. & Asano, M. (1990c) Evidence that pinacidil may promote the opening of ATP-sensitive K^+ channels yet inhibit the opening of Ca^{2+}-activated K^+ channels in K^+-contracted canine mesenteric artery. *British Journal of Pharmacology* **100**, 143–149.

Miyata, N., Tsuchida, K., Kaneko, K., Tanaka, M. & Otomo, S. (1990a) Mechanisms of inhibitory effects of CD-349 and K^+-channel activators on noradrenaline-induced contraction and changes in levels of cyclic GMP in rat aorta. *General Pharmacology* **21**, 665–669.

Miyata, N., Tsuchida, K. & Otomo, S. (1990b) Functional changes in potassium channels in carotid arteries from stroke-prone spontaneously hypertensive rats. *European Journal of Pharmacology* **182**, 209–210.

Moncada, M., Palmer, R. M. J. & Higgs, E. A. (1989) Biosynthesis of nitric oxide from L-arginine. A pathway for the regulation of cell function and communication. *Biochemical Pharmacology* **38**, 1709–1715.

Mondot, S., Mestre, M., Caillard, C. G. & Cavero, I. (1988) RP 49356: a vasorelaxant agent with potassium channel activating properties. *British Journal of Pharmacology* **95** (Suppl.), 831P.

Nagao, T. & Vanhoutte, P. M. (1992) Hyperpolarization as a mechanism for endothelium-dependent relaxations in the porcine coronary artery. *Journal of Physiology* **445**, 355–367.

Nakao, K. & Bolton, T. B. (1991) Cromakalim-induced potassium currents in single dispersed smooth muscle cells of rabbit artery and vein. *British Journal of Pharmacology* **102**, 155P.

Nakao, K., Okabe, K., Kitamura, K., Kuriyama, H. & Weston, A. H. (1988) Characteristics of cromakalim-induced relaxations in the smooth muscle cells of guinea-pig mesenteric artery and vein. *British Journal of Pharmacology* **95**, 795–804.

Nakashima, M., Li, Y. J., Seki, N. & Kuriyama, H. (1990) Pinacidil inhibits neuromuscular transmission indirectly in the guinea-pig and rabbit mesenteric arteries. *British Journal of Pharmacology* **101**, 581–586.

Nakayama, K., Fan, Z., Marumo, F. & Hiraoka, M. (1990) Interrelation between pinacidil and intracellular ATP concentrations on activation of the ATP-sensitive K^+ current in guinea pig ventricular myocytes. *Circulation Research* **67**, 1124–1133.

Nedergaard, O. A. (1989) Effects of pinacidil on sympathetic neuroeffector transmission in rabbit blood vessels. *Pharmacology and Toxicology* **65**, 287–294.

Nelson, M. T., Huang, Y., Brayden, J. E., Hescheler, J. & Standen, N. B. (1990) Arterial dilations in response to calcitonin gene-related peptide involve activation of K^+-channels. *Nature* **344**, 770–773.

Newgreen, D. T., Bray, K. M., McHarg, A. D., Weston, A. H., Duty, S., Brown, B. S., Kay, P. B., Edwards, G., Longmore, J. & Southerton, J. S. (1990) The action of diazoxide and minoxidil sulphate on rat blood vessels: a comparison with cromakalim. *British Journal of Pharmacology* **100**, 605–613.

Newgreen, D. T., Bray, K. M., Southerton, J. S. & Weston, A. H. (1988) The action of glyceryltrinitrate and sodium nitroprusside on rat aorta: a comparison with nicorandil and BRL 34915. *British Journal of Pharmacology* **93**, 17P.

Nielsen, C. B., Mellemkjaer, S. & Nielsen-Kudsk, F. (1989) Pinacidil uptake and effects in the isolated rabbit heart. *Pharmacology and Toxicology* **64**, 14–19.

Nielsen-Kudsk, J. E. & Thirstrup, S. (1991) Antidiabetic sulfonylureas relax isolated rabbit coronary arteries. *European Journal of Pharmacology* **209**, 273–275.

Nielsen-Kudsk, J. E., Nielsen, C. B. & Mellemkjaer, S. (1992) Influence of osmolarity of solutions used for K^+ contraction on relaxant responses to pinacidil, verapamil, theophylline and terbutaline in isolated airway smooth muscle. *Pharmacology and Toxicology* **70**, 46–49.

Noack, Th., Deitmer, P., Edwards, G. & Weston, A. H. (1992a) Characterization of potassium currents modulated by BRL 38227 in rat portal vein. *British Journal of Pharmacology* **106**, 717–726.

Noack, Th., Deitmer, P., Edwards, G., Weston, A. H. & Golenhofen, K. (1991) Effects of BRL 38227 on whole-cell currents in vascular smooth muscle. *Pflügers Archiv* **419**, R85.

Noack, Th., Edwards, G., Deitmer, P., Greengrass, P., Morita, T., Andersson, P-O., Criddle, D., Wyllie, M. G. & Weston, A. H. (1992b) The involvement of potassium channels in the action of ciclazindol in rat portal vein. *British Journal of Pharmacology* **106**, 17–24.

Noma, A. (1983) ATP-regulated K^+ channels in cardiac muscle. *Nature* **305**, 147–148.

Noma, A. & Shibasaki, T. (1985) Membrane current through adenosine-triphosphate-regulated potassium channels in guinea-pig ventricular cells. *Journal of Physiology* **363**, 463–480.

Notsu, T., Tanaka, I., Tokano, M. & Norma, A. (1992) Blockade of the ATP-sensitive K^+ channel by 5-hydroxydecanoate in guinea pig ventricular myocytes. *Journal of Pharmacology and Experimental Therapeutics* **260**, 702–708.

Ohno-Shosaku, T., Zünkler, B. J. & Trube, G. (1987) Dual effects of ATP on K^+ currents of mouse pancreatic β-cells. *Pflügers Archiv* **408**, 133–138.

Ohta, H., Jinno, Y., Harada, K., Ogawa, N., Fukushima, H. & Nishikori, K. (1991) Cardioprotective effects of KRN2391 and nicorandil on ischemic dysfunction in perfused rat heart. *European Journal of Pharmacology* **204**, 171–177.

Okabe, K., Kajioka, S., Nakao, K., Kitamura, K., Kuriyama, H. & Weston, A. H. (1990) Actions of cromakalim on ionic currents recorded from single smooth muscle cells of the rat portal vein. *Journal of Pharmacology and Experimental Therapeutics* **252**, 832–839.

Olesen, S-P., Clapham, D. E. & Davies, P. F. (1988) Haemodynamic shear stress activates a K^+ current in vascular endothelial cells. *Nature* **331**, 168–170.

Olsson, R. A. (1970) Changes in content of purine nucleoside in canine myocardium during coronary occlusion. *Circulation Research* **26**, 301–306.

Ono, K., Kihosue, T. & Arita, M. (1989) Isoproterenol, DBcAMP, and forskolin inhibit cardiac sodium current. *American Journal of Physiology* **256**, C1131–C1137.

Osterrieder, W. (1988) Modification of K^+ conductance of heart cell membrane by BRL 34915. *Naunyn-Schmiedeberg's Archives of Pharmacology* **337**, 93–97.

Osterrieder, W. & Waterfall, J. F. (1989) Therapeutic potential of K^+-channel modulation in heart. In Cook, N. S. (ed.) *Potassium Channels: Structure, Classification, Function and Therapeutic Potential.* Ellis Horwood Ltd, Chichester, pp. 337–347.

Paciorek, P. M., Burden, D. T., Burke, Y. M., Cowlrick, I. S., Perkins, R. S., Taylor,

J. C. & Waterfall, J. F. (1990) Preclinical pharmacology of Ro 31-6930, a new potassium channel opener. Journal of Cardiovascular Pharmacology 15, 188–197.

Parsons, A. A., Ksoll, E., Mackert, J. R. L., Schilling, L. & Wahl, M. (1990) Effect of sulfonylureas on cromakalim-induced relaxation of KCl pre-contracted rabbit, cat, and rat cerebral arteries. British Journal of Pharmacology 100, 331P.

Parsons, A. A., Ksoll, E., Mackert, J. R. L., Schilling, L. & Wahl, M. (1991a) Comparison of cromakalim-induced relaxation of potassium precontracted rabbit, cat, and rat isolated cerebral arteries. Naunyn-Schmiedeberg's Archives of Pharmacology 343, 384–392.

Parsons, A. A., Schilling, L. & Wahl, M. (1991b) Analysis of acetylcholine-induced relaxation of rabbit isolated middle cerebral artery—effects of inhibitors of nitric oxide synthesis, Na,K-ATPase, and ATP-sensitive K-channels. Journal of Cerebral Blood Flow Metabolism 11, 700–704.

Pilsudski, R., Rougier, O. & Tourneur, Y. (1990) Action of cromakalim on potassium membrane conductance in isolated heart myocytes of frog. British Journal of Pharmacology 100, 518–587.

Pratz, J., Mondot, S., Montier, F. & Cavero, I. (1991) Effects of the K^+ channel activators, RP 52891, cromakalim and diazoxide, on the plasma insulin level, plasma renin activity and blood pressure in rats. Journal of Pharmacology and Experimental Therapeutics 258, 216–222.

Prieto, D., Benedito, S., Nielsen, P. J. & Nyborg, N. C. B. (1991) Calcitonin gene-related peptide is a potent vasodilator of bovine retinal arteries in vitro. Experimental Eye Research 53, 399–405.

Quast, U. (1987) Effect of the K^+ efflux stimulating vasodilator BRL 34915 on $^{86}Rb^+$ efflux and spontaneous activity in guinea-pig portal vein. British Journal of Pharmacology 91, 569–578.

Quast, U. & Baumlin, Y. (1988) Comparison of the effluxes of $^{42}K^+$ and $^{86}Rb^+$ elicited by cromakalim (BRL34915) in tonic and phasic vascular tissue. Naunyn-Schmiedeberg's Archives of Pharmacology 338, 319–326.

Quast, U. & Baumlin, Y. (1991) Cromakalim inhibits contractions of the rat isolated mesenteric bed induced by noradrenaline but not caffeine in Ca^{2+}-free medium: evidence for interference with receptor-mediated Ca^{2+} mobilization. European Journal of Pharmacology 200, 239–249.

Quast, U. & Cook, N. S. (1989b) In vitro and in vivo comparison of two K^+ channel openers, diazoxide and cromakalim, and their inhibition by glibenclamide. Journal of Pharmacology and Experimental Therapeutics 250, 261–271.

Quast, U., Scholtysik, G., Weir, S. W. & Cook, N. S. (1988) Pertussis toxin treatment does not inhibit the effects of the potassium channel opener BRL 34915 on rat isolated vascular and cardiac tissues. Naunyn-Schmiedeberg's Archives of Pharmacology 337, 98–104.

Rademacher, C., Ehring, T. & Thamer, V. (1990) BRL 34915 ameliorates oxygen supply in ischaemic myocardium by a simultaneous enhancement of coronary blood flow and a reduction of myocardial function. Journal of Cardiovascular Pharmacology 15, 808–815.

Rand, V. E. & Garland, G. J. (1992) Membrane hyperpolarization is not essential for endothelium-dependent relaxation to acetylcholine in the rabbit basilar artery. British Journal of Pharmacology 106, 143–150.

Richer, C., Mulder, P., Doussau, M. P., Gautier, P. & Giudicelli, J. F. (1990a) Systemic and regional haemodynamic interactions between K-channel openers and the sympathetic nervous system in the pithed SHR. British Journal of Pharmacology 100, 557–563.

Richer, C., Mulder, P., Doussau, M. P. & Giudicelli, J. F. (1989) Agonistes potassiques:

profil vasodilateur régional chez le rat. *Archives des Maladies du Coeur et des Vaisseaux* **82**, 1333–1337.

Richer, C., Pratz, J., Mulder, P., Mondot, S., Giudicelli, J. F. & Cavero, I. (1990b) Cardiovascular and biological effects of K$^+$ channel openers, a class of drug with vasorelaxant and cardioprotective properties. *Life Sciences* **47**, 1693–1705.

Robertson, D. W. & Steinberg, M. I. (1990) Potassium channel modulators: scientific applications and therapeutic promise. *Journal of Medicinal Chemistry* **33**, 1529–1541.

Rubio, R., Berne, R. M. & Katori, M. (1969) Release of adenosine in reactive hyperemia of the dog heart. *American Journal of Physiology* **216**, 56–62.

Ruiz-Ceretti, E., Ragault, P., Leblanc, N. & Zumino, A. Z. (1983) Effects of hypoxia and altered K$_o$ on the membrane potential of rabbit ventricle. *Journal of Molecular and Cellular Cardiology* **15**, 845–854.

Ruiz-Petrich, E., de Lorenzi, F. & Chartier, D. (1991) Role of the inward rectifier I_{K1} in the myocardial response to hypoxia. *Cardiovascular Research* **25**, 17–26.

Sakamoto, S., Liang, C., Stone, C. K. & Hood, W. B. (1989) Effects of pinacidil on myocardial blood flow and infarct size after acute left anterior descending coronary artery occlusion and reperfusion in awake dogs with and without a coexisting left circumflex coronary artery stenosis. *Journal of Cardiovascular Pharmacology* **14**, 747–755.

Sanguinetti, M. C., Scott, A. L., Zingaro, G. J. & Siegl, P. K. S. (1988) BRL 34915 (cromakalim) activates ATP-sensitive K$^+$ current in cardiac muscle. *Proceedings of the National Academy of Sciences USA* **85**, 8360–8364.

Scholtysik, G. (1987) Evidence for inhibition by ICS 205-930 and stimulation by BRL 34915 of K$^+$ conductance in cardiac muscle. *Naunyn-Schmiedeberg's Archives of Pharmacology* **335**, 692–696.

Schwörer, H. & Kilbinger, H. (1989) Effects of cromakalim on acetylcholine release and smooth muscle contraction in guinea-pig small intestine. *Naunyn-Schmiedeberg's Archives of Pharmacology* **339**, 706–708.

Seltzer, H. S. & Allen, E. W. (1965) Inhibition of insulin secretion in 'Diazoxide diabetes'. *Diabetes* **14**, 439.

Shapiro, B. I. (1977) Effect of strychnine on potassium conductance of the frog node of Ranvier. *Journal of Physiology* **68**, 897–914.

Shen, A. C. & Jennings, R. B. (1972) Myocardial calcium and magnesium in acute ischemic injury. *American Journal of Pathology* **67**, 417–440.

Shoji, T., Aki, Y., Fukui, K., Tamaki, T., Iwao, H. & Abe, Y. (1990) Effects of cromakalim, a potassium channel opener, on regional blood flow in conscious spontaneously hypertensive rats. *European Journal of Pharmacology* **186**, 119–123.

Siegel, G., Mironneau, J., Schnalke, F., Schröder, G., Schulz, B-G. & Grote, J. (1990) Vasodilation evoked by K$^+$ channel opening. *Progress in Clinical Biological Research* **327**, 299–306.

Siegl, P., Wolleben, C., Zingaro, G. & Sanguinetti, M. (1989) Effects of the ATP-sensitive potassium channel modulators, glyburide and BRL 34915 on ischemia-induced fibrillation in isolated rat hearts. *FASEB Journal* **3**, A847.

Silberberg, S. D. & van Breemen, C. (1990) An ATP, calcium and voltage sensitive potassium channel in porcine coronary artery smooth muscle cells. *Biochemical and Biophysical Research Communications* **172**, 517–522.

Smallwood, J. K. & Steinberg, M. I. (1988) Cardiac electrophysiological effects of pinacidil and related pyridylcyanoguanidines: relationship to antihypertensive activity. *Journal of Cardiovascular Pharmacology* **12**, 102–109.

Smallwood, J. K., Ertel, P. J. & Steinberg, M. I. (1990) Modification by glibenclamide of the electrophysiological consequences of myocardial ischemia in dogs and rabbits. *Naunyn-Schmiedeberg's Archives of Pharmacology* **342**, 214–220.

Smith, J. M., Sanchez, A. A. & Jones, A. W. (1986) Comparison of rubidium-86 and potassium-42 fluxes in rat aorta. *Blood Vessels* **23**, 297–309.

Somlyo, A. P., Somlyo, A. V., Devine, C. E., Peters, P. D. & Hall, T. A. (1974) Electron microscopy and electron probe analysis of mitochondrial cation accumulation in smooth muscle. *Journal of Cell Biology* **61**, 723–742.

Southerton, J. S. & Weston, A. H. (1987) Some effects of Ca^{2+} and K^+ channel blocking agents on responses to BRL34915 and pinacidil in the isolated rat portal vein. *Journal of Physiology* **391**, 77P.

Southerton, J. S., Taylor, S. G. & Weston, A. H. (1987) Comparison of the effects of BRL 34915 and of acetylcholine-liberated EDRF on rat isolated aorta. *Journal of Physiology* **382**, 50P.

Southerton, J. S., Weston, A. H., Bray, K. M., Newgreen, D. T. & Taylor, S. G. (1988) The potassium channel opening action of pinacidil; studies using biochemical, ion flux and microelectrode techniques. *Naunyn-Schmiedeberg's Archives of Pharmacology* **338**, 310–318.

Standen, N. B., Quayle, J. M., Davies, N. W., Brayden, J. E., Huang, Y. & Nelson, M. T. (1989) Hyperpolarizing vasodilators activate ATP-sensitive K^+ channels in arterial smooth muscle. *Science* **245**, 177–180.

Stanfield, P. R. (1983) Tetraethylammonium ions and the potassium permeability of excitable cells. *Reviews in Physiology and Pharmacology* **97**, 1–67.

Steinberg, M. I., Ertel, P., Smallwood, J. K., Wyss, V. & Zimmermann, K. (1988) The relation between vascular relaxant and cardiac electrophysiological effects of pinacidil. *Journal of Cardiovascular Pharmacology* **12** (Suppl. 2), S30–S40.

Strong, P. N., Weir, S. W., Beech, D. J., Hiestand, P. & Kocker, H. P. (1989) Effects of potassium channel toxins from *Leiurus quinquestriatus hebraeus* venom on responses to cromakalim in rabbit blood vessels. *British Journal of Pharmacology* **98**, 817–826.

Sumimoto, K., Domae, M., Yamanaka, K., Nakao, K., Hashimoto, T., Kitamura, K. & Kuriyama, H. (1987) Actions of nicorandil on vascular smooth muscles. *Journal of Cardiovascular Pharmacology* **10** (Suppl. 8), S66–S75.

Suzuki, H. & Chen, G. (1990) Endothelium-derived hyperpolarizing factor (EDHF): An endogenous potassium channel activator. *News in Physiological Sciences* **5**, 212–215.

Taira, N., Satoh, K., Yanagisawa, T., Imai, Y. & Hiwatari, M. (1979) Pharmacological profile of a new coronary vasodilator drug, 2-nicotinamidoethyl nitrate (SG-75). *Clinical and Experimental Pharmacology and Physiology* **6**, 301–316.

Takano, M. & Noma, A. (1990) Selective modulation of the ATP-sensitive K^+ channel by nicorandil in guinea-pig cardiac cell membrane. *Naunyn-Schmiedeberg's Archives of Pharmacology* **342**, 592–597.

Tare, M., Parkington, H. C., Coleman, H. A., Nield, T. O. & Dusting, G. J. (1990) Hyperpolarization and relaxation of arterial smooth muscle caused by nitric oxide derived from the endothelium. *Nature* **346**, 69–71.

Taylor, S. G. & Weston, A. H. (1988) Endothelium-derived hyperpolarizing factor: a new endogenous inhibitor from the vascular endothelium. *Trends in Pharmacological Sciences* **9**, 272–274.

Taylor, S. G., Southerton, J. S., Weston, A. H. & Baker, J. R. J. (1988) Endothelium dependent effects of acetylcholine in rat aorta. A comparison with sodium nitroprusside and cromakalim. *British Journal of Pharmacology* **94**, 853–863.

Thoolen, M. J. M. C., Van Meel, J. C. A., Wilffert, B., Timmermans, P. B. M. W. M. & van Zweiten, P. A. (1983) Haemodynamic characteristics of pinacidil in rats: comparison with hydralazine. *Pharmacology* **27**, 245–254.

Thuringer, D. & Escande, D. (1989) Apparent competition between ATP and the potassium channel opener RP-49356 on ATP-sensitive K$^+$ channels of cardiac myocytes. *Molecular Pharmacology* **36**, 897–902.

Tilton, R. G., Williamson, E. K., Cole, P. A., Larson, K. B., Kilo, C. & Williamson, J. R. (1985) Coronary vascular hemodynamic and permeability changes during reperfusion after no-reflow ischemia in isolated diltiazem treated rabbit hearts. *Journal of Cardiovascular Pharmacology* **7**, 424–436.

Trezise, D. J. & Weston, A. H. (1991) Vasorelaxant properties of a group of structurally diverse potassium channel openers in rabbit isolated basilar artery. *British Journal of Pharmacology* **102**, 199P.

Trube, G. & Hescheler, J. (1984) Inward-rectifying channels in isolated patches of the heart cell membrane. *Pflügers Archiv* **401**, 178–184.

Trube, G., Rorsman, P. & Ohno-Shosaku, T. (1986) Opposite effects of tolbutamide and diazoxide on the ATP-dependent K$^+$ channel in mouse pancreatic β cells. *Pflügers Archiv* **407**, 493–499.

Tseng, G. N. & Hoffman, B. F. (1990) Actions of pinacidil on membrane currents in canine ventricular myocytes and their modulation by intracellular ATP and cAMP. *Pflügers Archiv* **415**, 414–424.

Turner, N. C., Dollery, C. T. & Williams, A. J. (1989) Endothelin-1-induced contractions of vascular and tracheal smooth muscle: effects of nicardipine and BRL 34915. *Journal of Cardiovascular Pharmacology* **135**, S180–S182.

Uchida, Y., Yoshimoto, N. & Murao, A. (1978) Effect of 2-nicotinamidoethyl nitrate (SG75) on coronory circulation. *Japanese Heart Journal* **19**, 112–124.

Uchida, Y., Nakamura, F., Tomaru, T., Sumino, S., Kato, A. & Sugimoto, T. (1986) Phasic contractions of canine and human coronary arteries induced by potassium channel blockers. *Japanese Heart Journal* **27**, 727–740.

Van der Laarse, A., Holaar, L. & Van der Volk, L. J. M. (1979) Release of alpha hydroxybutyrate from neonatal rat heart cell cultures exposed to anoxia and reoxygenation. Comparison with impairment of structure and function of damaged cardiac cells. *Cardiovascular Research* **13**, 345–353.

Venkatesh, N., Lamp, S. T. & Weiss, J. N. (1991) Sulfonylureas, ATP-sensitive K$^+$ channels, and cellular K$^+$ loss during hypoxia, ischemia, and metabolic inhibition in mammalian ventricle. *Circulation Research* **69**, 623–637.

Videbaek, L. M., Aalkjaer, C., Hughes, A. D. & Mulvany, M. J. (1990) Effect of pinacidil on ion permeability in resting and contracted resistance vessels. *American Journal of Physiology* **259**, H14–H22.

Videbaek, L. M., Aalkjaer, C. & Mulvany, M. J. (1988) Pinacidil opens K$^+$-selective channels causing hyperpolarisation and relaxation of noradrenaline contractions in rat mesenteric resistance vessels. *British Journal of Pharmacology* **95**, 103–108.

Vogel, W. M., Cerel, A. W. & Apstein, C. S. (1986) Post-ischemic cardiac chamber stiffness and coronary vasomotion: The role of edema and effects of dextran. *Journal of Molecular Cell Cardiology* **18**, 1207–1218.

Vrobel, T. R., Ring, W. S., Anderson, R. W., Emery, R. W. & Bache, R. J. (1980) Effect of heart rate on myocardial flow in dogs with chronic left ventricular hypertrophy. *American Journal of Physiology* **239**, H621–H627.

Walsh, K. B., Begenisch, T. B. & Kass, R. S. (1989) Beta-adrenergic stimulation of cardiac ion channels. Differential temperature sensitivity of potassium and calcium currents. *Journal of General Physiology* **93**, 841–854.

Wang, X. & Fiscus, R. R. (1989) Calcitonin gene-related peptide increases cAMP, tension, and rate in rat atria. *American Journal of Physiology* **256**, R421–R428.

Wang, Z., Kimitsuki, T. & Noma, A. (1991) Conductance properties of the Na$^+$-activated K$^+$ channel in guinea-pig ventricular cells. *Journal of Physiology* **433**, 241–257.

Weir, S. W. & Weston, A. H. (1986a) Effect of apamin on responses to BRL 34915, nicorandil and other relaxants in guinea-pig taenia caeci. *British Journal of Pharmacology* **88**, 113–120.

Weir, S. W. & Weston, A. H. (1986b) The effects of BRL34915 and nicorandil on electrical and mechanical activity and on ^{86}Rb$^+$ efflux in rat blood vessels. *British Journal of Pharmacology* **88**, 121–128.

Weiss, J. & Shine, K. I. (1982) Extracellular K$^+$ accumulation during myocardial ischemia in isolated rabbit heart. *American Journal of Physiology* **242**, H619–H628.

Weston, A. H. & Edwards, G. (1991) Recent progress in potassium channel opener pharmacology. *Biochemical Pharmacology* **43**, 1, 47–54.

Weston, A. H. & Edwards, G. (1991) Latest developments in K-channel modulator pharmacology. *Zeitschrift für Kardiologie* **80** (Suppl. 7), 1–8.

Wickenden, A. D., Grimwood, S., Grant, T. L. & Todd, M. H. (1991) Comparison of the effects of the K$^+$-channel openers cromakalim and minoxidil sulphate on vascular smooth muscle. *British Journal of Pharmacology* **103**, 1148–1152.

Wilson, C., Buckingham, R. E., Mootoo, S., Parrott, L. S., Hamilton, T. C., Pratt, S. C. & Cawthorne, M. A. (1988a) *In vivo* and *in vitro* studies of cromakalim (BRL 34915) and glibenclamide in the rat. *British Journal of Pharmacology* **93**, 126P.

Wilson, C., Coldwell, M. C., Howlett, D. R., Cooper, S. M. & Hamilton, T. C. (1988b) Comparative effects of K$^+$ channel blockade on the vasorelaxant activity of cromakalim, pinacidil and nicorandil. *European Journal of Pharmacology* **152**, 331–339.

Winquist, R. J., Heaney, L. A., Wallace, A. A., Baskin, E. P., Stein, R. B., Garcia, M. L. & Kaczorowski, G. J. (1989) Glyburide blocks the relaxation response to BRL 34915 (cromakalim), minoxidil sulphate and diazoxide in vascular smooth muscle. *Journal of Pharmacology and Experimental Therapeutics* **248**, 149–156.

Wolleben, C. D., Sanguinetti, M. C. & Siegl, P. K. S. (1989) Influence of ATP-sensitive potassium channel modulators on ischaemia-induced fibrillation in isolated rat hearts. *Journal of Molecular Cell Cardiology* **21**, 783–788.

Yamada, H., Yoneyama, F., Satoh, K. & Taira, N. (1990) Specific but differential antagonism by glibenclamide of the vasodepressor effects of cromakalim and nicorandil in spinally-anaesthetized dogs. *British Journal of Pharmacology* **100**, 413–416.

Yanagisawa, T., Hashimoto, H. & Taira, N. (1988) The negative inotropic effect of nicorandil is independent of cyclic GMP changes: a comparison with pinacidil and cromakalim in canine atrial muscle. *British Journal of Pharmacology* **95**, 393–398.

Yanagisawa, T., Teshigawara, T. & Taira, N. (1990) Cytoplasmic calcium and the relaxation of canine coronary arterial smooth muscle produced by cromakalim, pinacidil and nicorandil. *British Journal of Pharmacology* **101**, 157–165.

Yoshitake, K., Hirano, K. & Kanaide, H. (1991) Effects of glibenclamide on cytosolic calcium concentrations and on contraction of the rabbit aorta. *British Journal of Pharmacology* **102**, 113–118.

Zhang, H., Stockbridge, N., Weir, B., Krueger, C. & Cook, D. (1991) Glibenclamide relaxes vascular smooth muscle constriction produced by prostaglandin F$_{2\alpha}$. *European Journal of Pharmacology* **195**, 27–35.

Chapter 15
The pharmacology of potassium channel modulators in airways smooth muscle: relevance to airways disease

R. C. Small, J. L. Berry, R. W. Foster, K. A. Green
and M. A. Murray

Introduction

The past decade has seen the emergence of a novel group of smooth muscle relaxant drugs collectively known as potassium (K)-channel openers (KCOs). The group includes benzopyran derivatives such as cromakalim (BRL 34915), SDZ PCO 400 and Ro 31-6930, cyanoguanidine derivatives such as pinacidil and tetrahydrothiopyrans such as RP 49356 (*see* Chapter 11). Ro 31-6930 contains no chiral centre. However, cromakalim, pinacidil and RP 49356 are racemates and, in each case, their biological activity resides in a single enantiomer.

Studies of the actions of these compounds on airways smooth muscle *in vitro* and their ability to cause bronchodilatation *in vivo* have prompted the suggestion (Allen *et al.*, 1986a; Buckle *et al.*, 1987; Arch *et al.*, 1988; Nielsen-Kudsk *et al.*, 1988; Small *et al.*, 1988) that K-channel openers may be worthy of investigation as chemotherapy in the treatment of bronchial asthma.

In vitro effects of KCOs

General features

Cromakalim, pinacidil, RP 49356 and Ro 31-6930 each cause concentration-dependent suppression of the spontaneous tone of guinea-pig trachealis (Allen *et al.*, 1986a; Bray *et al.*, 1987; Arch *et al.*, 1988; Nielsen-Kudsk *et al.*, 1988; Paciorek *et al.*, 1989; 1990; Berry *et al.*, 1991; Raeburn & Brown, 1991). In experiments of this kind the maximal relaxant effects of cromakalim, pinacidil and RP 49356 are equivalent to 75–100% of the maximal relaxation induced by isoprenaline or aminophylline (Allen et al., 1986a; Bray et al., 1987; Arch et al., 1988; Nielsen-Kudsk et al., 1988; Murray et al., 1989; Paciorek et al., 1990; Berry et al., 1991; see Figs 15.5, 15.6).

Potassium-channel openers can relax guinea-pig trachealis muscle when tone has been induced by prostaglandins E_2 or $F_{2\alpha}$, agonists at histamine H_1 receptors or agonists at muscarinic cholinoceptors (Allen et al., 1986a; Arch et al., 1988; Gillespie & Sheng, 1988; Nielsen-Kudsk et al., 1988; Paciorek et al., 1990; Raeburn & Brown, 1991). However, when K-channel openers are tested against tone induced by exogenous spasmogens, their relaxant potency is reduced compared with that observed against spontaneous tone. Muscarinic agonists cause a greater reduction in the relaxant potency of K-channel openers than do agonists at histamine H_1 receptors (Allen et al., 1986a; Nielsen-Kudsk et al., 1988; Taylor et al., 1988b; Paciorek et al., 1990; Raeburn & Brown, 1991; Table 15.1).

The tracheal relaxant potencies of alkylxanthines and agonists at β-adrenoceptors are also more greatly reduced when a muscarinic agonist rather than an agonist at histamine H_1 receptors is used to induce tracheal tone (Spilker & Minatoya, 1975; Karlsson & Persson, 1981; Allen et al., 1986b; Small et al., 1989; Paciorek et al., 1990). Accordingly, it is likely that the greater reduction in the relaxant potency of K-channel openers observed in the presence of muscarinic agonists reflects differences in the mechanisms by which muscarinic agonists and agonists at histamine H_1 receptors cause contraction of airways smooth muscle.

The relaxant effects of K-channel openers in airways smooth muscle extend to bovine trachealis, a tissue which, in vitro, is virtually devoid of spontaneous tone. Following induction of tone using KCl (25 mM), cromakalim and pinacidil each caused concentration-dependent relaxation of bovine trachealis (Gater, 1989; Longmore & Weston, 1989).

Potassium-channel openers including cromakalim and SDZ PCO 400 can also suppress the spontaneous tone of human bronchial smooth muscle in vitro (Taylor et al., 1988a,b; Chapman, 1990). The relaxant activity of cromakalim and BRL 38227 in human bronchial smooth muscle is retained when tone is raised by histamine or carbachol (Taylor et al., 1988a; Barnes et al., 1990). In guinea-pig trachealis the relaxant potency of cromakalim tested against carbachol-induced tone is more than 100-fold less than its potency tested against histamine-induced tone (Taylor et al., 1988a). However, in human bronchioles, the relaxant potency of cromakalim tested against carbachol-induced tone is only threefold less than its potency against histamine-induced tone (Table 15.1). This has prompted the suggestion (Taylor et al., 1988a) that the mechanism by which muscarinic receptor activation causes tension

Table 15.1. IC_{50} (μM) and intrinsic activity (in parentheses) of cromakalim relative to an isoprenaline (10_M^{-3}) maximum relaxation.

	Spontaneous tone	PGE$_2$ (10 nM)	Leukotriene D4 (3 μM)	Histamine (5 μM)	5HT (0.8 μM)	Carbachol (0.3 μM guinea pig; 5 μM human)
Guinea-pig trachea	1.1 (0.89)	0.9 (0.93)	1.2 (0.87)	3.2 (0.77)	0.53 (0.93)	>100 (0.21)
Human bronchioles	0.35 (0.93)	–	–	0.57 (0.93)	–	1.96 (0.82)

From Taylor *et al.* (1988a) with permission.

development in human airways smooth muscle may differ from the equivalent mechanism in guinea-pig trachealis. Accordingly, the relative impotency of K-channel openers against spasm induced by cholinomimetics in guinea-pig trachea may not be predictive of poor bronchodilator activity in the human.

Evidence that cromakalim and similar drugs open plasmalemmal K-channels

A variety of observations suggests that cromakalim and similar drugs open plasmalemmal K-channels in airways smooth muscle cells. Electrophysiological studies of guinea-pig trachealis have shown that the relaxant effects of cromakalim, BRL 38227 and RP 49356 are associated with the suppression of spontaneous electrical slow waves and with hyperpolarization of the plasmalemma to a value close to the calculated K-equilibrium potential (Allen et al., 1986a; Murray et al., 1989; Berry et al., 1991; Fig. 15.1). Bovine trachealis in vitro exhibits very little or no spontaneous electrical activity but the application of cromakalim induces cellular hyperpolarization, again to a value close to the K-equilibrium potential (Longmore & Weston, 1989; Longmore et al., 1990).

Ion flux studies have shown that cromakalim can promote the efflux of $^{86}Rb^+$ or $^{42/43}K^+$ from guinea-pig trachealis pre-loaded with the relevant isotope (Allen et al., 1986a; Foster, 1989; Fig. 15.2). The promotion of $^{86}Rb^+$-efflux is small in absolute terms (Allen et al., 1986a) and small relative to the promotion of $^{42/43}K^+$-efflux (Foster, 1989). Since the presence of $^{86}Rb^+$ reduced the efflux of $^{42/43}K^+$ (Foster, 1989), it may be that the use of $^{86}Rb^+$ as a marker yields an underestimate of the K^+-fluxes induced by cromakalim. In bovine trachealis, too, K-channel openers such as cromakalim and pinacidil promote the efflux of $^{86}Rb^+$ and $^{42}K^+$ (Gater, 1989; Longmore & Weston, 1989). Furthermore, cromakalim again causes a greater rise in $^{42}K^+$-efflux than in $^{86}Rb^+$-efflux (Longmore & Weston, 1989; Longmore et al., 1990). This finding lends support to the suggestion that cromakalim-like drugs open plasmalemmal K-channels whose permeability to K^+ exceeds that to Rb^+.

Several groups of workers have examined the ability of K-channel openers to relax KCl-induced spasm of airways smooth muscle in vitro. A common finding is that these agents can suppress spasm induced by low ($< 40\,mM$) concentrations of KCl but not that evoked by higher concentrations of KCl (Allen et al., 1986a; Bray et al., 1987; Taylor et al., 1988b; Brown et al., 1989; Gater, 1989; Raeburn & Brown, 1991; Fig. 15.3). This phenomenon may be explained as follows. By opening plasmalemmal K^+-channels, K-channel openers raise the membrane potential to a more negative value and thereby reduce the likelihood that plasmalemmal voltage-operated Ca^{2+}-channels (VOCs) will be open. Calcium influx is

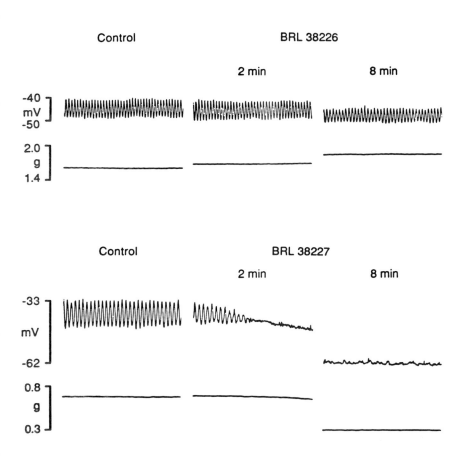

Fig. 15.1. Effects of the active (BRL 38227) and inactive (BRL 38226) enantiomers of cromakalim on the electrical and mechanical activity of guinea-pig isolated trachealis. In each row of recordings the upper trace represents membrane potential changes where all recordings were taken from the same cell. The lower trace represents the mechanical activity of a contiguous segment of trachea. Activity was recorded before (*control*) and 2 (*centre panel*) and 8 (*right panel*) min after application of the relevant enantiomer. Note that BRL 38226 (10 μM) was ineffective in suppressing the spontaneous tone of the trachea, which increased slightly during the experiment. BRL 38226 also had little or no effect on the electrical activity of the tissue. The mild hyperpolarization and reduction in slow wave activity evident here probably represent spontaneous changes in the activity of the impaled cell and were not observed in other cells challenged with BRL 38226. Note, in the lower row of recordings that BRL 38227 (10 μM) suppressed the spontaneous mechanical tone of the tissue, an effect accompanied by suppression of electrical slow wave activity and by marked cellular hyperpolarization. (M. A. Murray & R. C. Small, unpublished observations.)

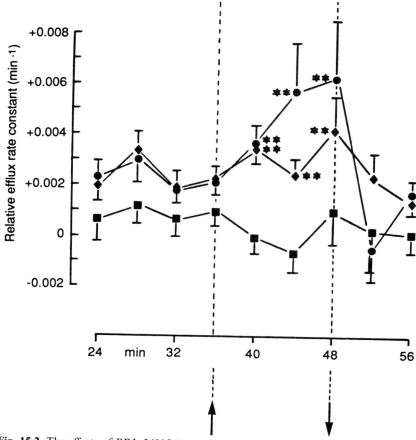

Fig. 15.2. The effects of BRL 34915 (cromakalim) on the efflux of $^{86}Rb^{+}$ from muscle-rich strips of guinea-pig isolated trachea. The abscissa scale indicates time (min) and the ordinate scale represents the relative efflux rate constant (/min). Drug (test tissues only) was present during the period between the arrows. Time-matched control tissues (■); test tissues treated with BRL 34915 1 μM (♦) or 10 μM (●). Data indicate means of values from eight tissues; vertical bars indicate SEM. ** indicates a significant ($P < 0.01$) difference from the corresponding point in the time-matched control tissues. (From Allen *et al.* (1986a) with permission.)

reduced and the tissue relaxes. This holds true for extracellular K^{+}-concentrations below 40 mM where the K-equilibrium potential lies at a value significantly more negative than the resting membrane potential of the cell. Plasmalemmal K-channel opening can therefore cause sufficient hyperpolarization to inhibit VOC opening. However, when the concentration of K^{+} in the extracellular fluid is raised above 40 mM the K-equilibrium potential adopts a value very close to the new resting membrane potential of the cell. In this circumstance the opening of plasmalemmal K-channels causes insufficient hyperpolarization to ensure that the opening of VOCs is inhibited. Calcium influx promoted by high external

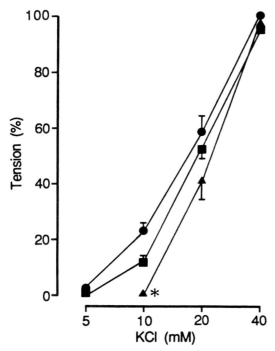

Fig. 15.3. The effect of BRL 34915 (cromakalim) on the log concentration/effect curve of KCl in guinea-pig isolated trachealis. The abscissa scale represents the concentration of KCl (mM) on a log scale. The ordinate represents tension as a percentage of the greatest tension achieved in the initial log concentration/effect curve of KCl. Pooled initial log concentration/effect curve for test and control tissues (●). Subsequent log concentration/effect curve constructed in control tissues after further incubation in Krebs' solution (■). Log concentration/effect curve constructed in test tissues treated with $10\,\mu M$ BRL 34915 (▲). Indomethacin ($2.8\,\mu M$) was present throughout these experiments. Data indicate the means of values from at least six tissues; SEM shown by vertical bars. * indicates a significant difference from the corresponding point for control tissues. (Adapted from Allen *et al.* (1986a) with permission.)

concentrations of K^+ is therefore not inhibited by the openers and they are accordingly unable to suppress the evoked spasm.

The effects of K-channel openers on the mechanical tone of trachealis muscle, on membrane potential and on ion fluxes can each be reduced by drugs believed to inhibit the opening of plasmalemmal K-channels. For example, the tracheal relaxant effects of cromakalim, pinacidil and RP 49356 are antagonized by compounds such as tetraethylammonium (TEA), procaine, 4-aminopyridine, glibenclamide and phentolamine (Allen *et al.*, 1986a; Brown *et al.*, 1989; Gater, 1989; Longmore & Weston, 1989; Murray *et al.*, 1989; McPherson & Angus, 1990; Nielsen-Kudsk *et al.*, 1990; Berry *et al.*, 1991; Raeburn & Brown, 1991). Tracheal hyperpolarization induced by cromakalim is reduced by TEA, procaine, glibenclamide or phentolamine (Allen *et al.*, 1986a; Longmore & Weston, 1989; Murray *et al.*, 1989). Furthermore, in bovine trachealis, cromakalim-induced stimulation of $^{86}Rb^+$ and $^{42}K^+$-efflux and pinacidil-induced stimulation of $^{86}Rb^+$-efflux can be inhibited by glibenclamide (Gater, 1989; Longmore & Weston, 1989). Not only does the effectiveness of these various K-channel inhibitors imply that the action of cromakalim-like drugs may depend on K-channel opening, but consideration of their selectivity in inhibiting the various types of plasmalemmal K-channel provides insight into the type of channel opened by the cromakalim-like drugs (*see below*).

In summary, electrophysiological studies, ion flux studies, spasmolytic effects against low but not high concentrations of KCl and antagonism by K-channel blockers all suggest that the actions of the cromakalim-like group of drugs depend on the opening of K-channels in the plasmalemma of the airways smooth muscle cell. It could be validly argued that most of this evidence is of an indirect kind. However, patch-clamp recording from airways smooth muscle (Collier *et al.*, 1990) is now beginning to yield direct evidence of cromakalim-induced K-channel opening in this tissue.

Antagonism of KCO-induced relaxation

The relaxant effects of cromakalim in airways smooth muscle are not antagonized by propranolol (Allen *et al.*, 1986a) and therefore do not depend on the activation of β-adrenoceptors. However, as mentioned above, cromakalim acting on guinea-pig trachealis can be antagonized by several agents with the ability to inhibit plasmalemmal K-channels. For example, procaine and TEA inhibit both the relaxant effects of cromakalim and the cellular hyperpolarization induced by cromakalim (Allen *et al.*, 1986a). Among the various types of K-channel known to be present in the plasmalemma, the inhibitor selectivity of procaine and TEA is poor (Yamanaka *et al.*, 1985; Cook, 1988). Accordingly, neither procaine nor TEA is helpful in identifying which of the various K-channels is involved in the actions of cromakalim-like drugs. However, the relaxant actions of K-channel openers in airways smooth muscle can be antagonized by the sulphonylurea, glibenclamide, and by phentolamine. The latter two antagonists are yielding clues as to the identity of the K-channel opened by cromakalim-like drugs.

Glibenclamide

In guinea-pig isolated trachea exhibiting spontaneous tone (Murray *et al.*, 1989; McPherson & Angus, 1990), Berry *et al.*, 1991) or tone induced by histamine (Nielsen-Kudsk *et al.*, 1990), glibenclamide antagonizes the relaxant action of K-channel openers such as cromakalim, pinacidil and

RP 49356. In the case of cromakalim and RP 49356, glibenclamide reduces the maximal relaxant effect (Murray *et al.*, 1989; McPherson & Angus, 1990; Nielsen-Kudsk *et al.*, 1990; Berry *et al.*, 1991) suggesting that the sulphonylurea produces insurmountable antagonism of the opener in each case. However, glibenclamide does not reduce the maximal relaxant effect of pinacidil. This may be a reflection of the fact that pinacidil possesses the ability to relax smooth muscle by more than one mechanism (Nielsen-Kudsk *et al.*, 1990).

There have been reports (Murray *et al.*, 1989; Berry *et al.*, 1991) that high (> 1 μM) concentrations of glibenclamide not only reduce the slope of the log concentration/relaxation curve of K-channel openers but also cause some leftward shift of the curve back towards the control position. The latter effect cannot be explained in terms of antagonism between the sulphonylurea and the opener. However, concentrations of glibenclamide of 5 μM or greater can cause some loss of tracheal tone (Lewis *et al.*, 1990; Berry *et al.*, 1991). Whether this relaxant action of glibenclamide is related to its action on K-channels remains to be determined. However, it may be that the relaxant effects of the sulphonylurea and the K-channel openers can be additive and this may mask the ability of glibenclamide to antagonize the opener.

In guinea-pig isolated trachealis, glibenclamide (1 μM) causes no change in mechanical tone, evokes very minor change (depolarization) in resting membrane potential and causes some reduction in the amplitude of spontaneous electrical slow waves. However, glibenclamide (1 μM) is able to inhibit both the relaxation induced by cromakalim and the cellular hyperpolarization and slow wave suppression caused by this agent (Murray *et al.*, 1989; Fig. 15.4). The ability of glibenclamide to inhibit cromakalim-induced hyperpolarization has also been observed in bovine trachealis (Longmore & Weston, 1989). In bovine airways smooth muscle cromakalim-induced stimulation of $^{86}Rb^{+}$- and $^{42}K^{+}$-efflux and pinacidil-induced stimulation of $^{86}Rb^{+}$-efflux can all be inhibited by glibenclamide (Gater, 1989; Longmore & Weston, 1989). It therefore would appear that glibenclamide can inhibit not only the mechanical effects of K-channel openers but also the electrophysiological changes and ion fluxes induced by these agents.

Glibenclamide antagonism of K-channel openers acting on guinea-pig isolated trachealis is selective (Fig. 15.5) in that the sulphonylurea does not antagonize the relaxant actions of agonists at β-adrenoceptors (Murray *et al.*, 1989; Neilsen-Kudsk *et al.*, 1990), theophylline (Murray *et al.*, 1989; Neilsen-Kudsk *et al.*, 1990; Berry *et al.*, 1991) or verapamil (Neilsen-Kudsk *et al.*, 1990). What does glibenclamide's selective antagonism of cromakalim tell us about the mechanism of action of the K-channel openers? There have been several reports (e.g. Schmid-Antomarchi *et al.*, 1987; Sturgess *et al.*, 1988) that glibenclamide can inhibit the opening of

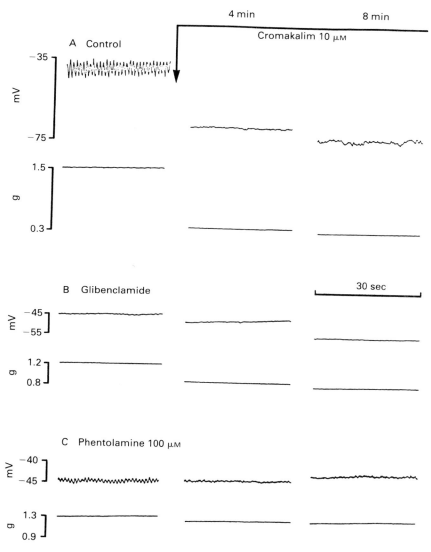

Fig. 15.4. Guinea-pig isolated trachealis: the electrical and mechanical effects of cromakalim (10 μM) and their antagonism by tissue pretreatment with glibenclamide or phentolamine. In each row of recordings the upper trace represents membrane potential changes recorded from a single cell, while the lower trace represents the mechanical activity of a contiguous segment of trachea. In each row the left-hand panel indicates control activity. The centre and right-hand panels indicate activity recorded 4 and 8 min, respectively, after tissue exposure to cromakalim (10 μM). A, no antagonist present. B and C, glibenclamide (1 μM) and phentolamine (100 μM), respectively, present throughout. Note that glibenclamide and phentolamine each reduced the ability of cromakalim to hyperpolarize and relax the trachealis muscle. (From Murray *et al.* (1989) with permission.)

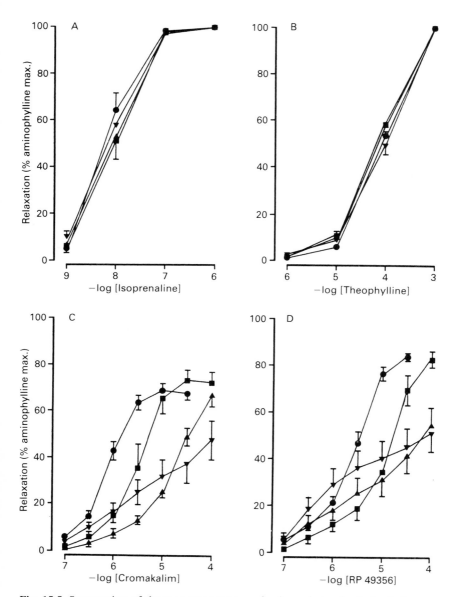

Fig. 15.5. Suppression of the spontaneous tone of guinea-pig trachealis by A, iso-prenaline, B, theophylline, C, cromakalim and D, RP 49356: the effects of glibencla-mide. In each panel (●) indicates the log concentration/effect curve of the relevant bronchodilator drug obtained in the absence of glibenclamide (time-matched control). Other log concentration/effect curves were obtained in the presence of 0.1 (■), 1.0 (▲) or 10 μM (▼) glibenclamide respectively. Each point represents the mean (± SEM) of at least six tissues. Note the ability of glibenclamide to antagonize cromakalim and RP 49356 without antagonizing either isoprenaline or theophylline. (Adapted from Murray *et al.* (1989) and from Berry *et al.* (1991) with permission.)

adenosine triphosphate sensitive K-channels (K_{ATP}) that are important for the regulation of insulin secretion in cell lines derived from pancreatic β-cells.

Such reports have prompted the suggestion (Newgreen *et al.*, 1989) that glibenclamide may block the K-channel opened by cromakalim in smooth muscle. However, in pancreatic cell lines glibenclamide can be effective against the K_{ATP} in concentrations as low as 0.1–20 nM (Schmid-Antomarchi *et al.*, 1987) whereas concentrations in the range 0.1–10 μM are required for antagonism of cromakalim in smooth muscle. This indicates that the cromakalim-opened K-channel in smooth muscle may not be identical to K_{ATP} in pancreatic cell lines.

Direct evidence for the existence of K_{ATP} in the plasmalemma of smooth muscle has been provided by the patch-clamp studies of rabbit mesenteric artery made by Standen *et al.* (1989). These authors showed that glibenclamide applied to the cytosolic surface of inside-out patches could inhibit cromakalim-induced opening of K_{ATP}. Evidence also exists that glibenclamide exhibits some selectivity as an inhibitor among the various types of plasmalemmal K-channel. For example, glibenclamide (10 μM) applied to the cytosolic or extracellular surfaces of plasmalemmal patches from cells of an insulin-secreting line failed to modify P_{open} of the large Ca^{2+}-activated K^+-channel (BK_{Ca}) (Sturgess *et al.*, 1988). When applied to the cytosolic surface of inside-out plasmalemmal patches from rabbit mesenteric artery (Standen *et al.*, 1989) or bovine trachealis (Berry *et al.*, 1991) glibenclamide again failed to modify P_{open} BK_{Ca}. It may therefore be that the effectiveness of glibenclamide against the relaxant actions of K-channel openers in airways smooth muscle is indicative that these agents act to open a plasmalemmal K-channel that is ATP-sensitive (*see below*).

Phentolamine

In guinea-pig trachea exhibiting spontaneous tone, phentolamine (1–100 μM) antagonizes the relaxant action of K-channel openers such as cromakalim and RP 49356 (Murray *et al.*, 1989; McPherson and Angus, 1990; Berry *et al.*, 1991; Fig. 15.6). Phentolamine in each case depresses the log concentration/relaxation curve and reduces the maximal response of these agents. Clearly, phentolamine antagonism of K-channel opener action on airways smooth muscle is insurmountable.

McPherson and Angus (1989) suggested that phentolamine antagonism of cromakalim acting on vascular smooth muscle was unrelated to the blockade of α-adrenoceptors. Evidence offered to support this suggestion included the fact that other antagonists at α-adrenoceptors (prazosin, rauwolscine and phenoxybenzamine) did not share the ability of phentolamine to antagonize cromakalim. In airways smooth muscle, too, phentol-

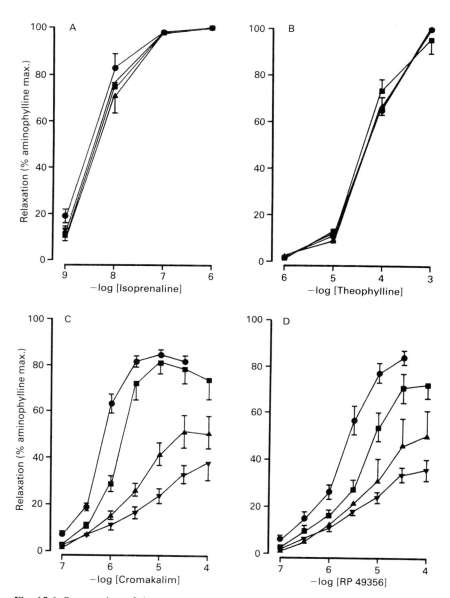

Fig. 15.6. Suppression of the spontaneous tone of guinea-pig trachealis by A, iso-prenaline, B, theophylline, C, cromakalim and, D, RP 49356: the effects of phentolamine. In each panel (●) indicates the log concentration/effect curve of the relevant bronchodilator drug obtained in the absence of phentolamine (time-matched control). Other log concentration/effect curves were obtained in the presence of 1 (■), 10 (▲) or 100 μM (▼) phentolamine respectively. Each point represents the mean (± SEM) of at least six tissues. Note the ability of phentolamine to antagonize cromakalim and RP 49356 without antagonizing either isoprenaline or theophylline. (Adapted from Murray *et al.* (1989) and from Berry *et al.* (1991) with permission.)

amine antagonism of K-channel openers seems unrelated to α-adrenoceptor blockade. Neither prazosin nor yohimbine share the ability of phentolamine to antagonize the tracheal relaxant action of cromakalim (Murray *et al.*, 1989).

In guinea-pig trachea, phentolamine (100 μM) causes no change in mechanical tone, evokes very minor change (depolarization) in resting membrane potential but may reduce the amplitude of spontaneous electrical slow waves. However, phentolamine (100 μM) is able to inhibit both the relaxation induced by cromakalim and the cellular hyperpolarization and slow wave suppression caused by this agent (Murray *et al.*, 1989; Fig. 15.4). Phentolamine therefore inhibits both the mechanical and electrophysiological responses of airways smooth muscle to cromakalim. It has yet to be reported whether phentolamine can inhibit the ion fluxes induced by K-channel openers in airways smooth muscle. Phentolamine antagonism of cromakalim acting on guinea-pig trachealis is selective (Fig. 15.6) in that phentolamine does not antagonize the relaxant actions of isoprenaline or theophylline (Murray *et al.*, 1989; Berry *et al.*, 1991). What does phentolamine's selective antagonism of cromakalim tell us about the mechanism of action of the K-channel opener? McPherson and Angus (1989) have suggested that phentolamine might antagonize cromakalim by blocking the K-channel that is opened by cromakalim. This suggestion has recently received support from patch-clamp studies of mouse pancreatic β-cells. The whole-cell recording mode was used to study $I_{K(ATP)}$. These currents were inhibited by phentolamine (20–100 μM), a finding which led to the proposal that phentolamine acts to inhibit K_{ATP} in the pancreatic β-cell (Plant & Henquin, 1990). Evidence is also emerging that phentolamine may exhibit some selectivity as an inhibitor among the various types of plasmalemmal K-channel. For instance, the application of phentolamine (100 μM) to the cytosolic surface of inside-out plasmalemmal patches from bovine trachealis did not significantly alter P_{open} of BK_{Ca} (Berry *et al.*, 1991). It may therefore be that the effectiveness of phentolamine against the relaxant actions of K-channel openers in airways smooth muscle is indicative that these agents act to open a plasmalemmal K-channel which is ATP-sensitive (*see below*).

Identity of the K-channel opened by cromakalim and similar drugs

More than 10 types of K-channel have been identified in the plasmalemmal membranes of excitable cells (Watson & Abbott, 1990). The various types of K-channel can be distinguished in terms of their conductance, the Ca^{2+}- and/or voltage-dependency of their activation and their susceptibility to inhibitors. Experimental evidence now accumulating allows us to reject certain of these K-channels as the site of action of the K-channel openers. The characteristics of the K-channel opened by cromakalim-like agents are beginning to emerge and we are beginning to form an impression of the role of this channel in determining the resting membrane potential and rectifying behaviour of the airways smooth muscle cell.

$SK_{Ca(Ap)}$

A Ca^{2+}-activated K-channel of small (6–14 pS) conductance ($SK_{Ca(Ap)}$: *see* Chapter 7) has been identified in some, though not all, types of mammalian smooth muscle. This channel is inhibited by apamin, a toxin exhibiting a high degree of selectivity as an inhibitor among the different types of K-channel (Cook & Quast, 1990). However, apamin failed to antagonize cromakalim-induced relaxation of guinea-pig isolated taenia caeci (Weir & Weston, 1986) and failed to inhibit cromakalim-induced hyperpolarization of smooth muscle cells from the guinea-pig urinary bladder (Foster *et al.*, 1988). Apamin did not reduce the ability of cromakalim to lower blood pressure in anaesthetized rats (Cook & Hof, 1988). Apamin (0.1 μM) also failed to antagonize cromakalim in suppressing the spontaneous tone of guinea-pig isolated trachea (Allen *et al.*, 1986a). Collectively these observations suggest that the smooth muscle relaxant actions of cromakalim do not depend on the opening of $SK_{Ca(Ap)}$.

BK_{Ca}

Large conductance (100–250 pS), Ca^{2+}-activated K-channels (BK_{Ca}: *see* Chapter 7) have been identified in many types of mammalian smooth muscle. Patch-clamp recording has been used to demonstrate their presence in airways smooth muscle from the dog (McCann & Welsh, 1986), guinea-pig (Hisada *et al.*, 1990; Small *et al.*, 1990), ox (Berry *et al.*, 1991; Green *et al.*, 1991), pig (Huang *et al.*, 1987) and rabbit (Kume *et al.*, 1990). The activation of K-channels of this type is dependent both upon the membrane potential and upon the concentration of free Ca^{2+} on the cytosolic side of the plasmalemma (McCann & Welsh, 1986; Berry *et al.*, 1991; Green *et al.*, 1991). In airways smooth muscle it has been shown that BK_{Ca} can be inhibited by the extracellular application of TEA (McCann & Welsh, 1986; Green *et al.*, 1991) or charybdotoxin (Green *et al.*, 1991; Fig. 15.7).

There have been reports that K-channel openers can promote the opening of BK_{Ca} in vascular smooth muscle. Application of cromakalim to the 'extracellular' surface of artificial lipid bilayers containing BK_{Ca} derived from rabbit aorta (Gelband *et al.*, 1989) or to the medium bathing whole-cell preparations from rat portal vein (Hu *et al.*, 1990) increased P_{open} of BK_{Ca}. However, cromakalim applied to the cytosolic surface of inside-out plasmalemmal patches from arterial muscle failed to modify P_{open} of BK_{Ca} (Standen *et al.*, 1989). Similar experiments have been

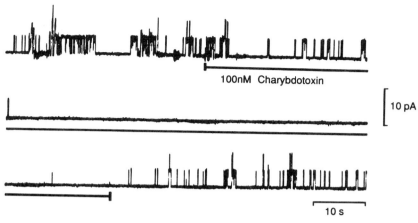

Fig. 15.7. The effects of charybdotoxin on the activity of large, Ca^{2+}-dependent K-channels in the plasmalemma of bovine trachealis muscle. The illustrated trace is a continuous unitary current recording from an outside-out plasmalemmal patch from bovine trachealis. The holding potential was 0 mV. The solution bathing the external surface of the patch contained 1.2 mM Ca^{2+} and 6 mM K^+ while that bathing the cytosolic surface contained 1 μM Ca^{2+} and 140 mM K^+. The bar underneath the trace indicates local perfusion of charybdotoxin (100 nM) by positioning a separate pipette near the patch. Note that the toxin abolished K-channel opening. Recovery of channel activity occurred as the toxin diffused away after removal of the application pipette. (From Green *et al.* (1991) with permission.)

performed with plasmalemmal patches from bovine trachealis (Berry *et al.*, 1991) and neither cromakalim (10 μM) nor RP 49356 (4–10 μM) modified P_{open} of BK_{Ca} (Fig. 15.8). If cromakalim has a site of action at the extracellular surface of the plasmalemma and penetrates the plasmalemma only very poorly, then it is possible that application of cromakalim to the intracellular surface of plasmalemmal patches will be ineffective. However, that cromakalim does not open BK_{Ca} in airways smooth muscle has also been indicated by the results of mechanical studies. In guinea-pig trachealis charybdotoxin (60 and 180 nM) antagonized isoprenaline-salbutamol- and aminophylline-induced relaxation without antagonizing cromakalim or pinacidil (Jones & Charette, 1990; Jones *et al.*, 1990). Similar experiments using charybdotoxin (100 nM) have confirmed that this agent can antagonize isoprenaline and theophylline without antagonizing cromakalim, SDZ PCO 400 and RP 49356 (Murray *et al.*, 1991; Small *et al.*, 1992).

In summary, when smooth muscle in general is considered, there is evidence both for and against the proposal that the actions of the KCOs involve promotion of the opening of BK_{Ca}. However, if airways smooth muscle alone is considered, the weight of evidence currently suggests that

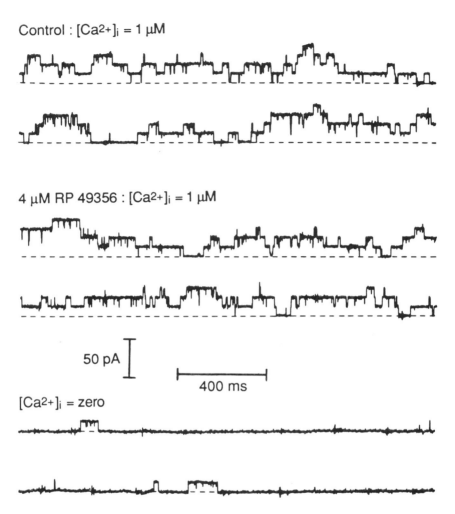

Fig. 15.8. Effects of RP 49356 and Ca^{2+} deprivation on the K-channel activity recorded from an inside-out plasmalemmal patch from bovine trachealis. All recordings were made from the same patch at a holding potential of $+60$ mV. The broken line indicates the position where no channels were open.

Upper panel: control activity recorded when free Ca^{2+} concentration in the internal solution was 1 μM.

Centre panel: activity recorded in the presence of RP 49356 (4 μM) and when free Ca^{2+}-concentration in the internal solution was 1 μM. Note failure of RP 49356 to modulate channel opening.

Lower panel: activity recorded in the absence of RP 49356 and when free Ca^{2+}-concentration in the internal solution was nominally zero. Note the marked reduction in channel activity caused by Ca^{2+}-deprivation. (From Berry *et al.* (1991) with permission.)

a channel other than BK_{Ca} is involved in the relaxant action of the K-channel openers.

K_{ATP}

Evidence is emerging (Standen et al., 1989) that the plasmalemma of vascular smooth muscle cells may contain ATP-regulated K-channels analogous to (but not identical with) those reported (Schmid-Antomarchi et al., 1987; Sturgess et al., 1988) in insulin-secreting cell lines. Such channels may also be present in airways smooth muscle. Recording from inside-out plasmalemmal patches from primary cultures of rabbit trachealis (Collier et al., 1990) revealed outward unitary currents with a reversal potential close to the calculated K-equilibrium potential. These currents were abolished by the addition of ATP (2 mM) to the solution bathing the cytosolic surface of the patches. Collier et al. (1990) concluded that their cells contained K_{ATP} and showed that such channels could be opened by the active enantiomer (BRL 38227) of cromakalim.

The use of K-channel blockers also suggests that cromakalim-like drugs may open K_{ATP} in airways smooth muscle. As mentioned above, glibenclamide can inhibit the opening of K_{ATP} in insulin-secreting cell lines (Schmid-Antomarchi et al., 1987; Sturgess et al., 1988) and can selectively antagonize cromakalim, pinacidil and RP 49356 acting on tracheal smooth muscle (Brown et al., 1989; Gater, 1989; Longmore & Weston 1989; Murray et al., 1989; Berry et al., 1991; Raeburn & Brown, 1991). Phentolamine, too, can inhibit the opening of K_{ATP} in insulin-secreting cells (Plant & Henquin, 1990) and can selectively antagonize cromakalim or RP 49356 in causing tracheal relaxation (Murray et al., 1989; McPherson & Angus, 1990; Berry et al., 1991).

In summary, direct (patch-clamp recording) evidence that K-channel openers act to open K_{ATP} in airways smooth muscle is currently to be found in a single, brief report (Collier et al., 1990). The use of antagonists known selectively to inhibit K_{ATP} in pancreatic β-cells, however, lends strong support to the idea that analogous (but not identical) K-channels are present in airways smooth muscle and can be activated by K-channel openers.

Physiological relevence

As stated above, concentrations of glibenclamide and phentolamine which provide antagonism of cromakalim, cause very minor depolarization of guinea-pig trachealis cells. Furthermore, these agents do not mimic the ability of TEA to convert electrical slow waves into regenerative action potentials and to induce tension development (Murray et al., 1989; Fig. 15.9). If it can be assumed that glibenclamide or phentolamine act to close

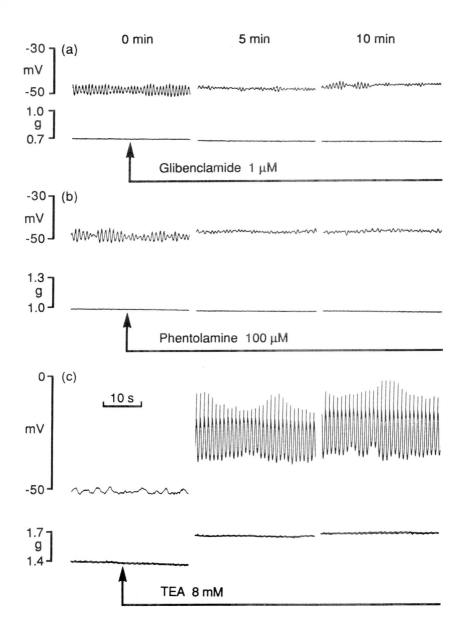

the cromakalim-sensitive K-channel, then it may be suggested (i) that the cromakalim-sensitive K-channel is not open under resting conditions and does not significantly contribute to the resting membrane potential and that (ii) the cromakalim-sensitive K-channel contributes very little to the marked rectifying behaviour of the airways smooth muscle cell.

The mechanism of K-channel opening by KCOs

The way in which cromakalim-like drugs open plasmalemmal K-channels is currently poorly understood. It is possible that these agents interact directly with the structure of the K-channel that they open. Alternatively, they may act at a site adjacent to the K-channel and may there initiate a series of biochemical changes that culminate in the channel opening.

It is widely accepted that the smooth muscle relaxant actions of agonists at β-adrenoceptors result from the activation of adenylate cyclase and the subsequent intracellular accumulation of cyclic adenosine monophosphate (cAMP). By activating protein kinase A, cAMP then triggers a variety of biochemical changes which result in relaxation. One such change may be the phosphorylation and subsequent opening of plasmalemmal K-channels. Kume *et al.* (1989) have shown in rabbit trachealis, that isoprenaline can increase the opening of Ca^{2+}-dependent K-channels and have attributed this effect to the phosphorylation of the channel (or a channel-related protein) by cAMP-dependent protein kinase.

Might K-channel openers evoke K-channel opening by increasing the intracellular concentration of cyclic nucleotides in smooth muscle? Several pieces of evidence suggest that this is not likely to be the case. Cromakalim ($0.1-1 \mu M$) was able to relax bovine retractor penis muscle precontracted with $1 \mu M$ guanethidine. However, cromakalim ($0.3-30 \mu M$) caused no changes in the tissue content of cAMP or cyclic guanosine monophosphate (cGMP; Gillespie & Sheng, 1988). Tested on vascular smooth muscle, cromakalim ($10-100 \mu M$) failed to increase the tissue content of cAMP or cGMP (Coldwell & Howlett, 1987; Taylor *et al.*, 1988c). Pinacidil

---

Fig. 15.9. (*Opposite*) Guinea-pig isolated trachealis: the effects of some antagonists of cromakalim on electrical and mechanical activity. In each row of recordings the upper trace represents membrane potential changes recorded from a single cell, while the lower trace represents the mechanical activity of a contiguous segment of trachea. In each row the left-hand panel indicates control activity and tissue exposure to the indicated drug commences at the arrow. The centre and right-hand panels show activity recorded at 5 and 10 min, respectively, after tissue exposure to the relevant drug. Note (in a and b respectively) that glibenclamide ($1 \mu M$) and phentolamine ($100 \mu M$) caused some suppression of spontaneous slow wave activity and very minor depolarization. These electrical changes were accompanied by little or no change in mechanical tone. In contrast (c) TEA ($8 mM$) evoked marked depolarization, promoted the discharge of regenerative action potentials and caused tonic tension development. (From Murray *et al.* (1989) with permission.)

Table 15.2. Effects of some drugs on the cyclic nucleotide content of muscle-rich strips of guinea-pig trachea.

Treatment	cAMP (pmol/mg protein)	cGMP (pmol/mg protein)
Control	12.16 ± 0.86 (24)	1.05 ± 0.08 (22)
Cromakalim		
3 μM	13.50 ± 1.80 (10)	0.87 ± 0.22 (8)
30 μM	14.91 ± 1.90 (10)	1.16 ± 0.16 (10)
75 μM	15.45 ± 2.60 (9)	1.14 ± 0.10 (10)
RP 49356		
3 μM	15.79 ± 1.65 (5)	1.07 ± 0.06 (5)
30 μM	13.36 ± 2.50 (5)	1.12 ± 0.05 (4)
75 μM	12.54 ± 0.92 (5)	1.22 ± 0.19 (5)
Forskolin		
160 nM	16.26 ± 2.40 (3)	1.20 ± 0.18 (3)
742 nM	84.30 ± 13.7 (9)*	1.31 ± 0.22 (9)
Sodium nitrite		
2.5 mM	8.70 ± 0.91 (9)	1.00 ± 0.07 (7)
25 mM	14.02 ± 1.10 (15)	2.09 ± 0.21 (15)*
Theophylline		
1 mM	13.00 ± 0.66 (5)	0.99 ± 0.13 (5)
1 mM theophylline + 160 nM forskolin	26.39 ± 3.70 (5)*	1.30 ± 0.22 (5)
30 μM cromakalim + 160 nM forskolin	16.64 ± 1.50 (5)	1.10 ± 0.16 (4)
30 μM RP 49356 + 160 nM forskolin	16.56 ± 2.10 (5)	0.81 ± 0.24 (5)

Data indicate mean ± SEM. Figures in parentheses indicate number of experiments.
* indicates a significant increase compared with controls.
From Berry *et al.* (1991) with permission.

(0.1–100 μM) did not increase the cAMP or cGMP content of rat aorta (Kauffman *et al.*, 1986). In guinea-pig trachealis muscle, relaxant concentrations of cromakalim and RP 49356 did not increase the tissue content of cAMP or cGMP. Furthermore, neither cromakalim nor RP 49356 was able to potentiate forskolin in increasing the tissue content of cAMP (Murray *et al.*, 1990; Berry *et al.*, 1991; Table 15.2).

The failure of cromakalim and RP 49356 to increase the intracellular content of cAMP or cGMP suggests that these two agents do not activate adenylate cyclase or guanylate cyclase. It may also be suggested that the actions of cromakalim and RP 49356 in relaxing airways smooth muscle do not involve the inhibition of cyclic nucleotide phosphodiesterases. This latter suggestion receives support from measurements of the phosphodiesterase activity in homogenates of muscle-rich strips of guinea-pig trachea. These measurements showed that RP 49356 was virtually devoid of phos-

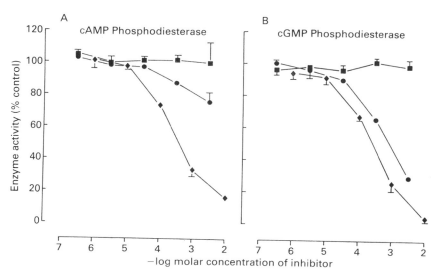

Fig. 15.10. Effects of cromakalim (●), RP 49356 (■) and theophylline (◆) on the activity of cAMP-phosphodiesterase, A and cGMP-phosphodiesterase, B, in homogenates of muscle-rich strips of guinea-pig trachea. *Abscissae:* − log molar concentration of inhibitor. *Ordinate scale:* enzyme activity (cAMP-PDE in A, cGMP-PDE in B) expressed as a percentage of control activity. Each data point indicates the mean of values from six experiments; vertical bars indicate SEM. (From Berry *et al.* (1991) with permission.)

phodiesterase inhibitory activity. Cromakalim was able to inhibit cAMP- and cGMP-phosphodiesterase activity, but only in a concentration greater than that required to produce full suppression of the spontaneous tone of the trachea (Berry *et al.*, 1991; Fig. 15.10). Pinacidil in concentrations as high as 1 mM did not inhibit cAMP-phosphodiesterase isolated from guinea-pig lung (Ho *et al.*, 1990).

Measurements of tissue cyclic nucleotide content and phosphodiesterase activity both suggest that the ability of K-channel openers to relax airways (and other) smooth muscle does not depend on the intracellular accumulation of cyclic nucleotides. It is conceivable, though, that these agents could directly activate protein kinase A. In that event they might phosphorylate and thereby open Ca^{2+}-dependent K-channels in a fashion similar to that utilized by the agonists at β-adrenoceptors. To our knowledge, however, no experiments have yet been performed to determine whether K-channel openers can directly activate protein kinase A.

In view of the evidence that K-channel openers may act to open an ATP-regulated K-channel in the plasmalemma, attention has recently been focused on the possibility that these agents may cause K-channel opening by altering the cellular content of ATP. In this respect it has been reported that the active enantiomer of cromakalim (BRL 38227) can

reduce the cellular content of ATP in vascular smooth muscle, an effect
inhibited by glibenclamide (Longman, 1989). The long incubation period
(120 min) used to achieve the cromakalim-induced reduction in intracellular ATP casts doubt on whether this effect is causally related to the
smooth muscle relaxant action of cromakalim (which is fully developed
within 10 min). However, the hypothesis that cromakalim reduces the
intracellular content of ATP and thereby opens ATP-regulated K-channels
may merit further investigation.

Relation of K-channel opening to the relaxant effects of KCOs in airways smooth muscle

Potassium channel openers could induce relaxation of airways smooth
muscle either by reducing the Ca^{2+} sensitivity or responsiveness of the
intracellular contractile machinery or by reducing the concentration of
free Ca^{2+} in the cytosol. The former has been tested in guinea-pig trachealis treated with the detergent Triton X-100 which very effectively destroys
the plasmalemma of trachealis cells (Cortijo et al., 1987) and the application of Ca^{2+} (0.1–10 μM) to the resulting skinned fibres evokes
concentration-dependent contraction (Cortijo et al., 1987, 1990). Pretreatment of skinned trachealis fibres with cromakalim (10 μM) failed to alter
the contractile response to Ca^{2+} (20 μM; Allen et al., 1986a). It may
therefore be suggested that cromakalim does not directly depress the Ca^{2+}
responsiveness of the intracellular contractile mechanisms. In this respect
cromakalim is similar to aminophylline and isoprenaline (Allen et al.,
1986b) but dissimilar to trifluoperazine (Cortijo et al., 1990). Whether
other openers are devoid of effects on the Ca^{2+} sensitivity or responsiveness of the intracellular contractile machinery of airways smooth muscle
remains to be determined. However, if the opening of K-channels indeed
underlies the relaxant effects of these compounds then they may be more
likely to reduce the cytosolic concentration of free Ca^{2+} than to reduce
directly the Ca^{2+} sensitivity or responsiveness of the intracellular contractile machinery.

How may K-channel opening result in a reduction in the cytosolic
concentration of free Ca^{2+}? The most important mechanism may involve
inhibition of Ca^{2+}-influx through the plasmalemma. Whatever the mechanism by which K-channel opening is achieved, the resultant elevation of
membrane potential to a more negative value reduces the likelihood of the
opening of VOCs in the plasmalemma and hence reduces Ca^{2+}-influx. This
explains the ability of cromakalim, pinacidil and RP 49356 (Allen et al.,
1986a; Bray et al., 1987; Taylor et al., 1988b; Brown et al., 1989; Raeburn
& Brown, 1991) to suppress tracheal spasm induced by KCl in concentrations less than 40 mM. As stated above, when the concentration of K^+ in
the bathing medium is 40 mM or greater, the relaxant activity of the

K-channel openers is virtually ablated. In this situation the K^+-equilibrium potential falls to a value less negative than that required for the opening of VOCs. Accordingly, K-channel opening drugs cannot evoke sufficient hyperpolarization to prevent the opening of VOCs induced by high ($\geqslant 40$ mM) concentrations of KCl.

Evidence exists to suggest that K-channel openers inhibit Ca^{2+}-influx through more than one type of voltage-dependent Ca^{2+}-channel in the trachealis plasmalemma. The spontaneous tone of guinea-pig trachealis depends upon the production of prostaglandins (Farmer et al., 1974) and is ablated in Ca^{2+}-free media (Foster et al., 1983, 1984). However, the spontaneous tone of guinea-pig trachealis is relatively little affected by inhibitors (e.g. nifedipine, verapamil) of Ca^{2+}-influx through L-type VOCs (Foster et al., 1984; Ahmed et al., 1985; Small & Foster, 1986; Arch et al., 1988). Accordingly, the maintenance of spontaneous tone in guinea-pig trachealis may involve Ca^{2+}-influx through channels discrete from those inhibited by dihydropyridines and verapamil. The effectiveness of the K-channel openers against spontaneous tone suggests that such channels are nevertheless voltage-dependent. It may be that the voltage-dependent plasmalemmal Ca^{2+}-channels that are resistant to organic inhibitors of Ca^{2+} influx are important in the filling of intracellular Ca^{2+} stores.

Some evidence that K-channel openers might interfere with Ca^{2+} loading of intracellular stores has been obtained in cells cultured from rabbit airways smooth muscle (Chopra et al., 1990). The plasmalemma in monolayers of the cultured cells was permeabilized by exposure to digitonin. Presumably the conditions of the permeabilization were such that intracellular structures such as the sarcoplasmic reticulum remained undamaged. The extent of the Ca^{2+} loading of the intracellular stores was assessed by loading the permeabilized cells with $^{45}Ca^{2+}$ and subsequent analysis of $^{45}Ca^{2+}$-efflux.

Preincubation of the permeabilized cells with BRL 38227 ($10\,\mu$M) slowed their subsequent uptake of $^{45}Ca^{2+}$ and reduced the Ca^{2+} content of the intracellular store by 26.6%. While allowing that the mechanism of the action of BRL 38227 in reducing store content was in need of further analysis, Chopra et al. (1990) suggested that BRL 38227 could produce its store depleting effect by acting at the level of K-channels in the sarcoplasmic reticulum.

In view of the possibility that dihydropyridine-resistant plasmalemmal Ca^{2+}-channels may be involved in the refilling of intracellular stores in airways smooth muscle (see above) and that digitonin treatment permeabilizes the plasmalemma, it could well be that the technique of Chopra et al. (1990) yields an underestimate of the inhibitory effect of K-channel openers on the filling of the intracellular Ca^{2+} store.

In summary, by opening plasmalemmal K-channels, cromakalim-like drugs move the resting membrane potential to a more negative value and hence reduce the likelihood of opening of both dihydropyridine-sensitive, VOCs and of other VOCs that are resistant to blockade by organic inhibitors of Ca^{2+}-influx. The latter Ca^{2+}-channels may be of importance in the filling of intracellular Ca^{2+} stores.

Potassium channel openers and neuroeffector transmission in the lung

Hall and MacLagan (1988) recorded intraluminal pressure changes from guinea-pig isolated trachea mounted in a medium containing in-domethacin (5 μM). The tracheal preparation was set up with the vagi and recurrent laryngeal nerves attached. Preganglionic stimulation of both vagi evoked a pressor response which could be reduced in a concentration-dependent way by cromakalim (0.1–6.4 μM). The administration of cro-makalim (2 μM) caused a slight rightward shift of the concentration/pres-sor–response curve for exogenous acetylcholine. Since cromakalim caused a greater (not more than 65%) reduction in responses to preganglionic vagal stimulation than in responses to exogenous acetylcholine, Hall and MacLagan (1988) concluded that the effect of cromakalim in reducing responses to vagal stimulation was due, at least in part, to an action on vagal neurones involving inhibition of neurotransmitter release.

Subsequent work has suggested that cromakalim may act at sites proximal to the postganglionic cholinergic nerve terminals. Using the tech-nique of intraluminal pressure recording in guinea-pig isolated trachea, McCaig and De Jonckheere (1989a,b) showed that cromakalim (0.1–10 μM) can inhibit pressor responses to preganglionic vagal stimulation without depressing the log concentration/pressor–response curve for exogenous acetylcholine (Fig. 15.11). These authors also performed experiments with field stimulation of intramural nerves. Pressor responses to this type of stimulation were resistant to hexamethonium but sensitive to atropine. The pressor responses to field stimulation were unaffected by cromakalim (0.2–10 μM). On the basis of these observations McCaig and De Jonck-heere (1989b) concluded that cromakalim did not inhibit acetylcholine release from postganglionic vagal nerve terminals. Instead they proposed that the action of cromakalim in inhibiting responses to preganglionic vagal stimulation might involve functional antagonism of the action of acetylcholine during ganglionic transmission. Alternatively, it was sug-gested that cromakalim might interfere with the conduction of neuronal action potentials in preganglionic nerve terminals.

An inhibitory effect of cromakalim on cholinergic neuroeffector trans-mission has also been demonstrated *in vivo*. Ichinose and Barnes (1990) anaesthetized guinea-pigs with urethane and subjected the animals to mechanical ventilation via a tracheal cannula. Airway opening pressure was monitored as an index of tracheobronchial resistance to airflow. The animals were bilaterally vagotomized and bilateral vagal stimulation was performed using electrodes applied to the peripheral ends of the sectioned vagi.

In animals pretreated with capsaicin, phentolamine and propranolol, cromakalim (33–400 μg/kg, i.v.) administered 1 min before bronchoconstrictor challenge reduced bronchoconstriction evoked by bilateral vagal stimulation in a dose-dependent manner. Similar doses of cromakalim also reduced bronchoconstrictor responses to exogenous acetylcholine (0.3–2 μg/kg, i.v.). However, the maximal effect of cromakalim against acetylcholine was smaller than that observed against vagal stimulation. On the basis of these observations, Ichinose and Barnes (1990) concluded that the action of cromakalim in inhibiting vagally mediated cholinergic bronchoconstriction involved both pre- and postjunctional sites of action. In this respect it should be borne in mind that the concentrations of cromakalim found to be effective against cholinergic nerve stimulation *in vitro* (Hall & MacLagan, 1988; McCaig & De Jonckheere, 1989a,b) were similar to those having direct relaxant activity on the trachealis muscle (Allen *et al.*, 1986a; Hall & MacLagan, 1988; Murray *et al.*, 1989). At present, therefore, it would be unwise to propose that the inhibitory effect of cromakalim on vagal cholinergic neural pathways might occur at concentrations lower than those having inhibitory effect on airways smooth muscle.

Evidence is emerging that K-channel openers can also depress the activity of excitatory peptidergic nerves supplying the lung. This action may be seen at KCO doses that do not depress the bronchoconstrictor responses to i.v. injection of the peptide neurotransmitter. For example, Ichinose and Barnes (1990) showed that, in anaesthetized guinea-pigs pretreated with atropine and propranolol, cromakalim (10–400 μg/kg, i.v.) administered 1 min before bronchoconstrictor challenge could reduce the non-adrenergic, non-cholinergic (NANC) bronchoconstrictor response to bilateral vagal stimulation in a dose-dependent fashion. However, similar doses of cromakalim did not attenuate bronchoconstrictor responses to substance P (5–25 μg/kg, i.v.; Fig. 15.12). The effect of cromakalim against NANC bronchoconstrictor responses to vagal stimulation was reduced by the prior administration of glibenclamide (25 mg/kg, i.v.) but not by the prior administration of phentolamine (2.5 mg/kg, i.v.). Ichinose and Barnes (1990) concluded that cromakalim could inhibit transmitter release from excitatory peptidergic neurones at doses that did not affect the direct action of the peptide neurotransmitter in the lung. Differential effects of cromakalim on peptidergic neuroeffector transmission and peptide action in guinea-pig lung have recently been confirmed by Lewis and Raeburn (1990). The latter authors also showed, that this action of cromakalim was shared by RP 49356 and its (−)-enantiomer (RP 52891).

Reports that K-channel openers can exert inhibitory effects on excitatory nervous pathways in the lung raise the possibility that such effects

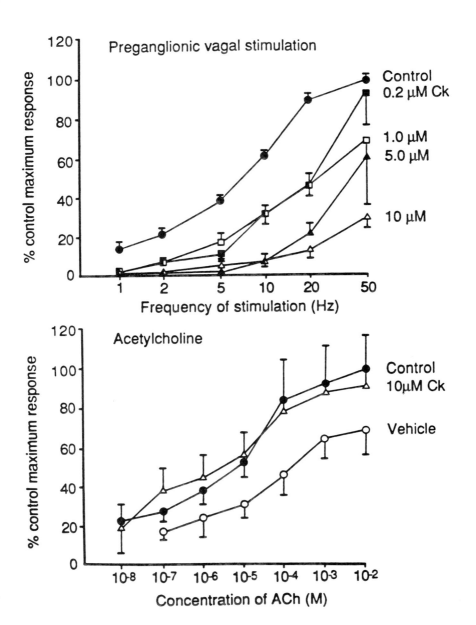

could contribute to the bronchodilator effects of these agents seen *in vivo* or could contribute to their ability to reduce or offset bronchial hyper-reactivity (*see below*).

Effects of KCOs on inflammatory cells in the lung

Few studies have yet been made of whether K-channel openers possess useful activity on cells involved in inflammatory processes in the lung. Tested in the guinea-pig, cromakalim has been reported to reduce platelet-activating factor (PAF)-induced airway hyperreactivity but not to reduce the numbers of eosinophils in lung lavage fluid from animals with idio-pathic bronchial eosinophilia (Sanjar *et al.*, 1989). In actively sensitized guinea-pigs the inhalation of allergen caused eosinophil migration into the airways lumen. The cromakalim analogue, SDZ PCO 400, failed to influence such eosinophil migration, whether administered orally or by inhalation (Chapman, 1990). Whether K-channel openers can influence mediator release from eosinophils remains to be determined.

Patch-clamp recording techniques have identified two types of Ca^{2+}-activated K-channels in human alveolar macrophages. Quinine inhibited both the opening of these K-channels and macrophage activation as assessed by chemiluminescence and leukotriene B_4 release (Kakuta *et al.*, 1988). This may suggest that the opening rather than the closure of plasmalemmal K-channels promotes macrophage activation. However, whether K-channel opening drugs have any influence on macrophage activation has yet to be reported.

Fig. 15.11. (*Opposite*) *Upper panel*: Guinea-pig isolated trachea: relationship between increase in intraluminal pressure, expressed as percentage control maximum response (ordinate scale) and frequency of stimulation (abscissa scale) of the vagus nerve in the absence (●) and presence of cromakalim, (Ck), $0.2\,\mu$M (■), $1\,\mu$M (□), $5\,\mu$M (▲) and $10\,\mu$M (△). Values are the mean of five to eight observations; vertical lines show SEM. All values (except the response at 50 Hz in the presence of $0.2\,\mu$M cromakalim) were significantly different from the corresponding control ($P < 0.05$, paired t-test).

Lower panel: Guinea-pig isolated trachea; relationship between increase in intra-luminal pressure, expressed as percentage of the initial control maximum (ordinate scale) and concentration of applied acetylcholine (ACh; abscissa scale) in the absence (●) and presence of cromakalim (Ck) $10\,\mu$M (△) and in time-matched controls (○). Values are mean of five observations; vertical lines show SEM. Res-ponses in time-matched controls at ACh 1 and 10 mM were significantly reduced ($P < 0.05$, t-test) compared with the corresponding responses in the initial curve. Responses in the presence of cromakalim were not significantly different from either the initial control or the time-matched control at any concentration of ACh. (Adapted from McCaig and De Jonckheere (1989b) with permission.)

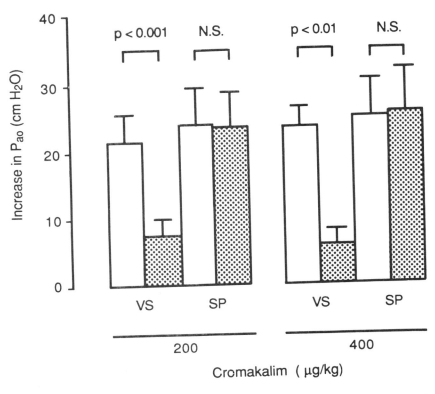

Fig. 15.12. The anaesthetized guinea-pig pretreated with atropine (1 mg/kg, i.v.) and propranolol (1 mg/kg, i.v.): effect of cromakalim (200–400 mg/kg, i.v.; stippled bars) on bronchoconstriction (increase in airway-opening pressure; P_{ao}) evoked by vagal stimulation (VS) and by substance P (SP; 5–25 μg/kg, i.v.). Open bars represent control responses before cromakalim. Data are mean ± SEM of five animals. Differences between means were analysed by Student's paired t-test. (From Ichinose & Barnes (1990) with permission.)

Bronchodilator activity of KCOs observed *in vivo*

General profile of action

Studies in conscious animals

Orally administered cromakalim or Ro 31-6930 have been shown to prolong the time to respiratory distress in conscious guinea-pigs challenged with an aerosol of histamine or ovalbumin (Arch *et al.*, 1988; Paciorek *et al.*, 1990). Ro 31-6930 (1–3 mg/kg) and cromakalim (3–10 mg/kg) provided dose-dependent protection against histamine challenge and the protective effects of the K-channel openers were of 1.5–2 h duration (Paciorek *et al.*, 1990). Ho *et al.* (1990) showed, in ovalbumin-sensitized, pyrilamine-treated guinea-pigs, that pinacidil (3–10 mg, p.o) reduced the severity of the respiratory distress induced by exposure of the animals to an aerosol of ovalbumin (10 mg/ml). That cromakalim administered by inhalation can delay the onset of histamine-induced respiratory distress has also been demonstrated in guinea-pigs (Bowring *et al.*, 1989).

Studies in anaesthetized animals

Ho *et al.* (1990) subjected anaesthetized, ovalbumin-sensitized guinea-pigs to whole body plethysmography and measured airways resistance (R_{aw}) and dynamic lung compliance (C_{dyn}). Exposure of the animals to an aerosol containing a low dose (50 μg/ml) of ovalbumin induced a gradually developing bronchoconstriction. Pinacidil (3 mg/kg, p.o.) markedly reduced the changes in R_{aw} and C_{dyn} induced by the ovalbumin aerosol. Bowring (1990) also measured R_{aw}, C_{dyn} and systemic blood pressure in anaesthetized guinea-pigs. In these experiments, BRL 38227 (50 μg/kg, i.v.) was administered 5 min prior to bronchoconstrictor challenge with i.v. injected histamine. The K-channel opener reduced the histamine-induced changes in R_{aw} and C_{dyn} by 45–50%. The i.v. injection of glibenclamide (20 mg/kg) 15 min prior to injection of BRL 38227 did not itself alter parameters of lung function, but markedly reduced the protective effect of BRL 38227 against the histamine-induced bronchoconstriction. This is consistent with the ability of glibenclamide to antagonize the actions of cromakalim and its enantiomer on airways smooth muscle *in vitro*.

Paciorek *et al.* (1990) anaesthetized guinea-pigs using urethane. The animals were then pithed, vagotomized and ventilated mechanically. Lung resistance changes were measured by a modification of the Konzett and Rossler (1940) technique. In these experiments Ro 31-6930 or cromakalim were injected intravenously, in a cumulative fashion, 10 min prior to bronchoconstrictor challenge with 5-hydroxytryptamine (5-HT) (1.5–8.0 μg/kg, i.v.) or histamine (1–4 μg/kg, i.v.). Dose-dependent attenuation of bronchoconstrictor responses was provided both by Ro 31–6930 (1–100 μg/kg) and cromakalim (10–1000 μg/kg). Since the animals had been pithed they exhibited a low resting diastolic blood pressure (13.8 $\pm$ 0.8 mmHg) and this was little affected by the administration of the K-channel openers.

In anaesthetized guinea-pigs which were not pithed, K-channel openers such as cromakalim inhibited bronchoconstriction induced by the i.v. injection of 5-HT (Fig. 15.13). However, the doses of the K-channel openers required for this effect also reduced diastolic blood pressure by 20–40% (Arch *et al.*, 1988; De Souza *et al.*, 1989). The blood pressure changes seen with bronchodilator doses of the openers reflect the actions of these drugs on vascular smooth muscle and, in anaesthetized animals, are probably accentuated by the suppression of baroreceptor reflexes.

The active enantiomer of cromakalim (BRL 38227), administered by

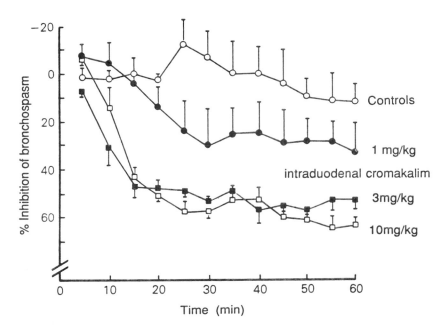

Fig. 15.13. The effects of intraduodenal administration of cromakalim on 5HT-induced bronchospasm in anaesthetized guinea-pigs. Cromakalim was given at 0.5 min at dose levels of 1 ($\bullet$, $n = 4$), 3 ($\blacksquare$, $n = 4$) or 10 ($\square$, $n = 6$) mg/kg. Controls (○, $n = 40$) were given the vehicle. The points are arithmetic means with vertical lines showing SEM. The effect of the 10 mg/kg dose was significant ($P < 0.05$) at the 10 min time point. The effects of both the 3 and 10 mg/kg dose levels were significant at the $P < 0.001$ level from 15 to 60 min. (Adapted from Arch *et al.* (1988) with permission.)

inhalation, protects against histamine-induced bronchoconstriction in anaesthetized guinea-pigs without causing significant change in blood pressure (Bowring *et al.*, 1989). This suggests that administration of K-channel openers by inhalation can minimize the likelihood of their lowering blood pressure. In any event, Arch *et al.* (1988) have argued that, since cromakalim has little hypotensive activity in normotensive human subjects, changes in blood pressure should not prevent the use of the substances such as bronchodilator agents in the treatment of asthma. This argument seems to be borne out by the limited amount of clinical data currently available (*see below*).

Effects of KCOs in animal models of airways hyperreactivity

Guinea-pigs subjected to an i.v. infusion of PAF (600 ng/kg per h) developed airways hyperreactivity. The i.v. infusion of sodium cromoglycate, dexamethasone, aminophylline, ketotifen or AH 21-132 prevented the development of PAF-induced hyperreactivity in a dose-dependent manner. The i.v. infusion of cromakalim (1 mg/kg per h) also inhibited the development of PAF-induced airways hyperreactivity (Sanjar *et al.*, 1989).

The ability of cromakalim to inhibit the development of airways hyper-reactivity is shared by SDZ PCO 400. The latter agent has been reported to suppress the development of airways hyperreactivity induced by the i.v. infusion of immune complexes, PAF or isoprenaline. In this respect PCO 400 was most potent against the hyperreactivity induced by immune complexes and least potent against that induced by isoprenaline. PCO 400 was also observed to reduce airways hyperreactivity already established in guinea-pigs following allergic reactions (Chapman, 1990). Interestingly, the effects of SDZ PCO 400 against airways hyperreactivity were seen at doses that did not induce overt relaxation of airways smooth muscle (Chapman, 1990). It could therefore be that, when K-channel openers are used in the treatment of bronchial asthma, suppression of airways hyper-reactivity will prove to be a more important feature of their activity than direct relaxation of airways smooth muscle (*see below*).

Studies of the bronchodilator activity of KCOs in the human

Tested in healthy volunteers, cromakalim administered as a single oral dose (2 mg) significantly increased the concentration of histamine causing a 40% fall in the partial expiratory flow rate. This effect was apparent 5 h after dosing and was accompanied by minor reduction in diastolic blood pressure and minor increase in heart rate (Baird *et al.*, 1988).

Trials of KCOs in the treatment of nocturnal asthma

In a two-centre study of patients with nocturnal asthma, single oral doses of cromakalim or placebo were administered at 23:30 h according to a randomized, double-blind, cross-over design. Forced expiratory volume in 1 s (FEV_1) was measured before dosing and at 06:00 h the following morning. The results of the study suggested that cromakalim, in doses of 0.25 and 0.5 mg, reduced the morning fall in FEV_1 by approximately 50%. In contrast, an oral dose of 1.5 mg of cromakalim did not significantly reduce the morning dip in lung function (Williams *et al.*, 1989, 1990a; Fig. 15.14).

The potential of cromakalim in the treatment of nocturnal asthma has also been demonstrated in a repeat-dose study. This comprised a random-ized, double-blind, placebo-controlled trial in which 12 patients with bronchial asthma were studied for a 3-week period. For 5 consecutive nights in each week patients received oral doses of cromakalim (0.25 or 0.5 mg) or placebo at 23:30 h. On the sixth and seventh nights of each week, the patients received placebo. On the fifth night FEV_1 was measured at 23:30 h. Forced expiratory volume in 1 s was measured again at 06:00 h

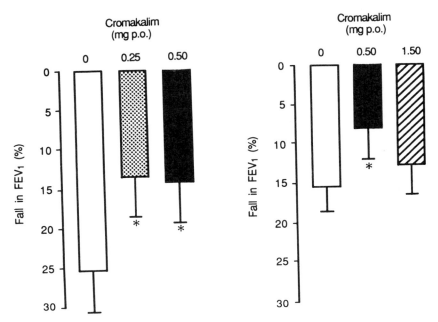

Fig. 15.14. Two-centre, single dose clinical trial of cromakalim in nocturnal asthma. Falls in FEV₁ from 23:00 to 06:00 h in patients with nocturnal asthma.

Left panel: percentage fall in FEV₁ after placebo or 0.25 mg cromakalim or 0.5 mg cromakalim (*n* = 7).

Right panel: percentage fall in FEV₁ after placebo or 0.5 mg cromakalim or 1.5 mg cromakalim (*n* = 16).

Empty columns = placebo; filled = 0.5 mg cromakalim; stippled = 0.25 mg cromakalim; hatched = 1.5 mg cromakalim. Bars describe SEM. * $P < 0.05$ compared with placebo. (Adapted from Williams *et al.* (1990a) with permission.)

the following morning. Compared with placebo, the percentage fall in FEV₁ (morning dip) was significantly reduced after dosing with either 0.25 or 0.5 mg cromakalim (Owen *et al.*, 1989; Williams *et al.*, 1990a).

In these trials of cromakalim against nocturnal asthma, oral doses of the drug up to 1.5 mg caused no significant changes in heart rate, systolic or diastolic blood pressure. However, the 1.5 mg oral dose caused headache in 10 of 23 subjects tested. Headache may have prevented these subjects from achieving their full value of FEV₁, and this possibility has been advanced to explain why the 1.5 mg dose of cromakalim failed to improve the morning dip in lung function (Williams *et al.*, 1990a).

A recent study (Williams *et al.*, 1990b) has shown that, in healthy volunteers, doses of up to 1 mg of cromakalim can be inhaled without causing significant changes in pulse rate, systolic or diastolic blood pressure. In the majority of the volunteers no headache was observed even following the inhalation of 1 mg of cromakalim. It remains to be seen whether the administration of cromakalim by the inhaled route will provide a beneficial effect in nocturnal asthma which is less limited by the occurrence of unwanted effects such as headache.

Site and mechanism of action of KCOs in nocturnal asthma

Gill *et al.* (1989) have measured the peak plasma concentrations of the active and inactive enantiomers of cromakalim following their oral administration in a dose of 1 mg to healthy adult males. The peak plasma concentration of the active enantiomer was reached 3.1 ± 1.5 h after drug administration and had a value of 6.8 ± 2.8 ng/ml ($0.024 \mu M$). In trials of cromakalim in patients suffering from nocturnal asthma (Williams *et al.*, 1990a) a single 0.25 mg oral dose of cromakalim administered on retiring attenuated the early morning dip in lung function. Presumably the peak plasma concentration of the active enantiomer of cromakalim achieved in these subjects was much less than $0.024 \mu M$.

In vitro studies with human bronchioles have shown that cromakalim can suppress spontaneous tone. The threshold concentration of cromakalim is $0.1 \mu M$ and the IC_{50} is $0.36 \mu M$ (Taylor *et al.*, 1988b). The peak plasma concentration of cromakalim achieved during effective treatment of nocturnal asthma is therefore at least 10 times less than that required to cause relaxation of human airways smooth muscle *in vitro*. How can this concentration difference be explained? It may be that cromakalim is concentrated in airways smooth muscle following its oral administration. It may be that airways smooth muscle exhibits reduced sensitivity to cromakalim once it is removed from the body. Alternatively, it could be proposed that the utility of cromakalim in nocturnal asthma does not result from its direct relaxant effects in bronchial smooth muscle. There is some experimental evidence that may support this latter proposal. As indicated above, Chapman (1990) has reported that, in laboratory animals, the cromakalim analogue SDZ PCO 400 can inhibit the development of airways hyperreactivity or reduce established hyperreactivity at doses that do not exert direct bronchodilator effects. It may therefore be that the most important effect of K-channel openers in alleviating nocturnal asthma involves the resolution of airways hyperreactivity and that this effect occurs at dose levels that do not directly relax airways smooth muscle.

Acknowledgements

The authors' work reported in this manuscript has been supported by the British Lung Foundation, the National Asthma Campaign, SmithKline Beecham Pharmaceuticals, Rhone Poulenc plc, Sandoz AG and the Wellcome Trust. The assistance of all colleagues who have contributed to our work is gratefully acknowledged.

References

Ahmed, F., Foster, R. W. & Small, R. C. (1985) Some effects of nifedipine in guinea-pig isolated trachealis. *British Journal of Pharmacology* **84**, 861–869.

Allen, S. L., Boyle, J. P., Cortijo, J., Foster, R. W., Morgan, G. P. & Small, R. C. (1986a) Electrical and mechanical effects of BRL 34915 in guinea-pig isolated trachealis. *British Journal of Pharmacology* **89**, 395–405.

Allen, S. L., Cortijo, J., Foster, R. W., Morgan, G. P., Small, R. C. & Weston, A. H. (1986b) Mechanical and electrical aspects of the relaxant action of aminophylline in guinea-pig isolated trachealis. *British Journal of Pharmacology* **88**, 473–483.

Arch, J. R. S., Buckle, D. R., Bumstead, J., Clarke, G. D., Taylor, J. F. & Taylor, S. G. (1988) Evaluation of the potassium channel activator cromakalim (BRL 34915) as a bronchodilator in the guinea-pig: comparison with nifedipine. *British Journal of Pharmacology* **95**, 763–770.

Baird, A., Hamilton, T., Richards, D., Tasker, T. & Williams, A. J. (1988) Cromakalim, a potassium channel activator inhibits histamine-induced bronchoconstriction in healthy volunteers. *British Journal of Clinical Pharmacology* **25**, 114P.

Barnes, P. J., Armour, C. L., Alouhan, L., Johnson, P. & Black, J. L. (1990) Potassium channel activation in human airway smooth muscle *in vitro*. *Thorax* **45**, 308–309.

Berry, J. L., Elliott, K. R. F., Foster, R. W., Green, K. A., Murray, M. A. & Small, R. C. (1991) Mechanical, biochemical and electrophysiological studies of RP 49356 and cromakalim in guinea-pig and bovine trachealis muscle. *Pulmonary Pharmacology* **4**, 91–98.

Bowring, N. E. (1990) Temporal differences in the effect of glibenclamide on pulmonary and cardiovascular responses to the K^+-channel activator lemakalim (BRL 38227) *British Journal of Pharmacology* **100**, 476P.

Bowring, N. E., Taylor, J. F., Francis, G. F. & Arch, J. R. S. (1989) Evaluation of inhaled cromakalim and its active enantiomer BRL 38277 as bronchodilators in the guinea-pig. *British Journal of Pharmacology* **98**, 805P.

Bray, K. M., Newgreen, D. T., Small, R. C., Southerton, J. S., Taylor, S. G., Weir, S. W. & Weston, A. H. (1987) Evidence that the mechanism of the inhibitory action of pinacidil in rat and guinea-pig smooth muscle differs from that of glyceryl trinitrate. *British Journal of Pharmacology* **91**, 421–429.

Brown, T. J., Sweetland, J. & Raeburn, D. (1989) Comparison of the effects of RP 49356, BRL 34915 and nifedipine on guinea-pig trachea *in vitro*. *Pflügers Archiv* **414** (Suppl. 1), 5188–5189.

Buckle, D. R., Bumstead, J., Clarke, G. D., Taylor, J. F. & Taylor, S. G. (1987) Reversal of agonist-induced bronchoconstriction in the guinea-pig by the potassium channel activator BRL 34915. *British Journal of Pharmacology* **92**, 744P.

Chapman, I. D. (1990) PCO 400. Abstract 4 in Proceedings of *New Drugs for Asthma*, Official Satellite Symposium, Davos, Switzerland, of XIth International Congress of Pharmacology.

Chopra, L. C., Twort, C. H. C. & Ward, J. P. T. (1990) Effects of BRL 38227 on calcium uptake by intracellular stores in cultured rabbit airway smooth muscle cells. *British Journal of Pharmacology* **100**, 368P.

Coldwell, M. C. & Howlett, D. R. (1987) Specificity of action of the novel antihypertensive agent, BRL 34915, as a potassium channel activator. Comparison with nicorandil. *Biochemical Pharmacology* **36**, 3663–3669.

Collier, M. L., Twort, C. H. C., Cameron, I. R. & Ward, J. P. T. (1990) BRL 38227 and ATP-dependent potassium channels in airway smooth muscle cells. Abstract P4 in Proceedings of *New Drugs for Asthma*, Official Satellite Symposium, Davos, Switzerland, of the XIth International Congress of Pharmacology.

Cook, N. S. (1988) The pharmacology of potassium channels and their therapeutic potential. *Trends in Pharmacological Sciences* **9**, 21—28.

Cook, N. S. & Hof, R. P. (1988) Cardiovascular effects of apamin and BRL 34915 in rats and rabbits. *British Journal of Pharmacology* **93**, 121–131.

Cook, N. S. & Quast, U. (1990) Potassium channel pharmacology. In Cook, N. S. (ed.), *Potassium Channels: Structure, Classification, Function and Therapeutic Potential.* Ellis Horwood Ltd, Chichester, pp. 181–231.

Cortijo, J., Dixon, J. S., Foster, R. W. & Small, R. C. (1987) Influence of some variables in the Triton X-100 method of skinning the plasmalemmal membrane from guinea-pig trachealis muscle, *Journal of Pharmacological Methods* **18**, 253–266.

Cortijo, J., Foster, R. W., Small, R. C. & Morcillo, E. J. (1990) Calcium antagonist properties of cinnarizine, trifluoperazine and verapamil in guinea-pig normal and skinned trachealis muscle. *Journal of Pharmacy and Pharmacology* **42**, 405–411.

De Souza, R. N., Gater, P. R. & Alabaster, V. A. (1989) Bronchodilators and tracheal relaxant effects of potassium channel openers in the guinea-pig. *British Journal of Pharmacology* **98**, 803P.

Farmer, J. B., Farrar, D. G. & Wilson, J. (1974) Antagonism of tone and prostaglan-din-mediated responses in a tracheal preparation by indomethacin and SC-19220. *British Journal of Pharmacology* **52**, 559–565.

Foster, C. D., Fujii, K. & Brading, A. F. (1988) The effects of potassium channel antagonists and cromakalim on membrane activity and K fluxes in smooth muscle from the guinea-pig urinary bladder. *Journal of Muscle Research and Cell Motility* **9**, 458–459.

Foster, K. A. (1989) Cromakalim activation of potassium channels in guinea-pig trachea: effects of extracellular rubidium. *British Journal of Pharmacology* **96**, 233P.

Foster, R. W., Okpalugo, B. I. & Small, R. C. (1984) Antagonism of Ca^{2+} and other actions of verapamil in guinea-pig isolated trachealis. *British Journal of Pharmacology* **81**, 499–507.

Foster, R. W., Small, R. C. & Weston, A. H. (1983) Evidence that the spasmogenic action of tetraethylammonium in guinea-pig trachealis is both direct and dependent on the cellular influx of calcium ion. *British Journal of Pharmacology* **79**, 255–263.

Gater, P. R. (1989) Effects of K^+-channel openers on bovine tracheal smooth muscle. *British Journal of Pharmacology* **98**, 660P.

Gelband, C. H., Lodge, N. J. & Van Breemen, C. (1989) A Ca^{2+}-activated K^+-channel from rabbit aorta: modulation by cromakalim. *European Journal of Pharmacology* **167**, 201–210.

Gill, T. S., Karran, M. A., Davies, B. E., Allen, G. D. & Tasker, T. C. G. (1989) Lack of an effect of atenolol on the stereochemical pharmacokinetics of cromakalim in healthy male subjects. *British Journal of Clinical Pharmacology* **27**, 112P.

Gillespie, J. S. & Sheng, H. (1988) The lack of involvement of cyclic nucleotides in the smooth muscle relaxant action of BRL 34915. *British Journal of Pharmacology* **94**, 1189–1197.

Green, K. A., Foster, R. W. & Small, R. C. (1991) A patch-clamp study of K^+-channel activity in bovine isolated tracheal smooth muscle cells. *British Journal of Pharmacology* **102**, 871–878.

Hall, A. K. & MacLagan, J. (1988) Effect of cromakalim on cholinergic neurotransmission in the guinea-pig trachea. *British Journal of Pharmacology* **95**, 792P.

Hisada, T., Kurachi, Y. & Sugimoto, T. (1990) Properties of membrane currents in isolated smooth muscle cells from guinea-pig trachea. *Pflügers Archiv* **416**, 151–161.

Ho, P. P. K., Towner, R. D., Esterman, M. & Bertsch, B. (1990) Pinacidil, N'-cyano-N-4-pyridinyl-N'-(1,2,2-trimethylpropyl) guanidine, is a potent bronchodilator. *European Journal of Pharmacology* **183**, 2132–2133.

Hu, S., Kim, H. S., Okolie, P. & Weiss, G. B. (1990) Alterations by glyburide of effects of BRL 34915 and P 1060 on contraction, ^{86}Rb and the maxi-K$^+$-channel in rat portal vein. *Journal of Pharmacology and Experimental Therapeutics* **253**, 771–777.

Huang, H. M., Dwyer, T. M. & Farley, J. M. (1987) Patch clamp recording of single Ca^{2+}-activated K$^+$-channels in tracheal smooth muscle from swine. *Biophysical Journal* **51**, 50a.

Ichinose, M. & Barnes, P. J. (1990) A potassium channel activator modulates both excitatory noncholinergic and cholinergic neurotransmission in guinea-pig airways. *Journal of Pharmacology and Experimental Therapeutics* **252**, 1207–1212.

Jones, T. R. & Charette, L. (1990) Inhibition of relaxation of guinea-pig trachea by the K$^+$-channel antagonist, charybdotoxin (CHTX). *European Journal of Pharmacology* **183**, 2131–2132.

Jones, T. R., Charette, L., Garcia, M. L. & Kaczorowski, G. J. (1990) Selective inhibition of relaxation of guinea-pig trachea by charybdotoxin, a potent Ca^{2+}-activated K$^+$-channel inhibitor. *Journal of Pharmacology and Experimental Therapeutics* **255**, 697–706.

Kakuta, Y., Okayama, H., Aikawa, T., Kanno, T., Ohyama, T., Sasaki, H., Kato, T. & Takishma, T. (1988) K$^+$-channels of human alveolar macrophages. *Journal of Allergy and Clinical Immunology* **81**, 410–468.

Karlsson, J. A. & Persson, C. G. A. (1981) Influence of tracheal contraction on relaxant effects *in vitro* of theophylline and isoprenaline. *British Journal of Pharmacology* **74**, 73–79.

Kauffman, R. F., Schenk, K. W., Conery, B. G. & Gohen, M. L. (1986) Effects of pinacidil on serotonin-induced contractions and cyclic nucleotide levels in isolated rat aortae: comparison with nitroglycerin, minoxidil and hydralazine. *Journal of Cardiovascular Pharmacology* **8**, 1195–1200.

Konzett, H. & Rossler, R. (1940) Versuchsanordnung zur üntersuchungen an der Bronchialmuskulatur. *Naunyn-Schmeideberg's Archiv für Pharmakologie und Experimentelle Pathologie* **195**, 71–74.

Kume, H., Takagi, K., Satake, T., Tokuno, H. & Tomita, T. (1990) Effects of intracellular pH on calcium-activated potassium channels in rabbit tracheal smooth muscle. *Journal of Physiology* **424**, 445–457.

Kume, H., Takai, A., Tokuno, H. & Tomita, T. (1989) Regulation of Ca^{2+}-dependent K$^+$-channel activity in tracheal myocytes by phosphorylation. *Nature* **341**, 152–154.

Lewis, P. E., Growcott, J. W. & Wilson, C. (1990) Potassium channel blockade: effects on cromakalim-induced relaxation of the guinea-pig tracheal chain. *British Journal of Pharmacology* **99**, 194P.

Lewis, S. A. & Raeburn, D. (1990) Preferential pre-junctional site of inhibition of non-cholinergic bronchospasm by potassium channel openers (KCOs) *British Journal of Pharmacology* **100**, 474P.

Longman, S. D. (1989) Potassium channel activation in smooth muscle cells may be associated with decreases in intracellular ATP. *British Journal of Pharmacology* **98**, 888P.

Longmore, J. & Weston, A. H. (1989) Effects of cromakalim and glibenclamide on isolated strips of bovine tracheal smooth muscle. *British Journal of Pharmacology* **98**, 804P.

Longmore, J., Weston, A. H. & Tresize, D. (1990) The effects of cromakalim and diazoxide on potassium and rubidium permeability in bovine tracheal smooth muscle. *European Journal of Pharmacology* **183**, 675.

McCaig, D. J. & De Jonckheere, B. (1989a) Effect of cromakalim on bronchoconstriction induced by stimulation of the vagus nerve in isolated guinea-pig trachea. *British Journal of Pharmacology* **96**, 252P.

McCaig, D. J. & De Jonckheere, B. (1989b) Effect of cromakalim on bronchoconstriction evoked by cholinergic nerve stimulation in guinea-pig isolated trachea. *British Journal of Pharmacology* **98**, 662–668.

McCann, J. D. & Welsh, M. J. (1986) Calcium-activated K^+-channels in canine airway smooth muscle. *Journal of Physiology* **372**, 113–127.

McPherson, G. A. & Angus, J. A. (1989) Phentolamine and structurally-related compounds selectively antagonise the vascular actions of the K^+-channel opener, cromakalim. *British Journal of Pharmacology* **97**, 941–949.

McPherson, G. A. & Angus, J. A. (1990) Characterization of responses to cromakalim and pinacidil in smooth and cardiac muscle by use of selective antagonists. *British Journal of Pharmacology* **100**, 201–206.

Murray, M. A., Berry, J. L., Cook, S. J., Foster, R. W., Green, K. A. & Small, R. C. (1991) Guinea-pig isolated trachealis: the effects of charybdotoxin on mechanical activity, membrane potential changes and the activity of plasmalemmal K^+-channels. *British Journal of Pharmacology* **103**, 1814–1818.

Murray, M. A., Boyle, J. P. & Small, R. C. (1989) Cromakalim-induced relaxation of guinea-pig isolated trachealis: antagonism by glibenclamide and by phentolamine. *British Journal of Pharmacology* **98**, 865–874.

Murray, M. A., Foster, R. W. & Small, R. C. (1990) Effects of the K^+-channel openers cromakalim and RP 49356 on the cyclic nucleotide content of guinea-pig isolated trachealis. *British Journal of Pharmacology* **100**, 367P.

Newgreen, D. T., Longmore, J. & Weston, A. H. (1989) The effect of glibenclamide on the action of cromakalim, diazoxide and minoxidil sulphate on rat aorta. *British Journal of Pharmacology* **96**, 116P.

Nielsen-Kudsk, J. E., Bang, L. & Bronsgaard, A. M. (1990) Glibenclamide blocks the relaxant action of pinacidil and cromakalim in airway smooth muscle. *European Journal of Pharmacology* **180**, 291–296.

Nielsen-Kudsk, J. E., Mellemkjaer, S., Siggaard, C. & Nielsen, C. B. (1988) Effects of pinacidil on guinea-pig airway smooth muscle contracted by asthma mediators. *European Journal of Pharmacology* **157**, 221–226.

Owen, S., Church, S., Stone, P., Bosch, B., Webster, S., Lavender, E., Williams, A. & Woodcock, A. (1989) Randomised, double blind, placebo controlled, crossover (RDBPCC) study of a potassium channel activator (KCA) in morning dipping. *Thorax* **44**, 852.

Paciorek, P. M., Cowlrick, I. S., Perkins, R. S. & Taylor, J. C. (1989) Actions of Ro 31-6930, a novel potassium channel opener, on guinea-pig tracheal smooth muscle preparations. *British Journal of Pharmacology* **98**, 720P.

Paciorek, P. M., Cowlrick, I. S., Perkins, R. S., Taylor, J. C., Wilkinson, G. F. & Waterfall, J. F. (1990) Evaluation of the bronchodilator properties of Ro 31-6930, a novel potassium channel opener, in the guinea-pig. *British Journal of Pharmacology* **100**, 289–294.

Plant, T. D. & Henquin, J. C. (1990) Phentolamine and yohimbine inhibit ATP-sensitive K^+-channels in mouse pancreatic β-cells. *British Journal of Pharmacology* **101**, 115–120.

Raeburn, D. M. & Brown, T. J. (1991) RP 49356 and cromakalim relax airway smooth muscle *in vitro* by opening a sulphonylurea-sensitive K^+-channel: a comparison with nifedipine. *Journal of Pharmacology and Experimental Therapeutics* **256**, 492–499.

Sanjar, S., Morley, J., Chapman, I. & Kings, M. (1989) K^+-channel activation in tests for prophylactic anti-asthma drug efficacy in the guinea-pig. *American Reviews of Respiratory Disease* **139**, A467.

Schmid-Antomarchi, H., De Weille, J., Fosset, M. & Lazdunski, M. (1987) The receptor for antidiabetic sulphonylureas controls the activity of the ATP-modulated

K^+-channel in insulin-secreting cells. *Journal of Biological Chemistry* **262,** 15 840–15 844.

Small, R. C. & Foster, R. W. (1986) Airways smooth muscle: an overview of morphology, electrophysiology and aspects of the pharmacology of contraction and relaxation. In Kay, A. B. (ed.), *Asthma: Clinical Pharmacology and Therapeutic Progress.* Blackwell Scientific Publications, London, pp. 101–113.

Small, R. C., Berry, J. L., Foster, R. W., Blarer, S. & Quast, U. (1992) Analysis of the relaxant action of SDZ PCO 400 in airway smooth muscle from the ox and guinea-pig. *European Journal of Pharmacology* (in press).

Small, R. C., Boyle, J. P., Duty, S., Elliott, K. R. F., Foster, R. W. & Watt, A. J. (1989) Analysis of the relaxant effects of AH 21-132 in guinea-pig isolated trachealis. *British Journal of Pharmacology* **97,** 1165–1173.

Small, R. C., Boyle, J. P., Foster, R. W. & Good, D. M. (1990) Airways smooth muscle: electrophysiological properties and behaviour. In Agrawal, D. K. & Townley, R. G. (eds), *Airways Smooth Muscle: Modulation of Receptors and Response.* CRC Press, Boca Raton, FL, pp. 69–94.

Small, R. C., Foster, R. W. & Boyle, J. P. (1988) K^+-channel opening as a mechanism for relaxing airways smooth muscle. In O'Donnell, S. R. & Persson, C. G. A. (eds) *Directions for New Anti-Asthma Drugs. Agents and Actions* Supplements, vol. 23. Birkhauser-Verlag, Basel, pp. 89–94.

Spilker, B. & Minatoya, H. (1975) The role of broncho-constrictors in evaluating smooth muscle relaxant activity. *Archives Internationales de Pharmacodynamie* **27,** 201–217.

Standen, N. B., Quayle, J. M., Davies, N. W., Brayden, J. E., Huang, Y. & Nelson, M. T. (1989) Hyperpolarizing vasodilators activate ATP-sensitive K^+-channels in arterial smooth muscle. *Science* **245,** 177–180.

Sturgess, N. C., Kozlowski, R. Z., Carrington, C. A., Hales, C. N. & Ashford, M. L. J. (1988) Effects of sulphonylureas and diazoxide on insulin secretion and nucleotide-sensitive channels in an insulin-secreting cell line. *British Journal of Pharmacology* **95,** 83–94.

Taylor, S. G., Bumstead, J., Morris, J. E. J., Shaw, D. J. & Taylor, J. F. (1988a) Cromakalim inhibits cholinergic-mediated responses in human isolated bronchioles but not in guinea-pig airways. *British Journal of Pharmacology* **95,** 795P.

Taylor, S. G., Shaw, D. J. & Taylor, J. F. (1988b) A comparison of the effects of cromakalim (BRL 34915) and verapamil on human and guinea-pig airways. *Journal of Muscle Research and Cell Motility* **9,** 457–458.

Taylor, S. G., Southerton, J. S., Weston, A. H. & Baker, J. R. J. (1988c) Endothelium-dependent effects of acetylcholine in rat aorta: a comparison with sodium nitroprusside and cromakalim. *British Journal of Pharmacology* **94,** 853–863.

Watson, S. & Abbott, A. (1990) TIPS receptor nomenclature. *Trends in Pharmacological Sciences,* **11** (Suppl.)

Weir, S. W. & Weston, A. H. (1986) Effect of apamin on responses to BRL 34915, nicorandil and other relaxants in the guinea-pig taenia caeci. *British Journal of Pharmacology* **88,** 113–120.

Williams, A. J., Hopkirk, A., Lavender, E., Vyse, T., Chiew, V. F. & Lee, T. H. (1989) Inhibition of nocturnal asthma by relaxation of airway smooth muscle with a potassium channel activator. *American Reviews of Respiratory Disease* **139** (Suppl.), A140.

Williams, A. J., Lee, T. H., Cochrane, G. M., Hopkirk, A., Vyse, T., Chiew, F., Lavender, E., Richards, D. H., Owen, S., Stone, P., Church, S. & Woodcock, A. A. (1990a) Attenuation of nocturnal asthma by cromakalim. *Lancet* **336,** 334–336.

Williams, A. J., Verden, P. & Lavender, E. (1990b) Inhalation of a potassium channel activator, cromakalim, is well tolerated in healthy volunteers. *European Journal of Pharmacology* **183,** 1045–1046.

Yamanaka, K., Furukawa, K. & Kitamura, K. (1985) The different mechanisms of action of nicorandil and adenosine triphosphate on potassium channels of circular smooth muscle of the guinea-pig small intestine. *Naunyn-Schmiedeberg's Archives of Pharmacology* **331,** 96–103.

Chapter 16
Potassium channel modulators: urogenital pharmacology

P-O. Andersson and M. G. Wyllie

Introduction

The interest in the action of K-channel openers on urogenital smooth muscle started soon after the mechanism of action of cromakalim had been elucidated (Hamilton *et al.*, 1986; Weir & Weston, 1986). The results from studies of the effects of K-channel openers in urogenital smooth muscle have been briefly summarized in a number of recent reviews on the action of K-channel openers in smooth muscle (e.g. Cook, 1988; Weston, 1989; Robertson & Steinberg, 1989, 1990; Cook & Quast, 1990; Duty & Weston, 1990; Friedel & Brogden, 1990). This chapter aims to provide a comprehensive review of the actions of K-channel openers on urogenital smooth muscle and their therapeutic potential.

The main focus of the studies in the urogenital system of these agents has been on their potential in the treatment of bladder dysfunction. Therefore, this review will mainly deal with the effects of K-channel openers on the urinary bladder. To a lesser extent, interest has also been shown for the potential of these agents as treatment of preterm labour, impotence and ureteric spasm and this will also be reviewed together with studies performed in other urogenital tissues.

The urinary bladder

The function of the urinary bladder is to store and, at appropriate times, empty its content of urine. The filling and expulsion phases of this process are regulated by activities in afferent and efferent pathways (Torrens & Morrison, 1987).

In most animal species, bladder contraction is mediated by both cholinergic and non-adrenergic, non-cholinergic excitatory mechanisms ($NANC_e$) whereas in humans it is widely accepted that normal bladder contraction is mediated almost exclusively by an activation of muscarinic receptors, i.e. via cholinergic pathways (Brading, 1987).

In the urinary bladder, resting tone, as well as spontaneous and agonist-induced contractions, has been shown to be dependent on extracellular calcium (Andersson & Forman, 1986). Although release of Ca^{2+} from intracellular stores might also be involved in agonist-induced contraction (Mostwin, 1985; Fovaeus et al., 1987), the predominant source of Ca^{2+} is extracellular and enters the cell through voltage-operated Ca-channels (Fovaeus et al., 1987).

Urinary incontinence

Urinary incontinence, urgency and frequency of urination are common problems especially in older age. These conditions may arise from involuntary contractions of the detrusor smooth muscle. One can distinguish between different types of overactive detrusor function, which may be important in the diagnoses and treatment of these conditions. The two main forms are detrusor instability and detrusor hyperreflexia (International Continence Society Committee on Standardisation of Terminology, 1988). Detrusor instability is when the detrusor contracts spontaneously, or on provocation (e.g. in clinical urodynamic evaluation), during the filling of the bladder when the patient is trying to inhibit micturition. This type of bladder dysfunction is often found in patients with partial outflow obstruction (e.g. due to benign prostatic hyperplasia) and secondary bladder hypertrophy, but is also seen in patients with no underlying pathology (idiopathic form).

Detrusor hyperreflexia is defined as detrusor overactivity due to an obvious perturbation of the nervous control mechanism, particularly in patients with spinal lesions, diabetes and multiple sclerosis.

There is no concrete evidence to indicate that the neurogenic control of bladder smooth muscle in patients with detrusor overactivity is different from normal individuals. Intriguingly, some degree of atropine resistance (20–50%), representing a considerable increase in apparent $NANC_e$ control over normals, has been found in bladder strips from patients with bladder hypertrophy secondary to outflow obstruction (Sjögren et al., 1982; Sibley, 1984a). However, as these contractions were also resistant to tetrodotoxin, Sibley (1984a) suggested that the morphological changes in these bladders led to a non-specific increase in membrane excitability.

The ideal drug for the treatment of detrusor overactivity should abolish the involuntary contractions but not affect the normal emptying of the bladder. At present no such drug is available and the results of treatment with the currently-used drugs, mainly antimuscarinics and smooth muscle relaxants, are often unsatisfactory (Wein, 1987; Andersson, 1988; Andersson & Mattiasson, 1988) due to incomplete efficacy or untoward anticholinergic side effects (e.g. dry mouth, constipation, blurred vision and tachycardia).

Effects of K-channel openers on isolated detrusor muscle

Spontaneous activity

Cromakalim and pinacidil have been shown to dose-dependently inhibit spontaneous activity and basal tone in detrusor strips from guinea-pig, rat, pig and humans (Fig. 16.1; Andersson *et al.*, 1988; Restorick & Nurse, 1988; Foster *et al.*, 1989a,b; Fovaeus *et al.*, 1989; Malmgren *et al.*, 1990;

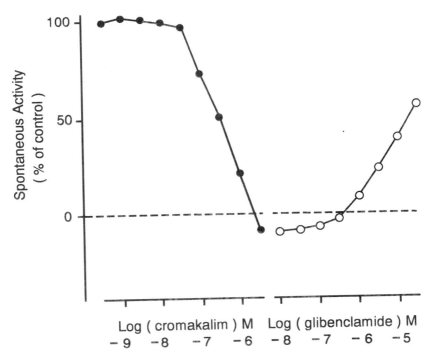

Fig. 16.1. Relaxant effect of cromakalim (●) on the spontaneous activity in rat urinary bladder *in vitro* and its reversal by glibenclamide (○).

Nurse *et al.*, 1991). The threshold for this effect is approximately 0.1 μM for both drugs.

Potassium-induced contractions

Characteristically, agents which relax smooth muscle via opening of K-channels block contractions induced by low ($\leqslant 40$ mM) but have virtually no effect on high ($\geqslant 80$ mM) concentrations of K^+ (Hamilton *et al.*, 1986). Cromakalim and pinacidil abolish contractions induced by 20 mM K^+ in the rat and human detrusor (Fovaeus *et al.*, 1989; Malmgren *et al.*, 1990) and markedly depress 25 mM-induced contractions in the guinea-pig, and pig (Foster *et al.*, 1989a,b). At high concentrations ($\geqslant 10$ μM) these agents also reduced contraction by 90–125 mM K^+ but only by 20–25%, indicating that their predominant effect at low concentrations is on K-channels, but that there may be some additional relaxant mechanism(s) at high concentrations.

Agonist-induced contractions

The effect of a range of concentrations of pinacidil on carbachol-induced contractions has been investigated in the human urinary bladder *in vitro* (Fovaeus *et al.*, 1989). This study showed that pinacidil produced a right-ward shift of the concentration–response curve and, at concentrations greater than 3 μM, a depression of the maximum. In rat, pig and human strips, cromakalim (10 μM) induced a right-ward shift of the concentration–response curve with a slight reduction of the maximum. Pinacidil had a similar effect on rat bladder strips (Malmgren *et al.*, 1990). Conversely, in the guinea-pig, cromakalim, at this concentration, had no effect on carbachol-induced contractions (Foster *et al.*, 1989a). The reason for this difference cannot currently be rationalized.

The action of pinacidil and cromakalim on the detrusor has been further investigated using electrical field stimulation. Both drugs caused a concentration-dependent inhibition of a supramaximal field stimulation-induced contractions in the rat bladder (Malmgren *et al.*, 1990).

Potassium efflux

In order to determine if this decrease in spontaneous myogenic activity produced by cromakalim and pinacidil is associated with an opening of sarcolemmal K-channels, ion efflux studies have been performed using $^{42}K^+$ or $^{43}K^+$ or utilizing $^{86}Rb^+$ as markers for K^+. In the studies where $^{42}K^+$- or $^{43}K^+$-efflux has been measured, cromakalim and pinacidil induced a clear-cut increase in the efflux with a threshold of $\geqslant 10$ μM (Foster *et al.*, 1989a,b; Edwards & Weston 1989; Edwards *et al.*, 1991).

When $^{86}Rb^+$ has been used as a marker the results are more equivocal, with observations of only small increases in flow rates (Edwards *et al.*, 1900, 1991) or no detectable increase at all (Foster *et al.*, 1989a). Similar discrepancies between $^{42}K^+$- and $^{86}Rb^+$-efflux have been reported in other tissues (Quast & Baumlin, 1988; Videbæk *et al.*, 1988). A recent study using a dual-labelling technique showed that the measured increase in $^{42}K^+$ and $^{86}Rb^+$-efflux was qualitatively similar using a range of K-channel openers but that the increase in Rb-efflux was approximately half of that seen using $^{42}K^+$ (Edwards *et al.*, 1991; Fig. 16.2). Overall, therefore, the flux studies are entirely consistent with an action of both agents on detrusor K-channels.

Electrophysiological studies

The electrophysiological effects of cromakalim have been investigated in both guinea-pig and pig urinary bladder by Brading and coworkers (Foster *et al.*, 1989a,b; Fujii *et al.*, 1990). Using microelectrode techniques in the guinea-pig bladder, they found an average membrane potential of $-60.6 \pm 3.2\,mV$ and most cells showed spontaneous spike activity, generated either continuously or in periodic bursts. Cromakalim reduced spike frequency at $0.1\,\mu M$ and caused a membrane hyperpolarization with a threshold at $1\,\mu M$ and achieving $22\,mV$ at $10\,\mu M$, i.e. bringing the membrane potential close to the theoretically calculated K-equilibrium potential. The magnitude of this cromakalim-induced hyperpolarization is similar to that recorded in pancreatic β-cells (Dunne *et al.*, 1990) and in vascular smooth muscle (Weir & Weston, 1986; Hamilton *et al.*, 1986).

In rat bladder Creed and Malmgren (1992) showed that cromakalim-induced a much smaller change in membrane potential. Cromakalim at $10\,\mu M$ hyperpolarized the tissue from -50.5 to $-54.8\,mV$ (i.e. $< 5\,mV$). The reason for the discrepancy between these data and those obtained in the guinea-pig (Foster *et al.*, 1989a; Fujii *et al.*, 1990) is not known. It is pertinent to note that complete smooth muscle relaxation in response to K-channel openers is seen in some other tissues such as the uterus (Hollingsworth *et al.*, 1987; *vide infra*) and the mesotubarium (Lydrup, 1991; Lydrup & Hellstrand, 1991; *vide infra*) despite a hyperpolarization of only 5–7 mV. Further, it has recently been shown that in bovine tracheal smooth muscle contracted with $25\,mM\,K^+$, BRL 38227 ($5\,\mu M$) caused full relaxation with a membrane hyperpolarization of only about $7\,mV$ (Longmore *et al.*, 1991).

Double sucrose-gap studies in the guinea-pig bladder have also shown that cromakalim has only a small effect on the excitatory junction potential (EJP) indicating little if any effect of the drug on transmitter release (Foster *et al.*, 1989a), suggesting that the activity of K-channel openers in the bladder is on the smooth muscle alone.

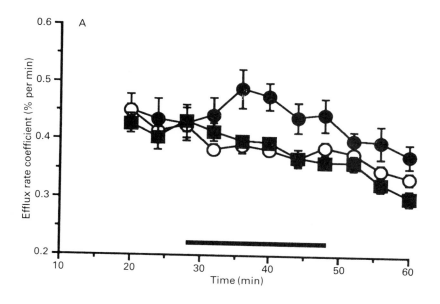

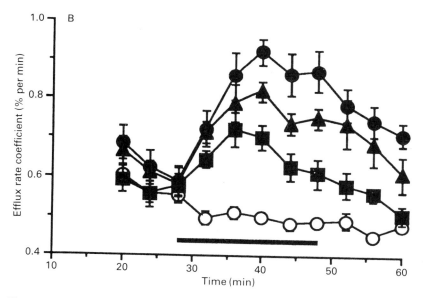

Fig. 16.2. Effect of BRL 38227 (5 μM; ●) on ^{86}Rb-efflux, A, and ^{42}K-efflux, B, using a dual-labelling technique, and the inhibition of the response by 1 μM (▲) or 3 μM (■) glibenclamide; (○) indicates vehicle control. The horizontal bar indicates the time of exposure to BRL 38227 or vehicle. Glibenclamide was present for 28 min before and during the exposure to BRL 38227. (From Edwards *et al.*, 1991, with permission.)

Investigations on strips from unstable bladders

In order to investigate the properties of overactive, hypertrophic bladder muscle, several animal models of bladder hypertrophy secondary to outflow obstruction have been developed. The two most commonly-used are those in the pig (Jørgensen *et al.*, 1983; Sibley, 1984b, 1985) and the rat (Mattiasson & Uvelius, 1982; Malmgren *et al.*, 1987). These models show many of the phenomena seen in patients with bladder dysfunction secondary to severe outflow obstruction, in particular bladder hypertrophy, detrusor instability, increased bladder capacity and residual urine.

Cromakalim and pinacidil abolish the spontaneous activity in strips from rat, pigs and humans with detrusor instability (Andersson *et al.*, 1988; Restorick & Nurse, 1988; Foster *et al.*, 1989b; Malmgren *et al.*, 1990).

In the only published functional comparative study in the rat, the effect of cromakalim and pinacidil on contractions induced by low K^+-concentrations as well as submaximal electrical field stimulation were more pronounced in hypertrophic than in normal bladder muscle (Fig. 16.3; Malmgren *et al.*, 1990).

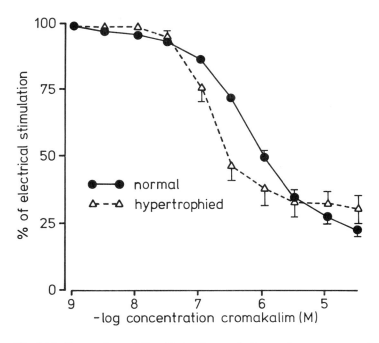

Fig. 16.3. Comparison of the effects of cromakalim on the response to electrical field stimulation of bladder strips from normal rats and from rats with bladder hypertrophy and detrusor instability secondary to outflow obstruction. Bladders from rats with detrusor instability were significantly more sensitive to cromakalim than those from normal rats. (From Malmgren *et al.*, 1990, with permission.)

In two studies, the effects of K-channel openers on K^+-efflux have been compared in strips from normal rats and from rats with unstable, hypertrophic, bladders secondary to outflow obstruction. In one study, measuring $^{43}K^+$-efflux in bladder from the mini-pig Forster *et al.* (1989b), strips from obstructed animals were more sensitive to cromakalim than strips from control animals. However, in a similar study in the rat, using $^{86}Rb^+$ as a marker, Malmgren *et al.* (1990) found no significant difference in the sensitivity to cromakalim or pinacidil between normal and hypertrophic tissue with regard to efflux. Whether this is due to differences in the permeability of the channels opened by these K-channel openers for K^+ and Rb^+ (*vide supra*; also Edwards *et al.*, 1991) in normal and hypertrophic bladder or due to species or experimental differences cannot be determined from current data.

In a study investigating the electrical properties of normal and hypertrophic rat bladder muscle, Creed and Malmgren (1992) demonstrated no difference in resting membrane potential, -47.2 ± 6.1 ($n = 29$) and -47.6 ± 6.0 mV ($n = 21$), respectively (mean $\pm$ S.D.) Further, there was no significant difference between the hyperpolarization induced by cromakalim (10 μM) in the two types of bladder muscle; in normal bladders cromakalim produced a mean change from -50.5 to -54.0 mV and in hypertrophic bladders from -45.0 to -51.8 mV.

Thus, at least in the rat bladder, the increased sensitivity of the hypertrophic, unstable, detrusor muscle does not seem to be caused by a different resting membrane potential in hypertrophied bladder muscle or a more pronounced hyperpolarization by cromakalim. It is of course possible that the hypertrophic bladder smooth muscle is more sensitive to low concentrations of cromakalim but, due to the magnitude of hyperpolarization, this is difficult to quantify.

Since opening of K-channels leads to a closure of voltage-operated Ca-channels thereby causing smooth muscle relaxation (Chiu *et al.*, 1988) another potential mechanism for the apparent increased sensitivity to K-channel openers in hypertrophic bladder muscle is indirect via changes in the properties of voltage-operated Ca-channels or in the sensitivity to intracellular Ca^{2+}. This has been invoked for bladder (Yamaguchi *et al.*, 1987) and vascular smooth muscle (Bruner & Webb, 1990).

Overall, therefore, it can be concluded that the mechanism underlying the increased sensitivity of hypertrophic smooth muscle to K-channel openers is unknown. Intriguingly, however, a similar observation of increased sensitivity for cromakalim has recently been reported in carotid arteries from stroke-prone spontaneously hypertensive rats (Miyata *et al.*, 1990). There are other interesting pathophysiological changes in K-channel opener sensitivity, e.g. the increased sensitivity to cromakalim and SDZ PCO 400 in airways hyperreactivity in the guinea-pig (Chapman *et al.*, 1991) and the decreased sensitivity for cromakalim in aortae from streptozotocin-diabetic rats (Katama *et al.*, 1989).

Whatever the cause, the increased sensitivity of the unstable, hypertrophic bladder to K-channel openers could have important implications for the potential of these agents in the treatment of detrusor instability.

Potassium-channel blockers

The effects of a range of K-channel blockers on the action of cromakalim have been investigated in the guinea-pig bladder with respect to mechanical response, K^+-efflux and membrane potential (Fujii *et al.*, 1990). Procaine abolished all effects of cromakalim, whereas quinidine and high concentrations of tetraethylammonium (TEA; 10 mM), and to some extent 4-aminopyridine had only partial effects. The sulphonylurea compounds, glibenclamide and tolbutamide, known to block adenosine triphosphate (ATP)-dependent K-channels (K_{ATP}) in the pancreas (Sturgess *et al.*, 1985; Trube, *et al.*, 1986; Schmid-Antomarchi *et al.*, 1987), reversed the relaxant effects of cromakalim on the bladder, as shown in Fig. 16.1, but effects on membrane potential and K^+-efflux have not been investigated.

It has recently been reported that glibenclamide reversed cromakalim- or pinacidil-induced $^{42}K^+$-efflux from rat bladder strips (Edwards *et al.*, 1991; Fig. 16.2), a finding similar to that previously reported in studies using vascular tissue (Newgreen *et al.*, 1990). In addition, glibenclamide competitively inhibited the relaxant effects of cromakalim and pinacidil on rat bladder strips precontracted with 20 mM K^+, with a pA_2 of 6.6–6.9, again similar to the observations in vascular smooth muscle (Corsi *et al.*, 1990; Edwards *et al.*, 1990, 1991).

Phentolamine and structurally-related analogues have been shown to block the hyperpolarization and relaxant effects of cromakalim in the rat femoral artery (McPherson & Angus, 1989). No data on the effect of these compounds, with respect to the bladder, have been published but, consistent with the vascular actions, results from our laboratory indicate that phentolamine antagonizes the cromakalim-induced relaxation in the rat bladder *in vitro*.

Intriguingly, the thermogenic agent ciclazindol (Rothwell *et al.*, 1981) has recently been shown to antagonize the actions on BRL 38227 on bladder as well as vascular smooth muscle both with regard to relaxation and to the stimulation of $^{42}K^+$-efflux (Morita *et al.*, 1992). The interaction with BRL 38227 in the bladder was non-competitive in nature thereby differing from the competitive antagonism seen with glibenclamide (Corsi *et al.*, 1990; Morita *et al.*, 1991). This observation, together with the inability of ciclazindol to displace ^3H-glibenclamide binding suggests that the sites of action of glibenclamide and ciclazindol are different (Noack *et al.*, 1992).

Comparison with effects in vascular smooth muscle

The limited *in vitro* studies on bladder smooth muscle, indicate that cromakalim and pinacidil in this tissue have all the characteristics of agents acting on plasmalemmal K^+-channels (as defined by phenomena observed in vascular smooth muscle). These agents produce membrane hyperpolarisation, an increase in K-conductance, inhibition of both spontaneous activity and contractions induced by low K^+-concentrations but only minor effects on the maximal contraction induced by agonist or high K^+-solution as well as glibenclamide sensitivity.

In two recent studies, the effect of a range of K-channel openers, cromakalim, its two enantiomers, BRL 38227 and BRL 38226, pinacidil, S 0121 and minoxidil sulphate, on the urinary bladder has been compared directly with those on vascular preparations *in vitro* (Corsi *et al.*, 1990; Edwards *et al.*, 1990, 1991). The data show that these agents generally are three to 10 times more potent on the rat portal vein than on the bladder. In fact, minoxidil sulphate was even more active on the rat portal vein (IC_{50} 1.0 μM) compared with the bladder (IC_{50} 23.5 μM).

Thus, the existing K-channel openers are vascular over bladder selective whereas, therapeutically, an agent with bladder over vascular selectivity is needed. As discussed previously, it should be emphasized that the unstable, hypertrophic, bladder smooth muscle is more sensitive to cromakalim and pinacidil than normal bladder muscle. This indicates that K-channel openers could be more potent in inhibiting unstable bladder contractions and thus less vascular-selective than indicated from the comparative *in vitro* studies cited above.

Effects of K-channel openers *in vivo*

Effects on normal bladder function

Malmgren and coworkers (1989) have investigated the effects of cromakalim and pinacidil on bladder function in conscious rats using an infusion of saline into the bladder during measurements of bladder pressure and micturated volume of urine, i.e. a situation mimicking clinical urodynamic evaluations (Torrens, 1987). This enabled not only the determination of bladder pressure, micturition pressure and bladder capacity, but also evaluation of residual volume and spontaneous bladder contraction. Figure 16.4 shows original recordings of the effects of cromakalim and pinacidil (1 mg/kg, p.o.) in normal rats. The K-channel openers had virtually no effect on bladder function in these experiments. A slight decrease in micturition pressure was seen but no effect on bladder capacity and no development of residual urine was observed. Even at 5 mg/kg, p.o. pinacidil has been shown to have no effect on bladder function in the conscious normal rat (Andersson *et al.*, 1988).

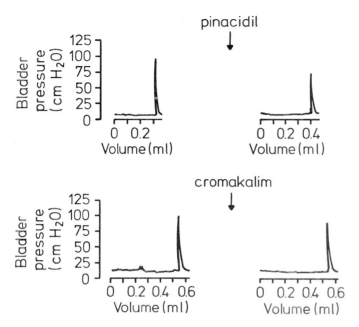

Fig. 16.4. Original recordings of cystometries performed in conscious normal rats. Pinacidil or cromakalim (1 mg/kg, p.o.) was given 1 h before the second cystometry. Note that the K-channel openers were virtually devoid of effect on normal bladder function in the normal rat. (From Malmgren *et al.*, 1989, with permission.)

The finding that cromakalim and pinacidil do not affect normal bladder function is potentially of great importance, since it indicates that effects on the bladder such as urinary retention are not likely to be a side-effect associated with the use of K-channel openers for other indications (e.g. in the treatment of hypertension or asthma).

Effects in animal models of detrusor instability

To test the therapeutic potential of K-channel openers in the treatment of bladder dysfunction, cromakalim and pinacidil have been tested in conscious rats and pigs with infravesical outflow obstruction (Malmgren *et al.*, 1989; Foster *et al.*, 1989b), models previously shown closely to resemble detrusor instability secondary to outflow obstruction in humans (Sibley, 1984b, 1985; Malmgren *et al.*, 1987).

In the obstructed mini-pig, Foster and coworkers (1989b) showed that cromakalim at 0.3 mg/kg, i.v. completely abolished the detrusor instability without inhibiting the animal's ability to void. However, this dose of cromakalim was reported to decrease blood pressure by 30 mmHg.

Malmgren and coworkers (1989) compared the effects of pinacidil and cromakalim on bladder function in both obstructed and normal rats. Both

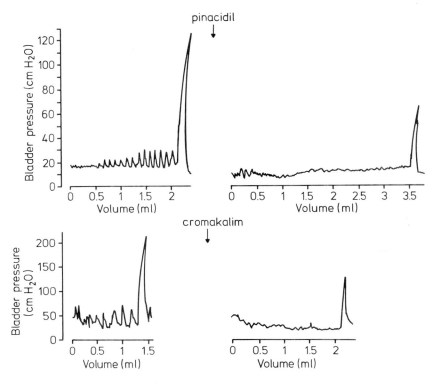

Fig. 16.5. Original recordings of cystometries performed in conscious rats with detrusor instability secondary to outflow obstruction. The detrusor instability is evident as the fluctuations in bladder pressure prior to micturition (*left panels*), not seen in normal animals (cf. Fig. 16.4). Pinacidil or cromakalim (1 mg/kg, p.o.) was given 1 h before the second cystometry. Note that the K-channel openers virtually abolished the detrusor instability. Pinacidil, and to a lesser extent cromakalim, also reduced micturition pressure. (From Malmgren *et al.*, 1989, with permission.)

agents (1 mg/kg, p.o.) inhibited the detrusor instability and lowered micturition pressure in rats with bladder hypertrophy, but did not change the bladder capacity or the animal's ability to void (Fig. 16.5). At this dose the effect of cromakalim on bladder instability would be associated with substantial changes in blood pressure and heart rate (*see* Chapter 12).

The cardiovascular effects of K-channel openers such as cromakalim can also be reversed by glibenclamide also *in vivo* (Buckingham *et al.*, 1989; Cavero *et al.*, 1989; Quast & Cook, 1989), but no such data are available on the effects of cromakalim on the bladder.

It seems clear from these studies that K-channel openers can abolish the detrusor instability in clinically-relevant animal models. With the agents presently available these effects are seen at doses which also affect the cardiovascular system. However, K-channel openers, selective for the urinary bladder, would offer a new therapeutic alternative in the treatment of bladder dysfunction.

Clinical experience with K-channel openers

Only two preliminary reports on the effects of K-channel openers in patients with detrusor overactivity have been published. In a single-blind study using cromakalim at 0.5–1 mg daily for 4 weeks, six of 17 patients (30%) reported an improvement in symptoms of urinary frequency (Restorick & Nurse, 1988; Nurse *et al.*, 1991). Four of these patients continued on treatment after the trial. Three of these had idiopathic detrusor instability and one neuropathic instability secondary to multiple sclerosis. The main side-effects were headache and skin rash. No data on cardiovascular parameters such as blood pressure and heart rate were offered.

The second study (Hedlund *et al.*, 1991) was a double-blind placebo controlled cross-over study with pinacidil (25 mg daily) in patients with detrusor instability secondary to outflow obstruction. In eight of 10 patients pinacidil was without effect on urodynamic variables whereas in two no detrusor instability could be detected at the end of the 2-week treatment period and they were also subjectively improved. However, in the overall assessment of the study no statistically significant beneficial effect of treatment could be shown. Blood pressure and heart rate were reported to be stable during the study and there were no drug-related side effects.

Based on the results from these pilot studies it cannot be concluded that an effect on detrusor instability can be achieved with cromakalim or pinacidil in the absence of obtrusive cardiovascular side-effects. The true therapeutic promise of K-channel openers in this condition awaits the discovery of bladder selective agents.

The uterus

The main indication for smooth muscle relaxants acting on the uterus is premature labour. Currently, β-adrenoceptor agonists e.g. salbutamol, are widely used for this indication. However, in addition to affecting the uterus, β-agonists also act on cardiac, vascular and skeletal muscle causing dose-limiting tachycardia, hypotension and tremor (Liggins & Vaughan, 1973; Lippert, 1983). Furthermore, in some women treated with β-agonists for preterm labour the relaxation of the uterus diminishes despite continued infusion, suggesting a tolerance to this type of agent with continued treatment (Liggins & Vaughan, 1973).

As in other smooth muscles, contractions in uterine smooth muscle are dependent on extracellular Ca^{2+} entering the cells through Ca-channels

(Edman & Schild, 1962) and Ca-antagonists have been shown to inhibit uterine contractions in humans (Forman *et al.*, 1981). At uterine-relaxing doses, Ca-channel blockers, such as nifedipine, produce less tachycardia but a greater vasodilatation than salbutamol (Abel & Hollingsworth, 1985) and may, therefore, offer a clinical alternative.

Obviously, present therapy for preterm labour is less than ideal and there is a medical need for an agent that selectively relaxes uterine smooth muscle.

Effects of K-channel openers on isolated uterine tissue

Diazoxide, a smooth muscle relaxant drug recently shown to act, at least partly by opening K-channels (Quast & Cook, 1989; Newgreen *et al.*, 1990) has long been known to relax uterine smooth muscle (Caritis *et al.*, 1979). The effects of pinacidil have been investigated on a variety of smooth muscle preparations (Cohen & Colbert, 1986). These workers showed that pinacidil (10–100 μM) inhibited oxytocin-induced contractions of the rat uterus but had little effect on the basal tone of the uterus.

The action of cromakalim on the uterus has been extensively investigated by Hollingsworth and co-workers. In the initial study (Hollingsworth *et al.*, 1987) cromakalim was found to relax spontaneous contractions (pIC_{50} 6.7 $\pm$ 0.2 M) in the isolated uterus from a full-term pregnant rat and also contractions induced by low (<20 mM) but not high concentrations (>40 mM) of KCl. Cromakalim was also active on oxytocin-induced contractions (Fig. 16.6). The functional effects were reversed by glibenclamide (Piper *et al.*, 1990). However, intracellular microelectrode

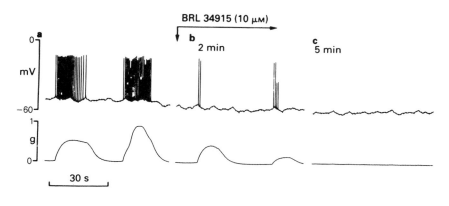

Fig. 16.6. Effects of cromakalim (BRL 34915). 10 μM, on the electrical (*upper trace*) and simultaneously recorded mechanical (*lower trace*) activity of the uterus of the term-pregnant rat. The tissue was stimulated with oxytocin (0.2 nM) throughout the experiment. Note that cromakalim totally abolished the mechanical activity suppressed spikes and caused a small hyperpolarization. (From Hollingsworth *et al.*, 1987, with permission.)

recordings showed that although cromakalim $(10\,\mu\text{M})$ inhibited action potentials induced by oxytocin this was associated with a hyperpolarization of only 5 mV (Fig. 16.6; Hollingsworth *et al.*, 1987), an effect much less than that observed in vascular tissue (Hamilton *et al.*, 1986; Weir & Weston, 1986). Furthermore, cromakalim did not alter $^{86}\text{Rb}^+$- or $^{42}\text{K}^+$-efflux (Hollingsworth *et al.*, 1987, 1989). This has led the authors to suggest that cromakalim (and other K-channel openers) act in the uterus by opening K-channels preferentially on pacemaker cells and indicates therefore the potential for achieving target organ selectivity.

These *in vitro* studies have recently been extended by Piper *et al.* (1990). Pinacidil and RP 49356 exert effects similar to cromakalim on the uterus whereas minoxidil sulphate shows low potency. The effects of this pyridine derivative are not modified by glibenclamide, which must raise questions as to the precise mechanism of action of this agent at least in the uterus.

Effects of K-channel openers *in vivo*

Studies by Hollingsworth and his group have shown that cromakalim (Downing *et al.*, 1989), and RP 49356 (Piper *et al.*, 1990), relax uterine smooth muscle *in vivo* (Fig. 16.7). Cromakalim induced a dose-dependent decrease in uterine contractility in ovariectomized, non-pregnant rats at the two doses tested (0.1 and 1 mg/kg, i.v.). An associated, dose-dependent decrease in blood pressure was also seen (Fig. 16.7) and there was no evidence for uterine selectivity. Cromakalim preferentially inhibited the frequency, rather than the amplitude, of the uterine contractions and the uterine activity tended to reappear in bursts with quiescent periods between. These *in vivo* effects of cromakalim and RP 49356 on the rat uterus were attenuated by pretreatment with glibenclamide (20 mg/kg, i.v.).

As indicated above, tolerance is a major clinical problem associated with the use of salbutamol in the treatment of preterm labour. Downing and coworkers (1989) have shown that tolerance in the rat also occurs with cromakalim, resulting in a 25-fold decrease in the sensitivity to the drug after three large bolus doses of cromakalim (1 mg/kg, i.v.) at 8 h intervals. However, in a recent preliminary study (Downing & Hollingsworth, 1989), using the same experimental protocol, tolerance was seen also to the cardiovascular effects of cromakalim, although to a smaller degree (fivefold).

Potentially, therefore, tolerance to the uterine effects might be a clinical problem with K-channel openers in the treatment of preterm labour. However, a recent preliminary study (Downing & Hollingsworth, 1990) showed that there was no cross-tolerance between salbutamol and cromakalim. Theoretically therefore, K-channel openers could be useful in conditions of tolerance to β-adrenoceptor agonists.

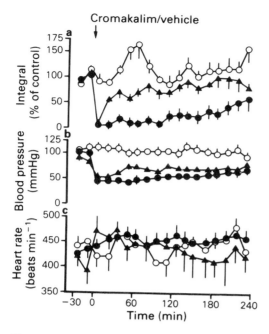

Fig. 16.7. Effects of a bolus i.v. injection of cromakalim (0.1 mg/kg; 1 mg/kg) or vehicle (↓) on integrated uterine contractions (*upper panel*), blood pressure (*middle panel*) and heart rate (*bottom panel*) in conscious non-pregnant rats. Uterine and cardiovascular effects were measured in different animals. Note that cromakalim clearly suppressed uterine activity at both doses but also significantly lowered blood pressure. (From Downing *et al.*, 1989, with permission.)

Clinical studies with K-channel openers

Diazoxide has achieved a limited use in the treatment of preterm labour but the effects are short-lasting (Baxi & Petrie, 1987). Apart from the studies using diazoxide no clinical studies on the effects of K-channel openers on preterm labour have been presented.

In summary, K-channel openers relax uterine smooth muscle, possibly by a preferential effect on pacemaker cells. Based on currently-available K-channel openers, there is no evidence for any selectivity for the uterus over vascular tissues. It is likely, therefore, that effects such as tachycardia, headache and fall in blood pressure would be seen at doses effective in relaxing human uterine smooth muscle. These agents apparently do not have any major advantage over current therapy for preterm labour. However, a K-channel opener selective for the uterus, would be a useful addition to the therapeutic arsenal.

Other genitourinary tissues

Erectile tissues

The primary event leading to penile erection is a decrease in arterial resistance leading to an increased arterial inflow to the penis and a subsequent filling of the erectile tissues (Sjöstrand & Klinge 1979; Andersson *et al.* 1984; Lue & Tanagho, 1987). Any vasoactive drug, i.e. one which relaxes penile vascular smooth muscle, can, when injected into the penis, induce erection in humans (Virag, 1982; Brindley, 1983). Intracavernosal injections of vasoactive substances, e.g. papaverine, phentolamine and prostaglandin E_1 are in fact now used regularly in the diagnosis and treatment of erectile impotence (Lue & Tanagho, 1987; Jünemann & Alken, 1989), although none is approved for this indication.

Gillespie and Sheng (1988) studied the effects of cromakalim on the histamine or noradrenaline (guanethidine)-induced contractions of the bovine retractor penis muscle *in vitro*. Cromakalim relaxed this preparation with an IC_{50} of 0.3 μM using either agonist, compared with values of 0.5 and 0.7 μM for noradrenaline- and histamine-induced contractions of the rabbit aorta, respectively. The relaxant effect of cromakalim in the retractor penis muscle was not affected by haemoglobin, an agent known to inhibit the non-adrenergic, non-cholinergic inhibitory (NANC) response to nerve stimulation in this tissue.

The effects of pinacidil and cromakalim have been investigated on isolated corpus cavernosum from pig, rabbit, monkey and humans (Giraldi & Wagner, 1990; Holmquist *et al.*, 1990a,b). In the rabbit penis, cromakalim and pinacidil relaxed noradrenaline-induced contractions with IC_{50} values of 0.46 and 1.9 μM, respectively. Both compounds relaxed contractions induced by low, but not high, concentrations of K^+ and increased the efflux of $^{86}Rb^+$ from the tissues, observations consistent with an action on K-channels.

In the human corpus cavernosum, pinacidil relaxed noradrenaline-induced contractions (IC_{50} 1.1 μM) and relaxed tissues contracted by low but not high K^+-concentrations. The drug also inhibited nerve stimulation-induced contractions and increased $^{86}Rb^+$-efflux (Holmquist *et al.*, 1990b). In addition, in the monkey pinacidil (5 mg) elicited an erectile response when injected intracavernosally (Giraldi & Wagner, 1990).

These data clearly indicate that cromakalim and pinacidil relax erectile smooth muscle and that K-channel openers can induce erection in animals after intracavernosal injection. No clinical studies have so far been published. Thus, at present it is not known if K-channel openers, alone or in combination with other vasoactive agents, will have utility in the diagnosis and treatment of erectile dysfunction.

Ureter

Ureteric colic is a common and painful condition which is usually treated with powerful analgesics or with prostaglandin synthetase inhibitors such as diclofenac. It has been known for a number of years that diazoxide relaxes ureteric smooth muscle. When given i.v. (1–4 mg/kg) diazoxide inhibits ureteric peristalsis in anaesthetized as well as conscious dogs (Boyarsky & Laby, 1972; Mayo & Halbert, 1981; Stower et al., 1986).

Recently, a preliminary study has been published on the effects of a range of K-channel openers on the ureter (Klaus et al., 1990a,b). In this study, the effects of cromakalim, pinacidil and nicorandil were compared with the Hoechst compounds, S 4010 and S 0121, and BRL 38226, the less active enantiomer of cromakalim. (For details of the chemical structures of these agents, see Chapter 13.)

Cromakalim, pinacidil, nicorandil, S 4010 and S 0121 relaxed the rhythmic contractions elicited in the guinea-pig ureter contracted by 40 mM K$^+$ whereas the (+)-enantiomer of cromakalim, BRL 38226, was virtually inactive.

Using electrophysiological techniques, it has been shown that both cromakalim and S 0121 cause hyperpolarization. Cromakalim (0.5 μM) hyperpolarized rabbit pulmonary artery and ureter by 20.5 and 11.3 mV, respectively, whereas the effects of S 0121 were less pronounced (13.0 and 3.8 mV, respectively). Further, both compounds were shown to relax contractions induced by high (80 mM) K$^+$ solution in human ureter and renal pelvis.

The finding that S 0121 relaxes the ureter, whereas BRL 38226 is inactive, is surprising since both drugs share the same configuration (see Chapter 13). However, while it is known that BRL 38226 is much less potent than cromakalim on both the ureter (Klaus et al., 1990a,b) and vascular tissues (Ashwood et al., 1986; Hof et al., 1988) recent studies suggest that S 0121 is also surprisingly active in vascular smooth muscle (Edwards et al., 1991). The reason why introduction of a 5′-methyl moiety into the benzopyran nucleus should yield a molecule of surprisingly high potency (like S 0121) remains to be established.

No clinical studies of the effect of K-channel openers in the ureter have been reported.

Vas deferens

As a component of a study on the effects of pinacidil on a variety of non-vascular smooth muscle, Cohen and Colbert (1986) investigated the effects of this agent on the rat vas deferens. Pinacidil was found to dose-dependently inhibit the contractile response to electrical field stimulation with an IC$_{50}$ of 1 μM.

Only one preliminary study has so far been published on the effects of cromakalim on the vas deferens. Eltze (1989) showed, in the rabbit, that cromakalim concentration-dependently inhibited the electrically-induced twitch contractions with an IC_{50} of $0.4 \pm 0.25\,\mu M$ and that this effect could be blocked by glibenclamide ($pA_2 = 7.2 \pm 0.4$). It was further shown that the effect of cromakalim could be reversed by Bay K 8644, suggesting that the relaxation involves reduction of Ca^{2+}-influx via voltage-dependent Ca-channels as previously postulated for vascular smooth muscle (Hamilton et al., 1986).

Mesotubarium

The mesotubarium is the smooth muscle structure surrounding the Fallopian tube and the uterine horn, containing some strands running longitudinally between the ovary and the uterus. The contractile pattern of the mesotubarium consists of long-lasting (5–6 min) contractions separated by relaxed periods of approximately 9 min duration (Hellstrand & Lydrup, 1988). Besides exerting a possible direct modulating effect on the contractility of the tubal wall, the mesotubarium may modify gross movements of the Fallopian tube which are associated with the capture of ova.

Modulation of the activity of the mesotubarium has no obvious clinical importance. However, because of the very regular pattern of activity, the guinea-pig mesotubarium is useful as a model tissue for the study of spontaneously active urogenital smooth muscle.

It has been shown that pinacidil ($10\,\mu M$) inhibits spontaneous contractions in the guinea-pig mesotubarium in vitro (Lydrup, 1991; Lydrup & Hellstrand, 1991). This is accompanied by a hyperpolarization of $7.0 \pm 0.6\,mV$ and a 1.4-fold increase in $^{86}Rb^+$ permeability. The relaxant effect of pinacidil ($10\,\mu M$) was not inhibited by $10\,mM$ TEA, $1\,\mu M$ apamin, or $10\,nM$ charybdotoxin (Lydrup, 1991), but was reversed by addition of $0.1\,\mu M$ glibenclamide (Lydrup & Hellstrand, 1991).

Glibenclamide $0.1\,\mu M$ had no effect on the spontaneous mechanical or electrical activity of the guinea-pig mesotubarium in normal Krebs' solution. However, this spontaneous activity disappeared on exposure to Krebs' solution containing cyanide and β-hydroxybutyrate instead of glucose, to block aerobic and glycolytic metabolism, respectively (Lydrup & Hellstrand, 1991). Since addition of glibenclamide restored electrical and mechanical activity, these workers concluded that K_{ATP} was present in the mesotubarium. If the conclusion is correct, the channel is probably closed under normal conditions and is only open in adverse metabolic circumstances.

References

Abel, M. H. & Hollingsworth, M. (1985) The potencies and selectivities of four calcium antagonists as inhibitors of uterine contractions in the rat *in vivo*. *British Journal Pharmacology* **85**, 263–269.

Andersson, K-E. (1988) Current concepts in the treatment of disorders of micturition. *Drugs* **35**, 477–494.

Andersson, K-E. & Forman, A. (1986) Effects of calcium channel blockers on urinary tract smooth muscle. *Acta Pharmacologica et Toxicologica* **58** (Suppl. II), 193–200.

Andersson, K-E. & Mattiasson, A. (1988) Drug treatment of the overactive detrusor. *Drugs of Today* **24**, 337–348.

Andersson, K-E., Andersson, P.O., Fovaeus, M., Hedlund, H., Malmgren, A. & Sjögren, C. (1988) Effects of pinacidil on bladder muscle. *Drugs* **36** (Suppl. 7), 41–49.

Andersson, P-O., Bloom, S. R. & Mellander, S. (1984) Haemodynamics of pelvic nerve induced penile erection in the dog: possible mediation by vasoactive intestinal polypeptide. *Journal of Physiology* **350**, 209–224.

Ashwood, V. A., Buckingham, R. E., Cassidy, F., Evans, J. M., Faruk, E. A., Hamilton, T. C., Nash, D. J., Stemp, G. & Willcocks, K. (1986) Synthesis and antihypertensive activity of 4-(cyclic amido)-2H-1-benzopyrans. *Journal of Medicinal Chemistry* **29**, 2194–2201.

Baxi, L. V. & Petrie, R. H. (1987) Pharmacologic effects on labor: effects of drugs on dystocia, labor, and uterine activity. *Clinical Obstetrics and Gynecology* **30**,1.

Boyarsky, S. & Laby, P. C. (1972) *Ureteral Dynamics*. Williams and Wilkins, Baltimore.

Brading, A. (1987) Physiology of bladder smooth muscle. In Torrens, M. & Morrison, J. F. B. (eds), *The Physiology of the Lower Urinary Tract*. pp. 161–191. Springer-Verlag, Berlin.

Brindley, G. S. (1983) Cavernosal alpha-blockage: a new technique for investigation and treating erectile impotence. *British Journal of Psychiatry* **143**, 332–337.

Bruner, C. A. & Webb, C. R. (1990) Increased vascular reactivity to Bay K 8644 in genetic hypertension. *Pharmacology* **40**, 24–35.

Buckingham, R. E., Hamilton, T. C., Howlett, D. R., Mootoo, S. & Wilson, C. (1989) Inhibition of glibenclamide of the vasorelaxant action of cromakalim in the rat. *British Journal of Pharmacology* **97**, 57–64.

Caritis, S., Edelstone, D. L. & Mueller-Heubach, E. (1979) Pharmacological inhibition of preterm labour. *American Journal of Obstetrics and Gynecology* **133**, 557.

Cavero, I., Mondot, S. & Mestre, M. (1989) Vasorelaxant effects of cromakalim in rats are mediated by glibenclamide-sensitive potassium channels. *Journal of Pharmacology and Experimental Therapeutics* **248**, 1261–1268.

Chapman, I. D., Kristersson, A., Mazzoni, L., Almsler, B. & Morley, J. (1991) Reversal of induced airway hyperreactivity by potassium channel openers: PCO 400 and cromakalim. *British Journal of Pharmacology* **102**, 355P.

Chiu, P. J. S., Tetzloff, G., Ho-Sam, A. & Sybertz, E. J. (1988) Effects of BRL 34915, a putative K channel opener, on transmembrane ^{45}Ca movements in rabbit aortic smooth muscle. *European Journal of Pharmacology* **155**, 229–237.

Cohen, M. & Colbert, W. E. (1986) Comparison of the effects of pinacidil and its metabolite, pinacidil-N-oxide, in isolated smooth and cardiac muscle. *Drug Development Research* **7**, 111–124.

Cook, N. S. (1988) The pharmacology of potassium channels and their therapeutic potential. *Trends in Pharmacological Sciences* **9**, 21–28.

Cook, N. S. & Quast, U. (1990) Potassium channel pharmacology. In Cook, N. S. (ed.), *Potassium Channels: Structure, Classification, Function and Therapeutic Potential*. Ellis Horwood Ltd., Chichester, pp. 181–255.

Corsi, M., Bettelini, L., Pietra, C., Toson, G. & Trist, D. (1990) The antagonism by glibenclamide of the effects of cromakalim and pinacidil on the isolated urinary bladder and aorta. *European Journal of Pharmacology* **183**, 267–268.

Creed, K. E. & Malmgren, A. (1992) Cromakalim — effects on the bladder. *Acta Physiologica Scandinavica* (in press).

Downing, S. J. & Hollingsworth, M. (1989) Cardiovascular tolerance to cromakalim in the rat *in vivo: British Journal of Pharmacology* **98,** 886P.

Downing, S. J. & Hollingsworth, M. (1990) Uterine tolerance to relaxants *in vivo*: lack of cross tolerance between relaxin, salbutamol and cromakalim. *British Journal of Pharmacology* **100,** 488P.

Downing, S. J., Miller, M. & Hollingsworth, M. (1989) Tolerance to cromakalim in the rat uterus *in vivo. British Journal of Pharmacology* **96,** 732–738.

Dunne, M. J., Yule, D. I., Gallacher, D. V. & Petersen, O. H. (1990) Comparative study of the effects of cromakalim (BRL 34915) and diazoxide on membrane potential. $[Ca^{2+}]_i$ and ATP-sensitive potassium currents in insulin-secreting cells. *Journal of Membrane Biology,* **114,** 53–60.

Duty, S. & Weston, A. H. (1990) Potassium channel openers. Pharmacological effects and future uses. *Drugs* **40,** 785–791.

Edman, K. A. P. & Schild, H. O. (1962) The need for calcium in the contractile responses induced by acetylcholine and potassium in the rat uterus. *Journal of Physiology* **161,** 424–441.

Edwards, G. & Weston, A. H. (1989) Effects of cromakalim on potassium and rubidium efflux rate following dual isotope labelling. *British Journal of Pharmacology* **98,** 926P.

Edwards, G., Henshaw, M., Miller, M. & Weston, A. H. (1991) Comparison of the effects of several potassium-channel openers on rat bladder and portal vein *in vitro*. *British Journal of Pharmacology*. **102,** 679–686.

Edwards, G., Henthorn, M. & Weston, A. H. (1990) Some effects of potassium channel openers on rat bladder and portal vein. *European Journal of Pharmacology* **183,** 2408–2409.

Eltze, M. (1989) Competitive antagonism by glibenclamide of cromakalim inhibition of twitch contractions in rabbit vas deferens. *European Journal of Pharmacology* **161,** 103–106.

Forman, A., Andersson, K-E. & Ulmsten, U. (1981) Inhibition of myometrial activity by calcium antagonists. *Seminars in Perinatology* **5,** 288–294.

Foster, C. D., Fujii, K., Kingdon, J. & Brading, A. F. (1989a) The effect of cromakalim on the smooth muscle of the guinea-pig urinary bladder. *British Journal of Pharmacology* **97,** 281–291.

Foster, C. D., Speakman, M. J., Fujii, K. & Brading, A. F. (1989b) The effects of cromakalim on the detrusor muscle of human and pig urinary bladder. *British Journal of Urology* **63,** 284–294.

Fovaeus, M., Andersson, K-E., Batra, S., Morgan, E. & Sjögren, C. (1987) Effects of calcium, calcium channel blockers and Bay K 8644 on bladder contractions induced by muscarinic receptor stimulation of isolated bladder muscle from rabbit and man. *Journal of Urology* **137,** 798–803.

Fovaeus, M., Andersson, K-E. & Hedlund, H. (1989) The action of pinacidil in the isolated human bladder. *Journal of Urology* **141,** 637–640.

Friedel, H. A. & Brogden, R. N. (1990) Pinacidil. A review of its pharmacodynamic and pharmacokinetic properties, and therapeutic potential in the treatment of hypertension. *Drugs* **39,** 929–967.

Fujii, K., Foster, C. D., Brading, A. F. & Parekh, A. B. (1990) Potassium channel blockers and the effects of cromakalim on the smooth muscle of the guinea-pig bladder. *British Journal of Pharmacology* **99,** 779–785

Gillespie, J. S. & Sheng, H. (1988) The lack of involvement of cyclic nucleotides in the smooth muscle relaxant action of BRL 34915. *British Journal of Pharmacology* **94,** 1189–1197.

Giraldi, A. & Wagner, G. (1990) Effects of pinacidil upon penile erectile tissue, *in vitro* and *in vivo*. *Pharmacology and Toxicology* **67**, 235–238.

Hamilton, T. C., Weir S. W. & Weston, A. H. (1986) Comparison of the effects of cromakalim and verapamil on electrical and mechanical activity in the rat portal vein. *British Journal of Pharmacology* **87**, 147–156.

Hedlund, H., Mattiasson, A. & Andersson, K-E. (1991) Effects of pinacidil on detrusor instability in men with bladder outlet obstruction. *Journal of Urology* **146**, 1345–1347.

Hellstrand, P. & Lydrup, M-L. (1988) Spontaneous electrical and contractile activity correlated to $^{86}Rb^+$ efflux in smooth muscle of guinea-pig mesotubarium. *Journal of Physiology* **407**, 587–597.

Hof, R. P., Quast, U., Cook, N. S. & Blarer, S. (1988) Mechanism of action of systemic and regional hemodynamics of the potassium channel activator BRL 34915 and its enantiomers. *Circulation Research* **62**, 679–686.

Hollingsworth, M., Amédée, T., Edwards, D., Mironneau, J., Savineau, Small, R. C. & Weston, A. H. (1987) The relaxant action of BRL 34915 in rat uterus. *British Journal of Pharmacology* **91**, 803–813.

Hollingsworth, M., Edwards, D., Miller, M., Rankin, J. R. & Weston, A. H. (1989) Potassium channels in isolated rat uterus and the action of cromakalim. *Medicinal Science Research* **17**, 461–463.

Holmquist, F., Andersson, K-E., Fovaeus, M. & Hedlund, H. (1990a) K^+-channel openers for relaxation of isolated penile erectile tissue from rabbit. *Journal of Urology* **144**, 146–151.

Holmquist, F., Andersson, K-E. & Hedlund, H. (1990b) Effects of pinacidil on isolated human corpus cavernosum penis. *Acta Physiologica Scandinavica* **138**, 463–469.

International Continence Society Committee on Standardisation of Terminology (1988) The standardisation of terminology of lower urinary tract function. *Scandinavian Journal of Urology and Nephrology* **114** (Suppl.), 5–19.

Jørgensen, T. M., Djurhuus, J. C., Jørgensen, H. S. & Sørensen S. S. (1983) Experimental bladder hyperreflexia in pigs. *Urological Research* **11**, 239–240.

Jünemann, K-P. & Alken, P. (1989) Pharmacotherapy of erectile dysfunction: a review. *International Journal of Impotence Research* **1**, 71–93.

Katama, K., Miyata, N. & Kasuya, Y. (1989) Functional changes in potassium channels in aortas from rats with streptozotocin-induced diabetes. *European Journal of Pharmacology* **166**, 319–323.

Klaus, E., Englert, H. C., Hropot, M., Mania, D. & Zwergel, U. (1990a) Inhibition of the rhythmic contractions of ureters by K^+ channel openers. *Naunyn-Schmiedeberg's Archives of Pharmacology* **340**, R59.

Klaus, E., Englert, H. C., Hropot, M., Mania, D. & Zwergel, U. (1990b) K^+-channel-openers inhibit the KCl-induced phasic-rhythmic contractions in the upper urinary tract. *European Journal of Pharmacology* **183**, 673.

Liggins, G. C. & Vaughan, G. S. (1973) Intravenous infusion of salbutamol in the management of premature labour. *Journal of Obstetrics and Gynecology British Commonwealth* **80**, 29–32.

Lippert, T. H. (1983) Tocolytic therapy for preterm labour. In Lewis, P. J. (ed.), *Clinical Pharmacology in Obstetrics.* John Wright & Sons, Bristol, pp. 182–218.

Longmore, J., Miller, M. & Weston, A. H. (1991) The relationship between the effects of lemakalim on tension and its effects on membrane potential and K permeability in bovine tracheal smooth muscle. *British Journal of Pharmacology* **102**, 26P.

Lue, T. F. & Tanagho, E. A. (1987) Physiology of erection and pharmacological management of impotence. *Journal of Urology* **141**, 54–57.

Lydrup, M-L. (1991) Role of K^+ channels in spontaneous electrical and mechanical activity of smooth muscle in the guinea-pig mesotubarium. *Journal of Physiology* **433,** 327–340.

Lydrup, M-L. & Hellstrand, P. (1991) Metabolic correlates to pacemaker activity in the smooth muscle of guinea-pig mesotubarium. *Acta Physiologica Scandinavica* **141,** 263–272.

McPherson, G. A. & Angus, J. A. (1989) Phentolamine and structurally related compounds selectively antagonize the vascular actions of the K^+ channel opener, cromakalim. *British Journal of Pharmacology* **97,** 941–949.

Malmgren, A., Andersson, K-E., Andersson, P-O., Fovaeus, M. & Sjögren, C. (1990) Effects of cromakalim (BRL 34915) and pinacidil on normal and hypertrophied rat detrusor *in vitro*. *Journal of Urology* **143,** 828–834.

Malmgren, A., Andersson, K-E., Sjögren, C. & Andersson, P-O. (1989) Effects of pinacidil and cromakalim (BRL 34915) on bladder function in rats with detrusor instability. *Journal of Urology* **142,** 1134–1138.

Malmgren, A., Sjögren, C., Uvelius, B., Mattiasson, A., Andersson, K-E. & Andersson, P-O. (1987) Cystometrical evaluation of bladder instability in rats with intravesical outflow obstruction. *Journal of Urology* **137,** 1291–1294.

Mattiasson, A. & Uvelius, B. (1982) Changes in contractile properties in hypertrophic rat urinary bladder. *Journal of Urology* **128,** 1340–1342.

Mayo, M. E. & Halbert, S. A. (1981) The effect of glucagon and diazoxide on the normal and obstructed upper urinary tract. *Urologica Internationalis* **36,** 100–109.

Miyata, N., Tsuchida, K. & Otomo, S. (1990) Functional changes in potassium channels in carotid arteries from stroke-prone spontaneously hypertensive rats. *European Journal of Pharmacology* **182,** 209–210.

Morita, T., Edwards, G., Andersson, P.O., Greengrass, P. M., Ibbotson, T., Newgreen, D. T., Weston, A. H. & Wyllie, M. G. (1992) Ciclazindol, a novel antagonist of the action of potassium channel openers in smooth muscle. *Journal of Physiology* **446,** 365P.

Mostwin, J. L. (1985) The action potential of guinea pig bladder smooth muscle. *Journal of Urology* **135,** 1299–1303.

Newgreen, D. T., Bray, K. M., McHarg, A. D., Weston, A. H., Duty, S., Brown, B. S., Kay, P. B., Edwards, G., Longmore, J. L., Southerton, J. S. (1990) The action of diazoxide and minoxidil sulphate on rat blood vessels: a comparison with cromakalim. *British Journal of Pharmacology* **100,** 605–613.

Noak, Th., Edwards, G., Deitmer, P., Greengrass, P., Morita, T., Andersson, P-O., Criddle, D., Wyllie, M. G. & Weston, A. H. (1992) The involvement of potassium channels in the action of ciclazindol in rat portal vein. *British Journal of Pharmacology* **106,** 17–24.

Nurse, D. E., Restorick, J. M. & Mundy, A. R. (1991) The effect of cromakalim on normal and hyper-reflexic human detrusor muscle. *British Journal of Urology* **68,** 27–31.

Piper, I., Minshall, E., Downing, S. J., Hollingsworth, M. & Sandraei, H. (1990) Effects of several potassium channel openers and glibenclamide on the uterus of the rat. *British Journal of Pharmacology* **101,** 901–907.

Quast, U. & Baumlin, Y. (1988) Comparison of the effluxes of $^{42}K^+$ and $^{86}Rb^+$ elicited by cromakalim (BRL 34915) in tonic and phasic vascular tissue. *Naunyn-Schmiedeberg's Archives of Pharmacology* **338,** 319–326.

Quast, U. & Cook, N. S. (1989) *In vitro* and *in vivo* comparison of two K^+ channel openers, diazoxide and cromakalim, and their inhibition by glibenclamide. *Journal of Pharmacology and Experimental Therapeutics* **250,** 261–270.

Restorik, J. & Nurse, D. (1988) The effect of cromakalim on human detrusor. An *in vitro* and *in vivo* study. *Neurourology and Urodynamics* **7,** 207–208.

Robertson, D. W. & Steinberg, M. I. (1989) Potassium channel openers: new biological probes. *Annual Reports in Medicinal Chemistry* **24**, 91–100.

Robertson, D. W. & Steinberg, M. I. (1990) Potassium channel modulators: scientific applications and therapeutic promise. *Journal of Medicinal Chemistry* **33**, 1529–1541.

Rothwell, N. J., Stock, M. J. & Wyllie, M. G. (1981) Sympathetic mechanisms in diet-induced thermogenesis: modification by ciclazindol and anorectic drugs. *British Journal of Pharmacology* **74**, 539–546.

Schmid-Antomarchi, H., DeWille, J., Fosset, M. & Lazdunski, M. (1987) The receptor for antidiabetic sulfonylureas controls the activity of the ATP-modulated K^+ channel in insulin-secreting cells. *Journal of Biological Chemistry* **262**, 15 840–15 844.

Sibley, G. N. A. (1984a) A comparison of spontaneous and nerve-mediated activity in bladder muscle from man, pig and rabbit. *Journal of Physiology* **354**, 431–443.

Sibley, G. N. A. (1984b) The response of the bladder to lower urinary tract obstruction. D. Phil. Thesis. University of Oxford.

Sibley, G. N. A. (1985) An experimental model of detrusor instability in the obstructed pig. *British Journal of Urology* **57**, 292–298.

Sjögren, C., Andersson, K-A., Husted, S., Mattiasson, A. & Møller-Madsen, B. (1982) Atropine resistance of transmurally stimulated human bladder muscle. *Journal of Urology* **128**, 1368–1371.

Sjöstrand, N. O. & Klinge, E. (1979) Principal mechanisms controlling penile retraction and protrusion in rabbits. *Acta Physiologica Scandinavica* **106**, 199–214.

Stower, M. J., Clark, A. G., Wright, J. W. & Hardcastle, J. D. (1986) The effect of various drugs on canine ureteric peristalsis. *Urological Research* **14**, 41–44.

Sturgess, N. C., Ashford, M. L. J., Cook, D. L. & Hales, C. N. (1985) The sulphonylurea receptor may be an ATP-sensitive potassium channel. *Lancet* ii, 474–475.

Torrens, M. (1987) Urodynamics. In Torrens, M. & Morrison, J. F. B. (eds), *The Physiology of the Lower Urinary Tract*, Springer-Verlag, Berlin, pp. 277–307.

Torrens, M. & Morrison, J. F. B. (eds) (1987) *The Physiology of the Lower Urinary Tract*. Springer-Verlag, Berlin.

Trube, G., Rorsman, P. & Ohno-Shosaku, T. (1986) Opposite effects of tolbutamide and diazoxide on the ATP-dependent K^+ channel in the mouse pancreatic β-cells. *Pflügers Archiv* **407**, 493–499.

Videbæk, L. M., Aalkjær, C. & Mulvaney, M. J. (1988) Pinacidil opens K^+-selective channels causing hyperpolarization and relaxation of noradrenaline contraction in rat mesenteric resistance vessels. *British Journal of Pharmacology* **95**, 103–108.

Virag, R. (1982) Intracavernous injection of papaverine for erectile failure. *Lancet* ii, 938.

Wein, A. J. (1987) Lower urinary tract function and pharmacologic management of lower urinary tract dysfunction. *Urological Clinics of North America* **14**, 273–296.

Weir, S. W. & Weston, A. H. (1986) Effect of apamin on the responses to BRL 34915, nicorandil and other relaxants in the guinea-pig taenia caeci. *British Journal of Pharmacology* **88**, 113–120.

Weston, A. H. (1989) Smooth muscle potassium channel openers; their pharmacology and clinical potential. *Pflügers Archiv* **414** (Suppl. 5), S99–S105.

Yamaguchi, O., Fukaya, Y., Yamaguchi, K. & Shiraiwa, Y. (1987) Response of chemically skinned bladder smooth muscle to calcium ion and its changes in obstructed bladder. *Neurourology and Urodynamics* **6**, 250–252.

Chapter 17
Potassium channel openers: clinical aspects
A. J. Williams

Introduction

The clinical effects of K-channel openers such as pinacidil and cromakalim have been studied in healthy volunteers and in patients with hypertension, angina pectoris and asthma. Nicorandil also possesses K-channel opening properties in addition to its ability to elevate intracellular cyclic guanosine monophosphate (cGMP) levels and has been extensively studied in angina pectoris. K-channel openers might also be useful in the treatment of a variety of other conditions, including peripheral vascular disease, and incontinence of urine due to bladder muscle instability. Undoubtedly, K-channel openers have potential in the treatment of all of these diseases, but at the present time their place in therapeutics has not been established and early clinical trials have concentrated upon establishing efficacy and patient tolerance in hypertension and asthma.

Pharmacokinetics

In humans pinacidil and nicorandil have short plasma half-lives (pinacidil 2–3 h, nicorandil 1 h; Ward *et al.*, 1984; DeLong *et al.*, 1988; Frydman *et al.*, 1989), whereas cromakalim and its active enantiomer, BRL 38227, have longer half-lives of about 24 h (Davies *et al.*, 1988; Gill *et al.*, 1988, 1990; Carey *et al.*, 1989; Bullman *et al.*, 1991). Pinacidil is excreted predominantly by hepatic metabolism and subsequent renal excretion of metabolites. Ward *et al.* (1984) administered pinacidil intravenously (i.v.) and McBurney *et al.* (1987a) gave a slow release formulation orally to healthy volunteers. During the 24 h after dosing only about 6% of the i.v. dose and 4% of the oral dose appeared in the urine as unchanged parent drug, whereas 32% after i.v. and 55% after oral dosing appeared in the urine as the major metabolite, pinacidil pyridine-N-oxide. This metabolite of pinacidil has been reported to have an antihypertensive effect of about one-quarter the potency of pinacidil in dogs (Eilertsen *et al.*, 1982). After acute dosing in humans the blood concentration of the N-oxide metabolite is found to be lower than that of pinacidil but the N-oxide has a longer plasma half-life (about 4 h; DeLong *et al.*, 1988) than pinacidil itself. Therefore during chronic dosing with pinacidil, the blood concentration of this metabolite accumulates relative to the parent drug, although its plasma concentration still remains lower than that of pinacidil (McBurney *et al.*, 1988). Pinacidil is about 40% bound to human plasma proteins at blood levels between 40 and 400 ng/ml (Ward *et al.*, 1984). Presumably because of its short plasma half-life, slow release formulations of the drug have been developed. McBurney *et al.* (1987a) compared the pharmaco-kinetics of a slow release capsule and a tablet formulation of pinacidil. After oral dosing the maximum plasma concentration of parent drug occurred 1.8 h after the tablet and only slightly later (at 2.5 h) after the capsule. In a separate study (McBurney *et al.*, 1987b), an increase in the bioavailability of a slow release tablet formulation of pinacidil was reported when coadministered with food. The clearance of pinacidil has been reported to be less in non-Caucasian ethnic groups, in elderly people and in smokers (Goldberg *et al.*, 1989a).

Nicorandil has a short plasma half-life (of about 1 h). This drug is linearly absorbed after oral dosing, is about 25% bound to human plasma proteins, and is extensively metabolized in humans with only about 1% of an administered dose appearing in the urine as parent drug (Frydman *et al.*, 1989). Its major metabolic pathway seems to be denitration followed by uptake into the nicotinamide pathway. Clinical studies of the pharmaco-dynamic effects of nicorandil have been reported after dosing sublingually (e.g. Kobayashi & Hakuta, 1987; Suryapranata & Surrey, 1989; Kashida *et al.*, 1990). However, no reports of the pharmacokinetics of nicorandil after sublingual administration could be found.

Cromakalim and its active enantiomer BRL 38227 have a long plasma half-life of about 24 h (Davies *et al.*, 1988; Gill *et al.*, 1988, 1990; Carey *et al.*, 1989; Bullman *et al.*, 1991). Cromakalim is metabolized in the liver and parent drug, the glucuronide and acyclic acid metabolites are excreted in human urine (Kudoh & Nakamura, 1990). After oral dosing it is linearly absorbed with increasing dose (0.5–2 mg cromakalim) reaching its peak plasma concentration between 2 and 4 h after dosing (Davies *et al.*, 1988). It is about 40% bound to plasma proteins (C. Kaye, personal communication). All drugs reach their steady-state plasma concentration after a dosing period of 5 half-lives and when dosing is stopped 5 half-lives are required for the drug to be cleared. Owing to its 24 h plasma half-life repeat dosing with cromakalim leads to achievement of steady-state levels after a 5-day period. Conversely, when dosing is stopped, it is 5 days before cromakalim is cleared from the human body.

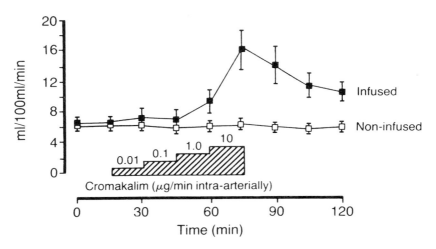

Fig. 17.1. Blood flow (ml/100 ml per min) in both the infused (■) and non-infused forearms (□) of eight subjects. Intrabrachial artery infusion of incremental doses of cromakalim (0.01–10 μg/min) preceded, and followed, by saline infusion. Values shown are mean ± SD. (From Webb *et al.*, 1989, with permission.)

Pharmacodynamics

In healthy volunteers, pinacidil and nicorandil have hypotensive effects (Ward, 1984; Belz *et al.*, 1985; Nicholls *et al.*, 1986). Cromakalim (up to 2 mg orally) has little or no hypotensive effect in healthy volunteers (Fox *et al.*, 1991). Singer *et al.* (1989) compared the effects on blood pressure of 1.5 mg cromakalim orally in healthy volunteers and hypertensive patients. Although the drug did not lower blood pressure and had only a mild effect on heart rate (increases of 8–10 beats/min), in healthy volunteers, at the same dose there was a significant reduction in blood pressure in the hypertensive patients. In contrast pinacidil (37.5 mg) given orally to healthy humans was reported to cause a reduction in blood pressure and a reflex tachycardia (Nicholls *et al.*, 1986). There is no doubt that cromakalim is a direct arterial vasodilator in healthy volunteers. Given orally to volunteers cromakalim (1 and 2 mg) increased forearm blood flow (Fox *et al.*, 1991) and this effect was confirmed by Webb *et al.* (1989) who infused cromakalim directly into the brachial artery (at doses between 0.01 and 10 μg/min; Fig. 17.1). In contrast cromakalim infused into the dorsal hand veins did not reduce noradrenaline-induced venoconstriction, thus demonstrating a clear arterial selectivity. Webb *et al.* (1989) suggest that this reflects the predominant membrane potential control of arteriolar smooth muscle tone. It is notable that a low plasma concentration (1.3 ± 0.5 ng/ml) of the (−)-enantiomer was associated with arteriolar dilation.

Both pinacidil and cromakalim cause reflex stimulation of the sympathetic nervous system and the renin–angiotensin axis (Byyny *et al.*, 1987; Ferrier *et al.*, 1989). For example, during a long-term dosing study in hypertensive patients, Byyny *et al.* found that plasma adrenaline and renin were consistently raised even after 9 months daily therapy with pinacidil. In this study, involving concomitant dosing with propranolol and hydrochlorothiazide, pinacidil was compared with hydralazine. Whereas the rise in plasma noradrenaline levels persisted during therapy with both vasodilators, the rise in plasma renin activity was only sustained during pinacidil therapy. The blood pressure lowering effect in the pinacidil and hydralazine groups was similar, suggesting a more pronounced effect on the renin–angiotensin axis by the K-channel opener in this study. However, Solomon and Weinberg (1987) and Abraham *et al.* (1987) found no elevation in plasma renin activity during chronic dosing with pinacidil in hypertensive patients. Abraham *et al.* also found a slight decrease in plasma aldosterone levels in their pinacidil treated patients and it has been suggested (Goldberg, 1988) that this may be due to sodium retention (secondary ultimately to vasodilation) suppressing aldosterone release.

During 5 days dosing in healthy volunteers Ferrier *et al.* (1989) found that cromakalim caused an increase in plasma renin, angiotensin II and noradrenaline levels with no change in blood pressure or plasma aldosterone, and only a small (8%) increase in heart rate. These workers also reported that cromakalim stimulated renin secretion from rat cultured juxtaglomerular cells. However, these findings were not confirmed in another laboratory (T. C. Hamilton, personal communication). Lijnen *et al.* (1989a) found that 6 days oral treatment with cromakalim (dose increasing from 0.5 to 2 mg daily) resulted in an increase in plasma renin activity, but had no effect on blood pressure or the plasma levels of angiotensin II, noradrenaline, aldosterone or atrial natriuretic peptide, in healthy volunteers. It is tempting to speculate that reflex stimulation of cardiac output and an effect on renin release might, in part, explain why cromakalim has only minimal effects on the blood pressure in normotensive subjects. There has been no study directly comparing the blood pressure lowering effects of pinacidil and cromakalim.

In contrast to pinacidil and cromakalim, nicorandil has been shown to reduce both arterial and venous tone. Both oral and sublingual dosing with nicorandil reduced both preload (reduction in venous tone) and afterload (reduction in arterial tone) in healthy volunteers (Belz *et al.*, 1984, 1985). This dual arterial and venous effect probably reflects the dual mechanism of action of nicorandil, affecting both K-channel opening and activation of guanylate cyclase.

In experimental animals K-channel openers have been shown to lower blood pressure by a mechanism susceptible to inhibition by high doses of glibenclamide (relative to its potency as a blocker of adenosine triphosphate (ATP)-sensitive K-channels and stimulator of insulin secretion in the pancreas). There have been few reports of the effects of K-channel openers on glucose metabolism in humans. However, pinacidil did not affect the release of insulin, or reduce plasma glucose concentration, in healthy volunteers (Neilsen-Kudsk *et al.*, 1990). There have been no published reports from clinical trials that K-channel openers have affected blood glucose levels after acute or chronic dosing. Similarly, there have been no reports that plasma K^+ levels are affected by these drugs. However, a slight fall in the concentration to K^+ within the red blood cell has been observed in healthy volunteers dosed for 6 days with cromakalim (Lijnen *et al.*, 1989b). This was associated with an increase in the number of Ca-dependent K-channels in the red cell membrane.

Pinacidil is now available, in a few countries, for treating hypertension. When given i.v. (0.2 mg/kg) to patients with essential hypertension, blood pressure was found to fall by an average of 30 mmHg, with a reduction in total peripheral vascular resistance of about 40% (Carlsen *et al.*, 1985). Concomitantly there was a fall in forearm vascular resistance, reflex tachycardia, an increase in cardiac muscle contractility (assessed by measurement of systolic time intervals) and cardiac output (measured by dye dilution). Similarly, Rijk and Thiem (1987) found that pinacidil given i.v. (at doses of 0.1–0.2 mg/kg) caused a fall in blood pressure in previously untreated hypertensives. The heart rate in these patients was increased by about 14 beats/min for every 10 mmHg fall in arterial blood pressure. The authors concluded that pinacidil (given i.v.) effectively lowered blood pressure but at the cost of a considerable increase in heart rate.

In a long-term dosing trial Carlsen *et al.* (1988) performed an oral dose titration study in hypertensives (increasing doses of pinacidil were given until diastolic blood pressure fell to 90 mmHg or a dose of 50 mg pinacidil twice daily was reached). Hydralazine was used as a comparator drug and cardiovascular haemodynamics were measured after 3 and 6 months treatment. Pinacidil and hydralazine both reduced blood pressure and caused similar increases in heart rate, stroke volume and cardiac output (forearm vascular resistance and pulmonary mean and wedge pressure were lower in the pinacidil treated group). In another trial in hypertensive patients Goldberg (1988) reported a clear reduction in blood pressure, with an accompanying tachycardia, in patients treated with pinacidil (142 patients given pinacidil, 142 given placebo in a double-blind study). However, the incidence of reported adverse events was high in the pinacidil-treated group, namely peripheral oedema (32% of patients), headache (28%), palpitations (12%) and tachycardia (9%). These are the side effects expected of a directly acting peripheral vasodilator. Although peripheral vasodilators might be expected to cause postural hypotension, there have been no reports of postural hypotension after oral dosing with pinacidil. Indeed, Caruana *et al.* (1985) found that tilt-testing produced no postural hypotension in hypertensives treated with oral pinacidil.

However, Ward *et al.* (1984) found that acute i.v. dosing with pinacidil was associated with distressing postural hypotension at serum concentrations above 300 ng pinacidil/ml.

Presumably the relatively high incidence of unwanted effects found in trials of pinacidil as monotherapy in hypertension, has led to studies of the drug in combination with diuretics (Goldberg & Offen, 1988; Goldberg *et al.*, 1989b). It seems unlikely that pinacidil will find a place as monotherapy for hypertension. Its use, like that of hydralazine (which has a similar cardiovascular pharmacodynamic profile; Carlsen *et al.*, 1985), will probably be confined to cotherapy with other agents (such as diuretics and β-adrenoceptor antagonists) which reduce its side-effect profile. Indeed the FDA Advisory Committee has recommended that pinacidil should be co-prescribed with a diuretic (*see Scrip*, 1987). Other unwanted effects with pinacidil include hypertrichosis (hair growth) on the face and arms (2% reported incidence in males and 13% reported incidence in females; Goldberg, 1988). This effect occurs only after prolonged treatment at high doses, and is reversible upon cessation of treatment.

Electrocardiographic T-wave flattening or inversion occurs in 20–30% of patients treated with pinacidil (Shub *et al.*, 1987). Both hypertrichosis and electrocardiographic T-wave inversion also occur during therapy with minoxidil (Linas & Nies, 1981; Zins, 1988) and one of the metabolites of minoxidil (minoxidil sulphate) in humans has K-channel opening properties. On a more positive note, Goldberg (1988), Rockhold *et al.* (1989) and Saku *et al.* (1990) reported a lowering of cholesterol (low density) and triglycerides, and an increase in high density lipoprotein cholesterol, during long-term treatment of hypertensive patients with pinacidil (*see* Fig. 17.2).

There are few reports of the effects of cromakalim and nicorandil on the blood pressure of hypertensive patients. Nicorandil (given as a single daily oral dose of 20 mg to 12 untreated patients with essential hypertension) caused a significant reduction in systolic and diastolic blood pressure, which was sustained for 24 h (Leonetti *et al.*, 1989). No reflex tachycardia was seen. Similarly, cromakalim (0.5–1.5 mg orally) lowered blood pressure when given acutely to patients with mild to moderate hypertension (Vandenburg *et al.*, 1986; Singer *et al.*, 1989). In an 8-day repeat dose study, cromakalim (1 and 1.5 mg) caused similar reductions in blood pressure after the first and the eighth doses. However, the increase in supine heart rate was smaller after the eighth dose (Vandenburg *et al.*, 1987). Adverse events attributable to cromakalim were typical of a vasodilator, the incidence of headache being dose related. There were no significant changes in body weight.

The effects of cromakalim (1.5 mg daily for 3 days) on renal haemodynamics were investigated in hypertensive patients (Lebel *et al.*, 1991). This K-channel opener reduced blood pressure while glomerular filtration

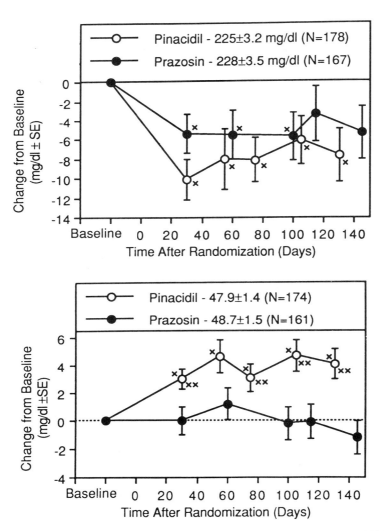

Fig. 17.2. Time-course of changes in total cholesterol (*upper panel*) and high density lipoprotein cholesterol (*lower panel*) produced by pinacidil and prazosin in hypertensive patients. $^{x}P < 0.05$, within that treatment group for that visit, mean change from baseline was significant. $^{xx}P < 0.05$, for that visit, mean change from baseline in the pinacidil group was significantly different from that in prazosin group. (From Rockhold *et al.*, 1989, with permission.)

rate was unchanged and effective renal plasma flow was slightly increased (reflecting reduced renal vascular resistance). An increase in urinary 6-keto-prostaglandin $F_{1\alpha}$ (the stable metabolite of prostacyclin) correlated with an increase in the effective renal plasma flow in some patients. There were no changes in parameters of the renin–angiotensin–aldosterone system or in plasma atrial natriuretic peptide levels (Lebel *et al.*, 1988).

In hypertensive patients whose blood pressure was inadequately controlled by the β-adrenoceptor antagonist, atenolol, addition of cromakalim was associated with a small additional fall in blood pressure but this effect appeared to be comparatively short-lived (Donnelly et al., 1990). Cromakalim had no effect on the pharmacokinetics of atenolol at steady state.

The clinical development of cromakalim has been halted in favour of its active ($-$)-enantiomer, BRL 38227. In a single dose tolerance study in hypertensive patients, BRL 38227 (0.25–3 mg) reduced blood pressure and increased heart rate, the peak fall in blood pressure occurring between 2 and 8 h with an effect persisting at 24 h after the higher doses ($>$ 1 mg; Jain et al., 1991). In a 28-day repeat dose study (Erwteman et al., 1991), BRL 38227 (0.75, 1 and 1.25 mg daily) reduced supine diastolic blood pressure at 4–5 h after the first dose and a significant effect was observed at 24 h after the last dose in the 1 and 1.25 mg dose groups.

Possibly because it reduces both preload and after-load (Belz et al., 1984, 1985; Kobayashi & Hakuta, 1987; Coltart & Signy, 1989), nicorandil has been investigated in both congestive heart failure and (more extensively) in angina. Given acutely to 11 patients with congestive heart failure nicorandil was reported to improve cardiac function (Solal et al., 1989). There was a reduction in pulmonary wedge pressure, mean arterial pressure, systemic vascular resistance and an increase in cardiac output. The improvement in cardiac function (assessed at cardiac catheterization) was not associated with a tachycardia. Similar results were obtained by Tice et al. (1990) in an acute study with nicorandil in 25 patients with congestive cardiac failure. There have been no reports of the clinical effects of nicorandil in heart failure during long-term dosing. However, both single and repeat doses of nicorandil have been reported to increase the duration of, and maximum exercise capacity reached, before the onset of chest pain or ECG changes in patients with angina (Kinoshita et al., 1986, 1989; Hayata et al. 1986; Camm & Maltz, 1989; Meany et al., 1989; Hughes et al., 1990). Nicorandil also increases coronary blood flow, by a direct vasodilating effect on coronary blood vessels (Aizawa et al. 1987; Suryapranta & Surrey, 1989; Kashida et al., 1990) which may contribute to its antianginal effect. However, the therapeutic benefits of nicorandil in angina are almost certainly due to actions in addition to the opening of K-channels. Certainly the haemodynamic effects of nicorandil differ markedly from those of cromakalim and pinacidil. In patients with ischaemic heart disease, single doses of nicorandil cause a reduction in preload and afterload and coronary vasodilation (Thormann et al., 1982; Aizawa et al., 1987; Kobayashi & Hakuta, 1987; Coltart & Signy, 1989; Kashida et al., 1990) whereas i.v. cromakalim (15 μg/kg infused over 10 min) produces only a reduction in afterload (Thomas et al., 1990).

Similarly, the haemodynamic effects of pinacidil are those of a peripheral arterial vasodilator (Goldberg, 1988).

Potassium-channel openers are smooth muscle relaxing agents and, therefore, have potential as bronchodilating agents in the treatment of asthma. Additionally, the pharmacological profile of the K-channel openers suggests that they may have other actions which might lead to therapeutic benefits in asthma. For example, cromakalim inhibits bronchoconstriction induced by stimulation of pulmonary non-adrenergic, non-cholinergic (NANC) excitatory nerves in the guinea-pig, possibly by means of prejunctional inhibition of release of peptidergic neurotransmitter(s) (Ichinose & Barnes, 1990). This latter finding suggests the possibility of an anti-inflammatory action of K-channel openers, since excitatory peptidergic NANC nerves may be involved in a neurogenic inflammatory pathway in asthma (*see* Barnes, 1987 for review). At the present time, the only reported studies of the effects of K-channel openers in human asthma have been with cromakalim and BRL 38227. In healthy volunteers, cromakalim was found to inhibit histamine-induced bronchoconstriction (Baird *et al.*, 1988). In this randomized, placebo-controlled, double-blind cross-over study, no differences were found between the effects of placebo, salbutamol or cromakalim (2 mg orally) on heart rate or blood pressure. However, Kidney *et al.* (1991) administered BRL 38227 (the active enantiomer of the racemic mixture cromakalim) at doses up to 0.5 mg (equivalent to 1 mg cromakalim) to normotensive patients with asthma. In randomized double-blind placebo-controlled cross-over studies, BRL 38227 did not inhibit histamine or methacholine-induced bronchoconstriction. Furthermore, there was a high incidence of headache (six of eight subjects, histamine study; seven of nine subjects, methacholine study).

Cromakalim has a long plasma half-life and for this reason it was investigated in patients with nocturnal asthma. This condition is common in asthmatics and is typified by nocturnal symptoms, and an accompanying deterioration in lung function which are the predominant features of their disease. Nocturnal asthma is often difficult to treat with currently-available drugs. In a pilot study, five patients with nocturnal asthma were given single oral doses of 0.5 and 1.5 mg of cromakalim (containing 0.25 and 0.75 mg of BRL 38227) at 23:00 h. In this randomized double-blind study, nocturnal asthma was assessed as the overnight fall in the forced expiratory volume in 1 s (FEV_1) measured at 06:00 h. There was a significant reduction in the overnight fall in FEV_1 after both doses of cromakalim compared with placebo (Williams *et al.*, 1988). This investigation was extended so that a total of 22 patients was studied. Again, the overnight fall in FEV_1 was significantly attenuated by 0.5 mg and 1.5 mg cromakalim (Williams *et al.*, 1989). Cromakalim has also been found to attenuate nocturnal bronchoconstriction (sometimes called 'morning dipping') after repeat dosing. Cromakalim was administered orally at 23:00 h for 5 days

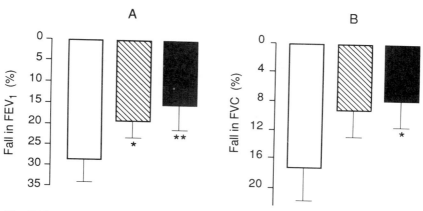

Fig. 17.3. Mean percentage fall in FEV_1, A, and forced vital capacity (FVC), B, from 23:00 h to 06:00 h on the fifth day of cromakalim repeat dose study. Empty columns = placebo; stippled = 0.25 mg cromakalim; filled = 0.5 mg cromakalim. Bars show SEM. *$P < 0.05$, **$P < 0.005$ compared with placebo. (From Williams et al., 1990a, with permission.)

so that the pharmacokinetic steady state was reached. In this randomized double-blind placebo-controlled cross-over study, patients were admitted to hospital on the fifth dosing day and FEV_1 was measured at 23:00 h and again at 06:00 h. There was a clear attenuation in the 06.00 h 'morning dip' in FEV_1 after both 0.25 and 0.5 mg doses of cromakalim compared with placebo (Owen et al., 1989). All these studies were initially reported on an 'intention to treat' basis. A single publication reported all the studies of cromakalim in which the data were analysed using only those patients who satisfied the protocols inclusion and exclusion criteria of the protocols (Williams et al., 1990a). In this analysis, cromakalim attenuated nocturnal asthma at all dose levels studied (see Fig. 17.3 for 0.25 and 0.5 mg cromakalim), but in 16 patients who received single doses of 1.5 mg cromakalim (containing 0.75 mg BRL 38227), this did not reach statistical significance. The authors suggest that this was due to the high incidence of headaches, which occurred in this group only, preventing the subjects performing a full FEV_1 manoeuvre. In these studies, cromakalim had no effect on the heart rate and blood pressure of the normotensive asthmatics.

In a randomized double-blind parallel group placebo-controlled study (Picot & de Vernejoul, 1991), BRL 38227 given orally (once daily for 28 days at doses in the range 0.125–0.75 mg) to patients with reversible bronchoconstriction did not affect FEV_1 measured 16 h after the final dose. However, a small improvement in FEV_1 was recorded at 4 h post-dose in the BRL 38227-treated groups. Thus in these patients, 66% of whom were also taking inhaled steroids, BRL 38227 conferred a modest, but short-lived, improvement in FEV_1. However, a high incidence of headache was also reported.

Cromakalim has been administered by inhalation to healthy volunteers up to a dose of 1 mg (Williams *et al.*, 1990b). The drug was well tolerated and no cardiovascular effects were seen (assessed by measurement of heart rate, blood pressure and ECG, together with stroke volume, cardiac output and cardiac inotropic state as measured by impedance cardiography). No reports have appeared of the effect of BRL 38227 or other K-channel openers given by inhalation.

The inhibitory actions of cromakalim and pinacidil on contractile activity in bladder preparations (including human detrusor muscle strips) has led to evaluation of their potential in the treatment of detrusor instability in patients. In a pilot single-blind study in 17 patients whose bladder dysfunction was unsatisfactorily controlled by other drugs, cromakalim (0.5 mg for 14 days, then 1 mg for a further 14 days) improved symptoms (urinary frequency) with an increase in mean voided volume (Nurse *et al.*, 1991). This suggests that further investigation of K-channel openers in such patients is warranted by means of double-blind protocols which should include urodynamic assessment. However, in a double-blind cross-over study in patients with bladder outflow obstruction secondary to benign prostatic hypertrophy, pinacidil (25 mg daily for 14 days) had no effect on urodynamic variables in eight out of 10 patients (Hedlund *et al.*, 1991).

Conclusions

The K-channel openers pinacidil, cromakalim and nicorandil have different pharmacokinetic and pharmacodynamic profiles in humans. Pinacidil is a peripheral arteriolar dilator, which has been shown to reduce blood pressure in formal therapeutic trials in hypertensive patients. When used as monotherapy for hypertension, however, there is a relatively high incidence of unwanted effects and these are predominantly secondary to its peripheral vasodilating action. Nicorandil has a haemodynamic profile that suggests that many of its major effects in humans are not due to opening of K-channels. This drug has utility in the treatment of angina pectoris. Cromakalim inhibits histamine-induced bronchoconstriction and nocturnal asthma at oral doses that do not affect heart rate and blood pressure in normotensive subjects. In hypertensive patients, cromakalim given acutely reduces blood pressure and causes a small reflex increase in heart rate. The active enantiomer of cromakalim, BRL 38227, is now undergoing formal assessment as monotherapy for once daily oral treatment for hypertension.

References

Abraham, P. A., Halstenson, C. E., Matzke, G. R. & Keane, W. F. (1987) Comparison of antihypertensive, renal haemodynamic and humoral effects of pinacidil and hydralazine monotherapy. *Journal of Clinical Hypertension* **3**, 439–451.

Aizawa, T., Ogasawara, K. & Kato, K. (1987) Effects of nicorandil on coronary circulation in patients with ischaemic heart disease: comparison with nitroglycerin. *Journal of Cardiovascular Pharmacology* **10** (Suppl. 8), 123–129.

Baird, A., Hamilton, T. C., Richards, D., Tasker, T. & Williams, A. J. (1988) Cromakalim, a potassium channel activator inhibits histamine-induced bronchoconstriction in healthy volunteers. *British Journal of Clinical Pharmacology* **25**, 114P.

Barnes, P. J. (1987) Airway neuropeptides and asthma. *Trends in Pharmacological Science* **8**, 23–27.

Belz, G. G., Matthews, J. H., Beck, A., Wagner, G. & Schneider, B. (1985) Haemodynamic effects of nicorandil, isosorbide dinitrate and dihydralazine in healthy volunteers. *Journal of Cardiovascular Pharmacology* **7**, 1107–1112.

Belz, G. G., Matthews, J., Heinrich, J. & Wagner, G. (1984) Controlled comparison of the pharmacodynamic effects of nicorandil (SG75) and isosorbide dinitrate in man. *European Journal of Clinical Pharmacology* **26**, 681–685.

Bullman, J. N., Davies, B. E., Gill, T. S., Taylor, A. C., Kaye, C. M. & Williams, A. J. (1991) The pharmacokinetics of BRL 38227 in healthy male volunteers. *British Journal of Clinical Pharmacology* **31**, 590P–591P.

Byyny, R. L., Nies, A. S., LoVerde, M. E. & Mitchell, W. B. D. (1987) A double blind randomized controlled trial comparing pinacidil to hydralazine in essential hypertension. *Clinical Pharmacology and Therapeutics* **42**, 50–57.

Camm, A. J. & Maltz, M. B. (1989) A controlled single-dose study of the efficacy, dose–response and duration of action of nicorandil in angina pectoris. *American Journal of Cardiology* **63**, 61J–65J.

Carlsen, J. E., Jensen, H. A., Rehling, M., Lund, J. O. & Trap-Jensen, J. (1988) Long-term haemodynamic effects of pinacidil and hydralazine in arterial hypertension. *Drugs* **36** (Suppl. 7), 55–63.

Carlsen, J. E., Kardel, T., Lund, J. O., McNair, A. & Trap-Jensen, J. (1985) Acute haemodynamic effects of pinacidil and hydralazine in essential hypertension. *Clinical Pharmacology and Therapeutics* **37**, 253–259.

Carey, O. J., Fleming, J. J., Ward, J. W. & Davies, B. E. (1989) Pharmacokinetics of cromakalim — a new antihypertensive agent, in patients with mild essential hypertension. *Xenobiotica* **19**, 93–95.

Caruana, M. P., Al-Khawaja, I., Royston, P. & Raftery, E. B. (1985) The effects of long acting pinacidil on intra-arterial blood pressure. *British Journal of Clinical Pharmacology* **20**, 140–143.

Coltart, D. J. & Signy, M. (1989) Acute haemodynamic effects of single dose nicorandil in coronary artery disease. *American Journal of Cardiology* **63**, 34J–39J.

Davies, B. E., Dierdorf, D., Eckl, K. M., Greb, W. H., Mellows, G. & Thomsen, T. (1988) The pharmacokinetics of BRL 34915, a new antihypertensive agent, in healthy volunteers. *British Journal of Clinical Pharmacology* **25**, 136P.

DeLong, A. F., Oldham, S. W., De Sante, K. A., Nell, G. & Henry, D. P. (1988) Disposition of ^{14}C pinacidil in humans. *Journal of Pharmaceutical Science* **77**, 153–156.

Donnelly, R., Elliott, J. L., Meredith, P. A. & Reid, J. L. (1990) Clinical studies with the potassium channel activator cromakalim in normotensive and hypertensive subjects. *Journal of Cardiovascular Pharmacology* **16**, 790–795.

Eilertsen, E., Magnussen, M. P., Peterson, H. J., Rastrup-Anderson, N., Sorensen, H.

& Arrigoni-Martelli. E. (1982) Metabolism of the new antihypertensive agent pina-cidil in rat, dog and man. *Xenobiotica* **12**, 187–196.

Erwteman, T., Blackwood, R. A. & Schrader, J. (1991) First clinical experience of BRL 38227 (K$^+$ channel activator) in hypertensive patients. *Journal of Hypertension* **9** (Suppl. 6), S440.

Ferrier, C. P., Kurtz, A., Lehner, P., Shaw, S. G., Pusterla, C., Saxonhofer, H. & Weidmann, P. (1989) Stimulation of renin secretion by potassium channel activation with cromakalim. *European Journal of Clinical Pharmacology* **36**, 443–447.

Fox, J. S., Whitehead, E. M. & Shanks, R. G. (1991) Cardiovascular effects of cro-makalim (BRL 34915) in healthy volunteers. *British Journal of Clinical Pharmacology* **32**, 45–49.

Frydman, A. M., Chapelle, P., Diekmann, H., Bruno, R., Thebault, J. J., Bouthier, J., Caplain, H., Ungethuem, W., Gaillard, C. & Le-Liboul, A. (1989) Pharmacokinetics of nicorandil. *American Journal of Cardiology* **63**, 25J–33J.

Gill, T. S., Bullman, J. N., Staniforth, D. H. & Davies, B. E. (1990) The pharmaco-kinetic and haemodynamic effects of intravenous cromakalim. *British Journal of Clinical Pharmacology* **29**, 617P.

Gill, T. S., Davies, B. E., Allen, G. D. & Greb, W. H. (1988) Stereospecific pharmaco-kinetics of cromakalim enantiomers in healthy male subjects. *British Journal of Clinical Pharmacology* **25**, 669P.

Goldberg, M. R. (1988) Clinical pharmacology of pinacidil. A prototype for drugs that affect potassium channels. *Journal of Cardiovascular Pharmacology* **12** (Suppl. 2), 41–47.

Goldberg, M. R. & Offen, W. W. (1988) Pinacidil with and without hydrochlorthiazide: dose–response relationships from results of a 4 × 3 factorial design study. *Drugs,* **36** (Suppl. 7), 83–92.

Goldberg, M. R., Rockhold, F. W., Offen, W. W. & Dornseif, B. E. (1989b) Dose–effect and concentration–effect relationships of pinacidil and hydrochlorthiazide in hyper-tension. *Clinical Pharmacology and Therapeutics* **46**, 208–218.

Goldberg, M. R., Rockhold, F. W., Thompson, W. L. & De Sante K. A. (1989a) Clinical pharmacokinetics of pinacidil, a potassium channel opener in hypertension. *Journal of Clinical Pharmacology* **29**, 33–40.

Hayata, N., Araki, H. & Nakamura, M. (1986) Effects of nicorandil on exercise tolerance in patients with stable effort angina; a double-blind study. *American Heart Journal* **112**, 1245–1250.

Hedlund, H., Mathiasson, A. & Andersson, K-E. (1990) Effect of pinacidil on detrusor instability in men with bladder outlet obstruction. *Journal of Urology* **146**, 1345–1347.

Hughes, L. O., Rose, E. L., Lakiri, A. & Raftery, E. B. (1990) Comparison of nicorandil and atenolol in stable angina pectoris. *American Journal of Cardiology* **66**, 679–682.

Ichinose, M. & Barnes, P. J. (1990) A potassium channel activator modulates both excitatory noncholinergic and cholinergic transmission in guinea-pig airways. *Journal of Pharmacology & Experimental Therapeutics* **252**, 1207–1212.

Jain, A. K., McMahon, F. G., Vargas, R. & Regel, G. (1991) A double blind (DB), randomised, single dose tolerance study of BRL 38227 in hypertensive patients. *Clinical Pharmacology and Therapeutics* **42**, 145 (Abstr. PI-87)

Kashida, H., Hata, N., Kusama, Y., Iwahora, S., Sasaki, Y., Mori, N., Yasutake, M., Kuomi, S., Takayama, M. & Munakata, K. (1990) Angiographic responses to a vasodilating drug, nicorandil, in patients with coronary artery disease. *Japanese Heart Journal* **31**, 135–143.

Kidney, J. C., Worsdell, Y. M., Lavender, E. A., Chung, K. F. & Barnes, P. J. (1991)

The effect of an ATP-dependent potassium channel activator BRL 38227 in asthmatics. *American Review of Respiratory Disease* **143**, A423 (Abstr.)

Kinoshita, M., Hachimoto, K., Ohbayashi, Y., Inoue, T., Taguchi, H. & Mitsunami, K. (1989) Comparison of antianginal activity of nicorandil, propranolol and diltiazem with reference to the antianginal mechanism. *American Journal of Cardiology* **63**, 71J–74J.

Kinoshita, M., Nishikawa, S., Sawamura, M., Yamaguchi, S., Mitsunami, K., Itoh, M., Motomura, M., Bito, K., Mashiro, I. & Kawakita, S. (1986) Comparative efficacy of high-dose versus low-dose nicorandil therapy for chronic stable angina pectoris. *American Journal of Cardiology* **58**, 733–738.

Kobayashi, K. & Hakuta, T. (1987) Effects of nicorandil on coronary haemodynamics in ischaemic heart disease: comparison of nitroglycerine, nifedipine and propranolol. *Journal of Cardiovascular Pharmacology* **10** (Suppl. 8), 109–115.

Kudoh, S. & Nakamura, H. (1990) Direct determination of the antihypertensive agent cromakalim and its major metabolites in human urine by high-performance liquid chromatography. *Journal of Chromatography* **515**, 597–602.

Lebel, M., Crose, J. H. & Lacourcière, Y. (1988) Effects of the novel antihypertensive agent BRL 34915 on endocrine sodium regulation in essential hypertension. *American Journal of Hypertension* **1**, 32A (Abstr. 1211)

Lebel, M., Grose, J. H. & Lacourcière, Y. (1991) Effect of short-term administration of cromakalim on renal haemodynamics and eicosanoid excretion in essential hypertension. *American Journal of Hypertension* **4**, 740–744.

Leonetti, G., Fruscio, M., Gradnik, R., Chianca, R., Bolla, G. B., Prandi, P. & Zanchetti A. (1989) Nicorandil, a new vasodilator drug, in patients with essential hypertension. *Journal of Hypertension* **7**, S292–293.

Lijnen, P., Fagard, R., Staessen, J., Weiping, T., Moerman, E. & Amery, A. (1989a) Humoral and cellular effects of the K(+) channel activator cromakalim in man. *European Journal of Clinical Pharmacology* **37**, 609–611.

Lijnen, P., Weiping, T., Fagard, R., Staessen, J. & Amery, A. (1989b) Changes in potassium content and membrane potassium channels in circulating cells from normal volunteers treated with cromakalim. *Journal of Hypertension* **7**, 403–407.

Linas, S. L. & Nies, A. S. (1981) Minoxidil. *Annals of Internal Medicine* **94**, 61–65.

McBurney, A., Farrow, P. R. & Ward, J. W. (1987a) Effects of formulation on the pharmacokinetics of orally administered pinacidil in humans. *Journal of Pharmaceutical Science* **76**, 940–941.

McBurney, A., Farrow, P. R. & Ward, J. W. (1987b) Effects of food on the bioavailability of sustained release pinacidil in humans. *Journal of Pharmaceutical Science* **77**, 68–69.

McBurney, A., Henry, J. A. & Ward, J. W. (1988) Accumulation of pinacidil-N-oxide during chronic treatment with pinacidil. *European Journal of Clinical Pharmacology* **35**, 93–95.

Meany, T. B., Richardson, P., Camm, A. J., Coltart, J., Griffith, M., Maltz, M. B. & Signy, M. (1989) Exercise capacity after single and twice daily doses of nicorandil in chronic stable angina pectoris. *American Journal of Cardiology* **63**, 66J–70J.

Neilsen-Kudsk, J. E., Mellemkjaer, S., Nielsen, C. B. & Siggaard, C. (1990) Lack of effect of the vasodilator pinacidil on insulin secretion in healthy humans. *Journal of Clinical Pharmacology* **30**, 409–411.

Nicholls, D. P., McNeill, J., Harron, D. W. & Shanks, R. G. (1986) Cardiovascular effects of pinacidil and propranolol alone and in combination in normal humans. *Journal of Cardiovascular Pharmacology* **8**, 51–54.

Nurse, D. E., Restorick, J. & Mundy, A. R. (1991) The effect of cromakalim on the normal and hyper-reflexic human detrusor muscle. *British Journal of Urology* **68**, 27–31.

Owen, S., Church, S., Stone, P., Bosch, P., Webster, S., Lavender, E., Williams, A. J. & Woodcock, A. A. (1989) A randomized double-blind placebo controlled crossover trial of a potassium channel activator in nocturnal asthma. *Thorax* **44**, 852P.

Picot, C. & de Vernejoul, D. (1991) Resultats d'une etudes multicentrique de recherche de posologie optimale du lemakalim (BRL 38227), per os pendant 28 jours chez 267 asthmatiques modéré. *Journées Nationales de la Société Française d'Allergologie*, 21–22 June, Abstract 47.

Rijk, M. C. & Thiem, T. (1987) Intravenous pinacidil in the acute treatment of hypertension. *Journal of Clinical Pharmacology* **27**, 468–474.

Rockhold, F. W., Goldberg, M. R. & Thompson, W. L. (1989) Beneficial effects of pinacidil on blood lipids: comparison with prazosin and placebo in patients with hypertension. Pinacidil–Prazosin and Pinacidil–Placebo Research Groups, Lilly Research Laboratories. *Journal of Laboratory Clinical Medicine* **114**, 646–654.

Saku, K., Ying, H. & Arakawa, K. (1990) Effects of pinacidil on serum lipid, lipoprotein and apolipoprotein levels in patients with mild to moderate hypertension. *Clinical Therapy* **12**, 132–138.

Scrip (1987), no. 1211, 22.

Shub, C., Zachariah, P. K., Ilstrup, D. M. & Tajik, A. J. (1987) Effects of pinacidil on the heart: serial electrocardiographic and echocardiographic observations. *Canadian Journal of Cardiology* **3**, 233–229.

Singer, D. R., Markandu, N. D., Miller, M. A., Sugden, A. L. & McGregor, G. A. (1989) Potassium channel stimulation in normal subjects and in patients with essential hypertension: an acute study with cromakalim (BRL 34915) *Journal of Hypertension* **7**, S294–S295.

Solal, A. C., Haeger, P., Bouthier, J., Juliard, J. M., Dahan, M. & Gourgon, R. (1989) Haemodynamic action of nicorandil in chronic congestive heart failure. *American Journal of Cardiology* **63**, 44J–48J.

Solomon, R. J. & Weinberg, M. S. (1987) Comparative effects of pinacidil and prazosin on blood pressure, weight plasma volume, the renin–angiotensin–aldosterone system and the renal kallikrein system in patients with essential hypertension. *Journal of Clinical Hypertension* **3**, 589–595.

Suryapranata, H. & Surrey, P. W. (1989) Coronary vasodilatory action after nicorandil: a quantitative angiographic study. *American Journal of Cardiology* **63**, 80J–85J.

Thomas, P., Dixon, M. S., Winterton, S. J. & Sheridan, D. J. (1990) Acute haemodynamic effects of cromakalim in patients with angina pectoris. *British Journal of Pharmacology* **29**, 325–331.

Thormann, J., Schlepper, M., Kramer, W. & Gottwick, M. (1982) Efficacy of nicorandil (SG-75) a substance with nitro-properties and long-term effects in coronary patients: improvement of LV-function and wall motility without pacing-induced myocardial ischaemia. *Zeitschrift für Kardiologie* **71**, 747–753.

Tice, F. D., Binkley, P. F., Cody, R. J., Moeschberger, M. L., Mohrland, J. S., Wolfe, D. L. & Leier, C. V. (1990) Haemodynamic effects of oral nicorandil in congestive heart failure. *American Journal of Cardiology* **65**, 1361–1367.

Vandenburg, M. J., Woodward, S. R., Hossain, M., Stewart-Long, P. & Tasker, T. C. G. (1986) Potassium channel activators lower blood pressure: an initial study of BRL 34915 in hypertensive patients. *Journal of Hypertension* **4** (Suppl. 6), S166–167.

Vandenburg, M. J., Woodward, S. M., Stewart-Long, P., Tasker, T., Pilgrim, A. J., Dews, I. M. & Fairhurst, G. (1987) Potassium channel activators: antihypertensive activity and adverse effect profile of BRL 34915. *Journal of Hypertension* **5** (Suppl. 5), S193–S195.

Ward, J. W. (1984) Pinacidil monotherapy for hypertension. *British Journal of Clinical Pharmacology* **18,** 223–225.

Ward, J. W., McBurney, A., Farrow, P. R. & Sharp, P. (1984) Pharmacokinetics and hypotensive effect in healthy volunteers of pinacidil, a new potent vasodilator. *European Journal of Clinical Pharmacology* **26,** 603–608.

Webb, D. J., Benjamin, N. & Vallance, P. (1989) The potassium channel opening drug cromakalim produces arterioselective vasodilation in the upper limbs of healthy volunteers. *British Journal of Clinical Pharmacology* **27,** 757–761.

Williams, A. J., Hopkirk, A., Vyse, T., Chiew, V. & Lee, T. H. (1989) Inhibition of nocturnal asthma by relaxation of airway smooth muscle with a potassium channel activator. *American Review of Respiratory Disease* **139,** 140 (Abstr.)

Williams, A. J., Lee, T. H., Cochrane, G. M., Hopkirk, A., Lavender, E., Richards, D. & Woodcock, A. A. (1990a) Attenuation of nocturnal asthma by cromakalim. *Lancet* **336,** 334–336.

Williams, A. J., Verdun, P. J. & Lavender, E. A. (1990b) Inhalation of a potassium channel activator cromakalim is well tolerated in healthy volunteers. *European Journal of Pharmacology* **183,** 1045 (Abstr.)

Williams, A. J., Vyse, T., Richards, D. H. & Lee, T. H. (1988) Cromakalim, a potassium channel activator, inhibits histamine-induced bronchoconstriction and nocturnal asthma. *New England Allergy Proceedings* **9,** 429 (Abstr.)

Zins, G. R. (1988) The history of the development of minoxidil. *Clinical Dermatology* **6,** 132–147.

Index

Page numbers in *italic* refer to figures; numbers in **bold** refer to tables.